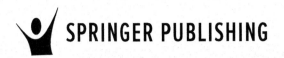 **SPRINGER PUBLISHING**

MW01052611

GET THE MOST FROM YOUR BOOK

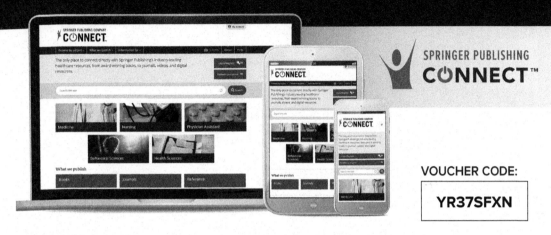

SPRINGER PUBLISHING
CONNECT™

VOUCHER CODE:

YR37SFXN

Online Access

Your print purchase of *Leadership in Practice: Essentials for Public Health and Healthcare Leaders*, includes **online access via Springer Publishing Connect**™ to increase accessibility, portability, and searchability.

Insert the code at http://connect.springerpub.com/content/book/978-0-8261-4924-4 today!

Having trouble? Contact our customer service department at cs@springerpub.com

Instructor Resource Access for Adopters

Let us do some of the heavy lifting to create an engaging classroom experience with a variety of instructor resources included in most textbooks SUCH AS:

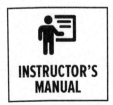

INSTRUCTOR'S MANUAL

POWERPOINTS

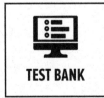

TEST BANK

Visit **https://connect.springerpub.com/** and look for the **"Show Supplementary"** button on your **book homepage** to see what is available to instructors! First time using Springer Publishing Connect?

Email **textbook@springerpub.com** to create an account and start unlocking valuable resources.

Leadership in Practice

Susan C. Helm-Murtagh, DrPH, MM (she/her/hers) is an assistant professor in the Department of Health Policy and Management at the Gillings School of Global Public Health at the University of North Carolina at Chapel Hill. She teaches strategic management and leadership in the DrPH program, and leadership/workforce management and U.S. healthcare system structure and policy in the Executive Masters' Program in Health Administration.

Helm-Murtagh has over a decade of experience in nonprofit leadership and board governance, health systems and health policy, and over 25 years of experience in healthcare financing. She is principal of DreamWork Consulting, LLC, a nonprofit leadership and strategic planning consulting firm, and co-founder and director of The Ellie Helm Foundation, a nonprofit organization dedicated to raising awareness of depression and preventing suicide among youth and bringing social engagement to older adults. She has served on several nonprofit boards and currently chairs the board of directors for The Davis Phinney Foundation for Parkinson's.

Helm-Murtagh holds a BS in psychology and management science from Duke University, an MM (with distinction) in marketing and finance from the Kellogg School of Management at Northwestern University, and a DrPH in health policy and management from the Gillings School of Global Public Health at the University of North Carolina at Chapel Hill.

Paul C. Erwin, MD, DrPH, is dean of the School of Public Health at the University of Alabama at Birmingham (UAB) and professor in the Department of Health Policy and Organization. Erwin earned a BS from the University of the South (Sewanee), an MD from the UAB Heersink School of Medicine, an MPH from Johns Hopkins University, and a DrPH from the University of North Carolina at Chapel Hill. He is board certified in internal medicine, public health, and preventive medicine, and is a fellow of the American College of Preventive Medicine.

Prior to his appointment as dean at the UAB School of Public Health, Dr. Erwin was a professor and department head for public health at the University of Tennessee for 11 years, where he established the department in order to grow the accredited public health program. Before that academic appointment, Dr. Erwin served with the Tennessee Department of Health for 16 years, with 12 years as the director of the East Tennessee Regional Health Office, overseeing 15 county health departments, mostly in rural Appalachia. From 1988-1990, Dr. Erwin was a fellow in international health in the Department of Community Health Sciences at the Aga Khan University in Karachi, Pakistan.

Erwin is an associate editor of the *American Journal of Public Health* and a member of the editorial boards for *Medical Education Cooperation With Cuba (MEDICC) Review* and the *Journal of Public Health Management and Practice*. He has authored over 100 peer-reviewed publications and served as the lead editor (with co-editor Dr. Ross Brownson) of the fourth edition of the textbook *Scutchfield and Keck's Principles of Public Health Practice*.

Leadership in Practice

Essentials for Public Health and Healthcare Leaders

Susan C. Helm-Murtagh, DrPH, MM

Paul C. Erwin, MD, DrPH

Editors

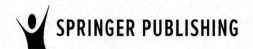

SPRINGER PUBLISHING

Springer Publishing Company, LLC
11 West 42nd Street, New York, NY 10036
www.springerpub.com
connect.springerpub.com/

Senior Acquisitions Editor: David D'Addona
Director, Content Development: Taylor Ball
Production Editor: Joe Stubenrauch
Compositor: Amnet Systems

ISBN: 978-0-8261-4923-7
ebook ISBN: 978-0-8261-4924-4
DOI: 10.1891/9780826149244

SUPPLEMENTS:
Instructor Materials:

A robust set of instructor resources designed to supplement this text is located at http://connect.springerpub.com/content/book/978-0-8261-4924-4. Qualifying instructors may request access by emailing **textbook@springerpub.com.**

Instructor's Manual ISBN: 978-0-8261-4925-1
Instructor's PowerPoints ISBN: 978-0-8261-4927-5

22 23 24 25 / 5 4 3 2 1

Library of Congress Cataloging-in-Publication Data

Names: Helm-Murtagh, Susan C. (Susan Cleland), editor. | Erwin, Paul C., editor.
Title: Leadership in practice : essentials for public health and healthcare
    leaders / Susan C. Helm-Murtagh, Paul C. Erwin.
Description: New York, NY : Springer Publishing Company, [2023] | Includes
    bibliographical references and index.
Identifiers: LCCN 2022020429 (print) | LCCN 2022020430 (ebook) | ISBN
    9780826149237 (paperback) | ISBN 9780826149244 (ebook)
Subjects: MESH: Public Health Practice | Leadership | Delivery of Health
    Care | United States
Classification: LCC RA971 (print) | LCC RA971 (ebook) | NLM WA 100 | DDC
    362.1068/4—dc23/eng/20220608
LC record available at https://lccn.loc.gov/2022020429
LC ebook record available at https://lccn.loc.gov/2022020430

Contact sales@springerpub.com to receive discount rates on bulk purchases.

Publisher's Note: **New and used products purchased from third-party sellers are not guaranteed for quality, authenticity, or access to any included digital components.**

Printed in the United States of America by Gasch Printing.

Contents

PART I: LEADERSHIP BASICS: SKILLS, TRAITS, AND BEHAVIORS

PART II: KEY LEADERSHIP THEORIES AND THEIR APPLICATION

PART III: THE CONTEXT AND CHALLENGES OF LEADERSHIP PRACTICE

PART IV: PUTTING IT ALL TOGETHER: YOUR LEADERSHIP PRACTICE

About the Contributors

Suzanne M. Babich, DrPH, MS

Suzanne Babich is associate dean of global health, acting chair of the Department of Global Health, and professor, global health, and health policy and management, at the Indiana University (IU) Richard M. Fairbanks School of Public Health in Indianapolis, Indiana. She joined IU in 2015 after 14 years on the faculty of the Department of Health Policy and Management and Department of Nutrition at the Gillings School of Global Public Health, University of North Carolina at Chapel Hill. She has worked in global health and international higher education for more than 20 years, following 20 years in nutrition practice and health journalism. She has a special interest in international, interdisciplinary education and applications of technology for progressive approaches to public health workforce education and leadership development. She directs the Doctoral Program in Global Health Leadership, a unique professional distance doctoral degree program for mid- to senior-level health practitioners working full-time around the world. She holds faculty positions in the School for Public Health and Primary Care, Maastricht University, the Netherlands, and the EHESP French National School of Public Health, Paris and Rennes. She is chair of the Board of Accreditation for the European Agency for Public Health Education Accreditation (APHEA) and served for 10 years on the U.S.-based Council on Accreditation of Health Management Education (CAHME). She holds a doctorate in public health from the Department of Health Policy and Management at the Gillings School of Global Public Health, University of North Carolina at Chapel Hill.

Stephanie B. C. Bailey, MD, MSHSA

Dr. Stephanie Bailey is a lifetime champion of community health excellence. Recently employed at MeHarry Medical College (2016 to 2021) as the senior associate dean for public health practice, Dr. Bailey previously served as the dean of the College of Health Sciences and director of public health initiatives at Tennessee State University (2013 to 2016). From 2006 to 2012 she served as the chief for public health practice at the Centers for Disease Control and Prevention (CDC) in Atlanta, Georgia. Dr. Bailey held the position of director of health for the City of Nashville/Davidson County (1985–2006). Dr. Bailey has been honored by local, state, and national governments and organizations; and has been invited to speak internationally and at all levels. Dr. Bailey is a published author; her book, *Remember, Recapture, Restore, Reclaim and Preserve: Principles for Living*, was released November 2021. Dr. Bailey is also a producer of a documentary entitled *Through My Father's Eye*. Dr. Bailey received her BA in psychology from Clark University, Worcester, Massachusetts (1972); her MD from MeHarry Medical College, Nashville, Tennessee (1976); and an MSHSA from the College of St. Francis, Joliet, Illinois (1993). Dr. Bailey is married to W. T. Bailey, Jr. and has three married children (six grandchildren). Her purpose in life is: "To lift people up so that they can soar." She is a member of Cornerstone Church, Nashville.

Edward L. Baker, MD, MPH, MSc

Dr. Baker has been a national leader in public health leadership development for over 30 years. In his role as a Centers for Disease Control and Prevention (CDC) center director and United States Public Health Service (USPHS) assistant surgeon general, he led the creation of the national Public Health Leadership Institute (PHLI; which he subsequently directed), and of state and regional public health leadership institutes, which trained over 7,000 public health leaders across the nation. In addition to these leadership development activities, Dr. Baker served as deputy director of the National Institute for Occupational Safety and Health (NIOSH), associate professor of occupational medicine at Harvard School of Public Health, and director of the North Carolina Institute for Public Health. Dr. Baker currently serves on the faculty of three schools of public health—University of North Carolina, Harvard University, and Indiana University—where he teaches courses on the theory and practice of leadership and is actively involved in leadership research. He is the editor of the Management Moment column in the *Journal of Public Health Management and Practice* (JPHMP) where he serves on the editorial board. Dr. Baker is a physician who is board certified in internal medicine and occupational medicine with specialty training in epidemiology in the CDC's Epidemic Intelligence Service (EIS). He was trained and certified as an executive leadership coach by the Center for Creative Leadership. Dr. Baker and his wife, Pam, recently celebrated 50 years of marriage and have three wonderful adult "children" and a grandson who are true delights. They live in two worlds: a small Tennessee town and the Peoples' Republic of Cambridge, Massachusetts.

Kaye Bender, PhD, RN, FAAN

Dr. Bender is the owner of Kaye Bender Consulting, LLC, where she works as an independent public health, organizational, and education consultant and strategist. She also serves as the executive director of the Mississippi Public Health Association. She is a part-time professor at the University of Mississippi Medical Center School of Nursing and the School of Health Related Professions. Dr. Bender served as the president and CEO of the Public Health Accreditation Board (PHAB) in Alexandria, Virginia, from 2009 to 2019. She was the dean of the University of Mississippi Medical Center School of Nursing prior to working for PHAB. She worked in local public health for several years in Mississippi and was the deputy state health officer for the Mississippi State Department of Health for 12 years. She has served as president of the American Public Health Association since October 2021. She is also a fellow in the American Academy of Nursing; a board member of the National Board of Public Health Examiners; the Public Health Foundation; and the Mississippi Public Health Institute. She has numerous publications and presentations related to governmental public health infrastructure improvement. Dr. Bender holds a BS in nursing from the University of Mississippi Medical Center; an MSN from the University of Southern Mississippi; and a PhD from the University of Mississippi Medical Center.

Angelina Casazza, MPH

Angelina Casazza is a senior leader at Children's National Hospital in Washington, D.C. She has led strategic planning, change management, and system implementation work in human resources, finance, and case management. Her current portfolio includes leading an organization-wide senior leadership talent and succession planning assessment and developing a strategic plan centered on promoting innovative healthcare career development opportunities, mission-centered leadership, and a compassion-driven organizational culture. Angelina has also led patient experience and family-centered care initiatives at Texas Children's Hospital, Boston Children's Hospital, and New York-Presbyterian Hospital. She graduated magna cum laude with a degree in medical anthropology from Princeton University and received her MPH from Columbia University.

Kathleen Colville, MSW, MSPH

Kathleen Colville is the president and CEO of the North Carolina Institute of Medicine (NCI-OM). The NCIOM is an independent agency chartered by the North Carolina General Assembly that works collaboratively with stakeholders from across the state to identify and build consensus around actionable solutions to the health challenges facing North Carolina (NC). This work ties together the throughlines of Kathleen's work and values, fostering policy and system change, integrating health and social care, and grounding it all in commitment to connected, inclusive, and caring communities. From 2014 to 2021, Kathleen led Cone Health's Department of Healthy Communities (Greensboro, North Carolina), working to connect clinical services and community assets to promote equity and access to the healthcare and living conditions that foster long and healthy lives. The healthy communities team led innovative work in urban and rural communities, including the first Centers for Disease Control and Prevention-recognized diabetes prevention program in NC, partnering with Greensboro Housing Coalition on the BUILD Health Challenge to promote healthy homes, and implementing the nation's first statewide electronic medical record-integrated closed-loop electronic referral system linking healthcare and social service organizations. Kathleen holds a bachelor's degree in comparative literature from Brown University and master's degrees in social work and public health from the University of North Carolina at Chapel Hill. She is a PhD candidate in public administration at North Carolina State University and a fellow in the Robert Wood Johnson Foundation's Interdisciplinary Research Leaders program.

W. Jack Duncan, PhD

Dr. Duncan is a professor of management emeritus and university scholar emeritus in the Collat School of Business and School of Public Health at the University of Alabama at Birmingham (UAB). He is author or co-author of a number of books including *Strategic Management of Health Care Organizations*, now in its 8th edition (with Peter M. Ginter and Lynda E. Swayne); *Management: Ideas and Actions;* and *Great Ideas in Management*, translated into seven languages. Dr. Duncan is also author of scholarly articles in leading management and healthcare journals including *Academy of Management Journal, Academy of Management Review, Academy of Management Perspectives, Academy of Management Learning & Education, Management Science, Journal of Management, Journal of Management Inquiry, Journal of Business Research, Strategic Organization, Public Health, Public Health Reports, Public Administration Review, Medical Care Research Review*, and others. Dr. Duncan is the former chair of the Management & Organization Department, associate dean of the Graduate School of Business, founding co-director of the PhD in Administration/Health Services program, and interim dean of the Collat School of Business at UAB. Dr. Duncan is a former member of the board of governors of the Academy of Management and chair of the Management Education & Development Division. He is the former president of the Southern Management Association and the Southwest Division of the Academy of Management. Dr. Duncan was elected fellow of the Academy of Management and is a former deputy dean of the fellows, fellow of the International Academy of Management, a founding fellow of the International Academy of Management, a founding fellow of the Southern Management Fellows, and former dean of the Southern Management Fellows. Dr. Duncan earned his PhD at Louisiana State University.

Michael R. Fraser, PhD, MS, CAE, FCPP

For over 20 years, Dr. Michael Fraser has served as a distinguished public health and healthcare leader. Dr. Fraser is currently chief executive officer of the Association of State and Territorial Health Officials (ASTHO). He assumed this role in August 2016 and ever since has led staff, members, partners, and public health leaders to further advance ASTHO's mission as an advocate, voice, and resource for state and territorial public health. He has worked tirelessly to transform ASTHO into a dynamic, relevant, and effective nonpartisan membership organization representing all state and territorial health agencies. Prior to joining ASTHO, he served as the executive vice president and CEO of the Pennsylvania Medical Society from 2013 to 2016. He served as CEO of the Association of Maternal and Child Health Programs from 2007 to 2013, where his leadership was recognized nationally by the Maternal and Child Health Bureau's Director's Award in 2014. Dr. Fraser was also the deputy executive director of the National Association of County and City Health Officials from 2002 to 2007 and served in several capacities at the U.S. Department of Health and Human Services, including positions at the Health Resources and Services Administration and the Centers for Disease Control and Prevention. In Spring 2015, he was admitted as a fellow in the College of Physicians of Philadelphia, one of just a handful on non-physician fellows in the nation's oldest professional society. Dr. Fraser has been featured in *The Washington Post, The New York Times, Politico, The Hill,* CNN, Bloomberg, MSNBC, Associations Now, Through the Noise, and other national and regional media outlets. He is a co-editor of *A Public Health Guide to Ending the Opioid Epidemic* and a co-editor and author of the *Handbook of Strategic Skills for Public Health Practice,* to be published in 2022. Dr. Fraser was also nominated for a 2018 CEO of the Year Award from *CEO Update* by his colleagues. Dr. Fraser is an affiliated faculty in the Departments of Health Administration and Policy and Global and Community Health at the George Mason University College of Health and Human Services. He is also a professorial lecturer in the Department of Health Policy and Management at the Milken Institute School of Public Health at George Washington University. His collaborative research and scholarship have been published in several academic journals including the *American Journal of Public Health,* the *Annals of Internal Medicine,* and the *Journal of Public Health Management and Practice.* Dr. Fraser received his doctorate in sociology and a master's degree in sociology from the University of Massachusetts Amherst. He also has a master's degree in management with a concentration on management, strategy, and leadership from the Eli Broad School of Management at Michigan State University. Dr. Fraser received his bachelor's degree in sociology from Oberlin College.

Sandro Galea, MD, DrPH, MPH

Sandro Galea, a physician, epidemiologist, and author, is dean and Robert A. Knox Professor at Boston University School of Public Health. He previously held academic and leadership positions at Columbia University, the University of Michigan, and the New York Academy of Medicine. He has published extensively in the peer-reviewed literature and is a regular contributor to a range of public media, about the social causes of health, mental health, and the consequences of trauma. He has been listed as one of the most widely cited scholars in the social sciences. He is past chair of the board of the Association of Schools and Programs of Public Health and past president of the Society for Epidemiologic Research and of the Interdisciplinary Association for Population Health Science. He is an elected member of the National Academy of Medicine. Dr. Galea has received several lifetime achievement awards. Dr. Galea holds a medical degree from the University of Toronto, graduate degrees from Harvard University and Columbia University, and an honorary doctorate from the University of Glasgow.

Peter M. Ginter, PhD

Dr. Ginter received his doctorate degree from the University of North Texas and MBA and BS degrees from Auburn University and is a professor in the Department of Health Policy and Organization in the School of Public Health at the University of Alabama at Birmingham (UAB). After 6 years at the University of Arkansas, Dr. Ginter joined the faculty in the Collat School of Business at UAB and moved to the UAB School of Public Health in 1997. In the UAB School of Public Health, Dr. Ginter served as interim dean in 2017 and 2018, as associate dean for Academic Affairs from 2015 through 2017, chair of the Department of Health Care

Organization and Policy from 1997 through 2012, and as interim chair of the Department of Environmental Health Sciences from 2018 through 2020. His academic areas of interest include strategic management, leadership, and organizational theory. He is co-author of 17 books including eight editions of *Strategic Management of Health Care Organizations*, with W. Jack Duncan and Linda E. Swayne, and *Public Health Leadership and Management: Cases and Context* with Stuart A. Capper and Linda E. Swayne. Dr. Ginter has published more than 160 peer-reviewed papers and case studies.

Claude A. Jacob, MPH

Claude Jacob is the health director of the San Antonio Metropolitan Health District. In this capacity, he oversees more than 30 programs of the Communicable Disease, Community Health, and Environmental Health & Safety divisions for a jurisdiction of over 2 million residents. Prior to joining Metro Health, Claude was chief public health officer for the City of Cambridge, Massachusetts, where he led the operations of the Cambridge Public Health Department (CPHD). Under Claude's direction, CPHD became one of the first local health departments in Massachusetts to meet the national standards as designated by the Public Health Accreditation Board (PHAB). Claude is a past president of the National Association of County and City Health Officials and serves on the PHAB Board of Directors. His previous work experiences include serving as a senior health administrator at the Illinois Department of Public Health, Baltimore City Health Department, and Sinai Health System in Chicago. He received a master of public health from the University of Illinois Chicago School of Public Health and is currently a doctoral candidate in health leadership at the University of North Carolina at Chapel Hill Gillings School of Global Public Health. He is the 2018 Curtis M. Hilliard Award recipient for outstanding achievement in public health given by the Massachusetts Health Officers Association.

C. William Keck, MD, MPH, FACPM

Dr. Keck is professor emeritus and chair emeritus of the Department of Community Health Sciences at the Northeast Ohio Medical University College of Medicine, and former director of health for the City of Akron. He holds an MD degree from Case Western Reserve University, and an MPH degree from the Harvard T.H. Chan School of Public Health. He is past president of the American Public Health Association, the Council on Education for Public Health, the Ohio Public Health Association, the Association of Ohio Health Commissioners, and the Summit County Medical Society. He is a past chair of the Council on Education for Public Health, currently chairs the Council on Linkages Between Academia and Public Health Practice, is the executive director of Medical Education Cooperation with Cuba (MEDICC), and is editor in chief of the journal *MEDICC Review*. Dr. Keck is board certified in Preventive Medicine/Public Health and is a fellow of the American College of Preventive Medicine. His career has been focused on providing quality public health services, teaching community health sciences to medical and other health professional students, and linking public health practice with its academic bases.

Cynthia D. Lamberth, MPH

Cynthia Lamberth serves as executive director of the Kentucky Population Health Institute (KPHI). She conducts leadership training and institutes for governmental and business clients, and is a certified facilitator, life coach, consultant, and author on leadership, mentoring, systems change, masterminds, and community engagement. She is recognized nationally for her knowledge and experience in community engagement and systems change and authored the "Community Health Assessment, Planning, and Implementation" chapter for the 4th edition of *Scutchfield and Keck's Principles of Public Health Practice*. Cynthia is considered a national expert in population health leadership and action learning and has over 40 years' experience in the health field, including positions in academia, consulting, and high-tech industries. Cynthia was previously associate dean for workforce development and community engagement at the University of Kentucky College of Public Health. She ranked in the top 50 funded researchers at the University of Kentucky. She also directed the Center of Excellence in Workforce Research and Policy, Kentucky Population Health Leadership Institute, Kentucky and Appalachia Public Health Training Center, and Center on Aging. She is also a graduate of the National Public Health Leadership Institute. She presented the American Public Health Association national conference closing session "Dying Too Soon," focusing on the high burden women experience from deaths of despair in the Appalachian region. She has traveled throughout the world delivering training seminars and consulting with managers on quality, leadership, team dynamics, performance management, strategic planning, Alzheimer's care, and crisis communication. Cynthia's experience also includes instructional design, curriculum development, strategic planning, and focus group facilitation.

Laura Magaña-Valladares, PhD, MS

Laura Magaña-Valladares brings over 35 years of experience and expertise in higher education and public health education, where she has delivered breakthrough results in international settings. She is an accomplished senior academic leader who has proven success in transforming and innovating educational organizations as an inspiring and motivational leader with the ability to move organizations forward. Dr. Magaña-Valladares is the president and CEO of the Association of Schools and Programs of Public Health (ASPPH), where she has led the association through significant organizational change and during multiple public health crises. Since beginning this position in 2017, she has instituted a strategic planning process to guide the work of the association; led the development of the Global Network for Academic Public Health, an alliance of regional associations for academic public health around the world; enhanced the voice of academic public health through advocacy efforts; and launched an institute to develop the leadership skills of new and upcoming academic public health leaders. In her previous position as the dean of the School of Public Health at the National Institute of Public Health (INSP) of Mexico, for over 12 years Dr. Magaña-Valladares led major innovation in education and technology at the institute and developed first-hand knowledge of the human resource and policy needs of Mexico's national health systems. She has over 35 years of teaching experience as a professor, lecturer, and guest speaker at private and public universities in Latin America, the United States, and Europe and has developed education software related to public health teaching. She regularly contributes to advancing conversations around higher education and public health issues by authoring books, book chapters, educational manuals, and articles in national and international peer-reviewed journals.

Barbara Alvarez Martin, DrPH, MPH

As a public health leader, researcher, and seasoned "implementer," Barbara Alvarez Martin has been bridging the worlds of science and practice for 30 years. She began her career specializing in public health advocacy and community organizing for policy change, leading state and local coalitions that successfully advocated for changes in policies to reduce tobacco use and underage drinking. Barbara then brought her experience to the world of research, when she directed an intervention for a large National Institutes of Health (NIH) community trial that succeeded in reducing alcohol-related consequences on college campuses. Since 2010, Barbara has led initiatives and teams at the University of North Carolina (UNC) Lineberger Comprehensive Cancer Center, where she currently serves on the center's senior leadership team and runs the Office of Community Outreach and Engagement. Throughout her career, Barbara has provided vision and leadership for diverse stakeholders to work together to address public health challenges. She leads teams through strategic planning and builds bridges across disciplines. Barbara continues to train and advise others in strategic planning, coalition building, and best practices to optimize health at a community level. Barbara received a master's in public health and a doctorate in health leadership from the UNC Gillings School of Global Public Health. Her dissertation research focused on how values-based framing can help public health organizations improve their messaging to be more effective in securing stakeholder buy-in and support in a politically polarized environment.

Daniel Martin, PhD

Danny Martin is an ecologically founded theologian. He is a principal creator of Mindfulness-Dialogue, which has been used worldwide to assist in leadership development, team building, and cultural enhancement. Danny's initial awareness of dialogue was through its absence in his conflict-ridden home of Belfast, Ireland. His early work with dialogue was as a Catholic priest in Kenya during the 1970s. Later he explored dialogue through the lens of transformation at the Pontifical Gregorian University in Rome. He brought dialogue to the United Nations (UN) as a religious advisor to the Environment Programme in the 1980s, helping create a program to engage the religions of the world in the environmental challenges. In 1988, Danny completed his doctorate in the field of environmental spirituality at Fordham University. Afterward he engaged environmental and religious leaders on every continent in the creation of an Earth Charter, which was presented at the UN Earth Summit in Brazil in 1992. In the 1990s Danny offered programs in dialogue to various institutions—including the Centers for Disease Control and Prevention and Jefferson Memorial Hospital. It was with the latter, in a program for addicted mothers, that mindfulness was added to dialogue, resulting in an integral method known today as Mindfulness-Dialogue. Danny is a founding member of many environmental initiatives, such as SoundWaters, in Connecticut, Green Belt Safaris with Wangari Maathai in Kenya, and The Thomas Berry Forum for Ecological Dialogue at Iona College. He consults with multiple groups, including Greenwich Psychotherapy and Associates and Transformative Educational Leadership. He is also the "spiritual advisor" of the "Leatherman's Loop," a popular trail-run in New York. Most recently, Danny co-founded a YouTube channel called "A New Global WE" to promote Mindfulness-Dialogue and showcase examples of this emerging WE: https://anewglobal-we.com/. Danny now resides in Cross River, New York, with his wife, Ann D'Elia.

Gene W. Matthews, JD

Gene Matthews is senior investigator at the North Carolina Institute for Public Health at the University of North Carolina (UNC) Gillings School of Global Public Health in Chapel Hill. He also teaches courses on leadership in health law and ethics for the UNC Executive Doctoral Program in Health Leadership (DrPH). Gene is the principal investigator of the Southeastern Regional Office of the Network for Public Health Law. Gene previously served as chief legal advisor to the Centers for Disease Control and Prevention in Atlanta from 1979 to 2004, directing a legal staff that grew to 30 persons. During that 25-year span, he handled a wide range of precedent-setting public health law issues and litigated key public health lawsuits and civil discovery cases. Gene has provided leadership for the founding and development of the modern public health law movement. Gene currently conducts legal research and provides technical assistance to public health practitioners on many legal topics. Gene is widely published and is frequently called upon to lecture on cutting-edge legal issues such as emergency preparedness, federalism, messaging, and future trends in public health leadership. Gene received the Distinguished Career Award of the Public Health Law Association "in recognition of a career devoted to using law to improve the public's health." He is a graduate of the University of North Carolina School of Law and is a member of the North Carolina Bar.

Lynn "Stevie" Sesslar McNeal, MBA

Stevie McNeal is a professor of the practice in consulting and healthcare at the Kenan-Flagler Business School (KFBS) at the University of North Carolina at Chapel Hill. Stevie holds a BA in history (summa cum laude and with university honors) from Texas Christian University in Fort Worth, Texas, and an MBA and Norman Block Award Recipient from KFBS. Prior to returning to KFBS, Stevie had a 35-year career in a variety of executive and leadership roles including as a consultant and senior engagement manager with McKinsey & Company. Over her career, Stevie has led both small and large healthcare organizations, served as president of multiple nonprofit organizations, and currently serves on several advisory boards. Through these experiences, Stevie has honed her leadership brand through trial and error along with an uncompromising commitment to help emerging leaders "be as wildly successful" as they aspire to be. Stevie and her musician husband John have four adult daughters—Paige, Abigail, Madeline, and Chloe. While Stevie and John reside in Chapel Hill with a menagerie of horses, donkeys, chickens, dogs, and cats, they take full advantage of the beauty and diversity of North Carolina by escaping to both the mountains and beaches when they can!

Donna J. Petersen, ScD, MHS, CPH

Dr. Petersen is senior vice president, University of South Florida (USF) Health, and professor and dean, College of Public Health at the University of South Florida. She earned her masters and doctoral degrees in maternal and child health from the Johns Hopkins University Bloomberg School of Public Health. She has held senior leadership positions at the Minnesota Department of Health and the University of Alabama at Birmingham School of Public Health and in several national organizations in academic public health including the National Board of Public Health Examiners, the Council on Education for Public Health, and the Association of Schools and Programs of Public Health. Locally she serves on the board of the Foundation for a Healthy St. Petersburg and of the Hillsborough County Health Care Plan. She has been honored for her work by the American Public Health Association, the Delta Omega National Public Health Honor Society, the National Healthy Mothers Healthy Babies Coalition, the Association of Maternal and Child Health Programs, and the U.S. Health Resources and Services Administration. In 2011 she was presented the Distinguished Alumna Award by Johns Hopkins University and in May 2021 was presented a USF President's Fellow Medallion for her work leading the USF COVID-19 Task Force. In October 2021, she received the Martha May Eliot Award from the American Public Health Association.

Eduardo Sanchez, MD, MPH, FAHA

Eduardo Sanchez serves as chief medical officer (CMO) for prevention for the American Heart Association (AHA). He is the principal investigator of the National Hypertension Control Initiative, jointly funded by the federal Office of Minority Health and the Health Resources and Services Administration (HRSA). He is one of the co-authors of the *2020 AHA Presidential Advisor: Structural Racism as a Fundamental Driver of Health Disparities*. Prior to joining the AHA, he served as vice president and CMO for Blue Cross and Blue Shield of Texas, and before that, he served as director of the Institute for Health Policy at the University of Texas (UT) School of Public Health. Dr. Sanchez served as commissioner of the Texas Department of State Health Services from 2004 to 2006 and commissioner of the Texas Department of Health from 2001 to 2004. He serves on numerous local, state, and national boards and advisory committees. Dr. Sanchez obtained his MD from the University of Texas Southwestern Medical School in Dallas, an MPH from the UT Health Science Center at Houston School of Public Health, and an MS in biomedical engineering from Duke University. He holds a BS in biomedical engineering and a BA in chemistry from Boston University. Dr. Sanchez is residency-trained in family medicine.

F. Douglas Scutchfield, MD

Dr. Scutchfield was the initial incumbent in the Peter P. Bosomworth Professorship in Health Services Research and Policy at the University of Kentucky. He held faculty appointments in the College of Public Health and the College of Medicine, where he became emeritus. At the time of contributing to this textbook he was a faculty fellow in the Lewis Honors College at the University of Kentucky. He received his MD degree from the University of Kentucky, where he was elected to the Alpha Omega Alpha Medical Honor Society. He completed post graduate medical education at Northwestern University, the Centers for Disease Control and Prevention, and the University of Kentucky. He held fellowships in both the American College of Preventive Medicine and the American Academy of Family Practice. He held honorary doctoral degrees from Eastern Kentucky University and the University of Pikeville. He was one of the founders of the College of Community Health Sciences at the University of Alabama and founded the Graduate School of Public Health at San Diego State University. He founded the school, now college, of public health at the University of Kentucky. Dr. Scutchfield has held many national positions in professional organizations, including president of the American College of Preventive Medicine, and received several awards from those organizations, including the American Medical Association's Distinguished Service Award and the American Public Health Association Sedgwick Medallion. Dr. Scutchfield passed away on May 23, 2022, as this book was in production.

James C. Thomas, PhD, MPH

Jim Thomas received his PhD in epidemiology at the University of California, Los Angeles, then worked as an epidemiologist for the Los Angeles County Health Department. He was a professor of epidemiology at the University of North Carolina (UNC) at Chapel Hill for more than 30 years. During that time, he also served as the associate dean for Academic Affairs at UNC's Gillings School of Global Public Health, and as director of the United States Agency for International Development-funded MEASURE Evaluation Project. As a social epidemiologist, he has studied organizational networks to effectively control infectious diseases and the unintended community health effects of mass incarceration. Dr. Thomas was the principal author of the first American Public Health Association (APHA) *Code of Ethics* and contributed to the 2019 revision of the code. For 3 years he served as an ethics advisor to the director of the Centers for Disease Control and Prevention. During the COVID pandemic, he created a website to guide policy makers in ethical pandemic control (pandemicethics.org). In 2021 he received the APHA Lifetime Achievement Award in ethics. Dr. Thomas has worked in over 40 countries as an epidemiologist or ethicist. He is presently a professor emeritus at UNC and an adjunct professor of global health at the École des Hautes Études en Santé Publique, and of public health ethics at Maastricht University in the Netherlands.

Trissa Torres, MD, MSPH, FACPM

Trissa Torres is a preventive medicine physician, healthcare leader, and change agent. Dr. Torres serves as the executive director for Population Health Improvement Partners, a small not-for-profit based in Raleigh, North Carolina, which coaches, facilitates, and supports organizations and communities to improve equitable population health outcomes. She leads her organization in applying equity-centering improvement methods to drive system transformation. Previously, Dr. Torres served as an executive leader at the Institute for Healthcare Improvement (IHI) in Boston, where she oversaw a portfolio of initiatives and associated resources in service of IHI's mission to improve health and healthcare worldwide. Before that, she served as a medical director at Genesys Health System in Flint, Michigan, for nearly 20 years, championing efforts to improve population and community health. While in Flint, Dr. Torres also held an appointment as an associate professor for the Department of

Family Medicine at the Michigan State University College of Human Medicine. Dr. Torres received her undergraduate degree from the University of Michigan, her medical degree from the University of Texas Health Science Center at San Antonio, and completed her preventive medicine residency at Meharry Medical College in Nashville, Tennessee. Dr. Torres is committed to partnering to advance antiracism and justice in all our improvement efforts.

Katherine L. Turner, MPH

Katherine Turner (she/her) is an internationally recognized executive consultant, coach, thought leader, public speaker, educator, author, and change agent who has led initiatives in English, French, and Dutch in more than 50 countries spanning five continents. Katherine is the founding president of Global Citizen, LLC, a consulting firm that works in the United States and internationally to strengthen inclusive leadership and effect organizational transformation and social impact by advancing diversity, equity, inclusion, public health, human rights, and global competence. She serves as adjunct professor at the University of North Carolina at Chapel Hill Gillings School of Global Public Health, where she teaches leadership, cultural humility, systems and design thinking, and global health topics and mentors the next generation of global leaders. Katherine graduated with honors from Duke University and earned a master of public health from the University of North Carolina at Chapel Hill. She served as a Peace Corps volunteer and national trainer in Togo, West Africa, and held leadership positions at the Durham County Health Department and Ipas, where she led health systems strengthening and innovated equity-focused programs. She founded her consulting firm in 2011. Current leadership roles include serving on the U.S. Global Leadership Coalition's North Carolina Advisory Committee, North Carolina Coalition for Global Competitiveness, and Duke LGBTQ+ Network Board. Katherine has founded and led the board of directors of nonprofit organizations and won awards for excellence in leadership, education, public health, and advocacy. Katherine and her family are proud to call Durham, North Carolina, their beloved hometown.

J. Bennet Waters, DHA, MPH

Bennet Waters has more than 20 years of senior leadership experience in operations, finance, and life-cycle mergers and acquisitions in Fortune 500 and privately held healthcare organizations as chief executive officer, chief operating officer, and in enterprise-wide roles with responsibility for strategy, marketing, and acquisition integration. He has led three private companies to successful liquidity events. Bennet also served in the U.S. Department of Homeland Security as chief of staff to the assistant secretary for health affairs and as counselor to the secretary and deputy secretary, where his counterterrorism portfolio included biodefense; emergency management; and aviation, border, and maritime security. In addition to his executive experience, Bennet has been a part-time assistant professor in the Department of Health Policy and Management of the University of North Carolina's Gillings School of Global Public Health since 2003. He maintains an active teaching load with masters and doctoral students and has served on numerous dissertation committees. Bennet is an honors graduate of Davidson College; received a masters in public health with a concentration in health law from the Boston University School of Public Health; and a doctorate in health administration from the Medical University of South Carolina (MUSC), where he was a dean's list graduate and inducted into the MUSC Honor Society. A native of Louisiana, Bennet resides in Durham, North Carolina, with his wife, three daughters, and golden retrievers Fenway and Beaux. He is an instrument-rated private pilot, novice golfer, avid sports fan, and enjoys cooking, travel, and spending time with his family in the North Carolina mountains.

John Wiesman, DrPH, MPH

John Wiesman was born and raised in the small midwestern town of Horicon, Wisconsin (population 3,000), and is the fifth of seven children of Lois and Leo. He attended public schools, hated physical education class as he was always picked last, loved swimming during the hot summers and playing tennis, and liked playing school and librarian in the basement of his home with his siblings and friends. John attended Lawrence University, a private liberal arts college in Appleton, Wisconsin, studying biology. His passion for public health was ignited by a July 4, 1983, *Time* magazine article highlighting the work of disease detectives. He received his MPH in chronic disease epidemiology from Yale University. It was during this time that John realized he is a gay man. Shortly after that, he met his now husband; they have been together for 35 years, married for 13, and chose not to have children. They reside in Durham, North Carolina. John has 30 years of governmental public health experience, working at four local health departments and serving as the Washington state secretary of health. In that job, he led the nation's response to the first case of COVID-19. John received his DrPH from the University of North Carolina at Chapel Hill Gillings School of Global Public Health where he now serves as a professor of the practice and director of the executive DrPH program.

Foreword

At no time in recent memory has the practice of public health leadership been more challenging. The challenges not only include the daunting leadership tasks associated with the COVID-19 pandemic crisis but also a companion crisis of mental health challenges experienced by frontline public health workers faced with "COVID fatigue" and potential burnout. Further, the widening range of public health issues requires that leaders must expand their horizons, enhance insights, and sharpen perspectives.

Coping with these wide-ranging challenges requires a well-developed leadership mindset, a comprehensive skill set, and a well-stocked tool kit of best practices. This up-to-date text offers you, the reader, fresh insights and concrete examples to sharpen your leadership mindset, to enhance your skills as a transformational leader, and to provide tested tools that you can immediately apply to your leadership practice.

Susan Helm-Murtagh and Paul Erwin offer this text as a "labor of love" to those who aspire to leadership practice. Both have studied a wide range of research-based theories of leadership practice, having graduated from the Doctoral Program in Health Leadership at the University of North Carolina at Chapel Hill (in which Susan and I still teach a course on this subject). In addition to their scholarly mastery of the research literature, both have practiced leadership within an organizational context and therefore "know whereof they speak." Their experiences include leading in a health insurance company, chairing boards of nonprofit organizations, leading a local health department, and serving as dean of an outstanding school of public health. Further, they have reached out to exceptional colleagues who are highly qualified to contribute chapters to the text based on their own "real-world" experience and areas of expertise. These colleagues are nationally known thought leaders in public health practice, academia, and healthcare who offer in these chapters their own "words of wisdom" and insights into leadership practice.

The components of the book represent a carefully crafted progression of topics from basic skills and theories leading to strategies and tactics needed to put these core concepts into practice. By adding a summary section on "Putting It All Together," the editors support the reader in developing a personal leadership framework to guide each learner over the course of their leadership journey. In this final section, practical guidance is provided on how to sustain growth over time by creating one's own "personal board of directors."

As a reader, you will be drawn to the personal stories of those who have practiced frontline leadership either during the COVID-19 pandemic or when facing other public health and healthcare threats and emergencies. As an important and timely addition to the text, the chapter on "Leadership Intangibles" will offer contemporary insights into foundational practices of mindfulness, self-restoration, and humility, which are essential contributors to deepening one's approach to leadership practice, particularly in these challenging times.

I'm confident that each of you will find many "pearls of wisdom" in these pages. You will no doubt incorporate the concepts and theories into your own leadership mindset. Further, you will build out your own set of leadership skills equipped with a "leadership tool set" which you can immediately put to use in your own practice of leadership. I wish you all the best in your leadership journey and know that those who share their ideas in this book will be your companions in that journey for years to come.

Edward L. Baker, MD, MPH, MSc
Assistant Surgeon General USPHS (retired)
Adjunct Professor, UNC Gillings School of Public Health,
Chapel Hill, North Carolina
Harvard Chan School of Public Health, Boston, Massachusetts

Preface

THE CONTEXT

Today's public health and healthcare leaders face an array of leadership contexts presenting formidable challenges, including the syndemics of COVID-19 and structural racism; an ageing population; unhealthy lifestyles; the rapid spread of infectious pathogens; national disasters, conflicts, and mass population movements; antimicrobial resistance; injuries; and the health impacts of climate change and environmental pollution.

As a result, effective public health and healthcare leaders must navigate in a world of unpredictability, complexity, ambiguity, and uncertainty. To do so, they need to be equipped with a set of practical, sustainable, and universal skills and abilities. This text, and its accompanying set of diverse and accessible learning experiences (interviews with notable leaders, case studies, self-assessments, reflection exercises, and the like), provides a solid foundation for the practice of leadership in organizations focusing on such leadership topics as strategic leadership, systems thinking, team leadership, change leadership, and the development of others. Further, the text exposes readers to the challenges, actions, and lessons learned from the COVID-19 pandemic and other public health and healthcare crises—from after-action reviews to interviews and insights from those on the front lines—culminating in the development of a leadership framework to inform leadership practice.

As our populations grow more diverse, public health and healthcare leaders are recognizing the value and the challenges that diversity brings. In recognition of the criticality of diversity, equity, access, and inclusion, in this book readers will hear from a wide range of voices. Leaders with different life and work experiences, perspectives, training, worldviews, and leadership styles were intentionally invited to contribute their wisdom, knowledge, and experience.

The intended audience for this textbook includes candidates for MHA, DrPH, and MPH degrees, as well as leaders in healthcare, health administration, and public health seeking to further develop their leadership practice.

IN THIS TEXT

Although key leadership theories will be explored and integrated, the primary focus of this book is on the practice of leadership. The key differentiating feature of the text is that it gives voice to those who *practice* leadership and have the credibility to discuss the popular as well as the academic literature on a topic—building on a solid foundation of theory, skills, behaviors, and lessons about the challenges leaders face and the contexts in which they must succeed. It also provides a wide and rich array of learning experiences that incorporate lessons and insights from public health and healthcare leaders.

This book is organized into four parts, each with a specific area of focus.

Part I: Leadership Basics: Skills, Traits, and Behaviors

Part I is divided into five chapters. Chapter 1 introduces readers to effective dialogue, the foundation on which communication, change leadership, building and maintaining trust, systems thinking, organizational learning, negotiation, problem-solving, and decision-making are built. Chapter 2 focuses on ethical leadership and moral courage; it provides students with tools and techniques to become role models for ethical behavior. Chapter 3 explores systems thinking, which enables leaders to better understand structural relationships and develop workable solutions to chronic problems. Chapter 4 addresses strategic thinking and analysis and provides tools to help leaders develop a clear set of goals, plans, and new ideas required to survive and thrive in a complex and changing environment. Finally, Chapter 5 provides an overview of emotional intelligence—the ability to understand and manage one's own emotions, as well as recognize and influence the emotions of others.

Part II: Key Leadership Theories and Their Application

Part II focuses on a subset of leadership theories that are particularly relevant to public health and healthcare leaders: the situational approach to leadership (Chapter 6); transformational leadership (Chapter 7); authentic leadership (Chapter 8); servant leadership (Chapter 9); and adaptive leadership (Chapter 10). Each chapter, written by a leader and practitioner within academia, public health, or healthcare, explores the history, evidence, and application of an extant leadership model. The authors enlighten readers through practical application by offering case studies and tools to build self-awareness through assessments and reflection.

Part III: The Context and Challenges of Leadership Practice

Part III introduces readers to the challenges that confront public health and healthcare leaders and discusses how the context for leadership is dynamic and evolving. Chapter 11 describes the process for leading change. Chapter 12 describes why diversity, equity, and inclusion (DEI) and intercultural competence are essential and how leaders can develop an equity mindset and equity leadership practices. Chapter 13 analyzes the sources and impact of conflict and describes how to effectively manage and resolve conflict at work. Chapter 14 discusses how leaders might effectively anticipate, prevent, prepare for, mitigate, respond to, and recover from complex organizational crises. Chapter 15 presents techniques and tools to facilitate team effectiveness. Chapter 16 outlines methods to identify, encourage, measure, evaluate, and improve employee performance. Chapter 17 addresses ways in which public health leaders can engage more deeply and meaningfully with communities burdened by poor health.

Part IV: Putting It All Together: Your Leadership Practice

Part IV focuses more specifically on the practice of leadership. Chapter 18 describes various stages in the evolution of a leader and development approaches at each stage. Chapter 19 addresses how to find a mentor, how to establish and maintain successful mentoring relationships, and how to serve as a mentor to others. Chapter 20 describes several traits and practices that facilitate leading through complexity and turbulence, such as mindfulness, self-restoration, courage, fallibility, compassion, gratitude, and resiliency. Chapter 21, which draws on the preceding chapters, guides readers through a structured, self-reflective process to aid in the development of leadership style and its application. Finally, Chapter 22 is a compendium of stories from leaders, in their own voices, about some of their more formative experiences and the lessons they gleaned from those experiences.

Having been in leadership positions for a combined 50+ years, and having taught leadership at the graduate level, this book has been our opportunity to intentionally reflect on and write about leadership. It is our hope that students, faculty, and leaders who use this textbook will be able to resonate with our experiences and those of the many co-authors who joined us in this endeavor.

Susan C. Helm-Murtagh, DrPH, MM
Paul C. Erwin, MD, DrPH

Acknowledgments

Paul. C. Erwin, MD, DrPH

Dr. F. Douglas Scutchfield, a contributing author to this textbook, passed away on May 23, 2022, prior to publication. A giant in the field of public health, "Scutch", as he was known by his many friends and colleagues, helped to establish two schools of public health (San Diego State University and the University of Kentucky), among his many accomplishments. He also founded the *Journal of Appalachian Health*, which remains a fitting legacy to a life's work of care and concern for the Appalachian region and its people. As a mentor of several decades to me, it is also a fitting tribute that he contributed to the chapter on mentoring in this textbook. Without his mentorship, I would not be where I am today, and with his passing away, I know my charge to "pay it forward." In Ulysses, Mentor, in responding to Telemakhos' questions about how he can approach his father, Odysseus, replies, "Reason and heart will give you words, Telemakhos; and a spirit will counsel others. I should say the gods were never indifferent to your life."

I am grateful to have been given this opportunity to work with my friend and colleague, Susan Helm-Murtagh, an exceptional leader, thinker, and outdoor enthusiast extraordinaire. And to my wife, Renee' Hyatt, who understands and gives to me the meaning of time.

Susan C. Helm-Murtagh, DrPH, MM

I would like to acknowledge the students in the University of North Carolina DrPH and MHA programs—you were the inspiration for this book.

I am indebted to those who have pulled me and pushed me along my life's journey: Mom and Dad; the many teachers and coaches who believed in me and helped me find my footing; the powerful women mentors and role models who showed me how to find my voice; and my partner in love, life, growth, and adventure, Rory Murtagh.

I am especially grateful to my friend, colleague, and co-editor, Dr. Paul Erwin; without his guidance, patience, and influence, this book would still be but a dream.

Finally, although I had the good fortune to get to know and work with Dr. Scutchfield only briefly, his wisdom and sense of service to others were apparent from our first interaction. The field of public health has indeed lost a champion, but his vision and purpose live on in those he has mentored, guided, and inspired. We are honored and grateful for his voice and presence in this book.

Instructor Resources

 A robust set of instructor resources designed to supplement this text is located at http://connect.springerpub.com/content/book/978-0-8261-4924-4. Qualifying instructors may request access by emailing **textbook@springerpub.com.**

Available resources include:

- **Instructor's Manual**
- **PowerPoint Presentations**

Chapter 1

Dialogue: A Foundational Skill for Effective Health Leadership

Daniel Martin and Edward L. Baker

INTRODUCTION

At no time in recent history has it been more difficult to effectively practice health and healthcare leadership. Whether at the organizational, local, state, or federal level, leaders are faced with a daunting set of external and internal challenges as they struggle to promote and protect the health of individuals and the public. Despite these overwhelming forces that beset the public health and healthcare landscapes, public health and healthcare leaders remain sources of inspiration for the communities they serve. However, as "COVID fatigue" becomes a central "occupational disease" among health workers, strategies and skills which served them in earlier "normal times" seem to be of less value than ever before.

The diverse set of challenges faced by public health and healthcare leaders are well noted in other chapters in this book. Within this context, a renewed emphasis on dialogue competency as a core public health and healthcare leadership skill is most timely. In that regard, this chapter offers a rationale for an enhanced emphasis on building dialogue competency and presents a range of guiding principles and best practices needed to enhance this core skill set.

OBJECTIVES

By the end of this chapter, the reader will be able to:

- Provide public health and healthcare leaders with an understanding of the context in which dialogue is to be practiced.
- Offer a conceptual foundation on which dialogue competency rests.
- Describe components of dialogue including skills of active listening and asking powerful questions.
- Summarize lessons learned by public health and healthcare leaders in the application of dialogue to practice.
- Explore future directions, including the benefits of mindfulness practice as a companion to dialogue.

FUNDAMENTAL CONCEPTS

It is important to first define what dialogue, in fact, means. The word "dialogue" comes from the Greek *dia,* which means "through," and *logos,* which refers to "meaning," and suggests a way of participating in the emergence of meaning. Often the word is conflated with similar but different words: "discussion" (from the Latin *discutere*—to "shake apart"), which refers to analysis and comparison; and "debate" (from the Latin *de-battere*—to "beat down"), which refers to refuting or convincing. Both have their place in creative interaction. In the face of unprecedented challenges, however, a more radical process like dialogue is required.

The practice of dialogue as participation in the emergence of meaning is based on two things: a new—expanded/expanding—way of seeing the world (a new story of life) and a new way of relating to each other and everything else that is founded on this new story. To effectively address public health and healthcare challenges, then, requires more than information or new technology. Rather, the deeper issue is one of story and relationship; the story of the universe and our place in it. Older societies related to the world and each other based on a realization (a story) of fundamental interdependence. More recent society developed a measure of control that redefined this relationship in a more utilitarian way. While this has led to many good things, including scientific knowledge and technological development, it has also resulted in the erosion of the fundamental relationship of interdependence that guided our ancestors. In time, this loss promoted increasing separation and hyperindividualism with its accompanying disparities and injustices that are the real foundation of many of the public health and healthcare challenges today.

Addressing this collective sense of loss and separation and the challenges it has created will require an approach that focuses on fostering collaboration not only between public health and healthcare officials and other parts of society—like education and government—but, even more importantly, between these officials and the communities they serve. Thomas Berry, in his work, *Universe Story,* puts it this way: "The universe is a communion of subjects, not a collection of objects."[1] The latter part of the statement reflects the assumptions of modern society and is the essential source of the many challenges faced today. To truly address these challenges, therefore, a change of this order is needed. Knowledge and skills certainly are important to this process, but a basic change of heart is primary and critical.

A growing awareness of life as interbeing—interconnected and interdependent—is impacting relationships and the systems they inform, from education to healthcare and from business to leadership. However, since these systems and their underpinning relationships have long been shaped and informed by a different awareness—of life as separate, competing units—new skills and new competencies will be required to assist with the implementation of our new awareness. Dialogue offers a framework for this aspect of transition. With its focus on connecting at a level that reflects a world of interbeing, this exploration may facilitate an appreciation for the challenges of relating to and understanding each other in an interconnected society, and lead to discoveries that reflect the continuous emergence of meaning from this constant communion of subjects.

If dialogue is "participation in the emergence of meaning," then it requires that participants (attempt to) connect at the most authentic level possible—to themselves, to each other, and to the moment—as the source and foundation of meaning. As noted in the text that follows, much conversation tends to fall into discussion (i.e., the comparison of perspectives) or debate (i.e., the competition between perspectives). In dialogue, the emphasis is on "participation," which suggests the discovery of something new.

Dialogue is an intentional, skillful interaction that leads to creative outcomes. As such, dialogue is "thinking together." The dialogue process works with, rather than against, differences in perspective, suggesting an alternative to our usual ways of interacting. By inviting the suspension of assumptions, dialogue welcomes different perspectives, listens deeply (to self and to others), and participates in building trust and making meaning. It is a crucial building block of creative leadership, just as it is the foundation on which communication, change leadership, building and maintaining trust, systems thinking, organizational learning, negotiation, problem-solving, and decision-making are built. Effective dialogue requires creating a safe and respectful environment which fosters listening to understand, asking powerful questions, and being open to new and different ideas and perspectives.

The essential and foundational conditions for dialogue are openness, equality, and empathy. One must be willing to be influenced by the perspectives of others and have a desire to change together with an attitude of humble inquiry.[2] Dialogue competency, in other words, requires being present to oneself and to others along with the intentional cultivation of presence. In doing so, one can create the conditions needed for the practice of dialogue.

STRATEGIC VALUE OF DIALOGUE AS A CORE LEADERSHIP SKILL—WHY IS IT IMPORTANT NOW?

Building mutually beneficial strategic partnerships is central to the practice of public health and healthcare.[3] As shown in the response to the COVID-19 pandemic, governmental public health leaders must engage with a widening range of partners to mobilize community-wide efforts needed to contain the menace of COVID-19. Often new (or renewed) partnerships are essential with elected officials, the faith community, the private sector, nongovernmental organizations, and others. Typically, these groups, who often do not see themselves as being part of the public health system, play a major role in policy development and in the implementation of public health measures (e.g., COVID immunization and mask wearing) required to protect community health. Unfortunately, these groups see the world through a lens different from the one used by the public health community. As a result, communication is challenging at best. Even the terms used by these disparate groups may be confusing to the public health mind (which has its own vocabulary that is in turn confusing to these other groups). Further, one result of this potential disconnect is that different parties "talk past each other" and fail to converge to build these much needed and mutually beneficial strategic partnerships.

In addition to COVID-19 pandemic challenges, public health practice over recent decades has broadened its scope significantly. Today the core public health role of protecting against the threat of infectious diseases has expanded to include the prevention of chronic disease, illness, and injury caused by occupational and environmental hazards (whether unintentional or intentional). Further, as public health leaders contemplate newer areas of emphasis, such as climate change and racism as a public health crisis, the collaboration skills of leaders will be tested in new and unimagined ways.

Along with these external challenges, public health leaders face internal collaboration challenges as the composition of the public health workforce evolves. As a result, broadening and strengthening the dialogue competency of the public health workforce will be central in attracting new talent with new skills and values (e.g., millenials in public health). Dialogue competency can play a strategic role in bridging the gap between the "boomers," millennials, and other generations that populate the workforce.

Part of the transgenerational communication/collaboration challenge relates to the evolving way that information is created and shared (e.g., the role of social media and rapidly changing technological environment; use of phones, tablets, and apps as central to our way of daily life). All too often, the use of the ever present "electronic aids" leads to "electronic fatigue syndrome" rather than enhanced connections across generations and between different mindsets and belief systems. As a result, public health leaders must struggle to manage attention and then adapt messages to the many new modes and manners of interaction. Dialogue practices, as noted in the text that follows, can help harness attention in more constructive and generative ways with the potential to advance the health of the public.

Furthermore, political polarization fueled both by issues related to the COVID-19 response, as well as in other polarizing public health issues (e.g., gun violence, reproductive health, and the opioid epidemic), has further complicated the communication and collaboration landscape. As noted elsewhere in this book,[4] crafting better messages to reach a broader spectrum of individuals who base their beliefs on a range of moral foundations has become central to providing effective public health leadership in these times.

BUILDING DIALOGUE COMPETENCY

For leaders to become more competent in the range of practices needed to incorporate dialogue as a foundational leadership skill, a few concepts should be understood. Development of the competency framework discussed here has been greatly influenced by the cogent thinking of Peter Senge[5] and William Isaacs[6] of the Massachusetts Institute of Technology (MIT) who in turn were greatly influenced by the seminal work of David Bohm,[7] the late theoretical physicist. The reader who wishes to deepen their insights into the nature and practice of dialogue should consult these very wise sources. Much of the following content derives from their work.

First, Bohm laid the intellectual foundation for the theory and practice of dialogue through a synthesis of two major intellectual currents: a holistic or systemic view of nature and life, along with a deeper understanding of our interactions, including our thinking processes and our internal models together with our perceptions and our actions. Bohm suggested that dialogue was "meaning passing through—a free flow of meaning between people, like a stream that flows between two banks."[7(p6)]. As noted by Senge, Bohm offered dialogue as a method for improving team learning—one of the five core disciplines of systems thinking leading to the creation of the "learning organization." Systems thinking requires calling attention to the fact that the consequences of our actions are guided by our perceptions and assumptions. Bohm draws the analogy between the behavior of elementary particles and the flow of thought as it emerges in a conversation. He then makes an important distinction between discussion and dialogue. The word "discussion," he notes, comes from the same root as the words "percussion" and "concussion." As such, a goal of a "discussion" is often to make a point (or even "score a point"). Dialogue, in contrast, allows a group to access a larger "pool of shared meaning" in which the whole may be greater than the sum of the parts. Central to the process of dialogue is to go beyond an individual's understanding to develop common meaning.[5]

Bohm identified three basic conditions necessary for dialogue:

1. All participants must "suspend" their assumptions; to hold them "as if suspended before us."
2. All participants must regard each other as colleagues.
3. There must be a "facilitator" who "holds the context" of dialogue. A dialogue facilitator functions as a process facilitator who influences the flow of the dialogue by modeling dialogue practices and steering the conversation away from the discussion modality as needed. Thus, the facilitator must help to balance the conversation between the modes of dialogue and discussion, both of which are needed to lead to a course of action.

Building upon Bohm's theoretical framework, Senge integrated these ideas into a development of ways in which dialogue might foster the creation of "learning organizations."[5] Systems thinking, he writes, is central to building a learning organization by cultivating five core disciplines: personal mastery, surfacing and challenging mental models, building shared vision, team learning, and systems thinking application. Senge notes that dialogue serves as a central tool in the process of team learning—"the process of aligning and developing the capacity of the team to create the results its members truly desire."[5 (p253)] He notes that often the process of dialogue allows participants to observe their thinking as an active process in which tension may arise because of individuals holding differing views. If a posture of dialogue can be established, individuals may come to separate themselves from their thoughts and thereby adopt a more creative and less reactive stance toward their thoughts.[5(p277)] Ideally, then, participants come to recognize that it is their thoughts which are in conflict rather than being in conflict as individuals. In this regard, suspending assumptions, and seeing them as such, provides an antidote to the delusion that "this is the way it is." To enter a space in which dialogue can be fostered, one must "suspend" assumptions. In other words, the process involves making implicit assumptions explicit. One might consider the image of being in a conversation with an assumption being suspended in space on the end of a string in full view. As a result, implicit assumptions can be examined by ourselves and others.

In his book *Dialogue: The Art of Thinking Together,*[6] Isaacs offers a range of techniques from the field of organizational development, such as balancing inquiry and advocacy while suspending assumptions, and the "four player model" of systems psychologist David Kantor that consists of "movers, opposers, followers, and bystanders." In this model, "movers" may express an idea while "followers" might say that they agree with the idea. In contrast, "opposers" may offer a different perspective and explain why. "Bystanders" may step back and summarize where the dialogue seems to be going. In a dialogue session, individuals may modulate between these roles over the course of the conversation.

Isaacs invites us to listen deeply and to actively "suspend our assumptions" and thereby allow ourselves to be influenced by the shared perspectives of others. Hopefully, by adopting new behaviors and skills, one can then cultivate a change in mindset which allows for new ways of seeing and enhanced awareness of one's own mental models. Thus, Isaacs' work provides both useful concepts and best practices for public health and healthcare leaders who wish to develop greater dialogue competency. As noted by these seminal thinkers, personal stories—the organizational and social contexts within which one lives, and how one thinks about the future—influence values, feelings, and actions. This frame of reference is self-reinforcing, such that one may tend to confirm the "rightness" of previously held values and beliefs and the actions that result. To change the results of these actions, therefore, one must begin by exploring underlying assumptions.

Another MIT professor, Chris Argyris, offered a tool that can help with this work of exploring one's assumptions and beliefs—The Ladder of Inference—that makes implicit thought processes more explicit and available for exploration.[8] One often "climbs the Ladder of Inference" very quickly, moving from data, through assumptions, conclusions, and reinforced beliefs, into what Argyris calls "noble certainties." This simple tool can help one determine "where we are on the ladder"—selecting data, adding meaning, or reinforcing old assumptions—and thereby better explore how one's position on the ladder shapes thinking and modes of communication (Figure 1.1).

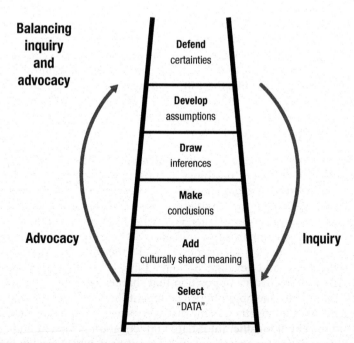

FIGURE 1.1: The Ladder of Inference.
Source: Reproduced with permission from Argyis C. *Reasoning, Learning, and Action.* Jossey-Bass; 1982.

THE STAGES OF DIALOGUE

In other recent applications, dialogue has evolved into a three-stage process: connecting, exploring, and discovering.[9] The stages can be viewed as a sequence in which each stage builds upon and reinforces the other.

CONNECTING STAGE

Connecting (through the sharing of life-changing stories) may foster the creation of the essential foundation for the radical process of dialogue—again, the emergence of meaning—to take place. The purpose of this stage, despite the name, is not simply to connect for the sake of connecting; rather, it more accurately is to create the space—or conditions—in which dialogue is more likely to happen. For when one connects deeply, all sorts of things happen: participants feel trust, feel safe, and feel heard. Participants may also feel a common cause if they have connected around something specific, like a purpose or challenge. What may happen in an interaction occurs beneath the surface in the sense that often it is what is not visible that is driving the process. Further, the stage of connecting may be fostered by the cultivation of skilled vulnerability (using vulnerability in the right way at the right time), which is developed over time through experience and practice.

EXPLORATION STAGE

The path of dialogue then proceeds with the stage of exploration that includes (a) a suspension of assumptions through internal listening, accepting differences, and further trust-building; (b) inquiry to explore each other's assumptions, reveal feelings, and build common ground; and (c) the ability to think as a group in a way that leads to new shared assumptions and the development of a new culture.

The exploration stage of dialogue benefits from the practice of many forms of listening and inquiry. It is important to emphasize that the purpose of this stage is mutual understanding, which is in keeping with the larger purpose of dialogue, which is to participate in the emergence of meaning. Mutual understanding allows differences to be held rather than simply dismissed, as is often the case in our interactions. This is a crucial point, for when differences are allowed in this way, the tension that is clearly still created can generate new insights in the form of shared understanding, as a kind of spontaneous process that is comparable to germination or musical composition. At times, dialogue participants may find themselves saying things like: "I never thought of it like this but..."; it is at this point that the dialogue stage of discovery begins.

DISCOVERY STAGE

In this stage, the interaction takes on a new energy. In the stage of discovery, the sense of "participation in the emergence of meaning" is most clearly experienced. Other skills can enhance this part of the process; skills that might be described as another form of listening: listening FOR. Here, participants are invited to pause and step away from the exploration process of listening and inquiry and to listen FOR what has been generated. This stage of dialogue has sometimes been compared to a kind of jazz where one participant—like the trumpet player in a jazz band—gives voice to a new thought; then another—like the clarinet player—picks up on the theme and develops it; then a third—like the trombone player—offers a counterpoint, like a little creative opposition that sharpens the idea. And so on, until yet another participant or band member offers a comment that weaves the pieces into a theme that the entire band takes up together. In the discovery stage of dialogue, then, new meaning is listened for and then built together into shared understanding. Shared understanding like this, in fact, is the foundation for agreement and commitment, which is what makes dialogue so critical and powerful as a process for addressing complex challenges.

LISTENING TO UNDERSTAND

Clearly, there are many obstacles to effective dialogue. A major obstacle may be that no one is really listening to what is being said; rather, they are composing what they plan to say in their mind. There may also be a lack of mutual respect or a low level of trust between the participants; then, simply advocating and defending positions may dominate. Other obstacles include the fast pace of life along with the pace of work life in which more is needed to be done with fewer resources; this dynamic is painfully apparent in the current public health world. As previously noted, our constant companions—those electronic distraction devices—may interfere with being really present and listening deeply.

In an increasingly complex and unpredictable world, the ability of leaders to avoid distractions and focus on the content and meaning of important conversations is increasingly challenging. Deliberate, or "active," listening presents the listener with the imperative of taking time to really listen. A basic precondition of doing so is to provide full attention to whoever is speaking. Certainly, putting aside obvious sources of distraction (e.g., cell phones) and making eye contact are first steps. As noted by Edgar Schein, the effective listener must also cultivate a mental posture of *humble inquiry and genuine curiosity*.[2] The listener must set aside premature judgments regarding what is being said and mentally surface and suspend assumptions that may obstruct one's ability to listen deeply. In one of the first essays ever written about listening, Sigmund Freud described what he termed "evenly hovering attention." He described the process as managing one's attention and focus by neither under-focusing (being distracted) or hyper-focusing (focusing on the wrong details or missing the meaning behind the words).[10]

Core components of effective listening include[10]:

1. **Listening for content:** The first step toward deepening the listening process is to listen for the content of what is being said. In this way, one can act like a voice recorder tracking key words or phrases. Here you are focusing on what is actually said, not on what you are imagining was said or what you would have preferred was said. This component requires focused attention and practice. Listening for content should call not only on the literal auditory processing ability to hear what is said, but also on intuitive capacity to hear what is not said. Sometimes those messages are conveyed indirectly and can be observed in a moment of "somatic leakage," where the speaker unintentionally communicates through nonverbal channels.

2. **Listening for meaning and intent:** A second aspect of deep listening is to listen for meaning and intent. In this aspect of deep listening, one is attempting to discern the underlying meaning of what is being said and the intention of the speaker. The intent could include simply informing the listener, attempting to influence the listener, or to enhance and deepen a relationship. This component requires not only focused attention but also the ability to step back and attempt to discern the underlying purpose of what is being said. Listening for meaning while listening for content is most challenging.

3. **Listening for feelings and values:** Feeling introduces affect into the skill mix. The affect is where the emotions and the power live. Being able to understand at the affective level enables a leader to know what to say and how to influence. It is what helps a leader connect to stakeholders. In this regard, one can infer much from the choice of words, tone, body language, and other aspects of the experience of effective listening as a way to better appreciate the underlying values of the speaker. This aspect of listening is reminiscent of the detective in the classic murder mystery "The Big Easy" commenting on interviewing a witness saying, "It's not what he says that's so important, it's what you hear that counts."

BENEFITS OF EFFECTIVE LISTENING

The most important benefits of effective listening are relationship building and the enhancement of trust. Effective listening can result in challenging one's own assumptions and thereby becoming more knowledgeable and even wiser. In the words of Stephen Covey (a quote originally from

St. Francis of Assisi): "Seek first to understand and then be understood."[11] One of the key lessons learned by senior leaders who work across cultural and national boundaries is that listening is the one skill that is universally effective at building trust and respect across borders. In an increasingly global world of diverse populations, good listening skills are a critical competency for leaders.

In contrast, poor listening may contribute to a range of negative reactions that have real consequences such as "they are not listening to me because they already have their mind made up." The impression (which is often true) may be that only people with certain attributes or credentials are really listened to. Poor listening may result in a misunderstanding (due to failure to properly listen for content), the listener being branded as lacking savvy (due to a failure to listen for meaning), or distrust (due to a failure to listen for feeling and values).

OBSTACLES TO EFFECTIVE LISTENING

One obstacle to effective listening is the emphasis on *telling* in contrast to *asking*.[2] In the Western culture, which is driven by a need to relate to what has just happened and what one wants to see happen, the dominant mode of conversation is telling, not asking. Perhaps the biggest obstacle to effective listening is constant internal dialogue and discomfort with silence. Asking (rather than telling) builds the curiosity needed to be an effective listener and helps to overcome these obstacles.

PRACTICAL APPROACHES TO BETTER LISTENING

Research from the Center for Creative Leadership[12] has identified certain approaches to overcoming obstacles to effective listening:

1. **Understand one's natural conversational style:** Each person has a range of conversational styles, from telling to asking. A telling style is often needed in short-term problem-solving situations while an "asking style" may be more desirable in long-term situations characterized by a need to challenge one's assumptions and patterns of thinking.
2. **Listen for specific words or phrases:** As noted in our description of "listening for content," one can listen for specific words or phrases that particularly capture the meaning of what is being said. Then, by practicing reflective listening, one can repeat back those exact words or phrases and ask, "Am I hearing you correctly?"
3. **Listen for embedded questions:** Often one may hear another say, "I'm wondering about something." When hearing this opening, one can explore further this line of inquiry.
4. **Maintain a posture of active inquiry and learning:** This can be achieved by avoiding common tendencies such as advocating for a position, problem-solving behaviors, and giving advice. One can also state what you have learned from the conversation.
5. **Maintain an awareness of one's own presence in the conversation:** To be able to listen effectively, one must be able to develop the capacity to monitor the quality of one's own presence in real time. This awareness includes an awareness of nonverbal cues such as eye contact, posture, tone, and facial expressions that impact the degree to which the other feels really listened to.
6. **Deepen the level of listening:** One can attempt to deepen the level of listening with a few probing questions such as "Why are you thinking this way?" or "What leads you to conclude that …?"

TIPS FOR EFFECTIVE LISTENING

This research[10] has also yielded a few concrete tips:

1. **Be attentive:** Lean forward and give nonverbal affirmation (e.g., a nod or a smile) while maintaining comfortable eye contact. Above all, be present!

2. **Clarify:** At some point, ask, "Am I clear about what you are saying?" or "Can you repeat what you said? I'm not sure I am following you."

3. **Paraphrase:** Using words or phrases that have been heard, one can paraphrase what they heard to signal an attempt to better understand. This step involves an analysis of the content and intent of what was said.

4. **Reflect:** In an attempt to step back and better understand what has been said and underlying dynamics and assumptions, one can reflect openly what they are understanding and their feelings about what has been said.

5. **Summarize:** As a way of demonstrating that one has been listening for content, meaning, and feelings of the person speaking, one can attempt to summarize one's understanding of what was said and then follow the summary with a question such as, "Am I understanding you?"

ASKING BETTER QUESTIONS

In addition to the core skill of listening to understand, leaders must also cultivate the skill of asking better, more powerful questions. As noted by Peter Drucker: "In the past, the leader was the person who came up with the right answers, in the future the leader will be the person who comes up with the right questions."[13]

Good questions help to focus attention on what is really important. In this world of information overload and constant electronic connectedness, leaders serve others by redirecting attention from "distraction devices" toward what those whom one is leading need to attend to. Better questions help to foster and deepen relationships; the central premise is that "relationships are primary—all else is derivative."[13]

Further, by developing the skill of asking better questions, leaders may learn to listen to themselves more effectively, even asking themselves the question, "What does it feel like to be really heard?" In this context, asking questions of the self can also be a buffer against cognitive bias.

As noted by Marquardt, better questions create confidence and improve team member competence.[14] As a result, teams may exhibit greater creativity and innovation. Better questions can also help to guard against the dangers of "group think," which undermines a team's ability to make effective decisions.

In many organizations (particularly ones with a strong technical orientation), leaders tend to hold themselves accountable for having all the "right answers"; this attitude is often developed as a result of acquiring deep technical knowledge in a particular area. As a result, these leaders don't want to show a lack of knowledge which seems to indicate "weakness." This tendency may cause some leaders to find it difficult to acknowledge that they don't have all the answers. In such stressful situations, a leader can easily misconstrue assumptions and conjecture as facts in an effort to appear competent and knowledgeable.

GUIDING PRINCIPLES

As leaders develop their skill in asking better questions, certain guiding principles may be useful.[15]

■ **Make questions open-ended:** Open-ended questions foster reflection, deep thought, and unexpected new ideas.

■ **Be a good listener:** Focus on what is being said (including body language) rather than composing your next thought or statement; and notice what is not being said, which can be extremely significant.

■ **Avoid questions which are "statements in disguise":** Make sure you are really engaging deep inquiry and not simply trying to make your point in a different way or reinforcing your biases or preconceptions.

■ **Make the process as conversational as possible:** Your tone and posture are very important in establishing trust and openness.

- **Allow questions to surface deeply held assumptions:** Assumptions drive beliefs and actions and are often implicit (not explicit).
- **Employ dialogue methods by balancing inquiry and advocacy**[6]: The process of asking better questions can be accompanied by expressing opinions and advocating for a position; however, we suggest that it is preferable to follow the maxim of Stephen Covey "Seek first to understand and then be understood."[11]

TACTICS

To put these principles into practice, one should consider a few tactics[15]:

- Keep questions short—five words or so.
- The use of "what," "how," or "why" questions gets the best responses.
- Avoid asking a string of questions—just ask one simple question at a time.
- Pace the asking and then wait PATIENTLY for an answer (and repeat as needed). Silence is golden.
- Keep the tone of voice soft.

LONG-TERM ORGANIZATIONAL IMPACT

Asking better questions (along with listening simply to understand) creates an environment which enhances commitment to accountability and community. Better questions can also reinforce shared values and beliefs and an awareness of strategic options and alternatives. Stronger teams with greater performance and enhanced creativity will develop and grow, leading to followers who say: "We didn't know what we could not do."

Further, there should be fewer expectations for leaders to "have all the answers," to feel pressured to respond to situations prematurely, and then to exert top-down control. Improved morale and greater staff satisfaction and retention may occur. Growth and development of leadership skills within the organization can be practiced regularly and also shared with others. Having permission for everyone to ask questions empowers everyone to lead and increases candor and commitment.

Better listening and better questions can result in a change in perspective leading to greater creativity.[15] Team members may develop the skills needed to surface and examine group assumptions and become more aware of their own assumptions. As a result, team functioning may improve, leading to a more meaningful engagement with a broader range of public health and healthcare partners. Ideally, development of these core leadership skills may contribute to a narrowing of the widening gap between the poles of strongly held views.

MINDFULNESS AND DIALOGUE

As a result of more recent work in applying dialogue practice to organizational and community health,[16] a decision was made to join dialogue techniques with the practice of mindfulness.[17] Dialogue, which is the art of creative interaction, and mindfulness, which is the art of presence and expanded awareness, are both wonderful tools for growth in their own right. Together, however, they create a powerful synergy that can inspire and inform the level of change being described here. Mindfulness enables one to be more present, compassionate, aware, and open to the world, while dialogue helps one connect, explore, and discover and build together new, shared meaning and commitment.

Mindfulness deepens the connecting stage of Dialogue, for Mindfulness is the discipline of being present. Being present keeps the neocortex engaged even as other parts of the brain react in fight or flight mode. Being present enables one to access a deeper self in stories — "the stranger who was myself," as the poet Derek Walcott puts it. Being present fosters empathy, teaches us to suffer, promotes vulnerability and surfaces an ever-expanding new story of life. All of which lead to deeper connection, not only with others and with oneself but, perhaps more importantly, with life itself. This deeper connection is the foundation of a what is sometimes called a 'container' where something new can happen. We've all experienced such a space: with a grandmother, a lover, a friend, a pet, even a place. And like those relationships, a container can be developed and strengthened so that we can access it easily the way we can turn to a good friend. The presence that Mindfulness brings is the glue that holds this container together.

Mindfulness also transforms the exploring stage of Dialogue, for the purpose of the exploring stage of Dialogue is simply understanding. In the Mindfulness–Dialogue format, a catalyst — an inspiring piece of poetry or music — serves as a bridge between connecting and exploring. It does this by maintaining the spirit of the connecting stage's container while at the same time, pointing towards how this spirit applies to the theme at hand. This brings to mind the religious practice of lectio divina which is a form of reflective, prayerful reading of a sacred text. A more mindful exploring can then happen by suspending — holding up for examination — our assumptions. Mindfulness helps us become more aware of our own assumptions as well as those of others which otherwise would create the same predictable outcomes as always. Mindfulness also helps us stay present to the moment: to listen without simply judging and reacting which unfortunately is the norm; and to hold the tension that exploring generates.

Finally, there is the stage of Discovering which we have described as a kind of jazz where individuals work with an inspiration. The inspiration, in this case, is born out of the tension that is generated by the attempt to work with our differences. The poet Rilke captures the essence of this mysterious process of creativity:

> *"I am the rest between two notes, which are somehow always in discord because Death's note wants to climb over— but in the dark interval, reconciled, they stay there trembling. And the song goes on, beautiful."*

We find it difficult to allow differences never mind hold the tension they generate. But when we do, something new always happens: the song goes on. In Dialogue terms, new meaning emerges which we then can build, as we've described previously, into shared understanding, which, of course, is the only foundation for commitment and accountability.

There is more to be said about — more that is in fact emerging out of — this fascinating marriage of Mindfulness–Dialogue, for it is still somewhat new in its applications. Already, though, we have found openings for it in a wide variety of fields, including healthcare where healing is generated; education where learning is generated; finances where wealth — certainly in a broader sense — is generated; and finally religion where faith is generated and expanded.

SUMMARY

To live creatively in a world that is essentially interconnected, even as the culture that continues to shape assumptions as well as institutions promotes the illusion of separateness and competition, leaders must practice connecting: to oneself, to each other, and to the things they encounter. It is the awareness of reality (and self) that this connection brings that will be the foundation for a way of living—both personal and public—that is good in every sense: healthy, balanced, joyful, and genuinely sustainable. Leaders can then bring the skills of dialogue to the exploration of old assumptions about the world and the health of the public, now inspired by this deepened awareness of reality. When leaders do this, they become more able to generate new—shared—meaning that more accurately reflects the reality of interconnectedness and interbeing. This shared meaning can become the foundation for new ways of living, personally and socially.

Einstein once spoke about the relationship between religion and science, which is analogous to this mindfulness-dialogue relationship. He said: "Science without religion is lame, religion without science is blind."[9] It might similarly be suggested that mindfulness without dialogue is lame, while dialogue without mindfulness is blind. They are both important methods for living life and addressing challenges, but they need each other to be truly effective.

Thomas Berry's statement, that it is not possible to have healthy people on a sick planet, provides the framework for this deeper approach to public health and healthcare.[1] Mindfulness–dialogue provides a method that can be applied as a personal practice as well as a model for interaction at every level from the interpersonal to the organizational. Together they can help us realize Berry's implied vision of healthy people on a healthy planet.

DISCUSSION QUESTIONS

1. What are the basic challenges facing public health and healthcare and why is dialogue important for addressing these challenges?.
2. What is dialogue: level 1 (referring to competency in communicating/collaborating)?
3. What is dialogue: level 2 (referring to participating in the emergence of meaning)?
4. Why and how do dialogue and mindfulness come together?

CASE STUDY: APPLICATION OF DIALOGUE TO THE PRACTICE OF PUBLIC HEALTH LEADERSHIP

In light of the realization that public health leaders might benefit from the development of dialogue competency, a pilot project involving several local public health agencies (one of which involved a coauthor [DM] of this chapter and the coeditor of this text [Dr. Paul Erwin]) and the Centers for Disease Control and Prevention (CDC) was undertaken several years ago.[18] In this effort, dialogue training was paired with the use of the MAPP process (Mobilizing for Action through Planning and Partnerships) and was designed to enhance the sharing of meaningful approaches to community health—the goal of the MAPP process. The MAPP process consists of six phases: (1) organizing for success and partnership development, (2) visioning, (3) community assessments, (4) identification of strategic issues, (5) formulation of goals and strategies, and (6) action. The National Association of County and City Health Officials (NACCHO) provides leadership and technical assistance in the implementation of the MAPP process at the community level. The process is now being updated in light of emerging public health issues.[19]

In the early 2000s, as MAPP was being implemented in several pilot locations, Paul Erwin saw the potential value of dialogue, as it had been used by the NACCHO workgroup in the process of developing MAPP, in creating a new level of communication and trust among the dozen county health department directors and health officers under his charge. Meetings with this group of leaders were too frequently experienced as *telling* from Paul Erwin, the regional director, with little *asking* on the part of either Erwin or the county leaders. There was certainly little sense of egalitarianism in this traditionally strict hierarchical organizational structure and culture. In one of the first facilitated dialogue sessions, Martin had the group play "The Name Game," in which each person simply states their full name and tells a story about their name. Following this, the group was encouraged to use the name that each person most desired for themselves. When it came to Mary Ruth's (a county health department director) time to speak, she addressed the regional director as Paul, not as Dr. Erwin, which was the first time in her career she had ever addressed a male physician director of the region by their first name. The *immediate* sense of equality permeated the room and led to what was then the most generative dialogue among this group that any had ever experienced. This internal use of dialogue was a necessary pre-condition for implementing MAPP, where the equality of community voice was paramount. This effort to develop dialogue competency revealed that leaders must focus not only on skills and the toolset needed to practice these skills but also the mindset needed to engage in a deeper form of communication which embraces a wider range of assumptions and beliefs than is often the case.[18] Among the lessons learned from the application of dialogue competency was that this practice can enhance the creation and development of mutually beneficial strategic partnerships needed to address a wide range of public health issues.

Evaluation of this pilot effort to promote dialogue competency building in public health agencies showed two things: One was a clear appreciation of these skills at both personal and professional levels[17]; the other was the resistance encountered to the changes implied in both behavior and policy. This is because promoting and integrating dialogue challenges our assumptions: personal assumptions in the form of habits of thinking and acting, but also collective assumptions in the form of policies, regulations, and even "org" charts: systems and institutions, in other words. Something more than presenting new skills is clearly required to realize the changes necessary to address challenges that are in large part based on assumptions of separation and competition, and rights in the form of policies and practices informed by these assumptions.

CASE STUDY QUESTIONS

1. In applying dialogue practice to addressing a public health issue, what is the role of the skilled facilitator in maintaining the dialogue process? What skills are required for the role of skilled facilitator?
2. In applying dialogue practice, how should dialogue participants act to "suspend their assumptions"?
3. How should the modalities of dialogue and discussion be balanced such that concrete actions are delineated, and specific steps are identified?

 A robust set of instructor resources designed to supplement this text is located at http://connect.springerpub.com/content/book/978-0-8261-4924-4. Qualifying instructors may request access by emailing textbook@springerpub.com.

REFERENCES

1. Berry T. Universe Story. https://thomasberry.org/life-and-thought/about-thomas-berry/a-universe-story

2. Schein E. *Humble Inquiry: The Gentle Art of Asking Instead of Telling*. Berrett-Koehler Publishers; 2003.

3. Johnson JH Jr. Civic entrepreneurship. In: Baker EL, Menkens AJ, Porter JE, eds. *Managing the Public Health Enterprise*. Jones & Bartlett; 2010:159–164.

4. Martin BA, Matthews G. Creating better messages. In: Helm-Murtagh S, Erwin P, eds. *Leadership in Practice: Essentials for Public Health and Healthcare Leaders*. Springer Publishing Company; 2022:Chapter 18.

5. Senge P. *The Fifth Discipline: The Art and Practice of the Learning Organization*. Doubleday/Currency; 1990.

6. Isaacs W. *Dialogue: The Art of Thinking Together*. Doubleday/Currency; 1999.

7. Bohm D. *On Dialogue*. Routledge Classics; 2004.

8. Argyris C. *Reasoning, Learning and Action*. Jossey-Bass; 1982.

9. Martin D. Dialogue and spirituality. In: Banathy BH, Jenlink P, eds. *Dialogue as a Means of Collective Communication*. Springer; 2007:71–103.

10. Baker EL, Dunne-Moses A, Calarco AJ, Gilkey R. Listening to understand: a core leadership skill. *J Public Health Prac Manag Pract*. 2019;25(5):508–510. doi:10.1097/PHH.0000000000001051

11. Covey SR. *The 7 Habits of Highly Effective People*. Free Press; 1989.

12. Center for Creative Leadership. Better Conversations Every Day™: Center for Creative Leadership, Greensboro NC, 2018. https://www.ccl.org/leadership-programs/better-conversations-every-day-coaching-culture/

13. Drucker P. *The Essential Drucker*. Harper Business; 2008.

14. Marquardt M. *Leading With Questions: How Leaders Find the Right Solutions by Knowing What to Ask*. Jossey-Bass; 2014.

15. Baker EL, Gilkey R. Asking better questions—a core leadership skill. *J Public Health Manag Pract*. 2020;26(6):632–633. doi:10.1097/PHH.0000000000001177

16. Abatemarco DJ, Gannon M, Hand DJ, Short VL, McLaughlin K, Martin D. The use of mindfulness dialogue for life in substance use disorder treatment in the time of COVID-19. *J Subst Abuse Treat*. 2021;122:108213. doi:10.1016/j.jsat.2020.108213

17. Martin D. *Mindfulness dialogue 21 day*. https://dannymartin.org/mindfulness-dialogue-21-day

18. Martin D. The role of dialogue in the NACCHO MAPP tool. *J Pub Health Manag Pract*. 2005;11(5):415–417. https://journals.lww.com/jphmp/Citation/2005/09000/The_Role_of_Dialogue_in_the_NACCHO_MAPP_Tool.7.aspx

19. National Association of County and City Health Officials. *Mobilizing for action through planning and partnerships (MAPP)*. https://www.naccho.org/programs/public-health-infrastructure/performance-improvement/community-health-assessment/mapp

Chapter 2

Moral Courage in Public Health Leadership

James C. Thomas

INTRODUCTION

Where there is power, there is ethics. With power there is a chance it can be abused. Ethics names those abuses and names measures to avoid them. In part because they can frustrate those in power, ethical measures often require courage.

Public health and healthcare leaders have power, and they are also subject to powers out of their control. Because public health programs and policies affect whole populations, public health practitioners and healthcare leaders need to be aware of their power. But many leaders in public health are most aware of the forces they must contend with to fulfill their responsibilities, and the limits of their power against those forces. The forces often include lack of funding, large and influential companies that value profit above public health, and other urgent population needs that render public health a lower priority.

During the COVID-19 pandemic, one of the forces to contend with was the politicization of common public health measures, such as wearing a mask or receiving a vaccine. Avoiding both became a badge of honor or a statement of belief. Moreover, some political leaders—mayors, governors, and legislatures—sought to undermine disease control measures, seeing them as governmental overreach, or denying the dangers of the epidemic. Acting as a public health or healthcare leader in this climate often required moral courage.

OBJECTIVES

By the end of this chapter, the reader will be able to:

- Describe moral courage and how it fits into the larger field of ethics.
- Explain how to engender moral courage in the workplace and equip people to practice it.
- Describe how public health ethics differs from medical ethics.
- Explain how ethics can be taught and modeled to equip students with the knowledge and skills to practice moral courage.

WHAT IS MORAL COURAGE?

Moral courage is the strength to do the right thing when there is a cost to doing so. This is simply enough stated, but this sentence is full of ambiguity. How do we know what is right? How do we know what the cost will be? And what if the cost is not direct, but indirect? What if it affects others whom we care about more than it affects us? To talk further about moral courage and to address these questions, it will be helpful to draw some distinctions between morals, ethics, justice, and courage. These overlap with each other, so clean distinctions are elusive.

Morals are generally considered values that are influenced by family, education, culture, and religion. Values include honesty and respect for others. The more philosophically oriented say morals stem from a sense of duty, deriving from Kantian philosophy. Ethics that focus on duty, or deontological ethics, is one of the three major schools of thought in ethics.[1] Another school focuses on outcomes, such as equal opportunity or the fair distribution of goods. Utilitarianism, or the greatest good for the greatest number, is an example of this school of thought. In philosophy, this school is called consequentialism.

Both deontology and consequentialism—or duty and outcomes—address the question of what is the right thing to do. The third school of ethics, called virtue ethics, answers the question, "What is a good person?" This too is influenced by family, education, culture, and religion. In many societies, a person is considered good if their qualities include faithfulness, generosity, and courage, for example.

In addition to being an umbrella term for major schools of thought in ethics, the term "ethics" also connotes systems of decision-making. Systems facilitate decision-making by incorporating duty, desired outcomes, and virtues into a set of principles, priorities, and processes. The American Public Health Association (APHA) provides these for common decisions in public health in its Code of Ethics, described more fully in the text that follows.[2]

Justice, like ethics, is a term with several uses and meanings. In the court system, justice is usually about deciding who has been wronged and determining the rightful compensation or punishment. This is called retributive justice. In contrast, distributive justice is concerned with a fair distribution of opportunities and goods. A just distribution, however, is often in the eyes of the beholder, depending on their values. Some, for example, will value an equal distribution of goods, while others will value an equal distribution of opportunity. The latter, commonly regarded as libertarianism, might assume that not all people take advantage of their opportunities, resulting in an unequal distribution of goods that is nonetheless just because the opportunity was available. Thus, when invoking the term "justice," one must specify the type of justice they are referring to.

Moral courage is a hybrid concept that draws from several of the concepts just described. "Moral" invokes a sense of duty. In this case, a duty to take action; to do something when a lack of morality, ethics, or justice is seen. "Courage" is one of the virtues required to take action. This chapter is framed around moral courage because knowing what is right is not enough; one must also work to right the wrongs. Stated more simply, ethics without action is something less than ethics.

THE FOUNDATION OF MORAL COURAGE

Courage is typically depicted in statues with a bold stance, chin up, and looking defiantly into a coming threat. The companion of courage that is absent from these depictions is fear. Acting in spite of fear is what makes an action courageous. Fear, in turn, stems from humility, which is also missing from most heroic statues. The humility that underlies courage is a recognition that one's perceptions of a threat, and one's capacity to respond, may be flawed or inadequate.

When leaders notice an injustice, they often wonder whether they have seen it clearly. If it is egregious, they may not believe that anyone would be so bold as to commit that act. Or they may wonder whether others know the whole story. Maybe there are extenuating circumstances that explain the action in part or whole. Leaders might wonder about which action to take. What will be effective in stopping or righting the wrong? And they often question their own effectiveness: "Do I, as a leader, have the kind of influence it will take to bring about the needed change?"

In wondering about their own effectiveness, leaders are demonstrating humility, the limits of their power. Even in wondering whether they know the whole story, leaders are acknowledging the limits of their information. Humility is key in preventing them from acting impulsively or out of self-righteousness. Because of humility, leaders seek more information and the perspectives of others. With humility, acts of courage are preceded by the thought, "I could be wrong, but." The rest of that sentence is also shaped by humility: "but I will

Box 2.1: Speaking Truth While Employed by Power

Bill Jenkins blew the whistle, but no one paid attention. In 1967, 22-year-old Bill had just graduated from Morehouse College with a degree in mathematics. The U.S. Public Health Service Commission Corps had begun a new program for recruiting African American graduates, and Bill became one of the program's first.

In his second year with the program, a Corps physician expressed concern to Bill about a study of untreated syphilis among African American sharecroppers in rural Alabama. Today we know of this study as the Tuskegee Study, in which the participants were not informed of the study goal and were misinformed that they were being treated. Actually, they were being studied to see if untreated syphilis affected Black patients the same way that it affected White patients studied at the turn of the century in Oslo, Norway. The Oslo study occurred before the advent of penicillin as an effective treatment for syphilis in the mid-1940s. But for the Alabama men to remain untreated, penicillin was withheld from them.

Bill asked his Corps advisor, a statistician, about the study. She explained that it was an important study but misunderstood and not to worry about it. (Bill later learned that she was the statistician for the study.) After talking with more people and reading articles published from the study, he decided it was grossly unethical.

Bill and a few of his African American colleagues had begun printing a newsletter called *The Drum* addressing racism in the Department of Health Education and Welfare. They wrote about the study in the newsletter and sent it, along with copies of the other study articles they had gathered, to well-known newspapers such as the *Washington Post*. They hoped the information would lead to a major expose, but nothing came of their whistleblowing.

A few years later, in 1972, a venereologist with the Public Health Service who had been concerned about the study since the mid-1960s shared information about the study with a reporter friend. That reporter in turn shared it with another who wrote an expose in the *Washington Star* newspaper. The article precipitated public outrage and the study was terminated within the year.

Source: Data from Stanley J. Tuskegee was 'the tip of the iceberg.' CHOICE/LESS, The Backstory, Episode 4. *Rewire News Group*. June 21, 2017. https://rewirenewsgroup.com/multimedia/podcast/choice less-backstory-episode-4-tuskegee-tip-iceberg; Bill Jenkins, epidemiologist who tried to end the Tuskegee syphilis study, dies at 73. *Washington Post*. February 17, 2019. https://www.washingtonpost .com/local/obituaries/bill-jenkins-epidemiologist-who-tried-to-end-tuskegee-syphilis-study-dies-at -73/2019/02/27/2319e142-3aa2-11e9-a06c-3ec8ed509d15_story.html

take action because I have the support of wise people I have conferred with." Humility is a foundational virtue in public health. The APHA Code of Ethics says, for example, "Humility about the limits of expertise is critical. Interpretation of community needs and interests by health professionals should not be given automatic precedence over conflicting points of view. Public health must remain in dialogue with the communities it serves."[2(p13)]

Moral courage can be instantaneous, as when the leader hears a racist or sexist comment, for example, and they challenge it in the moment. Often, though, leaders are confronted with complex, multilayered situations that require reflection and consultation. In those instances, courage requires action with the humility to call upon others (Box 2.1).

HOW DO LEADERS KNOW THE RIGHT THING TO DO?

Morals and ethics guide leaders toward the right thing. Generally speaking, morals are embedded in and promoted through culture, while ethics are encoded by institutions. Perhaps the most intimate cultural influence is family. Leaders first learn what is considered right and wrong when they observe our parents or guardians. In Harper Lee's classic story of moral courage, *To Kill a Mockingbird*, Atticus Finch, a White single father, serves as the defense lawyer for Jack Robinson, a low-income Black man unjustly accused of rape in an overtly racist small town. In the climactic scene, the children sneak into the courthouse balcony (where Blacks were relegated) to watch their father's closing defense. They witness him standing against the racist tide, presenting a forceful and eloquent defense of the accused man. Yet, in spite of Atticus Finch's argument, the jury finds Mr. Robinson guilty and sentences him to prison. The story is told through the eyes of Scout, one of the Finch children, who is so impressed by the moral courage of her father that she has to share the story with the world.

CAN MORALITY BE TAUGHT?

Culture shapes leaders in ways that can be hard to detect. But can morality be shaped through formal education? Ethics education in the health professions relies heavily on formal teaching. Ethics courses in this context are intended to socialize students to the profession, including values in the profession and systems to enact and maintain them. In some cases, the teaching is explicitly about ethics, while in others the ethical implications are more implicit and less obvious. Many courses, for example, promote evidence-based action. Reliance on evidence and the scientific method are values in public health. They stand in contrast to decisions based on hunches, rumors, or political favors. In courses on health economics, one learns about two particular types of evidence: cost-benefit and cost-effectiveness. These measures underscore the public health values of effectiveness and efficiency. Epidemiology and biostatistics are used to rank in importance health issues, causes, and interventions. How many people do they affect? Who is affected most? Measures such as rate differences are examples of determining how to benefit the most people or identify the people most in need. In philosophical terms, these measures reflect a utilitarian perspective. Seldom, however, do those teaching health economics, epidemiology, or biostatistics link their measures to an underlying ethical perspective.

When ethics are addressed explicitly in public health and healthcare, the topics often include concepts such as equity, human rights, and social justice. These concepts are important for understanding and addressing fundamental causes of health outcomes, which are central to a public health perspective. In describing health justice and equity as a core value of public health, the Code of Ethics states that "health justice does not pertain only to the distribution of scarce resources in transactions among individuals; it also involves remediation of structural and institutional forms of domination that arise from inequalities related to voice, power, and wealth."[2(p5)]

Racism is an important example of domination throughout the history of the United States. Attitudes of racial superiority formed the basis of white settlers' claim of their "manifest destiny" to populate and exploit all land between the east and west coasts. The racist dehumanization of Africans provided the justification for treating them as property ("chattle") to purchase for the support of a plantation economy or for use as domestic servants in cities. The echoes of these historical attitudes and actions remain powerful today. They were seen, for example, in the War on Drugs in the 1990s and 2000s, in which jail and prison sentences for cocaine possession were 10 times more severe for Blacks than they were for Whites. Blacks were six times more likely than Whites to be incarcerated, which greatly affected their ability to find employment upon release.[3] The effects on health were pervasive, through stress, a lack of health insurance, relegation to neighborhoods with poor housing and few nutritious foods, and more.

These structural forces are the fundamental causes of poor health in individuals and populations that healthcare and public health aim to address. Ethics courses in public health and healthcare can describe the magnitude of the inequities, the forces that maintain them, the reasons they are unjust, and approaches to ameliorating the injustices.

RESEARCH ETHICS

Although structural factors underlying health inequities are of central importance to public health, the ethics of addressing them is not the most commonly taught aspect of ethics in schools of public health. The most privileged topic is research ethics. This is because certification in research ethics is mandated for participation in the conduct of studies on human subjects. The emergence of the industry for teaching and monitoring research ethics stems from the Tuskegee syphilis study conducted by the U.S. Public Health Service and the Centers for Disease Control and Prevention from 1932 to 1972, mentioned in Box 2.1. The study was of untreated syphilis among low-income, low-education Black male sharecroppers in rural Alabama. In that study, an effective treatment for syphilis was withheld from the men to see what the "natural" outcome of the disease would be. Unfortunately, the infamous study was labelled with the name of a collaborating institution, the historically Black Tuskegee University, rather than the predominantly White institutions that conceived of and funded the study.[4]

An ethics commission created after the inglorious end of the study in 1972 identified three fundamental ethical principles to guide research on human subjects: respect for persons, beneficence (acting for the benefit of others), and justice, or nonpreferential treatment.[5] The commission met at the Belmont Conference Center in Maryland; thus, their report was called the Belmont Report. These three principles often translate practically into rules for the selection of study subjects, informing them of the study purpose and procedures, getting their consent to participate, extra cautions for vulnerable populations, and weighing the study risks and benefits. These concerns have been further codified into checklists to guide the review of study proposals by ethics committees, usually referred to in the United States as institutional review boards, or IRBs.[6]

Those conducting a study of human subjects, the researchers, and their assistants are to be trained in the rules and regulations; thus, the widespread occurrence of courses on research ethics in the health sciences, including public health. The institutional research ethics systems serve the purpose of preventing harm to research participants, but they also result in some unintended consequences. If not placed in the broader context of public health ethics, it can appear that research ethics is the whole substance of public health ethics, particularly if no other course teaches non-research ethics. In a crowded curriculum, once research ethics is covered, it can appear that the ethics box has been checked, and the rest of public health ethics loses leverage against other topics competing for space among the required courses. An ethics perspective beyond research is essential, however, because it elevates the profession and the mission beyond a technical pursuit. Ethics remind us of *why* we are engaged in protecting and improving the public's health.

PUBLIC HEALTH VERSUS MEDICAL ETHICS

Another unintended consequence of the pervasiveness of research ethics training is that, through the lens of research ethics, public health ethics is virtually indistinguishable from medical ethics; and yet there is a significant difference between the two. Medical ethics principles, made popular by the textbook authors Tom Beauchamp and James Childress, build upon those named in the Belmont Report,[5] but instead of "respect for persons," they name the autonomy of the patient; and in addition to beneficence, they add nonmaleficence, echoing the "do no harm" credo of the medical Hippocratic Oath.[7]

Ethics principles in medicine and public health stem from different power imbalances in each field. The prototypical setting for a power imbalance in medicine is the clinic examining room. In that room, the clinician can be considered the host and the patient the guest. The clinician is wearing symbols of power, such as a white coat and a stethoscope draped around the neck. Their licenses to exercise special skills are hanging on the wall, and their reinforcements—assistants and colleagues—are just outside the door. They have special knowledge and privileges that can ease the pain of the patient, and others that can increase the pain. Meanwhile, the patient may be partially debilitated by the pain that brought them in, seeking relief. They may be partially disrobed in an examination gown. Patients have very little power in the room, unless it is explicitly given to them, which is what the ethical principle of autonomy aims to do. With their autonomy, they can refuse medical advice and decline to participate in a medical study.

The power imbalance in public health resides in a different place. If pictured as a room, it would be a board room in the local health department. Instead of a clinician, those with the power are the health department staff. The party that lacks power is often not in the room at all. They are not an individual, but the entire population served by the health department—a county, city, state, or nation. Public health ethics thus includes provisions for representation and processes for group decision-making.

The health considerations for the same condition can also be different in public health and medicine. For an infectious disease, the clinician is seeking to make the patient better. In contrast, because the condition is infectious, a health department is also concerned with the risk that the infected person poses to others. For this reason, they may constrain the infected person's autonomy by asking (in rare cases, requiring) them to isolate themselves. Public health therefore balances autonomy with interdependence.

Public health ethics is thus distinct from medical ethics, but the distinction was recognized after medical ethics was already well-established. While public health ethics came into its own in the 1970s, much of contemporary medical ethics was formed in the 1940s as a reaction to the medical experimentation on Nazi prisoners. At that time, public health was often regarded as an extension of medicine, and physicians were seen as the ultimate keepers and purveyors of health knowledge. With this perspective, medical ethics stood in for all health-related ethics, including public health. Without a distinct set of ethical principles to articulate a unique public health perspective, ethics taught in schools of public health was usually framed in terms of medical ethics. In seeking to understand the right thing to do in a public health system, however, answers from another system, such as clinical medicine, may be informative but will miss important issues, such as governing whole populations and addressing historical social and economic forces that underlie many health concerns.

THE ARTICULATION OF A PUBLIC HEALTH ETHIC

The absence of a formal system of ethics stemming from and addressing the particular challenges of public health was noticed by a group of public health leaders in the late 1990s. Some felt that the greater good of the community, which is central in public health, was not in the forefront of medical ethics. And some sought an explicit ethics statement to help define the profession's values. They were a cohort of experienced professionals participating in advanced leadership training through the Public Health Leadership Society (PHLS). They were currently employed by institutions such as the Centers for Disease Control and Prevention, APHA, the Public Health Institute of the Center for Health Leadership and Practice (California), state and city health departments, and several universities. For a group project, they selected the creation of a public health code of ethics.

The group of public health practitioners drafted the code in progressively larger concentric circles. One of the group members wrote the first draft based on their training in ethics and their experience in public health. The rest of the PHLS group then made comments and suggested edits. They formed a broader group of advisors with expertise in ethics philosophy, public health law, and public health practice to comment on the second draft. The advisors suggested additional changes. At the next stage, the draft code was presented at an APHA annual meeting, followed by a period for comments from all APHA members. The PHLS group member who was working for APHA was on the Association's board of directors. She presented the final Code of Ethics to the board in early 2002, and they endorsed it.[8]

The Code was based on 11 values and beliefs. They included "Humans are inherently social and interdependent," "Identifying and promoting the fundamental requirements for health in a community are of primary concern to public health," and "The effectiveness of institutions depends heavily on the public's trust."[25(pp2-3)] The values informed 12 practical principles. The first was "Public health should address principally the fundamental causes of disease and requirements for health, aiming to prevent adverse health outcomes."[8(p1058)] With its emphasis on prevention, this principle stood in contrast to a medical, curative perspective.

Another of the principles states, "Public health policies, programs, and priorities should be developed and evaluated through processes that ensure an opportunity for input from community members."[8(p1058)] This principle puts a public health lens on what is called informed consent in medical ethics. However, communities are characterized by a complex mix of interests and preferences, and seldom is there unanimity. But community members and various stakeholders should have an opportunity to voice their views on public health programs and policies.

In 2019, after 17 years of experience with the first Code of Ethics, the APHA Ethics Section produced a revised and updated version (Box 2.2).

Box 2.2: Summary—The American Public Health Association Code of Ethics, 2019 Version

The APHA Code of Ethics is presented in four sections in the 2019 version.

The **introduction** explains the reason for a Code of Ethics (it is "like a promise to society"), and it names human flourishing as the overall goal. The public health profession is composed of many different disciplines. The Code for the overall profession does not aim to replace codes of ethics for individual disciplines, such as epidemiology or health education. Rather, it describes overarching values and principles that unify the profession.

Core values. Six core values are named: professionalism and trust, health and safety, health justice and equity, interdependence and solidarity, human rights and civil liberties, and inclusivity and engagement. Within each of these are further details. For example, the reliance on evidence for action is included under professionalism and trust.

Guidance for analysis of ethical actions identifies eight questions to consider.

- Is the action morally *permissible* and allowed by the law?
- Does the action show *respect* of individuals and communities?
- Does it incorporate *reciprocity* by offsetting the potential harms or losses?
- Will the action be *effective*?
- Is it a responsible use of scarce resources?
- Is the action *proportional* in scope to the issue it addresses?
- Is there *accountability and transparency* in how the action is carried out?
- Is there *public participation* in formulating the action?

The Code then provides **guidance for ethical action** in 12 domains, including "Investigate health problems and environmental public health hazards to protect the community." (p. 13) and "Evaluate and continuously improve processes, programs, and interventions." (p. 25) Each of the domains lists several specific ethical steps. For example, under "Evaluate and continuously improve" one sees the following:

- Involve a commitment to a continuous improvement process for all essential programmatic components.
- Engage a wide spectrum of stakeholders in the improvement process.
- Develop as appropriate strategic plans with measurable goals for essential program components.
- Incorporate regular reviews of all essential program aspects in the context of specifed goals.
- Assess the environment for improvements in evaluation approaches.
- Evaluate the quality improvement process on a regular basis.
- Involve an investment in relevant innovations in approaches to providing feedback through learning interventions. (pp. 25–26)

In the progression from values to analysis to action, the APHA Code of Ethics enables public health practitioners to identify ethical issues, as well as responses to those most commonly encountered in public health.

Source: Data from American Public Health Association. *Code of Ethics.* 2019. https://www.apha.org/-/media/Files/PDF/membergroups/Ethics/Code_of_Ethics.ashx

CREATING AN ENVIRONMENT FOR MORAL COURAGE

As previously stated, moral courage is the strength to do the right thing when there is a cost to doing so. Leaders learn what is considered right by their culture and by their institutions. But *knowing* what is right doesn't automatically translate into *doing* what's right. The courage to take action comes from a sense of one's integrity and one's obligations to others. Courage is often not tied to effectiveness, one of the values in public health. Rather, it is tied to the very real possibility of failure—of the courageous act not having its intended effect, or even backfiring into personal pain from retribution.

To take this risk, one must care about what they represent and what they are working toward. The factors that public health and healthcare leaders can attend to in the workplace, so their employees care about their work, extend beyond the scope of this chapter, but a few of the most critical are mentioned here.

Safety

The starting place for caring about work is feeling safe there. Although physical safety is important, the focus here is primarily *emotional safety*. Safety from sexual predation, from public shaming, from macro- and micro-aggressions, from unfair practices, and more. If one feels safe in the workplace, they can relax enough to be creative and courageous. Safety is important in every workplace, but especially in those with male leadership of a predominantly female staff. Women have been hurt too often by this historical power differential, including when the selection of leaders itself is unfair.

Respect

Leaders respect coworkers by honoring their time, trusting them, and keeping the workplace peaceful. People feel respected when requests for one-on-one meetings are fulfilled promptly, when group meetings start and end on time, and when timelines for group activities are kept. Leaders show trust by not micro-managing and giving each person space to be creative with their responsibilities. And leaders help keep the workplace peaceful, by not avoiding necessary, difficult conversations with individuals who are having a negative impact on the work of others.

Listening is also essential to respect. Can an employee ask questions and get prompt, thoughtful answers? Do they have an opportunity to make suggestions, and are the suggestions received with gratitude rather than resentment? Are suggestions seriously considered and sometimes implemented? Do they get credit for their helpful suggestions and other contributions? When a person believes they will be heard and they can influence practices or policies, they are more likely to share their thoughts.

Community in the Workplace

In a strong community, people bear one another's burdens. They are familiar with each other's strengths and struggles. They include coworkers where they can, while also respecting each other's boundaries. Small talk, or talk about things other than work, is essential to a sense of community, because to connect on a human level, people want to talk about their children, their search for the right pair of shoes, and their long wait at the Department of Motor Vehicles. If the community is strong, people will believe their coworkers will "have each other's backs" if they need to act courageously.

Meaning

Meaning comes from seeing the bigger picture that one is part of. An important part of leadership is helping each person to see how they are contributing to a worthy goal. The goal needs to be specific and credible, not just "saving lives" or "making the world a better place." A sense of meaning is helped by having clear roles and systems, so people know how their role helps others, and how they fit into the dance of each workday.

With such an environment—one that is safe, where a person feels respected, where there is a sense of being supported by a community, and the community is working together toward a worthy goal—employees are likely to care about their work and their shared goal. They will care that their work doesn't hurt anyone and that it has a good reputation for acting ethically. They will have a foundation for acting courageously.

ETHICS RESOURCES

To this environment that fosters a moral motivation, ethics resources are added that inform about the values, principles, actions, and practices that characterize healthcare and public health ethics. First among these is the *AMA Code of Medical Ethics* and the *APHA Code of Ethics*, the latter which was revised in 2019 (see Box 2.2).[2,9] Employees of healthcare organizations and public health agencies and organizations can learn about their respective Codes by having it included in their job training or on-boarding. Contributions to the ethical practice of public health and healthcare can be included in performance evaluations. The importance of the Code can be reinforced by occasionally discussing it as a group or referring to it in meetings when a new healthcare or public health challenge is being discussed.

Application of the APHA Code of Ethics to COVID-19, for example, can be found in publications[10] and the online *Pandemic Ethics Dashboard* (https://pandemicethics.org). The Dashboard (Box 2.3) is designed to guide viewers to relevant ethical guidance based on their institutional setting (e.g., a policy maker or a hospital employee) and the type of challenge they are wrestling with (e.g., engaging with stakeholders). The Dashboard then presents users with relevant guidance in the APHA Code of Ethics or other documents on ethical actions in a pandemic that were developed through consensus-making processes. These include documents from the Centers for Disease Control and Prevention (CDC) and WHO.

A series of free, brief *presentations on public health ethics* are available online.[11] Some of the topics are "Distinguishing public health ethics from medical ethics," "Values and beliefs inherent to a public health perspective," "The public health code of ethics," "Law and ethics in public health," "Decision-making in public health ethics," and "Barriers to the ethical

---

Box 2.3: The Pandemic Ethics Dashboard

A resource that brings together several ethics resources is the online Pandemic Ethics Dashboard (pandemicethics.org). It is designed to provide quick answers to policy makers about ethical actions in a pandemic. An illustrative example is the guidance on stakeholder engagement.

1. On the Dashboard home page, a public health official or policy maker would select the "Guidance for Government" option. There one finds 12 issues that government offices encounter in a pandemic. They include gathering evidence to inform policies, establishing ethical decision-making processes, and engaging stakeholders.

2. By selecting "Engage with stakeholders," the user is presented with five components of stakeholder engagement, such as "Seek input from those affected before, during, and after the implementation" and "Provide an opportunity for input from the full range of those affected."

3. If the latter is selected, there appears a list of nine statements of ethical guidance extracted from the APHA Code of Ethics, the CDC pandemic ethics guidance, and the Indiana University Center for Bioethics. Among the five excerpts from the APHA Code of Ethics, we read "Empower community members and stakeholders to be active participants in the decision-making process"[2(p15)] and "Be diligent in identifying communities and groups with a stake in public health planning and programming activities."[2(p18)]

TABLE 2.1: Resources for Establishing an Ethical Public Health Workplace

TOOL	DESCRIPTION
American Public Health Association Code of Ethics	A booklet produced by the Ethics Section of APHA delineating ethical principles in public health and their application in situations commonly encountered in public health (www.apha.org/-/media/Files/PDF/membergroups/Ethics/Code_of_Ethics.ashx).
Pandemic Ethics Dashboard	An online resource for quick navigation to established guidance from WHO, CDC, APHA, and others on how to respond to a pandemic ethically. One tab of the Dashboard presents tools for implementing the processes of public health ethics (https://pandemicethics.org).
Video clips on public health ethics	A series of short video clips that can be used for teaching public health ethics to students or for training employees (www.jcthomas.org/teaching).
Ethics and Public Health Model Curriculum	A set of chapters covering the core material of public health ethics that can be used in teaching students or training employees (https://repository.library.georgetown.edu/handle/10822/556779).
Public Health Ethics: Cases Spanning the Globe	A series of case studies that illustrate the application of public health ethics (http://link.springer.com/book/10.1007/978-3-319-23847-0).

APHA, American Public Health Association; CDC, Centers for Disease Control and Prevention; WHO, World Health Organization.

practice of public health." (The current versions require Flash technology. Non-Flash versions are being recorded and will appear on the same website.) The presentations can be used in classrooms, in workplace training, or as material to spark a discussion.

Shortly after the development of the first Public Health Code of Ethics, a group of people active in public health ethics developed a model curriculum. Entitled *Ethics and Public Health: Model Curriculum*, some of its chapters are, "The Legacy of the Tuskegee Syphilis Study," "Research Ethics in Public Health," "Ethics of Infectious Disease Control: STDs, HIV, TB," and "Ethics of Health Promotion and Disease Prevention."[12]

A case-based approach to ethics is available in an open access book entitled *Public Health Ethics: Cases Spanning the Globe*.[13] Forty cases are grouped into topics, including "Resource Allocation and Priority Setting," "Vulnerability and Marginalized Populations," and "International Collaboration for Global Public Health," among others.

Finally, the Pandemic Ethics Dashboard includes a list of links to tools for implementing public health ethics (Table 2.1). Listed there are tools for engaging stakeholders, collaborating, creating ethical decision-making processes, communicating with the public, allocating scarce resources, and more.[13]

WHEN A LEADER CARES ABOUT ETHICS

It takes leadership to create an environment and to embed ethics processes into a workplace. Individuals who are not in leadership positions can request changes to the workplace environment or introduce ethics resources, but they are unlikely to be implemented consistently or enthusiastically if not sanctioned and promoted by the leadership.

In the mid-2000s, well before the COVID-19 pandemic, the world was preparing for a pandemic of influenza. Part of the preparation was the identification of anticipated ethical issues and guidance on how to handle them. Expert committees produced ethics guidance documents at the WHO, the CDC, and some state health departments. At the same time, the states and territories of the United States were each writing their own plan for responding to the anticipated influenza pandemic. In a systematic review of all the plans, the authors found that only one in five states, on average, had identified an ethical framework.[14] Most often the framework applied to medical ethics for clinical settings. Other concerns, such as community engagement regarding plans for isolation and quarantine, were seldom addressed.

Seven states mentioned their intention to become more ethically prepared. Three years later, all but one had, indeed, followed through on their plans. As revealed in phone conversations between the researchers and those aware of their state's public health ethics in the seven states, there was an unambiguous and consistent reason for follow-through or its absence: having a leadership explicitly committed to ethics. That is, with a committed leader, ethics functions were strengthened; without a committed leader, ethics languished.

LEADING BY EXAMPLE

A workplace environment can enable moral courage when people care about their work and when the leadership informs them about values and practices for the ethical practice of public health and healthcare. However, nothing speaks as forcefully about moral courage as witnessing it, or the absence of it. In the example of Bill Jenkins (see Box 2.1), his colleagues had conversations with him as he grew aware of the syphilis study. They saw him grow uncomfortable and then agitated. They considered with him the steps one might take to voice an objection or even bring the study to a halt. Some may have said (as commonly happens) that speaking out would be a futile act; he would be risking his reputation for an action that was likely to go nowhere. They would have then watched as he mustered his courage to talk to CDC staff well above his pay grade. And then, when he shared his concerns with the media, his colleagues saw that it made no difference, at least to outside appearances.

But in watching Bill's knowledge grow into outrage, they could see that his ethics were more than theoretical, and how fury over an injustice signals that something really matters. It matters so much that one would risk their career in order to protect their integrity. Bill did not stand by idly; instead, he spoke out to those who could end the study. This willingness to experience personal pain in order to make things right will stay fixed in his colleagues' heads and hearts far longer than any training they might receive in a classroom.

Negative examples can also speak volumes. In one such instance, a university provost implemented an unpopular plan to bring students back to campus in the midst of rising COVID-19 case numbers in the state (Box 2.4). The provost may have viewed his decisions as moral courage. In his eyes, at the risk of failure, he pressed on against nay-sayers to achieve what he thought to be a laudable goal: a better learning experience for the students. If this is what he thought, however, his goals and methods did not align with the professional consensus on public health ethics. There is little ground in ethics to support a claim for his action as being moral. Rather than courage, his motivation was widely regarded by observers as fear of losing income from students' tuition and fees if the students didn't return to campus. This chain of events, then, was perceived as arrogance and economic interest rather than moral courage. To some, the breach of trust and lack of remorse that resulted in a campus catastrophe is a dark morality play. Such plays throw a spotlight on right morals and action through negative consequences when the morals are neglected. Especially when the result is a public failure, most observers will attribute the bad result to poor ethical practices, and surmise that ethical practices would have yielded a better result.

COURAGEOUS ACTION

Courage may be thought of as being flashy and dramatic: saving a child from a burning house, for example. There are also dramatic stereotypes of moral courage, like the civil rights marchers who crossed the Edmund Pettus Bridge in Selma, Alabama, in 1965, knowing they were walking into a beating by the police waiting with their billy clubs on the other side. Sometimes moral courage *is* dramatic and newsworthy. But much of the time it is not public and not flashy, just as much of the time leadership is done behind the scenes and invisibly.

Box 2.4: "I Don't Apologize"

The summer of 2020 was one of confusion over COVID-19. It had become clear that distancing and wearing masks reduce transmission. There was hope for an eventual vaccine, but hope remained distant. In the meantime, a number of cities were experiencing hospitalization rates that outstripped medical resources, and in some instances the deaths from COVID outstripped the capacity of the morgues, leading to the storage of corpses in refrigerator trucks.

In universities, students had been sent home from dormitories in the spring. During the summer of 2020, the question was whether to bring them back to campus in the fall. Some announced they would not: They would shift to all-remote teaching, with the hope that a vaccine would allow them to bring students to campus after the New Year.

At one university, the chancellor charged the provost (roughly the equivalent of a university chief operating officer) with managing the logistics of the university's response to the COVID-19 pandemic. The provost and his team of advisors were in communication with the local health department about this question because the influx of about 30,000 students could have a dramatic effect on transmission in the county.

Citing the deliberative process, the provost announced that all students would be brought back to campus in August. They would not be tested for infection before arriving because a negative test would only create a false sense of security, causing students to let down their guard. Many of the campus faculty, staff, and students objected strongly. The university, they said, was relying too much on an honor system in which students would wear masks and keep their distance.

In the week before the scheduled return of students, the county health department sent a letter to the chancellor and provost, saying, in effect, we don't think you were listening when we were talking about students in the fall. We can't force you to change your plan, but we advise against it. The provost chose not to share this communication with other stakeholder groups on campus, most notably, a faculty committee advising the chancellor and provost on COVID-19 plans. Then tens of thousands of students streamed into university town. Within days, outbreaks were occurring, and they quickly multiplied. Just 1 week after they had arrived, the provost decided the plan wasn't working and sent the students back home.

When it was revealed in a media story that the provost had ignored advice from the county health department, and had not been transparent about the advice, the faculty advisory committee was furious. In speaking to the committee, however, the provost said, "I do not apologize for trying" to bring students to campus. With their lack of regard for the safety of the campus faculty, staff, and students; their lack of transparency in decision-making; and their lack of remorse in having made a bad decision, the provost and chancellor lost a great deal of trust—perhaps the most valuable asset in a crisis.

For leaders, some of the most courageous acts are personal. It takes courage to yield control; to let others have their say, and to give them power to influence decisions. It takes courage to have a difficult conversation with an employee who is underperforming or having a negative effect on the workplace environment. And it takes courage to be humble by taking responsibility for a mistake or a failure, to apologize to those affected by it, and to make adjustments with a new approach.

COURAGEOUS SYSTEMS

Systems and procedures can also be morally courageous but not flashy. Democratic systems take away the power to act unilaterally, and thus they limit the power of individual leaders. However, they also often result in a decision that is embraced more broadly and implemented more effectively.

Ethical systems are called procedural ethics. They include systems for ensuring transparency and accountability. One of the most important is called fair process, in which stakeholders work together to identify an ethical issue and devise how to address it. Lists of the elements of good governance vary, but they include transparency and publicity about the reasons for a decision, rationales, and evidence that fair-minded parties would agree are relevant, as well as procedures for appealing and revising decisions in light of challenges by various stakeholders.[15]

These elements are incorporated into the following processes for ethical decision-making.[16]

1. **Define the problem:** Clarify the facts. When a problem is first identified, it is often incompletely understood. Although fact-finding is never complete, be sure that the most relevant questions are addressed. Don't assume that the problem raised is the key problem. With more information, it may disappear as a problem altogether, or a related concern may emerge as more important.

2. **Seek out relevant assistance, guidance, and support:** Who has information about the problem? What individuals or groups are affected by it and will potentially be affected by the action taken?

3. **Identify alternatives:** It is unlikely that a single course of action will emerge. To maximize creativity, let the ideas flow. Describe several potential courses of action.

4. **Evaluate the alternatives:** Examine them through ethical schools of thought, such as utilitarianism or human rights; or the perspectives of how each stakeholder is affected. The APHA Code of Ethics is an important reference to consult.

5. **Make the decision:** Compare the potential courses of action and decide which one, or which components of several, will best address the concern that was initially raised.

6. **Implement the decision:** In doing so, collect information that will help with an evaluation.

7. **Evaluate the decision:** After the action has had time to be implemented, engage the stakeholders in evaluating whether it was implemented as intended, and whether it achieved its intended purpose. Based on the evaluation, adjust the action as needed.

Following these steps, two different groups with the same initial ethical problem could identify different ethical issues to address, and different action steps to take. But because the relevant stakeholders were involved and the processes of the groups were fair, as previously described, they would both be ethical decisions. With this view, an ethical solution is less often about *the* right answer than it is about a fair process for arriving at *an* answer that can be honored.

The importance of a fair process was revealed in a comparison of ethical perspectives related to responses to an influenza pandemic.[17] The researchers conducted meetings in four regions of the world: Africa, Asia, Latin America, and the Middle East. In each region, the researchers brought together local public health practitioners, scientists, academics, ethicists, religious leaders, and other community members from throughout the region. They described how an epidemic of influenza would likely play out, and the ethical challenges that would arise. The ethical challenges included transparency and public engagement, allocation of resources, social distancing, obligations to and of healthcare workers, and international collaboration.

As anticipated, there were some regional differences in priorities. For example, in distributing scarce resources, the Africans expressed a greater importance of older adults than the other regions did. But the ethical concept that was consistently valued across regions was fair process. Such processes allow for values to vary by region, while arriving at solutions that can be widely endorsed and trusted.

COURAGEOUS OPTIONS

Systems for ethical decision-making are especially helpful for identifying the right thing to do. But what can be done when one has witnessed something wrong? What are the options for responding to, say, corruption among people higher up the chain? In the case of Bill Jenkins, he learned about research being done by his agency that was unethical for several reasons.

In the case of Bill Jenkins, start by noting the actions taken by others that did not display moral courage. These are the roads not taken for those seeking to be courageous. The physician who first informed Bill, who was troubled by the study, *avoided taking action himself*. Instead, he mentioned it to Bill, hoping Bill might do something. Others likely did still less. The physician was probably not the only one who was troubled by the study practices. Some who were involved may have *turned a blind eye* because they were benefiting from the study, or because they didn't want to make trouble. His advisor, the study statistician, *justified* the experiment, saying it was important. She advised him to "not worry about it," that is, to trust those who were involved and more senior.

Bill could have simply bad-mouthed the study within the Corps without taking a more decisive action. This would have allowed him to distance himself from the unethical study, and perhaps protect his integrity. He could have further distanced himself by quitting his job, either quietly or in protest to the study. Sometimes these are the right actions and require courage, but Bill felt he needed to stay in the agency to bring about change.

His first step was to *gather more information*. He *spoke with others* to get their perspectives, and he *read publications* from the study. Rather than acting alone, he relied on *a group of colleagues* whose insights and instincts he trusted. He *spoke with his direct supervisor*, but then discerned that she had a conflict of interest that kept her from seeing the study clearly. The action he eventually took was to *blow the whistle* by sending information to the media.

His action, though, was ineffective. He later concluded that he and his colleagues should have approached the media using their language, namely a press release. Conceivably, the media didn't pay attention to his concern because he lacked clout; he held a low-level position in the Public Health Service Commissioned Corps, he was not part of the study, he did not have a graduate degree, or perhaps it was because he was African American. Peter Buxton, whose whistleblowing was effective, was White and more senior. He was also better connected to the media. He told the story to a friend of his working in the media who, in turn, passed the story on to a colleague who could do something with it.

Bill Jenkins' ineffective whistleblowing does not make him any less courageous. But it does show that although the truth may be necessary to reveal the need for change, it may not be sufficient to bring the change about. Understanding the social and political dynamics of how change occurs is another needed element.

THE CONSEQUENCES OF COURAGE

At the beginning of this chapter, moral courage was described as the strength to do the right thing when there is a cost to doing so. For whistleblowing, the personal cost is often steep. The record is long of whistle-blowers who have been sidelined, passed over for a promotion, demoted, or even fired. Soon after his failed attempt, Bill Jenkins left the Corps to get a graduate degree in epidemiology so he could have more of a voice in addressing racism in public health. The consequences he might have experienced at work had he stayed, therefore, remain unknown.

However, the need for whistleblowing is relatively rare. Much more often, the need for moral courage is in the unflashy, daily actions in creating an ethical environment, and implementing ethical systems. There may be a cost of discomfort in having a difficult conversation, or embarrassment in admitting a mistake, but there are also benefits to these courageous actions. They result in trust, the most important asset in public health. There is trust among coworkers because they are included in processes, they are recognized for their contributions, and their leaders don't sweep their own mistakes under the rug. The population they serve trusts because processes are inclusive, the leaders are accountable, and again, they own up to their mistakes and make corrections.

Trust, in turn, is a key element to effectiveness in implementing public health. In a society that is not authoritarian and not coercive, moral authority is what can convince the general population to follow the policies and guidance of the public health agency. Moral courage, then, not only has costs—it also has substantial benefits. Indeed, where there is power there is ethics. But the opposite is also true, where there is ethics, there is power.

SUMMARY

Moral courage is the strength to do the right thing when there is a cost to doing so. This chapter emphasizes moral courage because simply a knowledge of ethics is not enough. To be meaningful, it must result in decisions and actions, which can be challenging and costly in terms of relationships and resources. Leaders seek to identify the right action through their personal morals, shaped by their families, cultures, and religions; and through systems of ethics that identify principles and practices for making decisions.

The courage to take action is influenced by the degree to which leaders care about their work and whether their workplace is supportive of acting ethically. The ways in which leaders in public health and health systems exercise courage are sometimes dramatic, but frequently quotidian. They include the courage to delegate, to listen to voices that express perspectives different from their own, and by supporting the systems that facilitate group decision-making rather than autocratic decisions.

The results of moral courage in public health can be push-back by those who disagree or who benefited from the problem being addressed. However, the daily practices that encourage caring about work, having a safe and supportive work environment, and empowering coworkers to act ethically can prevent the occurrence of unethical practices needing correction and build trust with the population served. Trust, in turn, can facilitate the implementation of public health policies and programs, thereby improving the health of the public.

DISCUSSION QUESTIONS

1. Where have you seen moral courage exhibited by a leader in public health or healthcare?
2. Where have you seen elements of the processes for ethical decision-making used?
3. Have you experienced a setting in which moral courage was facilitated or hampered? If so, in what way?
4. Describe your education in public health or healthcare ethics. Were there aspects that were covered insufficiently? If so, what were they?

CASE STUDY: USING EPIDEMIOLOGY TO REVEAL ENVIRONMENTAL INJUSTICES

The methods of epidemiology can be used to reveal inequalities. If the inequalities are tied to histories of systematic oppression, the combination of quantitative and qualitative evidence can put a spotlight on injustices. Steve Wing, an associate professor of epidemiology at the University of North Carolina in Chapel Hill, used epidemiology and community activism in this way.

Dr. Wing focused his expertise in occupational and environmental epidemiology in his home state of North Carolina. As a "right to work" state, North Carolina laws and policies favor employers over employees, and provide few means for workers to negotiate with their employers or hold them accountable. In part for this reason, the hog farm industry has a strong presence in the state. With their high numbers and concentrations of animals, industrial hog farms generate large quantities of waste, which is stored in ponds until it can be used on nearby land as fertilizer. The strong smell of the waste permeates the air of local communities. The communities have little recourse in getting the hog farms to relocate or change their practices. Their lack of power is the result of state laws that favor industries, but also because the communities are some of the poorer ones in the state, with fewer resources, including political connections, to draw upon.

Steve Wing documented the effects of the hog farms on the health of local communities and how they were systematically placed in poor communities.[18-21] He often used community based participatory research, which drew upon the expertise, insights, and networks of the local communities. This type of research requires the investment of a great deal of time in order to develop connections and establish trust with community members. Consequently, relatively few publications are generated from participatory research in comparison to (increasingly common) epidemiologic studies that rely on existing data and do not depend on bridge-building with the source population. Dr. Wing's publication rate thus did not reach the expectation of his department, and he was not promoted beyond the level of associate professor. Moreover, the hog industry objected to the articles that he did publish. They asked the dean of the UNC School of Public Health to pressure Dr. Wing into stopping his research or reframing his results (personal communication with Steve Wing). But he continued his research and writing undeterred. He passed away at the age of 64 in 2016.

CASE STUDY QUESTIONS

1. What values in public health did Steve Wing demonstrate in conducting his research on hog farms?
2. What other examples can you think of in which the quantitative sciences of public health—such as epidemiology, biostatistics, health economics, or laboratory sciences—were used intentionally to reveal an unethical act, an inequity, or an injustice?
3. Dr. Wing experienced a personal cost to his research in not being promoted to the rank of full professor. What benefits may he have accrued, nonetheless?

CASE STUDY: IMPLEMENTING PUBLIC HEALTH MEASURES IN THE CONTEXT OF RESISTANCE

The COVID-19 pandemic was first experienced broadly by American populations in March 2020, when cities and states began to "shelter-in-place" or impose social isolation mandates. Over the prior 3 years, the United States president, Donald Trump, had been a polarizing political and social figure. Political conservatism had traditionally resisted federal government intervention in personal lives. But under President Trump, this sentiment was enflamed and took expression, in part, as resistance to public health measures. Furthermore, over recent years, while political and social views became more entrenched, the rhetoric and actions toward those with opposing views became more strident and at times violent.

The resistance to public health measures, such as physical distancing and masks, was expressed as aggressive verbal challenges and intimidation of public health practitioners. Some received death threats. Already under stress themselves as they managed their own families during the pandemic, the aggressive resistance and threats they encountered in their jobs made their work lives not only stressful, but dangerous. Public health agencies across the country experienced a mass exodus of employees.[22]

When public health systems began to respond to COVID-19, Mimi Hall was the health services director of Santa Cruz County, California. In this role, she had the highest profile in the county's response to COVID-19. In response to the announcement of public health measures, she received a letter in which her family was threatened, and the writer wished her a slow death. In spite of this, Ms. Hall remained in her position and continued the public health messaging to protect her community.

Her colleague, Gail Newel, was the health officer for the county. Protestors gathered in front of her house to chant "Gail to Jail." She reported feeling intimidated to be out in the community. She too, however, continued with her work in implementing public health measures.

For continuing to provide public health messaging in the face of threats, and for making the threats known, Mimi Hall and Gail Newel were honored with a courage award by PEN America, a national organization supporting free expression and persecuted writers.[23,24]

CASE STUDY QUESTIONS

1. How do resources such as the APHA Code of Ethics and the Pandemic Ethics Dashboard assist professionals such as Mimi Hall and Gail Newel to implement public health measures in the face of resistance by some in the public?

2. The news stories don't report on the responses of those in higher positions, such as the mayor of the city of Santa Cruz, or the county board of health. But what could they have done to support the courageous actions of these two health department employees?

3. The urgency of the COVID-19 pandemic will wane, but political and social polarization will likely remain for years to come. There will be other public health threats to respond to in that time. What should the Santa Cruz County Health Department be doing to prepare its employees for public resistance to their responses to future emergencies?

 A robust set of instructor resources designed to supplement this text is located at **http://connect.springerpub.com/content/book/978-0-8261-4924-4.** Qualifying instructors may request access by emailing **textbook@springerpub.com.**

REFERENCES

1. Blackburn S. *The Oxford Dictionary of Philosophy.* 3rd ed. Oxford University Press; 2016.

2. American Public Health Association. *Public Health Code of Ethics.* 2019. https://www.apha.org/-/media/Files/PDF/membergroups/Ethics/Code_of_Ethics.ashx

3. Thomas JC. From slavery to incarceration: social forces affecting the epidemiology of STDs in the rural South. *Sex Trans Dis.* 2006;33(7 suppl):S6–S10. doi:10.1097/01.olq.0000221025.17158.26

4. Jones JH. *Bad Blood: The Tuskegee Syphilis Experiment.* Free Press; 1993.

5. U.S. National Commission of the Protection of Human Subjects of Biomedical and Behavioral Research. *The Belmont Report: Ethical Principles and Guidelines for the Protection of Human Subjects of Research.* U.S. Government Printing Office; 1978. https://www.hhs.gov/ohrp/regulations-and-policy/belmont-report/read-the-belmont-report/index.html

6. Thomas JC. Research ethics in public health. In: Jennings B, Kahn J, Mastroianni A, Parker L, eds. *Ethics and Public Health: Model Curriculum.* Association of Schools of Public Health; 2002. https://repository.library.georgetown.edu/handle/10822/556779

7. Beauchamp TL, Childress FC. *Principles of Biomedical Ethics*. 8th ed. Oxford University Press; 2019.

8. Thomas JC, Sage M, Dillenberg J, Guillory VJ. A code of ethics for public health. *Am J Public Health*. 2002;92:1057–1059. doi:10.2105/ajph.92.7.1057

9. American Medical Association. Code of Medical Ethics overview. https://www.ama-assn.org/delivering-care/ethics/code-medical-ethics-overview

10. Thomas JC, Dasgupta N. Ethical pandemic control through the lens of the public health code of ethics. *Am J Public Health*. 2020;110:1171–1172. doi:10.2105/AJPH.2020.305785

11. Thomas JC. Public health ethics free online lectures. http://www.jcthomas.org/teaching

12. Jennings B, Kahn J, Mastroianni A, Parker L. *Ethics and Public Health: Model Curriculum*. Association of Schools of Public Health; 2002. https://repository.library.georgetown.edu/handle/10822/556779

13. Barrett DH, Ortmann LW, Dawson A, Saenz C, Reis A, Bolan G, eds. *Public Health Ethics: Cases Spanning the Globe*. Springer Open; 2016. http://link.springer.com/book/10.1007/978-3-319-23847-0

14. Thomas JC, Young S. Wake me when there's a crisis: progress on state pandemic influenza ethics preparedness. *Am J Pub Health*. 2011;101:2080–2082. doi:10.2105/AJPH.2011.300293

15. Daniels N. Accountability for reasonableness. *Br Med J*. 2000;321:1300–1301. doi:10.1136/bmj.321.7272.1300

16. Ethics and Compliance Initiative. The PLUS ethical decision making model. https://www.ethics.org/resources/free-toolkit/decision-making-model

17. Lor A, Thomas JC, Barrett DH, Ortmann LW, Herrera Guibert DJ. Key ethical issues discussed at CDC-sponsored international regional meetings to explore cultural perspectives and contexts on pandemic influenza preparedness and response. *Int J Health Policy Manag*. 2016;5:653–662. doi:10.15171/ijhpm.2016.55

18. St. George DM, Wing SB, Lewis DL. Geographic and temporal patterns of toxic industrial chemicals released in North Carolina, 1988–1994. *N C Med J*. 2000;61:396–400.

19. Wing S, Horton R, Muhammad N, Grant G, Tajik M, Thu K. Integrating epidemiology, education, and organizing for environmental justice: community health effects of industrial hog operations. *Am J Public Health*. 2008;98:1390–1397. doi:10.2105/AJPH.2007.110486

20. Heaney CD, Wing S, Campbell RL, et al. Relation between malodor, ambient hydrogen sulfide, and health in a community bordering a landfill. *Environ Res*. 2011;111:847–852. doi:10.1016/j.envres.2011.05.021

21. Heaney CD, Wing S, Wilson SM, et al. Public infrastructure disparities and the microbiological and chemical safety of drinking and surface water supplies in a community bordering a landfill. *J Environ Health*. 2013;5(10):24–36. https://www.ncbi.nlm.nih.gov/pmc/articles/PMC4514614

22. Baker M, Ivory D. Why public health faces a crisis across the U.S. *New York Times*. October 18, 2021. https://www.nytimes.com/2021/10/18/us/coronavirus-public-health.html

23. Merzbach H. 'Standard bearers' Newel and Hall feted with courage award at NYC gala. *Santa Cruz Lookout*. October 5, 2021. https://lookout.co/santacruz/coronavirus/story/2021-10-05/santa-cruz-health-officials-gail-newel-mimi-hall-received-pen-america-courage-award

24. PEN America. 2021 PEN/Benenson Courage Award: Gail Newel and Mimi Hall. September 22, 2021. https://pen.org/2021-pen-benenson-courage-award

25. Public Health Leadership Society. *Principles of the Ethical Practice of Public Health*. Public Health Leadership Society; 2002. https://www.apha.org/-/media/files/pdf/membergroups/ethics/ethics_brochure.ashx

Chapter 3

Systems Thinking in Public Health

Kaye Bender

INTRODUCTION

Many healthcare and public health leaders emerge as leaders from the healthcare professions (e.g., physicians, nurses, nutritionists, or social workers). During their education, they are taught about systems as they relate to healthcare; that is, the basic human body systems, such as the integumentary system, skeletal system, muscular system, lymphatic system, respiratory system, digestive system, nervous system, endocrine system, cardiovascular system, urinary system, and reproductive systems. The study of these systems—which is basic to clinical training—introduces many individuals to the concepts of how diverse and complex systems within the human body work together to ensure a functional human being.[1] Similarly, epidemiologists and environmental health specialists enter public health with a scientific view related to their role, which is important but focused, and usually does not—at least initially—include a consideration of systems. Some graduate studies in healthcare professional education offer courses in systems thinking, but most of the basic healthcare professional education focuses on individuals rather than systems. Given their backgrounds, public health and healthcare leaders tend to view leadership as an extension of their healthcare education. This leads to a tendency to focus on the identification of problems within a single system, as opposed to assessing how the systems all work together and how they can be viewed in the larger context, which includes the environment in which they exist. Yet the role of public health and healthcare professionals in the 21st century is a complex one, requiring leadership to address complicated issues, from root causes of health status indicators to social determinants of health, to health equity in the midst of organizational and institutional racism. Further, the lessons learned from the COVID-19 pandemic—even as the pandemic continues while this chapter goes to press—have reinforced the notion that public health and healthcare leaders must be systems thinkers; they must blend their scientific and technical knowledge with intersectoral, collaborative, politically savvy leadership in a consistent and thoughtful manner if they are going to effect the changes in the systems that are needed to make a true impact on the health status of the populations they serve. It is not an easy role, but it is worthy of study and intentional execution. This chapter is designed as a resource for public health and healthcare leaders to consider deliberate actions to interject systems thinking into their leadership actions.

OBJECTIVES

By the end of this chapter, the reader will be able to:

- Review key elements of systems-level thinking, as applied to public health and healthcare.
- Identify models and frameworks for using systems-level thinking in public health and healthcare practice.
- Discuss application of systems thinking in two contemporary cases in public health and healthcare practice.

■ Describe guidance for public health practitioners based on the lessons learned from the two case studies.

■ Encourage dialogue among students and public health and healthcare practitioners about the application of systems thinking in 21st-century leadership.

EVOLUTION OF SYSTEMS THINKING

Although the concept of systems thinking in biology and engineering was described as early as the 1920s, it wasn't until the 1940s that Austrian biologist Ludwig von Bertalanffy formally developed a General Systems Theory (GST).[3] Bertalanffy identified three categories of systems thinking: systems technology, systems science, and systems philosophy. He later worked with Margaret Meade and Nobel Prize winners from economics, physiology, and physics to form the Society of General Systems Research, thus laying the groundwork for an evidence base for the concept that systems can be modeled and understood objectively.[2] At the same time, Dr. Jay Forrester from the Massachusetts Institute of Technology (MIT) identified a type of modeling to assist in the understanding of the nonlinear behavior of complex systems over time. This was applied to early work in computer modeling systems but had implications for application in other sectors.[3]

Shortly thereafter, in 1968, C. West Churchman defined five basic elements for thinking about systems approaches to solving complex problems. Those five elements were the objectives and performance of the entire system; the system's environment and fixed constraints; the resources of the system; the components of the system, their activities, goals, and measures of performance; and the management of the system. Building on this previous work, other systems thinking researchers emerged to further refine the application of systems thinking to problem-solving.[4]

However, it was not until the 1990s that public health and healthcare leaders began to focus on the work published by Peter Senge, another MIT scholar and researcher who wrote *The Fifth Discipline*, which combined systems thinking for management and organizational learning.[5] The textbook was widely used not only in academic settings, but also in the national Public Health Leadership Institute (PHLI), which had been formed to strengthen leadership skills for emerging public health leaders. In fact, systems thinking became one of the key concepts in the PHLI curriculum, and 67% of PHLI graduates reported having led or observed systems change that PHLI graduates themselves influenced directly or indirectly after their participation in the PHLI experience. An evaluation of the PHLI experiences from 1991 to 2006 revealed a general historical pattern of a group of "thought leaders who met at PHLI and worked together to reconceptualize how public health systems should be structured and should function, and also how public health leaders should work to improve them."[6]

Confident that that exposure to systems thinking for public health would result in changes in public health systems, graduates of the PHLI worked with and through established national public health organizations such as the American Public Health Association (APHA), the Association of State and Territorial Health Officials (ASTHO), the National Association of County and City Health Officials (NACCHO), and the Public Health Foundation (PHF) to devise and disseminate new tools to help state and local governments define and improve their public health infrastructure and systems. Examples of such tools include the ten Essential Public Health Services (EPHS), the National Public Health Performance Standards, health department accreditation systems, the Public Health Code of Ethics, an Operational Definition of Public Health, and many others.[6]

In *The Fifth Discipline*, Senge identified the five disciplines as[5]:

■ systems thinking
■ personal mastery

- mental models
- common vision
- team learning

Of these five disciplines, Senge identified systems thinking as the most important because it connects all the others together and leads to planned change within an organization. Senge also introduced the concept of a learning organization, which includes establishing a common vision for the future, leading to a common destiny. For many public health organizations, the application of systems thinking as a framework for complex system change was an approach worthy of adoption.

With regard to leadership, Senge also identified four core capabilities of effective systems leaders[7]:

- ability and willingness to "see" the system,
- commitment to fostering reflective and generative conversations,
- willingness to shift from reactive to co-creative problem-solving, and
- ability to identify, cultivate, and foster a network of diverse system leaders.

Senge, Scharmer, and others[8] further clarified the relationship between the five disciplines and the Theory U approach, which integrated them into collective learning and practice. The circular steps in the Theory U model are co-sensing (mental models, team learning, and systems thinking); co-presencing (moving from personal vision to shared vision); and co-realizing (team learning and systems thinking).[8]

Also building on the Theory U approach, Donella Meadows wrote extensively about systems thinking in the context of world events and the environment. Her book, *The Limits to Growth*, published in 1972 sold more than 9 million copies in 26 languages.[9] Her work continues today under the Academy for Systems Change and continues the legacy that she built when she stated:

> *We humans are smart enough to have created complex systems and amazing productivity; surely we are also smart enough to make sure that everyone shares our bounty, and surely we are smart enough to sustainably steward the natural world upon which we all depend.*[9]

A combination of Theory U and the five disciplines formed the initial foundation for the cross-sectoral work being done in public health today. For example, work being led by the Center for Sharing Public Health Services and the Public Health National Center for Innovations (PHNCIs) through a Cross-Sector Innovation Initiative, identified and supported public health, healthcare, and social services organizations striving to build stronger, sustainable connections to better meet the goals and needs of the people they serve and ultimately improve health equity. Using systems thinking as a framework, this project has further developed an understanding of the role of governmental public health departments in aligning efforts across the healthcare, public health, and social services sectors to improve population health. Through the work of 10 demonstration initiatives across the country, a deeper understanding about the practical dynamics and leadership characteristics associated with the complexities of working across sectors will be forthcoming and will be instructive to leaders who find themselves having to function in a cross-sectoral working environment. A few of the initiatives include operationalizing collaborative ideals through resource sharing in Spokane, Washington. Entitled "Better Health Together," this initiative brought together agencies in the county during the early days of the COVID-19 pandemic to share policies and procedures for telehealth; to group purchase personal protective equipment (PPE) and other supplies and equipment; and to coordinate spending for any of the Cares Act funding provided by Congress. In another initiative in Cleveland, Ohio, a collective impact consortium known as Health Improvement Partnership (HIP)-Cuyahoga, is working to accomplish health and equity goals that are most feasible through collaboration. HIP-Cuyahoga was established in 2009 and is a partnership with a membership of more than 300 community agencies and 1,000 individuals who are committed to transforming local health improvement through equity, racial inclusion, community engagement, and collective impact. Their goal is to "inspire, influence, and advance policy, environmental and lifestyle changes that foster health for everyone"[10(para4)] who lives in that county.

Another application of systems thinking involves the Iceberg Model, which grew from an early model of the theory of omission by writer and author Ernest Hemingway. The theory of omission assumes that a writer may omit things that he knows, and the reader will identify the omitted items as strongly as though the writer had stated them. The Iceberg Model moves the leader into systems thinking by encouraging inquiry into how various elements within a system influence one another. Applied to public health, the Iceberg Model moves the leader from thinking about the larger issues in the political, social, cultural, and business environments in which the organization functions into probing the factors within the organization that may contribute (positively or negatively) to the issue being analyzed. Such internal factors can be related to organizational performance, staff or team dynamics, policies and procedures, or facilities, for example.

According to the Iceberg Model, a systems thinking leader will be able to combine the observations about the external environment with the facts about the functioning of the internal environment to form conclusions about the system as a whole. Developing this systems-level perspective often allows the leader to engage in promoting solutions to problems that may not have otherwise been identified. It is a holistic picture of the way systems work. Figure 3.1 is a typical depiction of the Iceberg Model, as developed by the Donella Meadows Project and the Academy for Systems Change.[9]

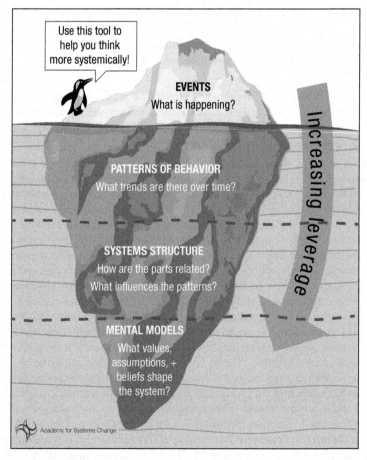

FIGURE 3.1: The Iceberg Model.

Source: Reproduced with permission from Academy for Systems Change. https://donellameadows
.org/systems thinking-resources/t.

Borrowing from the field of information systems, systems thinking can also be described in two large categories of activities: macro and micro. In the macro category, potential actions include the identification of system input/output boundaries for a system, as well as external systems variables that can and cannot be controlled; identification of subsystem component interactions; collection of data on system inputs and outputs; and analysis of the functioning of the system. A micro-level approach includes identification of system internal boundaries and interactions, processes, and flows; data collection; and modeling and analysis of the system. Systems thinking with both macro and micro connections provides a perspective that characterizes, synthesizes, and recognizes both patterns and anomalies of a contextualized system.[11] The next section of this chapter will provide selected examples of systems thinking and their applications in public health and healthcare at both the macro- and micro-levels.

SYSTEMS THINKING AT THE MACRO-LEVEL IN PUBLIC HEALTH AND HEALTHCARE

THE PUBLIC HEALTH SYSTEM

The 1988 landmark report, *The Future of Public Health*, defined public health as "what we, as a society, do collectively to assure the conditions for people to be healthy."[12(p19)] The objectives of the 2-year study were to define the mission of public health, describe the government's role in fulfilling that mission, and describe the detailed responsibilities of each level of government. The report defined public health as having three core functions: assessment, assurance, and policy development. It also depicted the public health system as being composed of a complex and broad range of federal, state, and local health agencies, laboratories and hospitals; nongovernmental public and private agencies; voluntary organizations; and individuals. While these other sectors were viewed as having their unique role in assuring healthy conditions, the emphasis on this report was on the responsibility of government. Governmental agencies, whether federal, state, or local, are arranged at the top and center of the pyramid because of their statutory leadership responsibilities for achieving a balance between individuals and equitable actions for the good of the entire population.[12] Figure 3.2, as published by the Centers for Disease Control and Prevention (CDC), depicts these components.

An update to the 1988 report, *The Future of the Public's Health in the 21st Century*, described the public health system in the broadest terms.[13] The report described the concept of an intersectoral public health system and charged the five broad systems that the report named as power brokers in effecting public health status improvement. Those five systems were the healthcare delivery system, employers and businesses, academia, the media, and communities and their organizations. The document described the governmental public health infrastructure as the "backbone" or the "conscience" of public health working with these five broad sectors. It is important to note that the 2003 report was being developed in the wake of the September 11, 2001 terrorist attacks in New York City and Washington, D.C., and the ensuing anthrax bioterrorist attacks. Many of the recommendations in the report were influenced by the work of the various sectors and systems in a dark time in America's history. The nation's public health system faced tremendous scrutiny in the wake of their lack of coordinated response (due to an historical lack of funding and training in the type of responses needed for terrorist attacks affecting health). In addition, the role of the other sectors—the media and law enforcement—were new partners to public health. The report, while containing public health in its title, focuses on the vital need for all sectors who work to ensure the public's health collaborate in order to strengthen the public health system as a whole.[13]

A systems thinking approach to public health was encouraged, with a basis being the 10 EPHS framework, which had originated in 1994. The 2003 report states "it is not just the health departments that play a role in carrying out the ten essential public health services . . . . Other sectors of society can contribute by transforming their impacts on the public's health

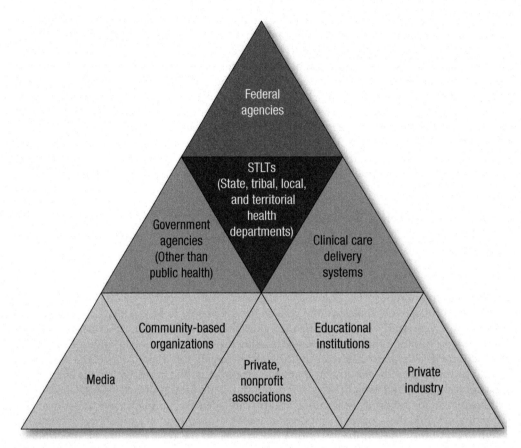

FIGURE 3.2: The Public Health System.
Source: Reproduced from Centers for Disease Control and Prevention. Components of public health system description. https://www.cdc.gov/publichealthgateway/funding/rfaot13/pyramid_description.html

so that they are no longer the result of random and unintentional actions but are the result of informed, strategic, and deliberate efforts to positively affect health."[13(p31)] This quote describes systems thinking at its core. Public health leaders are still encouraged to think about their work in the context of an intersectoral environment in which all of the players affecting the public's health have a significant role and responsibility. Building on work by Dahlgren and Whitehead in 1991, the 2003 IOM report also connected the concepts associated with multiple determinants of health to systems thinking for public health leaders. Figure 3.3 provides a model of those determinants of health, identifying both macro- and micro-level conditions.[13]

In 2002, the Public Health Practice Office at the CDC released a public health system diagram depicting the varied and diverse members of the macro-level public health system. This diagram (Figure 3.4) is still used today to teach new public health workforce members and their leaders how to view the collective work that is done to improve the health of a community, a state, or a nation.[14]

The CDC identifies the following as traits of a well-functioning public health system:

- strong partnerships, where partners recognize they are part of the public health system
- effective channels of communication
- system-wide health objectives
- resource sharing
- leadership by a governmental public health agency
- feedback loops among state, local, tribal, territorial, and federal partners

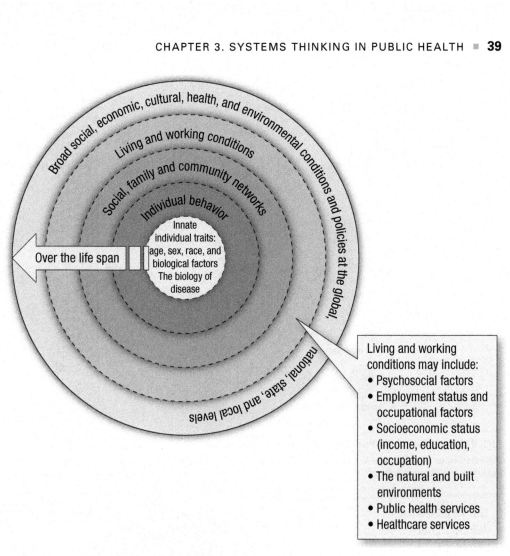

FIGURE 3.3: The Socioecological Model of Health.
Source: Reproduced from Institute of Medicine. *The Future of the Public's Health in the 21st Century*. National Academies Press; 2003. https://www.ncbi.nlm.nih.gov/books/NBK221239

Leaders who incorporate macro-level systems thinking into their routine strategy development are able to envision how all of these sectors can come together to fulfill the mission of supporting optimal health for their populations.[14]

REVISED 10 ESSENTIAL PUBLIC HEALTH SERVICES

Although the 1994 version of the 10 EPHS provided a roadmap of goals for carrying out the mission of public health in communities around the nation, that landscape has shifted dramatically. The Futures Initiative, a partnership between the de Beaumont Foundation, the PHNCI, and a Task Force of public health experts, was formed in Spring 2019 to better align the EPHS framework with current and emerging public health practice needs. The revised EPHS framework was released September 9, 2020 and is being used across the country to inform the public health system work that is needed in today's society (Figure 3.5). It is a strong model for envisioning the macro-level of the public health system in that these EPHS apply to both governmental and nongovernmental entities whose mission is to improve the health of the public and centers the EPHS on equity.[15]

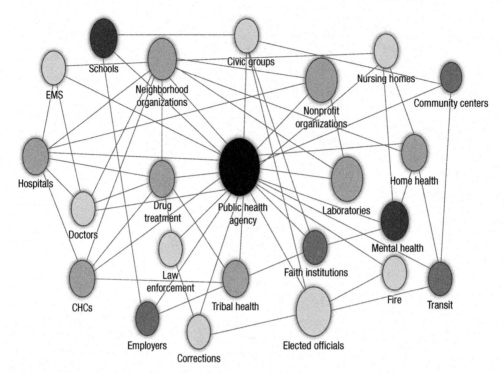

FIGURE 3.4: The CDC's Public Health System.
Source: Centers for Disease Control and Prevention. https://www.cdc.gov/publichealthgateway/zz-sddev/essentialhealthservices.html

THE 10 ESSENTIAL PUBLIC HEALTH SERVICES

To protect and promote the health of all people in all communities

The 10 essential public health services provide a framework for public health to protect and promote the health of all people in all communities. To achieve optimal health for all, the Essential Public Health services actively promote policies, systems, and services that enable good health and seek to remove obstacles and systemic and structural barriers, such as poverty, racism, gender discrimination, and other forms of oppression, that have resulted in health inequities. Everyone should have a fair and just opportunity to achieve good health and well-being.

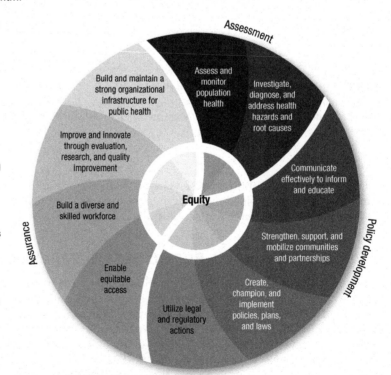

FIGURE 3.5: The 10 Essential Public Health Services.
Source: Public Health National Center for Innovations. https://www.cdc.gov/publichealthgateway/publichealthservices/essentialhealthservices.html

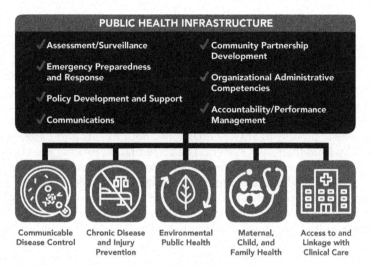

FIGURE 3.6: Foundational Public Health Capabilities.
Source: Public Health National Center for Innovations. http://phnci.org/national-frameworks/fphs

FOUNDATIONAL PUBLIC HEALTH CAPABILITIES

Another public health systems framework that should also be included in any macro-level systems thinking is the Foundational Capabilities framework. This framework is similar to the EPHS, but it was developed as a companion piece to identify the public health infrastructure needed to provide public health protections that offer fair opportunities for all to be healthy.[16] This framework includes seven capabilities:

1. Assessment/surveillance,
2. Emergency preparedness and response,
3. Policy development and support,
4. Communications,
5. Community partnership development,
6. Organizational administrative competencies, and
7. Accountability/performance management.

These capabilities were designed to reflect the public health services that should be present everywhere in order for the public health system to work anywhere. These capabilities align with the EPHS and the two can be used together to give public health leaders a pathway for how their public health system should work in its entirety (Figure 3.6).[16]

PUBLIC HEALTH SYSTEMS THINKING AT THE MICRO-LEVEL

As previously stated, public health systems thinking at the micro-level can be viewed through the identification of system internal boundaries and interactions, processes, and flows; data collection; and modeling and analysis of the system. It provides the public health leader with the impetus to look inside their organization and its workforce for answers to questions about how a system or a component of a system works. This micro-level view represents the Systems Structure and the Mental Models from the Iceberg Model. There are several compelling resources for public health leaders to use as they consider the internal operations of their part of the overall public health system.

PUBLIC HEALTH ACCREDITATION

Public Health Accreditation Board (PHAB) standards and measures for initial accreditation and for reaccreditation set forth the requirements for state, local, tribal, and territorial health departments to use to compare their work in a peer review process against national standards based on the EPHS.[17] The accreditation process provides a framework for a health department to apply systems thinking at the micro-level to an assessment of their work. A health department leader can use accreditation standards and measures and the peer review process to answer questions about Events and Patterns of Behavior (Iceberg Model) within their own system. The accreditation process goes further, however, to encourage and reward health departments for their work outside the walls of the health department as it relates to community engagement and stakeholder partnerships. Linking to the 10 EPHS provides the macro view while assessing the work within the health department provides the micro view. When put together, the public health leader can then apply additional systems thinking to seeking solutions to issues that should be addressed.[17]

PERFORMANCE MANAGEMENT AND QUALITY IMPROVEMENT SYSTEMS

Related to, but different from, the PHAB accreditation standards are models and frameworks for health departments and others to use to develop and implement quality improvement and performance management systems within their organizations. The results of these dedicated and formally organized efforts to assess the operations of the systems against planned goals is a component of internal or micro systems thinking. Whether a health department is accredited or not, it can learn much about its internal operations as well as the impact of its external practices through the use of a formalized performance management and quality improvement system. The PHF defines performance management as "a systematic process which helps an organization achieve its mission and strategic goals by improving effectiveness, empowering employees, and streamlining decision making."[18(para1)] Riley et al. defined "quality improvement" as

> the use of a deliberate and defined improvement process, such as Plan-Do-Check-Act, which is focused on activities that are responsive to community needs and improving population health. It refers to a continuous and ongoing effort to achieve measurable improvements in the efficiency, effectiveness, performance, accountability, outcomes, and other indicators of quality in services or processes which achieve equity and improve the health of the community.[19(p6)]

A health department leader who focuses on asking the tough questions about how their health department is doing and whether their work is actually accomplishing the stated goals is practicing micro-level systems thinking. Performance management and quality improvement, when combined, provide credible dashboards of how the governmental public health system is working.

INNOVATION IN PUBLIC HEALTH

With the establishment of the PHNCI in 2016, a new set of resources was added to the public health systems thinking cache. PHNCI defines "public health innovation" as "the creation and implementation of a novel process, policy, product, program, or system leading to improvements that impact health and equity."[20(para1)] Following the elements of systems thinking, PHNCI identifies tenets of public health innovation which include the following:

■ ongoing, systematic process that can generate incremental or radical change

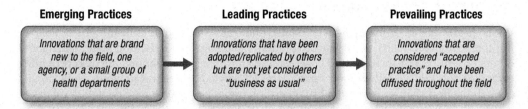

FIGURE 3.7: Public Health National Center for Innovation Model.
Source: Public Health National Center for Innovations. https://phnci.org/innovations/about-innovations

- collaboration with diverse team members and partners and co-production with people with lived experience who will be affected by the results of the innovation
- open process lending itself to adaptation or replication

PHNCI has not only tested these tenets in public health across the country, but they have also developed a model that depicts how the various elements of innovation work together to form a system that sparks a culture of innovation (Figure 3.7). PHNCI has also developed a roadmap that uses the innovation model and its tenets to effect public health systems change. A public health leader who wishes to move past the image that government cannot and will not improve itself can readily see how to dispel that image using the roadmap and other resources to test and implement changes in the system that move their work more efficiently and effectively toward population health improvement.[21]

THE CORE COMPETENCIES FOR PUBLIC HEALTH PROFESSIONALS

The Core Competencies for Public Health Professionals, developed by the Council on Linkages Between Academia and Public Health Practice, are a consensus set of skills for the broad practice of public health.[22] Building on the 10 EPHS, the Core Competencies describe a three-tiered approach to reflect skill areas of professionals engaging in the practice, education, and research of public health. Organized in eight domains, the Core Competencies identify leadership and systems thinking as one of the major areas:

- analytical/assessment skills
- policy development/program planning skills
- communication skills
- cultural competency skills
- community dimensions of practice skills
- public health sciences skills
- financial planning and management skills
- leadership and systems thinking skills

Leadership and systems thinking skills, as described in the Core Competencies, evolve based on the experience of the leader, from describing and "seeing" the system and its components to identifying opportunities to engage system partners to effect change. This domain also aligns the macro-level knowledge of systems thinking with the micro-level application of systems thinking within an organization. Emerging leaders can use the leadership and systems thinking section of the Core Competencies as a personal guide to assess their own actions regarding the use of systems thinking in their role as a leader.[22]

DIVERSITY, EQUITY, AND INCLUSIVITY

Public health has recently collectively stated that racism is a public health crisis. Following that statement, many public health leaders have engaged in issuing statements about diversity, equity, and inclusivity. Those leaders and their organizations are also providing examples of actions to follow their statements, acknowledging that statements alone are not enough to effect change. Intentionality regarding organizational change related to diversity, equity, and inclusivity is systems thinking at its finest. The APHA developed several resources on this topic, but two that are significant to systems thinking are a webinar series on advancing racial equity in organizations, institutions, and agencies[23] and a toolkit for organizations to use to assess their policies and practices at the organizational level.[24] The toolkit is very useful for leaders in nonprofit organizations to consider the systems level barriers to equity, diversity, and inclusion. The APHA toolkit states its change theory as "**IF** a small nonprofit governance board implements the E-D-I toolkit that operationalizes racial equity and inclusivity within their organizational structure **THEN** the organization will be better equipped to promote racial equity and justice within the communities they serve."[24(p3)] The toolkit is a valuable systems thinking resource for the emerging leader to use to address the complexities associated with institutional and structural racism.[23,24]

ALIGNMENT OF LEADERSHIP THEORY AND SYSTEMS THINKING

To further illustrate the usefulness of combining leadership theory with systems thinking theory, it is helpful to review them together in the simplest of terms. Table 3.1 presents the central components of leadership as defined by Peter Northouse alongside several key systems thinking elements described earlier in this chapter. Further, public health and healthcare applications of the elements are elucidated.

The emerging leader is encouraged to reflect on their own leadership skills and traits as they align with systems thinking in the public health and healthcare environments. Systems thinking, combined with leadership reflection, can lead us to challenge how our habitual assumptions and values affect our responses to the issues we are called to face, as well as how to identify those opportunities for systems change.

Two helpful case studies which describe systems change based on both macro- and micro-systems level thinking are included in this chapter to help the reader consider application of these constructs in a public health setting. The first case study is Healthy San Diego (HSD), a system which was designed and implemented 25 years ago and that remains in place today. The second case study is newer and focuses on systems change post COVID-19, using those lessons learned to impact the delivery of preventive health services for the future. Both case studies exemplify the concepts discussed in this chapter.

SUMMARY

This chapter strives to bring leadership based on systems thinking to bear on key challenges that relate to both the public health and the healthcare sectors' roles in improving the health of the populations they serve. Clearly there are unique roles for both public health and healthcare when it comes to their daily operational functions. This content, along with the two case studies, underscores the need for public health and healthcare systems to be viewed together as part of the greater public health system that serves an entire population. Leaders in both systems can use these frameworks as models to guide their thinking when challenges or new opportunities surface.

In their recent book, *Contemporary Public Health: Principles, Practices and Policy*, Scutchfield and Holsinger[25] discuss a major upgrade needed for public health.

TABLE 3.1: Alignment of Leadership, Systems Thinking, and Selected Public Health and Healthcare Concepts

LEADERSHIP COMPONENTS (NORTHOUSE)	(SENGE) SYSTEMS THINKING CONCEPTS (SENGE) AND ICEBERG MODEL (MEADOWS)	PUBLIC HEALTH AND HEALTHCARE APPLICATIONS OF FAMILIAR CONCEPTS
Leadership is a process.	Ability and willingness to "see" the system What is happening? What trends are there over time?	Essential public health services Foundational capabilities Performance management Quality improvement
Leadership involves influence.	Ability to identify, cultivate, and foster a network of diverse system leaders Are the parts related? What and who influences the patterns?	Social determinants of health Cross-sectoral partnerships Performance management Quality improvement Core competencies
Leadership occurs in groups.	Willingness to shift from reactive to co-creative problem-solving	Cross-sectoral partnerships Public health innovation Equity, diversity, and inclusivity
Leadership includes attention to common goals.	Commitment to fostering reflective and generative conversations What values, assumptions, and beliefs shape the system?	Public health innovation Public health accreditation Equity, diversity, and inclusivity

The upgrade includes an emphasis on cross-sector collaboration and policy, environmental, and systems-level actions that impact the social determinants of health. Public health leaders who imagine their role as a chief health strategist must embrace and practice routine and ongoing systems thinking to be successful in preventing disease and promoting the health of their populations. They reiterate the seven practices that high-performing public health departments will have to exhibit in the future if they are to be successful. Those seven practices, when viewed in the context of leadership for systems thinking, provide an effective, practical summary of the content of this chapter.[25]

- Adopt and adapt systems level strategies to combat the leading causes of illness, injury, and premature death.
- Develop effective systems-level strategies for promoting health and well-being.
- Identify, analyze, and distribute real-time information for a variety of systems.
- Build collaboration between clinical care and public health systems.
- Collaborate with a broad array of systems-level allies.
- Replace outdated organizational practices with systems-level practices.
- Work with systems-level federal partners.

Rowitz postulated that public health is a complex adaptive system and that the practice of public health takes place within this complex adaptive system.[26] The reflections in this chapter assume that the emerging leader begins with that premise and aligns leadership styles and traits with both macro-level and micro-level public health systems thinking. Doing this will give the emerging leader confidence that the decisions that are being made are done so with the whole system in mind, with multiple partners and stakeholders, and with consensus among the various players in the complex system called public health. The work is interesting and compelling, but not easy. However, there are many tools and resources to assist the emerging leader in being successful.[26]

DISCUSSION QUESTIONS

1. What is the potential role of systems thinking when public health and healthcare leaders are confronted with new challenges or opportunities to plan and implement programs and services to improve the health of the populations they serve?
2. What are some principles from the systems thinking frameworks described in this chapter that are of similar use in both public health and healthcare?
3. How does systems thinking promote considerations of the social determinants of health to advance health equity?

CASE STUDY: HEALTHY SAN DIEGO

HSD is the Medicaid-managed care oversight system for San Diego County. Organized 25 years ago, HSD identifies its values as: patient choice in selecting health plans, value added by ensuring local involvement in assuring quality and access to health services, and local oversight for problem-solving and continuous quality improvement. This initiative provides a compelling case study in complex system leadership that has been sustained over time despite changes in the medical, clinical, public health, political, and financial reimbursement landscapes. The case study also provides emerging leaders with informative guidance about leading change within and across systems.

BACKGROUND

Discussions about the implementation of managed care for the California Medicaid population in the early 1990s led five key organizations to come together to form a partnership that is now known as HSD. Leaders from the hospital association, the county health department, the medical society, legal aid, and the council of community clinics convened to assess the three potential options available to establish a managed care process for their Medicaid population.

■ A county organized health system
■ A two-plan model whereby the county would have one plan and the commercial interests would provide another one so that enrollees would have a choice of providers
■ A system whereby health plans would be certified to serve a specific geographical area (Geographic Managed Care, or GMC Model). Provision was made early on for two pilots. San Diego requested to be one of those two pilots.

After 2 years of planning, in October 1994, then California Governor Pete Wilson signed the landmark AB 2176 HSD Legislation. San Diego was selected as one of two pilot sites in the state to implement the GMC model.

Today, nearly one million individuals are enrolled in the model, and the initial partnerships that were established are still in place to ensure that HSD remains a strong and viable managed care initiative. A related component is the HSD Joint Consumer and Professional Advisory Committee, whose role is to monitor Medi-Cal managed care issues affecting San Diego County and to advise the director of the Health & Human Services Agency concerning those issues.

ROLE AND FUNCTION OF HEALTH SYSTEM PARTNERS IN LEADING SYSTEMS CHANGE

The early engagement of the public health and healthcare system representatives provided a forum of high trust for leading this massive system change. The five original organizational representatives mentioned earlier remain the core group, while other organizations, including the health plans, provide for a broad base of systems representation.

This case study highlights the importance of partnerships in a community coming together with a common goal of ensuring access to healthcare services for the most vulnerable members of its population. HSD was working across sectors and across disciplines even as early as the 1990s. More than 60 organizations, representing a broad array of systems, were engaged and remain engaged in the HSD efforts. Some of the examples of system members include:

- medicine
- community health centers
- public health
- health plans
- legal aid
- consumer advocacy
- other healthcare providers
- State Department of Health Care Services (DHCS)/Medi-Cal Managed Care Division
- County of San Diego Health and Human Services Agency (HHSA)

The system partner roles within the HSD structure include the following:

- State DHCS: Contracts for services directly with the health plans.
- Health Plans: Provide healthcare services.
- San Diego County HHSA: Provide day-to-day administration and presentations for Health Care Options enrollment. Identify issues and provide local forum for problem-solving and assistance.
- Consumers/Professionals: Provide advice to County HHSA through the HSD Consumer and Professional Advisory Committee.

The Consumer and Professional Advisory Committee was once comprised of two committees who met both separately and jointly. Over time, as the level of trust became stronger, the two committees merged into one committee. The committee operates subcommittees focused on such topics as quality improvement, behavioral health, COVID-19, and other pertinent topics. The structure continues to provide an open forum for all the system representatives and the consumers to work together to keep HSD strong.

RELATIONSHIP TO HEALTH EQUITY

The work to establish HSD was rooted in the values of equity. The organizing parties were committed from the beginning to ensuring that managed care for the San Diego Medicaid population was implemented according to the values mentioned earlier in this case study. The work was established with intentionality around fairness, transparency, and equality in terms of healthcare access. With attention to ongoing quality improvement and timely complaint resolution, HSD remains grounded in the commitment to monitoring services provided to this population to ensure equity across healthcare plans. At the present time, meetings of the HSD Joint Consumer and Professional Advisory Committee, which are held monthly, are open for members of the public to address the Committee on any issue within its assigned purview and not on the agenda. They also make provisions for special accommodations as may be needed.

ADVICE FOR OTHERS

When asked about their advice for others who are planning to effect major complex systems change, the HSD representatives interviewed provided the following observations based on their experience.

- Monitoring the changing healthcare landscape and the potential effect of the introduction of managed care on the Medicaid population provided an early opportunity for this initiative to be pilot tested.
- Relationships among the key systems representatives existed prior to their work together on this initiative. Those strong relationships provided an early atmosphere of trust as the planning ensued.
- A decision was made early on for the work to be apolitical. This commitment allowed the initiative to be developed and implemented with little to no political interference.
- The role of public health leadership, while official and supportive, was also subtle. This was intentional so that the team of partners and stakeholders would maintain ownership and commitment to HSD. It was not seen as a health department-driven initiative. Even today, public health supports HSD, but they do not set the agenda. It is still "owned" by the community.
- Sustained consumer engagement remains a challenge, but the HSD leaders continue to seek ways to ensure consumers have opportunities to be engaged with policy decisions that are made and as complaints are processed. This commitment requires constant vigilance.
- The leadership for HSD has been consistent over the 25 years. However, some turnover in that leadership is anticipated soon. Deliberate work has been done to ensure succession planning so that the initial values, goals, objectives, and systems relationships continue.

CASE STUDY QUESTIONS

1. What is the primary change in the public health system that occurred or will occur because of this initiative?
2. Who are the system partners in this initiative, and what aspects of systems thinking are reflected in its structure?
3. Where do you see examples of systems thinking in HSD?

CASE STUDY: MISSISSIPPI CONNECTED CARE PROGRAM

BACKGROUND

In 2020, the early effects of COVID-19 on the public health and healthcare systems in Mississippi were affected by a weak internet infrastructure to support both teleworking and virtually learning or working from home or elsewhere. Although the population of Mississippi is just under three million, the state reported 326,804 COVID-19 cases as of July 2021, with 7,465 deaths. As caseloads peaked during 2020, emergency rooms and intensive care units were overflowing with COVID-19 patients. For months, most businesses and schools were closed. The education system was ill-prepared for remote learning, not only because of the lack of teacher preparation for leading e-learning, but also because of the lack of reliable broadband internet services in rural parts of the state. Most of Mississippi's population is rural, and more than half of the physicians practice in four urban areas, and all or part of the 82 counties are considered to be medically underserved. This latter fact was not news to anyone working in public health or healthcare, but the COVID-19 pandemic exacerbated access issues. That is, until leaders in the state saw a window of opportunity to initiate a "no fail" access policy across systems to ensure that individuals and communities in which they live could receive much needed preventive health services online, in person (typically with an advanced practice nurse), or through a statewide, seamless system of telehealth.

On January 15, 2021, the Federal Communications Commission (FCC) formally announced that $26.6 million would be awarded to 14 pilot projects with over 150 treatment sites in 11 states under the umbrella program "Connected Care Pilot Program." The focus of the projects in both urban and rural areas of the country is to help the country better understand how telehealth can reduce costs and increase the quality of care in areas of greatest need across the country. The Pilot Program will use Universal Service Fund monies to help defray the costs of connected care services for eligible healthcare providers, providing support for 85% of the cost of eligible services and network equipment. These include: (a) patient broadband internet access services, (b) healthcare provider broadband data connections, (c) other connected care information services, and (d) certain network equipment.

ROLE AND FUNCTION OF HEALTH SYSTEM PARTNERS IN LEADING SYSTEMS CHANGE

One of the funded pilot projects is a partnership between the University of Mississippi Medical Center (UMMC) and the Mississippi State Department of Health (MSDH). With a budget of $2,377,875, the project will provide broadband internet access service to patients across the state. This will enable much-needed remote patient monitoring technologies and ambulatory telehealth visits to low-income patients suffering from chronic conditions or illnesses requiring long-term care. UMMC estimates the project would impact up to 237,120 patients across Mississippi, more than half of which are low-income. This systems change has been initiated and led by the vice chancellor for health affairs at the state's only academic health sciences center, the state health officer (who oversees a centralized public health system statewide), payors of health and public health services in the state (such as Medicaid and private insurance), the state's arm of the FCC, and Mississippi lawmakers.

A rural state long plagued with issues related to access to healthcare, Mississippi has leveraged the pandemic to expand its telehealth initiatives to include population health. Applying systems thinking to a budding Telehealth Center of Excellence (designated by the federal Health Resources and Services Administration in 2017 as one of only two such programs in the country to receive that designation), public health leaders, telehealth providers, and internet service providers have come together to develop the policies, protocols, and funding for the Connected Care Pilot Program. Furthermore, over 30% of the state's population lacks access to broadband internet service, making this kind of innovative program even more important.

An earlier, targeted version of this type of program was funded in 2014 by C Spire (one of the state's progressive providers of cellular service) and was aimed at testing the impact of remote patient monitoring for type 2 diabetics living in the Mississippi Delta. That pilot program showed that remote patient monitoring improves outcomes and reduces costs. Indeed, participants saw a 1.7% reduction in hemoglobin A1C (an indicator of blood sugar level). That may not sound like a lot, but studies show that a reduction in hemoglobin A1C of just 1% has been known to reduce cardiovascular death by 45%. It should also be noted that none of the participants of the study were readmitted to a hospital or emergency room for diabetes during the first 3 months. Policy makers readily understood that programs like remote patient monitoring could reduce costly readmission rates to the emergency room and decrease Medicare penalties to rural hospitals.

With the new initiative, public health programs such as early childhood screenings, HIV pre-exposure prophylaxis (PrEP) monitoring, tuberculosis directly observed therapy monitoring, perinatal high-risk management case conferences, family planning services, and many others will now be more readily available to the individuals in their communities via this statewide telehealth network. Lessons learned from the COVID-19 statewide centralized appointment system, testing and vaccine distribution, and contact tracing informed the application of this same type of system change to these other programs and services in a state where Mississippi Medicaid covers about 755,000 people, or about a quarter of the state's population.

RELATIONSHIP TO HEALTH EQUITY

Mississippi has a long history of struggles with health equity. The social determinants of health play such a significant role in the state that those who provide services aimed at improving health status are often overwhelmed with the need. For example, 118,698 (15.22%) families in Mississippi live below the poverty level. Of those families, 87,646 families (73%) have children. The unemployment rate is 7. 23%, and about a tenth of Mississippians have less than a high school education.

Leaders working on the systems change to bring preventive health services into all the homes in all the communities in the state adopted a "no fail" access value across all the systems engaged in this initiative. Currently, there are 82 different phone lines that people have to call to make a preventive health services appointment (one in each local health department); soon there will be one centralized system for individuals to call. Reimbursement barriers for these preventive health services have been removed. Intellectual power is centralized so that access to specialists is improved. Local clinics are utilized when lab services or other in-person services are needed. The intention for this entire initiative is to get preventive healthcare to everyone in the state who needs it, regardless of where they live. The ultimate goal is to positively impact the adage that "where you live determines how long you live."

ADVICE FOR OTHERS

Although this initiative is still in the early stages, when asked about their advice for others who are planning to effect major complex systems change, the individuals interviewed offered the following:

- Make the most of the existing systems infrastructure instead of feeling the need to start over. This not only potentially assists in the adoption of the systems change but can help enable its sustainability over time.

- Invest in partnerships with nontraditional public health sectors. In this initiative, some of the key partners were representatives from the information technology arena, such as experts in electronic billing and electronic health records.

- Invest time and money up front into data governance and compliance; that was the area identified as presenting the greatest risk to all the systems involved.

- Resist the temptation to wait for all the details to be perfect before you begin the initiative. Do as much planning as you can, but at some point, you just have to get started and adjust as you need to.

- Public health safety net providers, including the academic medical center clinics, must be willing to be flexible and, in some cases, to downscale, as telehealth visits took the place of former in-person clinic visits. Attention to the staff's engagement in the systems change was a vital component of the planning.

CASE STUDY QUESTIONS

1. What is the primary change in the public health system that has occurred or will occur as a result of the Mississippi Connected Care Program?
2. Who are the system partners in this initiative and how did they apply systems thinking to their planning efforts?
3. Where do you see examples of systems thinking in the Mississippi Connected Care Program?

ADDITIONAL RESOURCES

TOOLS FOR SELF-ASSESSMENT FOR SYSTEMS THINKING

There are two suggested tools for emerging leaders to use to assess their individual competencies and skills as they relate to systems thinking. Neither of these tools are unique to public health or heathcare, but the skills are the same and can be readily applied.

1. Assessing systems thinking: a tool to measure complex reasoning through ill-structured problems by Jacob R. Grohsa, Gary R. Kirka, Michelle M. Soledad, and David B. Knight, Virginia Tech, Blacksburg, VA. Available online 22 March 2018. https://www.sciencedirect.com/science/article/pii/S1871187117302511

2. *Systems Thinking Complete Self-Assessment Guide* Paperback—January 6, 2018 by Gerardus Blokdyk (Author). https://www.amazon.com/Systems thinking -Complete-Self-Assessment-Guide/dp/1489139087

 A robust set of instructor resources designed to supplement this text is located at **http://connect.springerpub.com/content/book/978-0-8261-4924-4.** Qualifying instructors may request access by emailing **textbook@springerpub.com.**

REFERENCES

1. Hall JE. *Guyton and Hall Textbook of Medical Physiology (Guyton Physiology).* 13th ed. Saunders; 2015.
2. von Bertalanffy L. *General Systems Theory.* Braziller; 1968.
3. Forrester J. *Industrial Dynamics.* Productivity Press; 1961.
4. Churchman CW. *The Systems Approach.* Laurel Books; 1970.
5. Senge PM. *The Fifth Discipline: The Art and Practice of the Learning Organization.* Doubleday; 1990.
6. Umble KE, Baker EL, Woltring C. An evaluation of the National Public Health Leadership Institute–1991-2006: part I. Developing individual leaders. *J Public Health Manag Pract.* 2011 May-Jun;17(3):202–213. doi: 10.1097/PHH.0b013e3181f1e3dc.
7. Senge PM. *The Fifth Discipline: The Art and Practice of the Learning Organization: Second Edition.* Doubleday; 2006.
8. Senge P, Scharmer CO, Jaworski J, Flowers BS. *Presence.* Society for Organizational Learning; 2004.
9. The Donella Meadows Project. Systems thinking resources. https://donellameadows.org/systems -thinking-resources
10. Health Improvement Partnership (HIP)-Cuyahoga. Tackling racism head-on. The Public Health National Center for Innovations. https://phnci.org/journal/tackling-racism-head-on
11. Zhu P. Macro vs micro level of systems analysis. Future of CIO BlogSpot. http://futureofcio.blogspot.com/2015/03/macro-vs-micro-level-of-systems-analysis.html
12. Institute of Medicine. *The Future of Public Health.* National Academies Press; 1988.
13. Institute of Medicine. *The Future of the Public's Health in the 21st Century.* National Academies Press; 2003.
14. The Public Health System & the 10 Essential Public Health Services. https://www.cdc.gov/publichealthgateway/zz-sddev/essentialhealthservices.html
15. The Public Health National Center for Innovations. Celebrating 25 years and launching the revised 10 Essential Public Health Services. http://phnci.org/national-frameworks/10-ephs
16. The Public Health National Center for Innovations. Revising the foundational public health services in 2022. http://phnci.org/national-frameworks/fphs
17. Public Health Accreditation Board. What is public health department accreditation? https://phaboard .org/what-is-public-health-department-accreditation
18. Public Health Foundation. Performance management. http://www.phf.org/focusareas/performance-management/Pages/Performance_Management.aspx
19. Bialek R, Beitsch, L, Cofsky, A, et al, unpublished data, 2009, as quoted in Riley W, Moran J, Corso L, Beitsch L, Bialek R, Cofsky A. Defining quality improvement in public health. *J Public Health Manag Pract.* 2010;16(1):5–7. doi:10.1097/PHH.0b013e3181bedb49
20. The Public Health National Center for Innovations. What is public health innovation? http://phnci .org/innovations/about-innovations
21. The Public Health National Center for Innovations. Innovation in governmental public health: building a roadmap. 2017. https://phnci.org/uploads/resource-files/Innovation-in-Governmental-Public -Health-Building-a-Roadmap.pdf

22. Public Health Foundation. Core competencies for public health professionals. Revised June 26, 2014. https://www.phf.org/resourcestools/Documents/Core_Competencies_for_Public_Health_Profes sionals_2014June.pdf

23. American Public Health Association. Racism and health. https://www.apha.org/Topics-and-Issues/ Health-Equity/Racism-and-health

24. Oyetunde T, Boulin A, Holt J. Equity diversity inclusion: action toolkit for organizations. American Public Health Association. https://www.apha.org/-/media/files/pdf/affiliates/equity_toolkit.ashx

25. Holsinger JW, Scutchfield FD. *Contemporary Public Health: Principles, Practices and Policy.* University Press of Kentucky; 2021.

26. Rowitz L. *Public Health Leadership.* 2nd ed. Jones & Bartlett; 2009.

Chapter 4

Strategic Thinking: Rationale, Process, and Behaviors

Peter M. Ginter and W. Jack Duncan

INTRODUCTION

Thinking strategically has been discussed throughout history, variously focusing on games, military and political advantage, business competition, planning, recognizing, and responding to change as well as organizational learning. Today, strategic thinking has become an essential leadership activity because there is no status quo and organizational leaders must continually cope with or initiate evolutionary, revolutionary, or disruptive change. Strategic thinking is the process for identifying, understanding, and addressing continuous external change.

Strategic thinking is essentially learning and may be viewed as occurring in several incremental stages: awareness, anticipation, analysis, interpretation, synthesis, and reflection. There are practical behaviors or habits that can initiate and operationalize strategic thinking at each stage and include such activities as nonjudgmental curiosity, visioning, data gathering, transformative thinking, developing strategic plans, and a reconsidering of beliefs and assumptions. Strategic thinking is the fundamental task of leaders but should be practiced throughout an organization.

OBJECTIVES

By the end of this chapter, the reader will be able to:

- Briefly describe the history and evolution of strategic thinking.
- Describe why strategic thinking is essential in today's dynamic public health and healthcare environments.
- Discuss how strategic thinking provides a process for coping with change.
- Describe the process, stages, and behaviors of strategic thinking.
- Describe the role of strategic thinking in leadership and identify who in an organization should be a strategic thinker.

THE EVOLUTION OF STRATEGIC THINKING

Dixit and Nalebuff, in their 1991 book *Strategic Thinking*, describe strategic thinking as the art of outdoing an adversary, knowing that the adversary is trying to do the same to you.[1(pix)] They go on to describe strategic thinking essentially as game theory. Game theory, originally based in mathematical models, considers the strategic interaction of rational decision-makers. For Dixit and Nalebuff, strategic thinking was mainly about competitive decision-making and winning and losing.[1] The strategic interaction of decision-makers has a long history in the management literature, often focusing on strategic planning, business competition, and decision-making techniques.

Prior to the 1990s, the focus of strategy in the management literature was on strategic planning and competition. Academic research and corporate offices were committed to developing the process and building models that were mostly linear and mechanical. The first systematic treatment of strategy was H. Igor Ansoff's 1965 book, *Corporate Strategy: An Analytical Approach to Business Policy for Growth and Expansion.*[2] Mintzberg praised Ansoff's book as representing "a kind of crescendo in the development of strategic planning theory, offering a degree of elaboration seldom attempted since."[3(p43)] Nakamura refers to Ansoff as the "Father of Strategic Management."[4(px)] Also influential, Michael Porter's books, *Competitive Strategy; Techniques for Analyzing Industries and Competitors*[5] and *Competitive Advantage: Creating and Sustaining Superior Performance,*[6] set the tone for the competitive nature of strategy and decision-making for many years.

Since the 1990s, the management literature has moved toward conceptualizing strategy in terms of thinking that is directly or indirectly allied to an organization's processes and context.[7] Dhir, Dhir, and Samanga more directly discuss the difference between strategic thinking (cognitive, integrative, conceptual) and strategic planning (systematic, decisive, documentative) concluding that they are distinct and work in tandem.[8(p273)] Another important contribution came from Schwartz, who reported on his work at Royal Dutch/Shell Group and the development of scenario planning.[9] He later expanded many elements of strategic thinking in *Inevitable Surprises: Thinking Ahead in a Time of Turbulence.*[10]

Of course, strategic thinking goes back much further in history than the early management literature. For instance, the underlying principles of strategy were discussed by Sun Tzu, Homer, Euripides, and many other early strategists and writers. Two of the most often cited early authors are Sun Tzu and Niccolo Machiavelli. For example, Sun Tzu's book *The Military Methods of Master Sun*, which in the West is generally known as the *Art of War*, was probably written around the fourth century B.C.E.[11] Wintzel notes that this book, along with Tzu's other writings, became the foundational texts of later strategic thinking for Chinese and Japanese military leaders.[12(p953)] He further notes that the book is required reading in most military academies. Machiavelli's work, although useful in the study of organizational power and leadership, has less to do with strategy and strategic thinking.

Although there are still competitive aspects to strategic thinking, today the concept goes beyond just winning or losing, head-to-head competition, military and political tactics, or strategic planning.[13] Strategic thinking, of course, is still about success; however, it also concerns innovation, transformation, invention, creativity, and, most importantly, organizational relevancy. More than just understanding, anticipating, and outmaneuvering the competition in an industry, strategic thinking now more broadly concerns identifying and understanding fundamental changes that will alter the "rules for success" not only in one industry, but—perhaps in many industries—the type of thinking that is fundamental to leadership. Moreover, Sohail and Dhir found in their meta-analysis of 45 empirical studies that strategic management and leadership are not likely to be successful without strategic thinking.[14] More broadly, research consistently reveals that strategic thinking is a critical component of leadership.[15]

Before precisely defining strategic thinking, examining its reasonably discrete stages, and exploring its underlyingly behaviors in detail, it is first useful to understand why strategic thinking is essential for most modern organizations. Understanding why strategic thinking is essential provides context and rationale for engaging in its unmistakably difficult and time-consuming behaviors.

WHY STRATEGIC THINKING IS ESSENTIAL

Most simply, strategic thinking is essential because of change. Strategic thinking is not particularly important when there is little change. If tomorrow will be much like today and today is similar to yesterday, then the conditions for success today will likely be the same conditions for success tomorrow. In contrast, if there is continuous change, the factors for success likely will change as well. Strategic thinking concerns anticipating, understanding, and coping with such change as well as determining the new conditions for success. In today's dynamic environment, all solutions and successful strategies are temporary.

Perhaps the simplest approach to describing change is to use the categories of evolutionary and revolutionary change and a special condition of revolutionary change called disruptive change. Evolutionary change is slow and incremental while revolutionary change is fast and punctuated. The third and most challenging category is disruptive change; most commonly, this type of change is the result of an innovation that completely disrupts and even displaces market leaders by creating new markets and value networks.[16,17] Public health and healthcare in general are experiencing such disruptive change. New approaches to vaccine development such as ribonucleic acid (RNA) biology promise to disrupt how health departments and healthcare providers manage the public's health, and developments such as gene therapy and subdermal implants, and—less esoteric—telemedicine will continue to disrupt the delivery of care.

Without exception, for organizations to be successful over time they must change. Whether it is the fundamental strategy of the organization or the latest human resource issue or policy, leaders must embrace the concept that all solutions are temporary and view their organizations to be in a constant state of renewal. They must proactively identify and cope with change and reinvent their organizations in real time. Determining just what that renewal might look like is the fundamental task of strategic thinking.

THE PROCESS AND BEHAVIORS OF STRATEGIC THINKING

When there is significant change, leaders must expect to learn and establish new directions as they progress. The new direction must be guided by some form of strategic sense—an intuitive, entrepreneurial sensing of the "shape of the future" that transcends ordinary logic.[18] That process is called "strategic thinking"—a process that senses change, strives to understand its implications, and incorporates new insights and learning into a new plan or direction. More specifically, "strategic thinking" is an intellectual activity that is hyperperceptive to emerging changes, puts meaning to the changes, considers its strategic implications, and develops innovative and transformative responses. At its most fundamental level, strategic thinking includes the states of awareness, anticipation, analysis, interpretation, synthesis, and reflection.[18] If strategic thinking can be approached in a disciplined way, then there will be an increased likelihood of establishing new successful directions. The states of strategic thinking and its iterative nature are shown in Figure 4.1.

Normatively, strategic thinking proceeds in incremental development slices beginning with awareness and progressing through reflection and back to awareness with each of these strategic thinking states providing additional information to the next. The entire strategic thinking process may happen in a flash or over a period of months. In flashes of the mind, these states might occur in any order and in combination with each other. Indeed, awareness and anticipation or analysis and interpretation might occur simultaneously.[18] For strategic thinking occurring over a longer period, there are a number of behaviors that can initiate and enhance the process. Goldman and Scott indicated that strategic thinking is associated with "behaviorally specific descriptors" at all steps of the strategic planning process from visioning to implementation.[19] Dhir, Dhir, and Samanta developed a scale to measure strategic thinking cognitive behaviors.[8] Therefore, to better understand what happens as strategic thinking takes place, we will discuss strategic thinking as a logical process occurring in repeated cycles progressing from one state to the next (as progressive stages) and fostered by specific practical behaviors. The strategic thinking states, their central concepts, and their information-generating behaviors are summarized in Table 4.1.

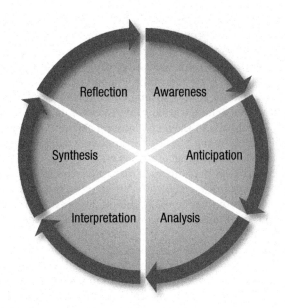

FIGURE 4.1: The Strategic Thinking Process.

TABLE 4.1: Strategic Thinking Behaviors

STRATEGIC THINKING STATES	CENTRAL CONCEPT	STRATEGIC THINKING BEHAVIORS IN ACTION
Awareness	External mindfulness and a hypersensitivity to external change	Taking time to think, systematic observation, nonjudgmental curiosity, active listening, and questioning
Anticipation	Imaginative extension of the signals of change into what might be next	Dreaming, visioning, storytelling and developing scenarios, optimism, passion, and hope
Analysis	Examining issues and adding additional data/information	Searching for more information, financial analysis and market research, application of strategic thinking tools and techniques, and viability conclusions
Interpretation	Deriving meaning and sensemaking framing of information	Understanding biases, skepticism, constructing meaning, transformative thinking, and visioning
Synthesis	Putting it all together, making judgments, and planning	Formulation of mission and vision, setting goals and objectives, developing strategic plans, and documenting the plan
Reflection	Reconsideration and assessment of the interpretations and synthesis	Performance evaluation, reconsideration of beliefs and assumptions, learning from doing, and adjusting the strategic plan

Each of the states of strategic thinking will be examined in detail focusing first on the central concepts and then on the applied behaviors and the expected results that will be passed on to the next state of thinking. This discussion should answer the questions: "How does one practically accomplish the state?" and "What should the state produce?" After completing this section, you should be able to systematically engage in strategic thinking. Once you have experience with the strategic thinking behaviors, strategic thinking will progress more intuitively, rather than in discrete stages.

STAGE ONE—AWARENESS

Strategic awareness is a hypersensitivity to the cues of external change that might best be described as externally oriented mindfulness. Fundamentally, mindfulness is thinking—paying attention—and being intensely aware of what one is sensing and feeling, without interpretation or judgment. More succinctly, mindfulness has been described as "the process of actively noticing new things"[20] and even more simply as being "fully in the moment."[21] Mindfulness is usually practiced through a period of quiet, thoughtful meditation and it is the central concept underlying awareness. Refer to Chapter 1, "Dialogue: A Foundational Skill for Effective Health Leadership," for more on mindfulness.

Research has shown that mindfulness can improve how we focus, think, and feel.[21] Mindfulness can enhance awareness, providing time and occasion to think and focus—focus on the wider world. With an outward focus, mindfulness can help us sense the consequences of external patterns, events, and trends and consider how seemingly unrelated data might connect and play out in the future.[22] Such mindfulness requires vigilance, openness, and nonjudgmental freedom. Mindfulness is essential for detecting environmental change and dealing with uncertainty. As a result, leaders should view strategic planning and mindfulness together.[23]

Awareness in Action

As shown in Figure 4.2, there are several practical behaviors that will help enable attentiveness and facilitate strategic thinking awareness. These behaviors are taking time for mindfulness, systematic observation, nonjudgmental curiosity, active listening, and questioning. Engaging in awareness behaviors should periodically produce tangible results that can be expanded and refined in the anticipation stage of strategic thinking. These results might be best described as inklings or clues of change that might reverberate through the industry or society itself.

To heighten awareness, leaders must consciously set aside time just to think (practice mindfulness). Understandably, leaders are busy and, at first, scheduling this time might

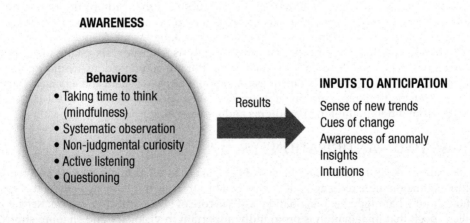

AWARENESS

Behaviors
- Taking time to think (mindfulness)
- Systematic observation
- Non-judgmental curiosity
- Active listening
- Questioning

Results

INPUTS TO ANTICIPATION

Sense of new trends
Cues of change
Awareness of anomaly
Insights
Intuitions

FIGURE 4.2: Awareness Behaviors and Inputs to Anticipation.

seem impossible, but what could be more important than preparing for the future? This time must be protected at all costs as it is all too easy to schedule other tasks by adopting the attitude that this is *only* thinking time. Once mindfulness habits are clearly established, other people will typically respect that time as "off limits" and schedule around it.

Practicing mindfulness by considering the entire external environment of an organization might seem overwhelming; however, systematic observation of smaller segments of the environment might be more feasible. Systems thinking can help break down such complexity, thus allowing focus on one subsystem of the environment at a time (see Chapter 3, "Systems Thinking in Public Health"). For example, rather than focusing on change in the entire external environment, one might first focus on a segment of the environment such as the technological or social subsystem. Breaking down complexity into smaller parts is a hallmark of systems thinking and makes the observational task more comprehensible. In addition, changes discovered in one subsystem might provide cues to changes in other subsystems. Thus, leaders practicing systematic observation must interconnect subsystems when possible.

Another important behavior in awareness is nonjudgmental curiosity. Nonjudgmental curiosity is more difficult than might be initially expected. Everyone has beliefs and values that influence their behaviors. These beliefs and values create paradigms or decision rules that govern how people think, shape their view of convention, and can block openness to new ideas. New perspectives, information, or processes that are counter to one's current ways of thinking may be difficult to comprehend or even see. Thomas Kuhn in his book *The Structure of Scientific Revolutions*, found that information that is counter to one's adopted paradigms or current way of seeing things is almost impossible to see.[24] In contrast, information that agreed with their current views and beliefs were easy to see. Thus, expectations tend to filter information. Kuhn concluded that "discovery commences with awareness of anomaly, i.e., with the recognition that nature has somehow violated the paradigm-induced expectations that govern normal science".[24(pp52–53)] Seeing anomalies requires an openness to change signals and a tolerance for ambiguity—a patience to not act or judge too quickly. Energetic creative thinking, a spark of intuition, a connection between different patterns of information, or a leap into the unexpected can help strategists think beyond what already exists to invent a genuinely new way of doing business—simply waiting for inspiration to strike is not the answer.[25]

Similarly, awareness and curiosity are not passive; rather, they imply a behavior of active listening; that is, seeking information, aggressively sensing transformative ideas, finding interconnections among systems, or picking up clues of significant change. Leaders can learn through listening to the opinions and ideas of others. Listening is also required in a broader sense, detecting changing preferences and lifestyles; therefore, leaders should actively seek a diversity of information sources outside of traditional industry outlets and gather opinions from a variety of people.[26]

Finally, questioning today's reality is key to awareness. Creativity involves reaching beyond precedents and known alternatives to ask questions that prompt the exploration of fresh ideas and approaches.[27] Asking questions can help expose signal blocking paradigms; therefore, strategic thinkers are always questioning—asking "what if" questions. For example, to break what Joel Barker calls "paradigm paralysis," he suggests asking the question: "What today is impossible to do in your business, but if it could be done would fundamentally change it?"[28(p147)] Such "what if" questions should be asked again and again as a normal part of strategic thinking. Additionally, asking; "What do you think?" can elicit opinions derived from different thinking paradigms and sensemaking frames.

STAGE TWO—ANTICIPATION

Anticipation concerns extending the signals of change to what might be next and requires informed imagination, or imagination informed by strategic thinking awareness. It is speculation about what might be. Imagination is at the core of successful anticipation. Reeves and Fuller[27] posit that imagination is profoundly important in visionary and shaping strategies and suggest that imagining things, situations, or products that don't yet exist is essential in understanding the change signals identified in the awareness stage.

Imagination converts insights, intuitions, and anomalies into possibilities for things and processes that do not yet exist. As Martin suggests: "'If you can't imagine it, you will never create it.' The future is about imagination . . . . To imagine a future, one has to look beyond the measurable variables, beyond what can be proven with past data."[29(para6)] Haque expressed it as "being able to see and then *believe in* a vastly different, radically better future."[30(para18)]

Anticipation in Action

As shown in Figure 4.3, exercising one's imagination requires some playful flights of fantasy, daydreaming, and visioning. These mental trips into the future can be enhanced by storytelling and developing scenarios and are fueled by optimism, passion, and hope for a better way, a better future. Anticipation behaviors nurture a new mindset or way of looking at things, new ideas, an emerging vision, new proposals, new processes, and new products and services prospects for analysis.

Imagining, flights of fancy, and daydreaming provide a starting point for anticipation and there are few rules in dreaming about the future. Dreaming and what appears to be daydreaming are not particularly valued in modern organizations. Yet how are we to get to previously improbable or unfathomable innovations, products, and solutions, if we do not suspend the rules and let our mind wander wonderfully out of control? Invention and organizational success start with visualization, which is then structured into stories and scenarios.

In many sports, athletes are taught to visualize success—to conceptualize how the game will play out or the physical act they are trying to master. For example, many professional golfers try to conceptualize their golf shot from the swing of the club to the flight of the ball, and through its landing and roll. This process of visualization alerts them to the possible hazards, but also to the opportunities for success. Visualization provides a possible path to success and defines what success looks like. The same is true for organizations: a leader must have some concept of the end game and how to get there, which is the yet untold story of success.

Storytelling and scenario development involve the creation and elaboration of a coherent description of the future, using the world of today as a starting point. Stories and scenarios "put meat on the bones" of intuitions and dreams. They can qualitatively assess and extend external trends identified in awareness; thus, creating probable visions or pictures of the future based on their likely (or unlikely) impact. The efficacy of stories and scenarios is due in large part to the inability of other, more quantitative forecasting methods to predict and incorporate major external shifts, surprises, and innovations and they provide a better context for strategic thinking.[18]

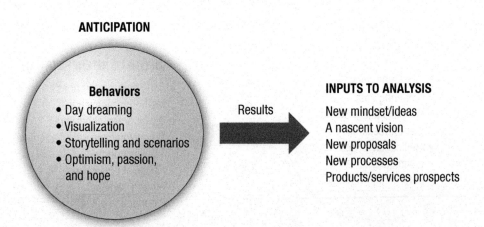

ANTICIPATION

Behaviors
- Day dreaming
- Visualization
- Storytelling and scenarios
- Optimism, passion, and hope

Results

INPUTS TO ANALYSIS

New mindset/ideas
A nascent vision
New proposals
New processes
Products/services prospects

FIGURE 4.3: Anticipation Behaviors and Inputs to Analysis.

Finally, anticipation takes optimism and a passion and hope for making things better. One must stay positive and believe that strategic thinking will provide some hints of the secrets of the future—hints that can be turned into opportunities or help the organization avoid coming threats. A passion to know and a hope for something better drive anticipation and provide the ideas to be assessed in the analysis stage of strategic thinking.

STAGE THREE—ANALYSIS

Analysis involves examining and organizing the new ideas, concepts, product prospects, and stories presented in anticipation, thereby adding information. Analysis can add structure, real-world application, and feasibility to promising proposals, processes, products, and their stories. Laura Alber, CEO of Williams-Sonoma, indicated that she found that the very best solutions came from blending art with science, ideas with data, and instinct with analysis.[31] Taking relatively unstructured ideas and concepts developed through storytelling in the anticipation stage of strategic thinking provides a framework for analysis. Bayer and Taillard advocate such framing, stating that stories enable an even more rigorous analysis of data by allowing the analysts to construct hypotheses, and the stories provide a guide for investigating the data.[32] Equally important, stories build trust in the leader by testifying to an understanding of the organization's history and demonstrate a coherence with values of followers.[33]

Analysis in Action

Analysis often adds a quantitative argument to previously qualitative scenarios; that is, giving substance to anticipation's optimism, passion, and hope. There are many types of strategic thinking analysis and examination behaviors; however, as shown in Figure 4.4, they may be broadly grouped as data gathering, financial analysis and market research, the application of various strategic thinking tools and techniques, and determining potential viability and practicality. The analysis stage will likely produce concept feasibility estimates such as consumer preferences, market attractiveness, development barriers, and technological and social adoption assessments as well as financial projections, growth potential, and introduction costs.

Analysis behaviors might begin with gathering more data. Searching for information has become easier with the internet and electronic databases available today. Literature searches are a common method to begin an analysis of an idea or concept to determine what has been written previously on the topic. Both primary and secondary data can provide valuable information in analysis. Primary data collection might include patient, employee, or stakeholder surveys, interviews, and focus groups. Secondary data are collected by someone else

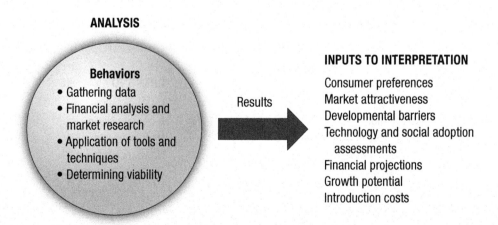

ANALYSIS

Behaviors
- Gathering data
- Financial analysis and market research
- Application of tools and techniques
- Determining viability

Results

INPUTS TO INTERPRETATION

Consumer preferences
Market attractiveness
Developmental barriers
Technology and social adoption assessments
Financial projections
Growth potential
Introduction costs

FIGURE 4.4: Analysis Behaviors and Inputs to Interpretation.

and may reside in databases, historical archives, scholarly journals, and trade publications. In addition, analytics and big data (analysis of multiple large datasets) can be used to uncover patterns and correlations that may not be apparent otherwise. Of course, knowing what information to collect is critical. Meckler and Boal urge that properly identifying and understanding the issue is key in successful data gathering.[34] Similarly, if the relationship among the elements of information is not properly understood, the information will be of little value.

Financial analysis and market research are a necessary part of the analysis stage of strategic thinking, even though specific proposals, products, services, or processes may not yet be fully articulated. Strategic decisions are influenced by the financial resources of the organization, and conversely, the financial resources of an organization are shaped through the implementation of its strategic plan.[35] Similarly, consumer preferences play a vital role in shaping the nature of products, services, or processes. At some point, ideas and proposals must be considered in light of their costs and benefits and market viability.

Often financial analysis and market research can only be "best guesses"; however, some financial and market perspective will be required in evaluating new ideas and proposals, and the more accurate the forecast the more likely a favorable outcome will result.[36] In evaluating proposals, market and internal data may be used in the development of an operating budget that will produce expected revenues and expenses. Such data can be used to produce a pro forma statement of activities (or income statement), which in turn informs a pro forma balance sheet and statement of cash flows.[37] These statements provide some preliminary perspective concerning the feasibility of the concept being considered. Other common financial and market analyses employed when possible are breakeven analysis, return on investment (ROI) projections and analysis, capital requirements forecasts, sensitivity analysis, ratio analyses, and consumer preference surveys and focus groups.

In addition to financial analysis and market research, there are several strategic thinking tools and techniques that can help organize thinking and uncover important variables for consideration. Some of these tools and techniques benefit from data mining and analysis, while some require collaboration and the engagement of others.[38] Describing each of these methods is beyond the scope of this chapter; however, several of the best known are summarized in Table 4.2. None of the tools can make the decision; these methods can only illustrate the interrelationships, organize the major components, and provide the framework for discussion. They are designed to initiate strategic thinking.

At the conclusion of the analysis stage of strategic thinking, decision-makers should have some sense of the potential viability of the concept, proposal, or product. Such a conclusion should consider the development of competing projects, financial feasibility, barriers to entry, internal resource demands, market potential, and adoption issues, thereby providing the information needed to interpret and add meaning to the diverse data and information.

STAGE FOUR—INTERPRETATION

Interpretation considers information gained through the awareness, anticipation, and analysis stages; incorporates divergent opinions, different perspectives, innovative ideas, and creative musings; and adds shape and detail to a concept, proposal, or product.[39] At the same time, interpretation takes place within a context bounded and influenced by experiences, socialization, and training. This context provides the sensemaking frame. As a result, data, information, opinions, and context (framing) are all influential in making practical sense of the information accumulated in the previous strategic thinking stages.

More specifically, interpretation involves obtaining, manipulating, assessing information, and assigning exact meaning. By contrast, Weick states that "sensemaking is about such things as placement of items into frameworks, comprehending, redressing surprise, constructing meaning, interacting in the pursuit of mutual understanding, and patterning."[40(p6)] Thus, sensemaking provides the context within which interpretation assigns meaning to acquired and manipulated information; therefore, individuals' opinions and biases play a role in constructing the situation they attempt to understand.[41]

TABLE 4.2: Strategic Thinking Tools and Techniques*

TOOL OR TECHNIQUE	BRIEF DESCRIPTION
BCG Portfolio Analysis	Evaluation of an organization's products and services in terms of relative market share and market growth rate
Benchmarking	A process of comparing an organization against a set of its peers or top performers on critical metrics for success
Competitive Analysis	Five forces framework for analyzing the attractiveness of a product/service category considering the threat of new entrants, intensity of rivalry among competitors, threat of substitute products/services, bargaining power of customers, and the bargaining power of suppliers
Forecasting	A process of extending trends and issues based on current data and trends to predict the future state of a phenomenon
Geographical Information System (GIS) Analysis	Software that captures, manages, analyzes, interprets, and creates visualizations of geographical data related to three-dimensional data (geospatial data)
Needs/Capacity Assessment	An evaluation method for developing strategy alternatives for not-for-profit and public organizations based on community need and the organization's ability to deliver programs that meet the need
Product Life Cycle Analysis	A method, and typically graphic representation, used to develop strategy alternatives based on the principle that all goods and services progress through the distinct stages of introduction, growth, maturity, and decline
SPACE Analysis	Acronym for Strategic Position and Action Evaluation—an analysis method and graphic depiction that indicates the appropriateness of strategic alternatives based on factors relating to the service category strength, external stability, the organization's relative competitive advantage, and the organization's financial strength
SWOT Analysis	A systematic investigation to consider an organization's internal strengths and weaknesses and its external opportunities and threats; often displayed in a two-by-two matrix

* Definitions adapted from Ginter PM, Duncan WJ, Swayne LE. *Strategic Management of Health Care Organizations.* 8th ed. John Wiley & Sons; 2018, Glossary of Strategic Management Terms.

The development of the "frame" within which interpretation takes place is personal, begins at a young age, and continues throughout life. As a result, accumulated learning and experience are extremely important in framing and interpretation.[42,43] Experienced decision-makers, when faced with uncertainty and ambiguity, can more readily interrupt the momentum and assign meaning to what has been happening over a period of time.[44] Meaning and context happen together and cannot happen in isolation.

Interpretation in Action

As shown in Figure 4.5, strategic thinkers engage in a variety of interpretation behaviors including understanding biases, skepticism, constructing meaning, transformative thinking, and envisioning. Interpretation brings specificity to what all the gathered information means, the vision, proposals, processes, and projected products and services.

When biases are conscious, well-intentioned decision-makers attempt to minimize, or at least recognize, the effects of stereotypes, opinions, and workplace culture on their thinking and actions. Unconscious bias is a more troublesome issue. Unconscious biases exist because each person "views the world from a unique vantage point, collecting information through physical senses, and interpreting it through their own beliefs."[45(p548)] This unique vantage point has been associated with various demographics such as age, gender, occupation, and related factors.[46(p17)] Understanding one's conscious and unconscious biases frees leaders to move past sensemaking framing barriers including those frames associated with structural bias, social inequities, and racism.

Informed strategic thinkers are skeptical of the information they receive and the sources supplying it. Skepticism can be functional or dysfunctional. For example, skepticism of science causes concern when it comes to disavowing the dangers of climate change or vaccine resistance.[47] Skepticism on the part of the strategic thinker, on the other hand, may be quite functional. Managers are often inundated with information (e.g., reports, graphs, tables, and white papers). The questions for the strategist are "Where do these numbers come from?" and "Who complied them?" Does the provider of this information have ulterior motives? The skeptical strategic thinker must carefully distinguish between "mitigable ignorance of pertinent but knowable information and immitigable indeterminacy."[48(p766)] Simply put, the strategic thinker must distinguish between what is not known, but can be known, and what cannot be known even with additional search. When additional information is deemed to be of little or no value, even the skeptical thinker must cease additional search.

To progress to the next strategic thinking stage, strategic thinkers must construct meaning. There is more to the construction of meaning than just acquiring and manipulating data. It is in the interpretation stage that the dream, its supporting story, and analysis come together in the form of a final detailed concept, product, or proposal. Interpretation infuses practical meaning into the results generated from the earlier strategic thinking stages and provides the "so what?" of strategic thinking; that is, the specific concept or proposal to be moved forward into the planning stage (synthesis).

In the interpretation stage, strategic thinkers embrace grand challenges and transformations. Such bold thinking does not mean that everyone who thinks strategically enables lasting changes in their industry; however, sometimes they do. Transformative thinking is basically "thinking out of the box," or going outside of convention. It involves pioneering

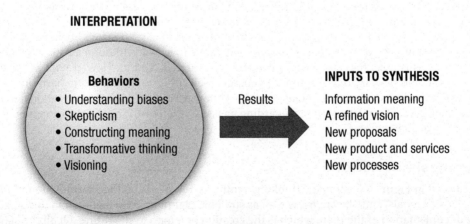

INTERPRETATION

Behaviors
- Understanding biases
- Skepticism
- Constructing meaning
- Transformative thinking
- Visioning

Results

INPUTS TO SYNTHESIS

Information meaning
A refined vision
New proposals
New product and services
New processes

FIGURE 4.5: Interpretation Behaviors and Inputs to Synthesis.

nontraditional solutions; pursuing unique original answers; introducing something new, better, or different; or the redefining of issues using a different perspective. Such flashes of insight can be transformative and can happen in most any environment. For example, researchers who focus on community-based enterprises or humanitarian aid providers have long sought "transformations in how their services can alleviate the suffering of vulnerable people and co-create value by influencing long-term uplifting changes" in a community.[49(p411)]

Finally, interpretation requires clear vision, a compelling and motivating picture of what can be. Vision provides an inspirational picture of future possibilities. Visionary thinkers inspire others to follow them or to "buy into" the vision. In fact, "visionary leadership is transformative in itself and based on the power to inspire."[50] The most effective visionaries are also committed to acquire the resources to achieve the goals.[51] Armed with a clear vision the strategic thinker can begin the development of strategic goals and a comprehensive strategic plan.

STAGE FIVE—SYNTHESIS

In its most visible form, synthesis involves the traditional tasks of leadership and management—the development of goals and strategic plans. In the synthesis stage, the leadership of an organization goes about the tasks of formulating mission, vision, goals, objectives, and a strategic plan. This process usually involves a group of leaders reaching consensus on a strategy for the interpretation of accumulated information, opinions, and perspectives.

Less obvious in the strategic thinking synthesis stage is the amalgamation of information, its consideration, and decision-making—the "go" or "no go" decision. The most important decisions in life as well as in organizations are qualitative; they cannot be fully quantified, and are often made based on intuition or "gut feeling." As Peter Drucker has stated, "A decision is a judgment. It is a choice between alternatives. It is rarely a choice between right and wrong .... much more often a choice between two courses of action neither of which is probably more nearly right than the other."[52(p470)] As a result, organizations are led and managed based largely on a synthesis of opinions, judgments, and consensus. Moreover, decision-making is often more than choosing between competing alternatives; it also concerns integrative thinking. Often leaders are able to creatively resolve the tension between alternatives by generating a new, better option that contains elements of two or more alternatives.[53] Synthesis is at the core of strategic innovation and creativity and involves pulling together seemingly unrelated concepts or alternatives. Sometimes it involves selecting a course of action among alternatives and other times it means charting a whole new direction. Thus, the synthesis stage of strategic thinking converts intuition, dreams, and hopes and their interpretation into practical goals, objectives, plans, and timelines.

As discussed in the interpretation stage of strategic thinking, information has context and is framed through sensemaking. Synthesis concludes this process and concerns reaching a consensus on how to move forward and documenting opinions, judgments, and intuitions into a workable plan. Consensus has the effect of temporarily "freezing" beliefs, assumptions, and frames so that strategic planning may move forward. Although a reasonable level of consensus is essential, it is also a powerful force and should be viewed with suspicion. Leaders should be wary of groupthink (members seek conformity and desire harmony even if it results in dysfunctional decisions) and the Abilene Paradox (where organizational members fail to reveal their true feelings regarding an issue, often resulting in a decision that none of the participants prefer).

Synthesis in Action

As shown in Figure 4.6, strategic thinking synthesis behaviors include formulation of mission, vision, goals, and objectives, as well as strategic planning. Also included in this stage is the documentation of the plan, which is the creation of a map to the future. Of all the stages of strategic thinking, synthesis creates the most tangible outputs. Much of what occurs in

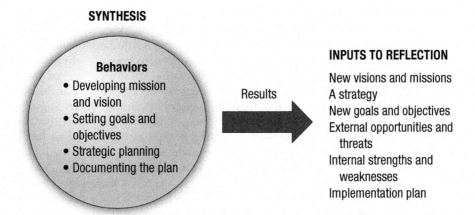

FIGURE 4.6: Synthesis Behaviors and Inputs to Reflection.

synthesis is documented and provides benchmarks for the reflection stage including the vision and mission, the strategy, and goals and objectives as well as the current view of the external opportunities and threats, internal strengths and weaknesses, and the implementation plan.

Creating a mission and vision as well as goals and objectives for emergent ideas or proposals to which interpretation has infused meaning provides organizational momentum. Missions are statements of distinctiveness and unique purpose. These statements serve as reminders to everyone of organizational focus. Vision statements, on the other hand, express a hope for the future and the dream of fulfilling the mission. These statements are important "stakes in the ground" for the organization and provide context, substance, and definition to the road forward. Effective mission and vision are only possible if strategic thinking has progressed through the awareness, anticipation, analysis, and interpretation and meaningful synthesis stages.

The setting of goals and objectives moves the strategic thinker from the relatively abstract to the specific and concrete. Ultimately, they translate the dream for the future into milestones and timelines. The planning process relies on a knowledge of the external environment and the types and pace of change taking place. Goals and objectives also indicate the activities that will be necessary to achieve them and move toward the vision or, essentially, the strategic plan. The resulting strategic plan should focus on maximizing the relevancy of the organization and will never be perfect. Nonetheless, the strategic plan will create organizational momentum. These activities require considerable strategic thinking. The strategic plan and its implementation require the synthesis of creativity, innovation, judgment, and consensus.

Finally, synthesis requires the documentation of the decisions made throughout the process. This documentation is called a strategic plan. Fundamentally, it is a map or guidebook to the future. Like all maps, however, it can become dated over time as things change; therefore, strategic plans must be updated constantly as change is happening around us all the time. The strategic plan properly conceived is a living document that is never complete. It is a journey not a destination requiring ongoing reflection. So, strategic thinkers must be prepared to adjust and understand that the strategy will always be in flux. Such a dynamic perspective encourages openness, innovation, and a preparedness to change.[54]

STAGE SIX—REFLECTION

Reflection is essentially a reconsideration and assessment of the results of interpretation and synthesis and reality testing of the strategic plan. This type of strategic thinking takes time and it is clear that most leaders do not systematically allow enough time to be reflective.[55]

Reflection requires quiet time and slow, deliberate thinking and is where retrospection on the past and awareness of the future intersect in the strategic thinking process. These two strategic thinking stages require protected time for contemplation and mindfulness. In these quiet times, reflection on "where we have been" moves to awareness of "where we are going" and back again to reflection. It involves a reconsideration or "unfreezing" of the beliefs and assumptions underlying the plan as well as a recognition of emergent changes. Reeves, Torres, and Hassan suggest; "In reflective thought, a person examines underlying assumptions, core beliefs, and knowledge, while drawing connections between apparently disparate pieces of information."[55(para2)] It is in thinking about the strategy today and connecting to the cues for change where creativity happens; however, leaders will not see the big picture, let alone a shapeable picture of the future, unless they stand back and reflect.[27] As Jennifer Porter states: "The most useful reflection involves the conscious consideration and analysis of beliefs and actions for the purpose of learning. Reflection gives the brain an opportunity to pause amidst the chaos, untangle and sort through observations and experiences, consider multiple possible interpretations, and create meaning."[56(para3)]

Although in practice, reflection and awareness are similar, there are differences. In reflection, there is a clear goal—an assessment, a relevancy test. Practicing mindfulness awareness is free flowing and not bound by any particular objective, other than discovery. In reflection, there is an evaluation of the goals and actions taken in light of "what we know now" or asking the question, "Have we got it right?" Through past actions, learning has taken place as to what is working and what is not. Adjustments have been made and, at the same time, change has once again put everything in question. Reflection is, therefore, focused more on the organization's current fit with its environment, its relevancy to society, and its connectivity to stakeholders.

Reflection in Action

As shown in Figure 4.7, reflection is the process of organizational renewal and performance evaluation, a reconsideration of beliefs and assumptions, learning and reframing, and adjusting the strategic plan, which make up the essential reflection strategic thinking behaviors. The conclusion of reflection provides a new beginning to strategic thinking. Reflection once again "unfreezes" context and the sensemaking frame for the next round of strategic thinking. Thus, reflection begins to shape the new reality of the organization. Strategic thinking awareness then may result in a search for new possibilities, insights, and perspectives, which propels one again through the strategic thinking process.

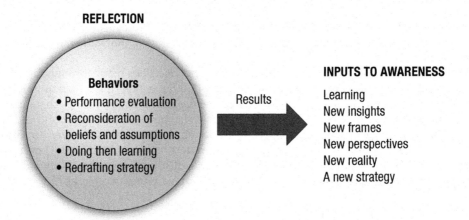

FIGURE 4.7: Reflection Behaviors and Inputs to Awareness.

Evaluation is at the heart of reflection. Performance evaluation provides a starting point for thinking about the strategy and its implementation. Although it is not all about the numbers, the numbers do provide some anchors to the reality of how well the organization is translating dreams into actions. Performance and success may be measured in many different ways—financial, human, societal, technological, and so on—however, leaders should be assessing the effectiveness of the strategy in some relevant way. Such measures are usually implicit or explicitly predetermined in the planning (synthesis) stage of strategic thinking. Evaluating "how we are doing" opens up a stream of reflective thinking.

Performance evaluation can also ignite a reconsideration of the fundamental beliefs and assumptions underlying the strategy. Leaders should identify the important beliefs and assumptions upon which the strategy was built and ask if these foundational supports are still sound. This reconsideration can take place in quiet meditation or in group discussions with key leaders. Methods to enrich strategic thinking, particularly reflection, are reviewed later in this chapter.

Learning is a key aspect of reflection. In schools we are taught to learn something, and then we try to do it. In other words, we learn and then do; however, in most situations throughout life, we do and then learn. As the strategy of an organization unfolds, we get a better understanding of how to make it work. A part of reflective thinking concerns what has been learned and incorporating that learning into a reformulation and reframing of the strategy.

Finally, the logical conclusion of reflection is to adjust the strategic plan to accommodate the new realities (e.g., external change, performance perspectives, underlying beliefs and assumptions, and the learning that has taken place). Such updates should be considered a normal part of leadership and do not require formal strategic planning retreats. Usable strategic plans that serve as guides to actions are preferable to formal bound plans that usually remain on the shelf. Our maps to the future should reflect the latest strategic thinking.

LEADERSHIP AND STRATEGIC THINKING

Wherever we look for leadership, we should find strategic thinking. There are a number of approaches and theories of leadership discussed in this book and elsewhere, including the Trait Approach, Behavioral Approach, Transformational Leadership, Authentic Leadership, Servant Leadership, and Cultural Leadership, to name a few. Although leadership is more than just strategic thinking, it is an explicit part of or strongly implied in all leadership theories. In fact, strategic thinking is central to effectively setting direction for an organization. The word "leadership" itself implies setting direction for others to follow. Strategic thinking is the clearest signal of the existence of leadership in an organization and it is the leaders in an organization who must be the initiators, keepers, and promoters of the vision of an organization.

Leadership and its central task of strategic thinking are now routinely practiced at every level in many organizations: in divisions, departments, and units. It is all a matter of defining the strategic thinking scope. For example, a department is situated within a larger organization which constitutes part of the department's changing environment. Furthermore, there are likely specific technologies, particular legislation, or special economics unique to a department's mission that must be considered. Strategic thinking in divisions, departments, and units is now an integral part of leading them, and strategic thinking habits can and should be instilled throughout the organization. Everyone in the organization should be encouraged to become a strategic thinker and to consider how to reinvent what they do. Everyone can and should be a leader.

SUMMARY

Doing seems to be more valued than *thinking* in Western societies; however, it is thinking that leads to learning and learning leads to better doing. Similarly, strategic plans are valued more than the strategic thinking that guided their development; however, it is strategic thinking that initiates as well as renews the process of developing strategy and the resultant strategic plans. Today, strategic thinking goes beyond just focusing on competitive issues: it has a broader focus on fundamental societal patterns and trends. Without strategic thinking, transformative strategic plans are never developed, and innovative implementation rarely happens.

Strategic thinking is now essential because of the external change that most all industries and socioeconomic sectors are experiencing. Public health and healthcare continue to have "white water" change constantly altering the factors for success. In few sectors is there more revolutionary and disruptive change than in health-related environments. Therefore, serious strategic thinking is required to create relevant strategic plans to guide organizational efforts.

Typically, strategic thinking progresses through six stages: awareness, anticipation, analysis, interpretation, synthesis, and reflection. Each of these stages initiates leadership behaviors and activities directed toward identifying, understanding, and acting on the subtle change cues taking place in the environment. As a result, effective strategic thinking, and the strategic plans it generates, are clear signals of engaged leadership. In organizations with a long-term history of success, strategic thinking is practiced throughout the organization.

Finally, strategic thinking requires concentrated effort and takes practice. Lasting change will be made only through a lifelong commitment to a continuing discipline. Lasting organizational change and organizational renewal comes from thinking strategically and adopting sound leadership principles that are practiced on a continuing basis. There are no quick fixes. Strategic thinking enables the organization to change itself, and potentially the world.

DISCUSSION QUESTIONS

1. Why has strategic thinking become crucial in today's dynamic public health and healthcare industry?

2. Why are conceptual models of management processes useful for leaders? More specifically, why is a model of strategic thinking (an intellectual process) helpful?

3. What is the difference between the terms "strategic thinking" and "strategic planning"?

4. How can knowing the behaviors that can initiate and enhance strategic thinking be helpful to leaders?

CASE STUDY: AN IDEA TAKES SHAPE

Rebecca E. Kennedy, Peter M. Ginter, and W. Jack Duncan

In December of 2020, the University of Alabama at Birmingham (UAB) was the first university in the United States to adopt the Okanagan Charter and become an internationally, formally recognized health promoting university (HPU). Shortly thereafter in 2021, UAB was named America's number one best large employer by Forbes, topping a list of more than 500 public and private corporations, hospitals, and universities. In addition, UAB had recently been named number four in the nation and the top higher education institution by Forbes among top employers for diversity. While UAB had always been focused on improving health and well-being, at the signing of the Okanagan Charter, UAB

President Dr. Ray L. Watts noted that adopting the Charter "aligns who we have always been as an institution with an internationally known framework and network."[57(para6)]

As detailed in the UAB Charter signing press release, an HPU is a university that strives to infuse health and well-being into everyday operations, business practices, and academics and to strengthen ecological, social, and economic sustainability, thus creating a culture of compassion, well-being, equity, and social justice (Okanagan Charter[a]). HPUs are guided by the Okanagan Charter—an international charter for health-promoting universities and colleges originally developed in the territory of the Okanagan Nation (British Columbia, Canada, and Washington state, United States).

UAB's impetus to adopt the Charter and move to become an HPU were initially the result of the inspiration and championing of Dr. Rebecca Kennedy, UAB assistant vice president for student health and well-being. After the signing of the Okanagan Charter, President Watts named Dr. Kennedy and the dean of the school of public health to lead a task force to guide the university's efforts to fully implement becoming an HPU.

Dr. Kennedy was introduced to the Okanagan Charter and the International HPU movement in 2017. Taking time to periodically think about changes taking place in higher education in the United States as well as the broader environment, Dr. Kennedy was convinced this was a framework that could improve the well-being of students, staff, and faculty not just in other countries but in the United States as well. Issues such as climate change, social justice, economic disparities, and environmental sustainability as well as several other social determinants of health were emerging as major issues on U.S. college campuses that university presidents were being challenged to address. Dr. Kennedy began a systematic observation of these phenomena, actively seeking out information, listening, and questioning. Through this externally oriented mindfulness, she became sensitive to the external changes bringing into focus the heightened importance of the overall health and well-being of students, staff, and faculty on college campuses. Through this process she also became aware of the Canadian and International HPU networks and the opportunity to start an HPU in the United States. Dr. Kennedy began reaching out to others who were interested in a U.S. HPU network and, as a result, gained valuable insights as to the requirements, conditions, and prospects of developing the first U.S. HPU.

Dr. Kennedy began to speculate on what might be next in the development of HPUs. She dreamed of what an HPU could be: a movement that could change the entire culture of a university from providing treatment and interventions with individuals who became ill or unhealthy, to using a settings and whole systems approach to create conditions for health, creating supportive environments in which all students, staff, and faculty could thrive. She imagined a university campus where every policy and initiative were considered and implemented based on how they might enhance student, employee, and community health and well-being. She visualized the perfect HPU and began developing a picture of what a university could be when fully implementing the Okanagan Charter. She embraced an optimistic view that such a vision was possible for UAB and became more and more passionate and hopeful that she could make it happen. She began to develop a mental scenario of an emerging HPU at UAB.

[a]https://static1.squarespace.com/static/56a801c4c21b869a7c0c8cb7/t/56b42432f8baf3b2377843ef/1454646350974/Okanagan_Charter_Oct_6_2015.pdf

Dr. Kennedy began methodically examining issues surrounding HPUs and searching for additional information. She began to think about the costs as well and benefits of UAB becoming an HPU and began discussing that with others. She concluded that the long-term benefits could be huge, not only for the university, but also for the community. Beyond improving health and the university's culture, a holistic approach to health and well-being on a college campus would serve as a model in the United States and would be very attractive to students interested in studying at UAB. She recognized that as a premier HPU, student enrollment, as well as retention and persistence, could increase. She also concluded that becoming an HPU could positively impact the culture for the faculty, staff, and healthcare workers. As an HPU, UAB would further boost employment opportunities and the community would also benefit from increasing the already annual $7 billion economic impact of the university. Indeed, an HPU might be very viable for multiple reasons.

Sitting in her office on the UAB campus, Dr. Kennedy stared at the Charter press release of President Watts signing the Okanagan Charter laying on the corner of her desk. Not really seeing it, she began asking herself: "What did my information gathering, and analysis mean?" "Am I letting my concern for students and their health, as AVP for Student Health and Wellbeing, influence me too much?" "Am I being objective?" "Could this effort be truly transformative for the university?" She continued thinking, realizing that: "Of course, it would not happen overnight." Then, she wondered; "Where do we go from here?" and "How should we proceed?"

CASE STUDY QUESTIONS

1. Has Dr. Kennedy been engaged in strategic thinking? If so, what makes you think so?
2. What should Dr. Kennedy do next?

 A robust set of instructor resources designed to supplement this text is located at http://connect.springerpub.com/content/book/978-0-8261-4924-4. Qualifying instructors may request access by emailing textbook@springerpub.com.

REFERENCES

1. Dixit AK, Nalebuff BJ. *Strategic Thinking*. W. W. Norton & Company; 1991.
2. Ansoff HI. *Corporate Strategy: An Analytical Approach to Business Policy for Growth and Expansion*. McGraw Hill; 1965.
3. Mintzberg H. *The Rise and Fall of Strategic Planning*. The Free Press; 1994.
4. Ansoff HI. *Strategic Management: Classic Edition*. Palgrave Publishing; 2007.
5. Porter ME. *Competitive Strategy: Techniques for Analyzing Industries and Competitors*. The Free Press; 1980.
6. Porter ME. *Competive Advantage: Creating and Sustaining Superior Performance*. The Free Press; 1985.
7. Gross R. Towards an understanding of the relationship between leadership style and strategic thinking: a small and medium enterprise perspective. *J Bus Stud Q*. 2016;8(2):22–39.
8. Dhir S, Dhir S, Samanta P. Defining and developing a scale to measure strategic thinking. *Foresight*. 2018;20(3):271–288. doi:10.1108/FS-10-2017-0059

9. Schwartz P. *The Art of the Long View: Planning for the Futue in an Uncertain World*. Currency Doubleday; 1991.

10. Schwartz P. *Inevitable Suprises: Thinking Ahead in a Time of Turbulence*. Gotham Books; 2003.

11. Griffiths SB. *The Art of War*. Oxford University Press; 1963.

12. Wintzel M. *The Biographical Dictionary of Management, Vol 2*. Thoemmes Press; 2001.

13. Andrevski G, Miller D. Forbearance: strategic nonresponse to competitive attacks. *Acad Manag Rev*. Published online January 10, 2022. doi:10.5465/amr.2018.0248

14. Sohail A, Dhir, S. A meta-analytical review of factors affecting the strategic thinking of an organization. *Forsight*. 2020;22(2):144–177. doi:10.1108/FS-08-2019-0076

15. Hunitie M. Impact of strategic leadership on strategic competitive advantage through strategic thinking and strategic planning: a bi-meditational research. *Bus Theory Pract*. 2018;19(2):322–330. doi:10.3846/btp.2018.32

16. Meier KJ. Additive manufacturing—driving massive disruptive change in supply chain management. *J Work-Appl Manag*. 2020;12(2):221–231. doi:10.1108/jwam-05-2020-0024

17. Christensen CM, Raynor ME, McDonald R. What is disruptive innovation. *Harv Bus Rev*. 2015;93(12): 44–53. https://hbr.org/2015/12/what-is-disruptive-innovation

18. Ginter PM, Duncan WJ, Swayne LE. *Strategic Management of Health Care Organizations*. 8th ed. John Wiley & Sons; 2018.

19. Goldman E, Scott AR. Competency models for assessing strategic thinking. *J Strategy Manag*. 2016;9(3):258–280. doi:10.1108/JSMA-07-2015-0059

20. Langer E, Beard A. Mindfulness in the age of complexity. *Harvard Business Review*. 2021, March 29. https://hbr.org/2014/03/mindfulness-in-the-age-of-complexity

21. Lyddy C, Good DJ. Bolino MC, Thompson PS, Stephens JP. Where mindfulness falls short. *Harvard Business Review*. March 18, 2021. https://hbr.org/2021/03/where-mindfulness-falls-short

22. Goleman D. The focused leader. *Harv Bus Rev*. 2013;91(12):51–60. https://hbr.org/2013/12/the-focused-leader

23. Butcher J. Mindfulness as a management technique goes back to at least the 1970s. *Harvard Business Review*. Updated May 8, 2018. https://hbr.org/2018/05/mindfulness-as-a-management-technique-goes-back-to-at-least-the-1970s

24. Kuhn TS. *The Strcture of Scientific Revolutions*. The University of Chicago Press; 1970.

25. Brandenburger A. Strategy needs creativity. *Harvard Business Review*. March-April 2019. https://hbr.org/2019/03/strategy-needs-creativity

26. Beausoleil E. Listening obliquely: listening as norm and strategy for structural justice. *Comtemp Political Theory*. 2021;20(6):23–47. doi:10.1057/s41296-020-00405-5

27. Reeves M, Fuller J. We need imagination now more than ever. *Harvard Business Review*. April 10, 2020. https://hbr.org/2020/04/we-need-imagination-now-more-than-ever

28. Barker JA. *Future Edge: Discovering the New Paradigms of Success*. William Morrow and Company; 1992.

29. Martin RL. Management by imagination. *Harvard Business Review*. January 19, 2010. https://hbr.org/2010/01/management-by-imagination-2

30. Haque U. How strategic imagination happens. *Harvard Business Review*. April 8, 2008. https://hbr.org/2008/04/how-strategic-imagination-happ-1

31. Alber L. The CEO of Williams-Sonoma on blending instinct with analysis. *Harv Bus Rev*. 2014;92(9): 41–44. https://hbr.org/2014/09/the-ceo-of-williams-sonoma-on-blending-instinct-with-analysis

32. Bayer J, Taillard M. Story-driven data analysis. *Harvard Business Review*. September 27, 2013. https://hbr.org/2013/09/story-driven-data-analysis

33. Auvinen T, Aaltio I. Blomqvist K. Constructing leadership by storytelling— the meaning of trust and narratives. *Leadersh Organ Dev J*. 2013;34(6):496–514. doi:10.1108/LODJ-10-2011-0102

34. Meckler M, Boal K. Decision errors, organizational iatrogenesis, and errors of the seventh kind. *Acad Manag Perspect*. 2020;34(2):266–284. doi:10.5465/amp.2017.0144

35. Smieliauskas W, Bewley K, Gronewold U, Menzefricke U. Misleading forecasts in accounting estimates: a form of ethical blindness in accounting standards. *J Bus Ethics*. 2018;152(2):437–457. doi:10.1007/s10551-016-3289-1

36. Kim HY, Lee YS, Jun DB. The effect of real life performane feedback on judgmental forecasting accuracy. *Manag Decis*. 2019;57(9):1695–1711. doi:10.1108/MD-06-2017-0549

37. Rucks AC. Health care organization accounting, finance, and performance analysis. In: PM Ginter, WJ Duncan, LE Swayne, eds. *Strategic Management of Health Care Organizations*. John Wiley & Sons, Inc; 2018:443–461.

38. Nogueira F, Borges M, Wolf JH. Collaborative decision-making in non-formal planning settings. *Group Decis Negot.* 2017;26(5):875–890. doi:10.1007/s10726-016-9518-2

39. Alvarez SA, Porac J. Imagination, inderterminacy, and managerial choice at the limit of knowledge. *Acad Manag Rev.* 2020;45(4):735–744. doi:10.5465/amr.2020.0366

40. Weick KE. *Sensemaking in Organizations.* Sage Publishers; 1995.

41. Glynn MA, Watkiss L. Of organizing and sensemaking: from action to meaning and back again in a half-century of Weick's theorizing. *J Manag Stud.* 2020;35(5):592–605. doi:10.1111/joms.12613

42. Mithani MA. Adaptation in the face of the new normal. *Acad Manag Perspect.* 2020;34(4):508–530. doi:10.5465/amp.2019.0054

43. Wenzel M. Taking the future seriously: from corporate foresight to "Future Making." *Acad Manag Perspect.* Published online January 21, 2021. doi:10.5465/amp.2020.0126

44. Konlechner S, Latzke M, Guttel WH, Hofferer E. Prospective sensemaking, frames and planned change interventions. *Hum Relat.* 2018;72(4):706–732. doi:10.1177/0018726718773157

45. Eyal T, Steffel M, Epley N. Perspective mistaking: accurately understanding the mind of another requires getting perspective, not taking perspective. *J Pers Soc Psychol.* 2018;114(4):547–571. doi:10.1037/pspa0000115

46. Vania B, Murhadi WR, Herlambang A. The effect of demographic factors on behavioral biases. *J Siasat Bisnis.* 2021;25(1):17–29. doi:10.20885/jsb.vol25.iss1.art2

47. Rutjens BT, Van der Linden S, Van der Lee R. Science skepticism in times of COVID-19. *Group Process Intergroup Relat.* 2021;24(2):276–283. doi:10.1177/1368430220981415

48. Packard MD, Clark BB. On the mitigability of uncertainty and the choice between predictive and non-predictive strategy. *Acad of Manag Rev.* 2020;45(4):766–786. doi:10.5465/amr.2018.0198

49. Obaze Y. The transformative community-based humanitarian service ecosystem. *J Humanit Logist Supply Chain Manag.* 2018;9(3):410–437. doi:10.1108/JHLSCM-06-2018-0039

50. Loh KL, Yusof SM, Lau DH. Blue ocean leadership in lean sustainability. *Int J Lean Six Sigma.* 2016;10(1):275–295. doi:10.1108/IJLSS-06-2016-0029

51. Benjamin GC. Visionary leadership, visionary goals: NPHW@25. *Am J Public Health.* 2020;110(4):427. doi:10.2105/AJPH.2019.305501

52. Drucker PF. *Management: Tasks, Responsibilities, Practices.* Harper & Row, Publishers; 1974.

53. Martin RL. How successful leaders think. *Harv Bus Rev.* 2007;85(6):60–67. https://hbr.org/2007/06/how-successful-leaders-think

54. Kenny G. Strategic plans are less important than strategic planning. *Harvard Business Review.* June 21, 2016. https://hbr.org/2018/04/your-strategic-plans-probably-arent-strategic-or-even-plans

55. Reeves M, Torres R, Hassan F. How to regain the lost art of reflection. *Harvard Business Review.* September 25, 2017. https://hbr.org/2017/09/how-to-regain-the-lost-art-of-reflection

56. Porter J. Why you should make time for self-reflection (even if you hate doing it). *Harvard Business Review.* March 21, 2017. https://hbr.org/2017/03/why-you-should-make-time-for-self-reflection-even-if-you-hate-doing-it

57. Thomason S. UAB becomes first Health Promoting University in the United States. December 15, 2020. https://www.uab.edu/news/campus/item/11756-uab-becomes-first-health-promoting-university-in-the-united-states

APPENDIX 4.1: SELF-ADMINISTERED STRATEGIC THINKING AUDIT EXERCISE

An important part of strategic thinking is to ensure engagement in each stage of the process. As a leadership exercise, leaders can assess their active participation in each stage of strategic thinking by evaluating their level of involvement in key activities for each stage. A score of less than 20 for any stage suggests that additional focus on the strategic thinking behaviors for that stage might enhance strategic thinking (an example score is shown in the Awareness stage). For the entire strategic thinking audit, a score of less than 150 suggests a lack of commitment to serious strategic thinking.

STRATEGIC THINKING BEHAVIORS	SELF-EVALUATION		
AWARENESS	**LOW**		**HIGH**
I take time to think about change (mindfulness).	1 2 3 4 5 6 7		
I practice systematic observation to reduce complexity then interconnect subsystems.	1 2 3 4 5 6 7		
I engage in nonjudgmental curiosity.	1 2 3 4 5 6 7		
I engage in active listening.	1 2 3 4 5 6 7		
I ask "what if?" questions.	1 2 3 4 5 6 7		
AWARENESS TOTAL			
ANTICIPATION	**LOW**		**HIGH**
I take time to dream about possibilities.	1 2 3 4 5 6 7		
I visualize how trends and patterns might appear in the future.	1 2 3 4 5 6 7		
I develop stories or scenarios of what the future will be.	1 2 3 4 5 6 7		
I am optimistic that we can turn change into opportunity.	1 2 3 4 5 6 7		
I have passion and hope to make a positive difference.	1 2 3 4 5 6 7		
ANTICIPATION TOTAL			
ANALYSIS	**LOW**		**HIGH**
I search for and gather additional information.	1 2 3 4 5 6 7		
I perform financial analysis to determine financial viability.	1 2 3 4 5 6 7		
I perform market research to assess consumer preferences.	1 2 3 4 5 6 7		
I employ strategic thinking tools and techniques.	1 2 3 4 5 6 7		
I assess project/concept viability.	1 2 3 4 5 6 7		
ANALYSIS TOTAL			
INTERPRETATION	**LOW**		**HIGH**
I try to understand my conscious and unconscious biases.	1 2 3 4 5 6 7		
I am skeptical and search for evidence.	1 2 3 4 5 6 7		
I try to construct meaning from cues and signals.	1 2 3 4 5 6 7		
I strive for transformative ideas and concepts.	1 2 3 4 5 6 7		
I try to pull it all together in a vision.	1 2 3 4 5 6 7		
INTERPRETATION TOTAL			

SYNTHESIS	LOW						HIGH
I develop clear and realistic missions.	1	2	3	4	5	6	7
I develop inspiring visions.	1	2	3	4	5	6	7
I set realistic goals and objectives.	1	2	3	4	5	6	7
I develop workable strategic plans.	1	2	3	4	5	6	7
I document the strategic plan to serve as map to the future.	1	2	3	4	5	6	7
SYNTHESIS TOTAL							
REFLECTION	LOW						HIGH
I conduct a performance evaluation on the project.	1	2	3	4	5	6	7
I reconsider the strategy's underlying beliefs.	1	2	3	4	5	6	7
I assess my assumptions.	1	2	3	4	5	6	7
I incorporate what we have learned into the strategic plan.	1	2	3	4	5	6	7
I adjust the strategic plan to the new realities.	1	2	3	4	5	6	7
REFLECTION TOTAL							
STRATEGIC THINKING TOTAL							

(Note: The deductive approach was taken to the design and development of this self-administered Strategic Thinking Audit exercise by the chapter authors to help leaders to consider their strategic thinking behaviors.)

Chapter 5

Emotional Intelligence

Susan C. Helm-Murtagh

INTRODUCTION

Emotional intelligence (EI) is a crucial leadership skill. While there are several models of EI with differing constructs, it is generally defined as the ability to understand and manage one's own emotions, as well as recognize and influence the emotions of others. Higher levels of EI have been positively associated with well-being, life satisfaction, mental and physical health, academic performance, psychological adjustment, workplace success, happiness, and relationship quality.[1-4] Being aware of one's emotions and managing them effectively and positively can, in fact, be more critical than intelligence or technical skills in determining success in many aspects of life, including leadership.[5,6]

OBJECTIVES

By the end of this chapter, the reader will be able to:

- Define EI.
- Understand the history, development, and four major models of EI.
- Know why EI is important to leadership.
- Identify resources and approaches to assess and develop one's EI.
- Apply EI knowledge to two case studies.

DEFINITIONS, HISTORY, AND MODELS OF EMOTIONAL INTELLIGENCE

The subject of human intelligence has been a matter of discussion and debate for centuries, dating back to at least Plato and Aristotle, who posited that there are three components of mind and soul: intellect, sentiment, and will.[7] Intelligence is an individual's ability to comprehend new or challenging situations, apply existing knowledge to manipulate one's surroundings or circumstances, or to apply abstract thinking.

For much of the 20th century, psychologists focused on modeling and measuring intelligence, which was generally described as an ever-expanding set of intellectual or mental abilities. Charles Spearman's two-factor theory of intelligence, developed in 1904, includes general intelligence (g) and the specific factor (s). "General intelligence," as the term implies, is the foundation for all forms of intellectual abilities, whereas the specific factor refers to the type of intelligence (such as mathematics) that a particular test measures.[8] In 1938, Louis L. Thurstone's "Primary Mental Abilities" (PMAs) model included seven primary cognitive abilities: (1) verbal understanding, (2) verbal flexibility, (3) number, (4) memory, (5) perceptual speed, (6) inductive reasoning, and (7) spatial visualization.[9] In 1955, Joy Paul Guilford expanded the concept of intelligence to include 120 different types of intelligence.[10]

In 1985, Robert Sternberg proposed a three-part intelligence model: analytical intelligence (problem-solving), creative intelligence (handling new situations), and practical intelligence (adapting to new challenges).[11]

During the 1980s, noting that intellectual prowess does not necessarily translate into success in educational or occupational settings, researchers began focusing on the role that other skill sets or types of intelligence play in human performance, including the ability to process emotional information. Building on the work of David Weschler, who in 1943 posited that nonintellectual abilities are essential for predicting one's ability to succeed in life, developmental psychologist Howard Gardner introduced the idea that different forms of intelligence encompass more than purely cognitive abilities. His theory of Multiple Intelligences (MI) originally included seven modalities of intelligence: linguistic intelligence, logical-mathematical intelligence, spatial intelligence, bodily-kinesthetic intelligence, musical intelligence, interpersonal intelligence, and intrapersonal intelligence.[12] In addition to including traditional forms of intelligence, such as logical-mathematical intelligence, Gardner's model notably introduces a form of physical intelligence, defines musical ability as a form of intelligence, and includes two forms of social intelligence, interpersonal intelligence (which he dubbed "people smart") and intrapersonal intelligence ("self smart"). Interpersonal intelligence is the capacity to understand the intentions, motivations, and desires of other people. Intrapersonal intelligence includes the ability to understand one's innermost feelings, as Gardner elaborates, "The core capacity at work here is access to one's own feeling life— one's range of affects or emotions: the capacity to label them to enmesh them in symbolic codes, to draw upon them as a means of understanding and guiding one's behavior."[13(p239)]

What, then, is "emotional intelligence"? EI is now commonly understood as the ability to understand, regulate, and use emotions positively, both one's own and those of others. The concept of EI has its roots in social intelligence, which was first introduced in 1920 by Edward Lee Thorndike, an American psychologist at Columbia University. He described social intelligence as "the ability to understand men and women, boys and girls—to act wisely in human relations."[14(p229)] Like Gardner's interpersonal and intrapersonal intelligences, the original concept of EI, largely attributed to American psychologists Peter Salovey and John Mayer, included an awareness of the self and others. In addition, Gardner's constructs of intrapersonal and interpersonal intelligence include the ability to recognize and understand feelings. However, EI involves much more than simply being able to accurately assess one's own feelings and the feelings of others; it includes the ability to solve problems and regulate behavior by understanding and using the emotional states of the self and others.[15]

There are four major models of EI: the Ability EI Model (Salovey and Mayer), the Trait EI Model (Petrides), the EI Model (Goleman), and the Emotional-Social Intelligence Model (Bar-On). Each model has different constructs and different bases, and each one contributes to the overall concept of EI. The following section summarizes the major constructs of each model, how each assesses EI, and potential applications.

THE ABILITY EI MODEL

Description

In 1990, Yale University psychology professor Peter Salovey and postdoctoral student John Mayer first identified EI as a subset or form of social intelligence. They defined it as "the ability to perceive emotions, to access and generate emotions so as to assist thought, to understand emotions and emotional knowledge, and to reflectively regulate emotions so as to promote emotional and intellectual growth."[15(p189)] Importantly, they defined emotions not as disruptions or disturbances of mental activity that needed to be controlled, which was the then-current thinking in the field of psychology, but instead as organized, adaptive responses with the potential to transform interactions with others into opportunities for growth. Their seminal work also included the first conceptual model of EI, which consisted of three "branches": appraisal and expression of emotion, regulation of emotion, and utilization of emotion. The latter construct was comprised of flexible planning, creative thinking, redirected attention, and motivation.[15]

Salovey and Mayer were the first to attempt to develop valid measures of EI, which subsequently led to the introduction in 1997 of their expanded *Four Branches of Emotional Intelligence* Model. This model, which both builds on and amplifies their original conceptual model, was further refined in 2002 with David Caruso. Their revised model is a process-oriented model that emphasizes the stages of development in EI, the potential for growth, and the contributions that emotions make to intellectual growth. The branches, which are arranged from more basic abilities (or psychological processes) to more advanced ones, include perceiving emotion, reasoning with emotion, understanding emotions, and, finally, managing emotions. Each branch has four subgroups and stages of EI skill.

1. The Perception, Appraisal, and Expression of Emotion
   a. Ability to identify emotion in one's physical states, feelings, and thoughts
   b. Ability to identify emotion in other people, designs, artwork, etc., through language, sound appearance, and behavior
   c. Ability to express emotions accurately, and to express needs related to those feelings
   d. Ability to discriminate between accurate and inaccurate, or honest vs. dishonest expressions of feeling
2. Emotional Facilitation of Thinking
   a. Emotions prioritize thinking by directing attention to important information.
   b. Emotions are sufficiently vivid and available that they can be generated as aids to judgment and memory concerning feelings.
   c. Emotional mood swings change the individual's perspective from optimistic to pessimistic, encouraging considerations of multiple points of view.
   d. Emotional states differentially encourage specific problem-solving approaches, such as when happiness facilitates inductive reasoning and creativity.
3. Understanding and Analyzing Emotions; Employing Emotional Knowledge
   a. Ability to label emotions and recognize relations among the words and the emotions themselves, such as the relation between liking and loving
   b. Ability to interpret the meanings that emotions convey regarding relationships, such as that sadness often accompanies a loss
   c. Ability to understand complex feelings: simultaneous feelings of love and hate or blends such as awe as a combination of fear and surprise
   d. Ability to recognize likely transitions among emotions, such as the transition from anger to satisfaction or anger to shame
4. Reflective Regulation of Emotions to Promote Emotional and Intellectual Growth
   a. Ability to stay open to feelings, including those that are pleasant and those that are unpleasant
   b. Ability to reflectively engage or detach from an emotion depending upon its judged informativeness or utility
   c. Ability to reflectively monitor emotions in relation to oneself and others, such as recognizing how clear, typical, influential, or reasonable they are
   d. Ability to manage emotion in oneself and others by moderating negative emotions and enhancing pleasant ones, without repressing or exaggerating information they may convey

---

THE FOUR BRANCHES, ILLUSTRATED

Mayra and Jorge are about to meet with a legislator to convince them to support a bill that would help provide funding for their agency. There is a lot riding on the meeting; this legislator is the "swing vote," and passage of the bill means that the agency's financial future is secure for the next 5 years.

Branch 1 (The Perception, Appraisal, and Expression of Emotion): Mayra is really excited about the meeting; she knows that she and Jorge have a solid pitch, backed by hours of hard work, good research, and sound logic. She notices that Jorge is unusually quiet, but Mayra expresses her enthusiasm for the meeting and optimism about the outcome.

Branch 2 (Emotional Facilitation of Thinking): Mayra starts to plan out the conversation with the legislator in her head, generating the various questions and objections they might get, and thinking through how she and Jorge can respond. Jorge's silence makes her realize that he is nervous about the meeting, and she begins to think about what might go wrong.

Branch 3 (Understanding and Analyzing Emotions; Employing Emotional Knowledge): Mayra tells Jorge that she is excited and optimistic about the meeting; after all, they worked hard to button down their facts and understand the legislator's position. Jorge remains pensive, and Mayra starts to worry that he might forget some of the important points she is counting on him to make or be too nervous to speak up when he is supposed to. Mayra realizes that she is becoming less optimistic about the meeting.

Branch 4 (Reflective Regulation of Emotions to Promote Emotional and Intellectual Growth): Mayra realizes that her optimism is actually making Jorge more nervous, so she tones it down a bit. She asks him how he is feeling about the meeting; when he expresses his concerns, she listens closely and turns her attention to addressing the issues he raises.

Source: Adapted from Ackley D. Emotional intelligence: a practical review of models, measures, and applications. *Consul Psychol J Pract Res.* 2016;68(4):269–286. doi:10.1037/cpb0000070

Mayer, Salovey, and Caruso believe that EI is an inborn form of intelligence, which means that it is a cognitive ability which can be measured. Measures of EI, or EQ (Emotional Quotient), they argue, predict one's ability to learn emotional skills just as Intelligence Quotient (IQ) predicts one's ability to learn cognitive skills. In their view, while emotional skills can be improved, the extent of that growth is limited by an individual's EQ. Hence, their model is commonly referred to as the Ability Model.

Measurement Tool

Salovey and Mayer's original EI assessment, the Multifactor Emotional Intelligence Scale (MEIS), was developed in 1999. In 2002, Salovey and Mayer developed a revised scale, the Mayer–Salovey–Caruso Emotional Intelligence Test (MSCEIT), which is an ability-based test designed to measure the four branches of their EI model. Each branch is measured with two objective, ability-based tasks using different response formats, including 5-point rating scales and multiple-choice responses. Like other intelligence tests, such as the IQ test, answers are considered correct or incorrect. The MSCEIT consists of a total of 141 items and typically takes 30–45 minutes to complete.[16]

Of the ability EI tests, the MSCEIT is the most researched and supported; it has been cited in more than 1,500 academic studies.[17]

Application

The MSCEIT is designed to measure inborn skill (EQ), in accordance with the Mayer–Salovey model. That inborn skill is a predictor of one's capacity for improving their EI skills, so the MSCEIT is most useful for determining how well someone can learn. It could, for example, reveal whether an individual could benefit from training or coaching. A high EQ would suggest that is the case; a low EQ may indicate there is little to no benefit to be gained.[18]

In addition, since the MSCEIT is an ability-based measure, it does not perform as well in predicting behavior as trait-based measures, but does have some validity in predicting several work-related measures, such as job satisfaction and job performance.[17]

THE TRAIT EMOTIONAL INTELLIGENCE MODEL

Description

In 2001, claiming that EI is not a form of intelligence but a set of personality traits, Konstantinos V. Petrides, a psychologist at the University College of London, developed the Trait Emotional Intelligence Model. EI, according to Petrides, cannot be assessed or graded as an intellectual capability. Instead, the Trait Model evaluates emotional self-perception, or how an individual perceives their emotional abilities (referred to as emotional self-efficacy). According to this model, once a person is able to recognize and utilize their own emotions and personality strengths, they will then be able to understand and regulate the emotions of others.[19]

Measurement Tool

The Trait EI Model uses a personality-based, self-reporting measurement tool (the Trait Emotional Intelligence Questionnaire, or TEIQue). For adults, there are 153 items and 15 subscales organized under four factors: well-being, self-control, emotionality, and sociability. The subscales include adaptability, assertiveness, emotion expression, emotion management of others, emotion perception (of self and others), emotion regulation, impulsiveness, relationships, self-esteem, self-motivation, social awareness, stress management, trait empathy, trait happiness, and trait optimism.[20] Descriptions of each of the facets, expressed as the self-perceptions of those who score themselves highly on the dimension in question, are provided in Table 5.1.

Application

Since the TEIQue is a trait-based assessment, it measures an individual's typical behavior, rather than providing an assessment of capability (as ability-based measures do). That means that it is more suitable for assessing the specific training and coaching needs for an individual than it is for personnel selection—in other words, it does a better job answering what an individual needs vs. what emotional skill capabilities or potential an individual has. It is widely used, is considered highly reliable and valid, and has been cited in more than 2,000 academic studies; however, the TEIQue is not available for free for commercial or personal use.

THE GOLEMAN EMOTIONAL INTELLIGENCE MODEL

Description

The concept of EI first gained popularity outside of academic circles with the 1995 publication of Daniel Goleman's book *Emotional Intelligence: Why It Can Matter More Than IQ*. Goleman, a writer and scientific journalist, suggested that EI is indispensable to leadership performance—even more so than intelligence and technical skills—because it enables leaders to maximize not only their own performance, but that of their followers.[6] Goleman's work has been simultaneously criticized as lacking scientific rigor and praised for making the concept of EI accessible outside of academic circles.

Goleman defines EI as "the capacity for recognizing our own feelings and those of others, for motivating ourselves, and for managing emotions effectively in ourselves and others. An emotional competence is learned capacity based on EI that contributes to effective

TABLE 5.1: The Sampling Domain of Trait EI in Adults

FACETS	HIGH SCORERS VIEW THEMSELVES AS...
Adaptability	...flexible and willing to adapt to new conditions.
Assertiveness	...forthright, frank, and willing to stand up for their rights.
Emotion expression	...capable of communicating their feelings to others.
Emotion management (others)	...capable of influencing other people's feelings.
Emotion perception (self and others)	...clear about their own and other people's feelings.
Emotion regulation	...capable of controlling their emotions.
Impulsiveness (low)	...reflective and less likely to give into their urges.
Relationships	...capable of maintaining fulfilling personal relationships.
Self-esteem	...successful and self-confident.
Self-motivation	...driven and unlikely to give up in the face of adversity.
Social awareness	...accomplished networkers with superior social skills.
Stress management	...capable of withstanding pressure and regulating stress.
Trait empathy	...capable of taking someone else's perspective.
Trait happiness	...cheerful and satisfied with their lives.
Trait optimism	...confident and likely to "look on the bright side" of life.

Source: Reproduced with permission from Chamorro-Premuzic T, von Stumm S, Furnham A. *The Wiley-Blackwell Handbook of Individual Differences*. Blackwell Publishing Ltd.; 2011.

performance at work."[21(p2)] He sees EI as a set of noncognitive skills, rather than personality traits, which can be further developed through experience and training. His model is composed of five clusters: self-awareness, self-regulation, motivation, empathy, and social skills.[6] Each of these clusters is briefly described in the text that follows, along with Goleman's characterizations of how leaders who display each cluster act.

Self-awareness means being able to accurately recognize and understand one's emotions, as well as how one's emotions, emotional states (or moods), and actions affect others. Critically, self-awareness includes the knowledge that feelings and actions are related. This awareness is developed through self-monitoring, observing others' reactions, being open to different ideas and experiences, and a keen interest in learning from social interactions. Self-awareness also includes a sense of one's own personal strengths and limitations. Self-aware leaders, according to Goleman, are self-confident, are capable of realistic self-assessment, have a self-deprecating sense of humor, and actively seek out constructive criticism.[22]

Self-regulation involves the appropriate expression of emotion. Specifically, it refers to the ability to control or redirect emotions and impulses that are disruptive. In addition to self-awareness, self-regulation also includes taking ownership of one's actions and the effect they have on others. According to Goleman, leaders who are proficient at self-regulation are trustworthy, have integrity, and are comfortable with ambiguity and change.[22]

In the context of EI, motivation refers to the quality of being driven to achieve to meet personal goals and needs (intrinsic motivation), as opposed to being motivated by external rewards such as recognition, acclaim, or money (extrinsic motivation). Given their need for achievement, intrinsically motivated individuals are more likely to demonstrate initiative, have a bias for action, and be highly committed and goal oriented. According to Goleman, motivated leaders display a passion for the work itself and for new challenges, have unflagging energy to improve, and display optimism in the face of failure.[22]

Displaying empathy means recognizing and considering others' feelings and responding appropriately, especially when making decisions. According to Goleman, empathic leaders are experts in attracting and retaining talent, are good at developing others, and demonstrate sensitivity to cross-cultural differences.[22]

Social skills refer to the ability to interact well with others, to find common ground and to build rapport. According to Goleman, leaders who are socially skilled are effective in leading change, are persuasive, and are proficient at building and leading teams.[22]

In 2000, Goleman further refined his model to focus on four key categories (self-awareness, social awareness, self-management, and relationship management), with supporting subcategories, as represented in Box 5.1.

Goleman believes that there is both a genetic component and an experiential component to EI; in other words, EI is driven both by nature and nurture. It also increases with age and training. He asserts that EI is housed in the limbic system, which governs emotion, behavior, long-term memory formation, and olfaction (the sense of smell).[23] According to Goleman, since successful EI training must focus on changing behavior, it can only be accomplished through motivation, extended practice, and feedback, suggesting an individualized and more protracted approach to training. Goleman further asserts that since most EI training, like other forms of leadership training, targets the neocortex, which governs analytical and thinking ability, it is ineffective and can even result in negative impacts on performance.

Goleman's EI model is often referred to as a mixed model, as it is seen as a blend of the trait and the ability models.

Box 5.1: Goleman's Emotional Intelligence Domains and Competencies

Self-Awareness

- Emotional self-awareness

Self-Management

- Emotional self-control
- Adaptability
- Achievement orientation
- Positive outlook

Social Awareness

- Empathy
- Organizational awareness

Relationship Management

- Influence
- Coach and mentor
- Conflict management
- Teamwork
- Inspirational leadership

Source: Adapted from Goleman D. *Working With Emotional Intelligence.* Bantam Books; 1998.

Measurement Tool

The Emotional and Social Competency Inventory (ESCI), developed by Daniel Goleman, Richard Boyatzis, and the Hay Group in 2011, is a 360-degree survey designed to assess 68 items that comprise the 12 competency scales. The ESCI replaced the original Emotional Competency Inventory (ECI) developed in 1996 and the ECI-2 developed in 2007. According to the Korn Ferry Research Guide and Technical Manual, "the ESCI measures the demonstration of individuals' behaviors through their perceptions and those of their raters, making it distinct from measures of EI that assess ability, self-assessments of ability, or personality preference."[24(p1)]

Application

The ESCI is designed to measure emotional competencies that differentiate work performance; as such, the items are generally written to reflect workplace scenarios. Of the four assessments included in this chapter, this instrument has been studied the least, so its reliability and validity are as yet poorly understood. It is also costly to administer and to evaluate the results; however, given its workplace orientation, it is considered a good option for that type of application.

THE BAR-ON MODEL OF EMOTIONAL-SOCIAL INTELLIGENCE (ESI)

Description

Israeli psychologist Reuven Bar-On's (2006) Emotional-Social Intelligence (ESI) Model was influenced by Darwin's observations of the role that emotional expression played in survival and adaptation. The ESI Model, which also draws on the work of Thorndike and Gardner (among others), views emotional and social intelligence as the keys to well-being and effective human performance. Bar-On defines emotional-social intelligence as "an array of interrelated emotional and social competencies, skills and behaviors that determine how well we understand and express ourselves, understand others and relate with them, and cope with daily demands, challenges and pressures."[5] He views EI and cognitive intelligence (IQ) as different, separate concepts, and, like Goleman, he suggests that the former is more important than the latter in predicting an individual's success in life. He also believes that EI can be learned and improved.

The ESI Model consists of five interrelated competencies, skills, and behavior clusters that were identified from academic literature. These clusters are:

1. Self-Perception
2. Interpersonal
3. Decision-Making
4. Self-Expression
5. Stress Management

The clusters are further broken down into a total of 15 factors, which are used as the basis for assessment.

Measurement Tool

The ESI Model now employs the EQ-i 2.0, which was published in 2011.[25] The EQ-1 2.0 can be administered as a self-report instrument or a full 360 assessment. The assessment takes 15 to 20 minutes to complete and generates a total EQ score, five composite (cluster) scores, and 15 specific subscale scores, organized as follows:

Self-Perception

- Self-Regard
- Self-Actualization
- Emotional Self-Awareness

Interpersonal

- Interpersonal Relationships
- Empathy
- Social Responsibility

Decision-Making

- Problem-Solving
- Reality Testing
- Impulse Control

Self-Expression

- Emotional Expression
- Assertiveness
- Independence

Stress Management

- Flexibility
- Stress Tolerance
- Optimism[25]

The EQ-i 2.0 also includes a well-being measure, which is not included in the overall EQ score.

Application

Like the ESCI, the EQ-i 2.0 measures personality traits, social skills, and emotional competencies (as opposed to cognitive constructs). The addition of the 360 assessment component, which provides information on others' perceptions, increases its application to workplace performance prediction and improvement. It is most widely used in workplace applications as a baseline assessment to identify an individual's areas for EI coaching, training, and development.

Table 5.2 presents a summary and comparison of the four major EI models.

TABLE 5.2: Comparison of Four Major Models of Emotional Intelligence

TYPE	ABILITY	TRAIT	MIXED	MIXED
Creators	Salovey, Mayer, and Caruso	Petrides	Goleman	Bar-On
Major Constructs or Elements	Perceiving emotion Reasoning with emotion Understanding emotions Managing emotions	Well-being Self-control Emotionality Sociability	Self-awareness Self-regulation Motivation Empathy Social skills	Self-Perception Interpersonal Decision-Making Self-Expression Stress Management
Measurement Tools	MSCEIT	TIEQue	ESCI	EQ-i
Innate or Acquired	Acquired	Innate	Both	Both

CAN EMOTIONAL INTELLIGENCE BE DEVELOPED?

According to the developers of the ability and mixed EI models, the answer is yes, and a growing body of evidence indicates that EI can, in fact, be developed and improved. For example, one study found that empirically derived EI training (lectures, role-play, group discussions, partner work, readings, and journaling) resulted in significant increases in participants' emotion identification and emotion management abilities; these improvements were still present 6 months later.[26] Other studies have demonstrated that EI training can not only raise EI assessment scores, but can lead to improved emotion-guided decision-making and can help sustain critical aspects of mental health during crises (in this case, the COVID-19 pandemic).[27,28]

A review of ability EI training studies found that EI improvements can occur through two training pathways. The first involved increasing emotional knowledge and related competencies through teaching and practice, using reflections, role-plays, and practice with other workshop participants. The second approach used brain-training principles to improve basic cognitive processes, such as executive control or emotional inhibition.[29]

In organizational settings, Cherniss et al. suggest that successful EI training programs must distinguish between and incorporate both cognitive learning and emotional learning. According to the authors, cognitive learning is critical to help participants grasp the concept of how to improve emotional abilities, while emotional learning involves unlearning old habits and relearning more adaptive ones. Their four-part process for developing EI in organizations, outlined in their paper "Bringing Emotional Intelligence to the Workplace," forms the basis for Goleman's approach to organizational training. (Goleman was one of the authors.)[30]

Dana Ackley is an EI coach, a two-time Fellow of the American Psychological Association, and author of the book *The EQ Leader Program* (2006); he has also written several journal articles on the subject, including a practical review of the various EI models, assessments, and how to apply them. Based on the 22 principles of good practice for developing EQ, as outlined by Cherniss et al., he offers the following approach for developing successful workplace EQ programs:

- Conduct an initial workshop with all participants.
- Perform an EQ assessment, along with a detailed interview, for each participant.
- Provide feedback in the form of the computer-generated reports associated with the assessment tool and a report for each individual that integrates test results, interview data, and any other information provided to him.
- Hold an individual debrief meeting that includes development planning.
- Perform individual and/or group coaching that includes exercises for the development of those EQ skills identified by the assessment as the best targets for development.
- Hold periodic meetings to review progress and align ongoing goals.[31]

THE IMPORTANCE OF EMOTIONAL INTELLIGENCE IN LEADERSHIP

EI is positively associated with overall leadership effectiveness, even more so than IQ or personality. In addition, EI has been strongly linked to both the transformational leadership and authentic leadership styles, both of which are considered effective leadership styles.[32]

As the name implies, transformational leaders are generally viewed as highly effective at leading people and organizations through change (see Chapter 7, "Transformational Leadership"). They accomplish this by empowering and nurturing their followers, serving as positive role models, listening and being open to new and opposing viewpoints, creating a vision for the organization, and serving as social architects. Transformational leadership is based on developing and maintaining effective working relationships by building trust, fostering collaboration, and celebrating accomplishments.[33] Several studies have found that EI, particularly the ability to understand and manage emotions, is strongly related to transformational leadership behaviors.[34]

Authentic leaders are purposeful, value centered, relationship-oriented, self-disciplined, and compassionate (see Chapter 8, "Authentic Leadership"). They also exhibit a desire to serve others, are mission-driven, and are focused on results and the long term.[35] A large meta-analysis, including more than 11 studies and more than 3,500 respondents, determined that EI/EQ and authentic leadership are strongly and positively associated. This finding extended to both men and women and was present in both male-dominated and female-dominated fields, indicating the extent to which EI plays a role in authentic leadership.[36]

In the first study to evaluate the effects of EI, personality, and IQ on overall leadership effectiveness, David Rosete and Joseph Ciarrochi found that higher EI was associated with higher leadership effectiveness.[32] Using both objective performance measures and 360-degree assessments of leadership performance, they determined that EI (as measured by the MSCEIT) was a better determinant of leadership effectiveness than personality (as measured by the 16PF5[a]) or cognitive ability (as measured by the WASI[b]). Their work validated an earlier finding that EI explained an individual's career progression to a greater degree than either cognitive intelligence or personality traits.[37]

Arguably, the most widely known and cited analysis of the relationship between EI and leadership effectiveness is Daniel Goleman's. In order to determine which capabilities drove leadership performance and to what degree, he evaluated competency models from 188 firms, grouping capabilities into three categories (technical skills, cognitive abilities, and EI). By calculating the ratio of each of the capabilities as determinants of performance, he found that EI was twice as important as cognitive abilities and technical skill for roles at all levels of the organizations he studied. He also found that EI increases in importance with rank; specifically, the vast majority (90%) of performance differences between senior leaders was attributable to EI.[38]

EI is also a determinant in who will emerge as the leader in a group. Psychologists Stéphane Côté, Paulo N. Lopes, Peter Salovey, and Christopher T. H. Miners studied small, leaderless groups to examine the association between EI and leadership emergence.[39] Their study found that group members with the highest EI were most frequently the ones who naturally emerged as leaders of the group over time. Like earlier studies, EI was more strongly associated with leadership emergence than personality traits and cognitive intelligence. (In this case, EI was also found to play a bigger role than gender.) In particular, the EI component of emotional awareness and understanding was most strongly associated with leadership emergence.[39]

EI also affects team performance. Prati et al., in a review of EI literature related to teams, team processes, and team effectiveness, propose that EI can improve team effectiveness by aiding in team leader and member role identification and adherence, moderating the effect of individual personality traits on leader and team interactions, raising the levels of team cohesion, increasing levels of team trust and creativity, improving decision-making abilities, and maintaining motivation levels.[40]

THE ROLE OF EMOTIONAL INTELLIGENCE IN PUBLIC HEALTH AND HEALTHCARE LEADERSHIP

Emotionally intelligent leaders are more effective leaders. A summary of the research literature suggests that, among other things, they are better equipped to cope with uncertainty (adaptation), lead with empathy, make better decisions under pressure, lead people and organizations through change (transformational leadership), lead with authenticity, build trust, and maintain motivation levels. These are all invaluable leadership capabilities, particularly for public health and healthcare.

---

[a] The 16PF5 refers to the Sixteen Personality Factor Questionnaire (fifth edition), a personality trait assessment that measures 16 personality constructs as identified by Dr. Raymond Cattrell in the 1940s.

[b] WASI is the Wechsler Abbreviated Scale of Intelligence, which measures cognitive ability in clinical, educational, and workplace settings.

Public health settings can be stressful, emotional, and political. In the *Oxford Textbook of Public Health*, William H. Foege, a physician, epidemiologist, former director of the Centers for Disease Control and Prevention, and the architect of the strategy that led to the eradication of smallpox in the 1970s, identifies more than 20 challenges that public health leaders routinely face. These range from the persistent public health challenges of prevention, equity, prioritization, and resource inadequacy to the reality that public health leaders must often make decisions with incomplete information—decisions which, if made incorrectly, can result in harm to hundreds, thousands, or even millions. Other challenges on the list include the changing public perceptions of public health, disease importation, and privacy issues. Finally, in his discussion of the challenges of utilizing the political structure, Foege notes that "public health improvements ultimately depend on a political decision."[41(p671)] Public health leaders work in a fragmented, chronically underfunded system and in an increasingly politicized function.

Healthcare leaders in the United States must navigate through one of the most complex and fragmented delivery systems in the world. These challenges are compounded by the sweeping changes brought about by the Affordable Care Act (ACA), the resulting regulatory uncertainty as successive administrations adopt different positions on it, the proliferation of new payment models, increasing pressure to reduce costs, an aging and sicker population, changing consumer expectations, and healthcare workforce shortages. These challenges are wrapped around the very real consideration that the decisions that healthcare leaders make can and do impact human lives.

On top of this already challenging leadership landscape, public health and healthcare leaders have faced the unparalleled crisis of COVID-19. This global pandemic exacted a heavy toll worldwide—in human lives, job losses, financial hardship, illness, and levels of stress, fear, anxiety, and depression. Public health and healthcare leaders and workers were at the heart of the crisis, caring for patients, responding to rapidly changing public health and medical care paradigms, dealing with critical equipment and supply shortages, developing strategies to reduce the spread of the infection, educating the public, and navigating a precarious social and political landscape. Healthcare workers experienced emotional and physical exhaustion and burnout from extreme workloads, high patient death rates, fear of exposure to the virus, and added childcare responsibilities due to school closures. Public health officials found themselves caught in the crossfire between politics, public health, and economic recovery. Many faced harassment and/or death threats, felt undermined by the elected officials and residents of the communities they serve, and were frustrated and exhausted by the ongoing battle between mis- and dis-information and science. As a result, between April 1 and December 15, 2020, 181 state and public health leaders in 38 states had resigned, retired, or been fired, the largest exodus of public health leaders in history.[42]

In addition, emotionally intelligent leadership will be key in the dismantling of systemic racism in public health and healthcare that has resulted in grave health inequities. Action must be taken at the micro (individual), meso (group or institutional), and macro (the public health and healthcare systems) levels; this will require authentic, transformational, empathic, and adaptive leaders and followers. At the individual level, emotionally intelligent leaders can more effectively identify when emotional information is skewed by implicit bias; employing self-awareness and self-regulation can result in more equitable and empathic leadership actions and decisions. At the group or institutional level, emotionally intelligent leaders can leverage their authentic and transformational leadership traits to lead their organizations through the difficult tasks of examining, challenging, and discarding systems, processes, and beliefs that institutionalize discrimination. Finally, if the people and the institutions that comprise the public health and healthcare systems are centering equity, then so too will those systems.

DEVELOPING EMOTIONAL INTELLIGENCE

There are a number of EI developmental resources, ranging from books, online courses, coaching services, and guided exercises. Several of these resources are included at the end of the chapter.

SUMMARY

EI is considered a form of social intelligence; it is now commonly understood as the ability to understand, regulate, and use emotions positively, both one's own and those of others. There are four major models of EI: the Ability Model (Salovey and Mayer); the Trait Model (Petrides): the Goleman Model; and the Bar-On Model. Each has different constructs and methods of assessment, but each contributes valuable insights to the field.

EI has been linked to leadership effectiveness and has been characterized as being more critical than technical skill or intellectual capabilities in determining a leader's performance. There is an emerging body of evidence highlighting EI's role in decision-making, trust-building, team performance, career progression, and overall workplace performance. It is also strongly associated with the transformational and authentic leadership styles. Given the complex, dynamic, stressful, and often emotional contexts in which public health and healthcare leaders must operate, EI can and should be considered a critical leadership competency.

DISCUSSION QUESTIONS

1. What are the key differences between the ability and trait models of EI? Why are these differences important from a leadership perspective?
2. How is EI related to transformational and authentic leadership?
3. Identify two examples of great leaders who you have worked with or for. How did EI contribute to their effectiveness? (Please frame your answer using one of the models outlined in the chapter.)
4. Identify two examples of ineffective leaders who you have worked with or for. How did the lack of EI contribute to their ineffectiveness? (Please frame your answer using one of the models outlined in the chapter.)
5. What are some of the ways in which EI contributes to leader effectiveness?

CASE STUDY: B-KIND

MS is the executive director for a United States-based, national nonprofit organization, B-Kind, that provides anti-bullying programming to youth. The past 2 years had been difficult for the organization and highly stressful for MS. The pandemic had forced the cessation of all in-person activities; since B-Kind collected a fee for each of those activities, all sources of earned revenue had dried up for 18 months. Thanks to deep reserves, conservative spending, and government assistance in the form of the Paycheck Protection Program (PPP) and Economic Injury Disaster Loans (EIDL), the organization had weathered the financial storm.

As programming began to resume, however, new issues were emerging. B-Kind has chapters in 48 states and the District of Columbia; each is run by a volunteer director and staff, and events are supported by armies of community volunteers. B-Kind's national headquarters provides programming support, training and certification of volunteer counselors, financial assistance through its development operation, risk management, and operating standards for each of its chapters. The geographic diversity of B-Kind's chapters had always meant that the headquarters was constantly walking a fine line between maintaining an inclusive environment for the youth it served and respecting the local socio-political culture, particularly when it came to policy development. However, while policy issues, such as the recognition and inclusion of transgender youth, had created some intraorganizational tensions in the past, most had been resolved over time.

Even during the COVID-19 pandemic, headquarters delegated decision-making regarding how and when to both modify and resume in-person programming to each chapter, advising them to adhere to local public health guidelines, the organizations' safety and risk management requirements, and the judgment of its directors. That had resulted not only in each chapter being in charge of its own destiny, but had actually generated new programming ideas, many of which had persisted even after the pandemic began to wane.

In the late summer and early fall of 2021, the divides over matters like mask mandates and vaccination requirements began to percolate in B-Kind, mirroring what was happening across the country. These divides existed both within the chapters and between the chapters and headquarters; they finally came to a head in a videoconference in September. These calls were held on a regular basis between headquarters staff and chapter directors to exchange information, provide updates on programming or projects at headquarters, troubleshoot problems, and build community. Given the size of the staff and the number of chapter directors, anywhere from 35 to 50+ people could be in the videoconference.

Early in the call, MS noted that any headquarters staff members that were beginning to travel on behalf of B-Kind were subject to a vaccine requirement, explaining that this was being done to reduce the risk to the employee and their coworkers, families, and communities. The organization had previously not adopted a stance on this topic, he explained, since all employees were working remotely, and all travel had been banned. With the resumption of in-person events and employee travel, he felt compelled to make a decision on the matter, noting that the policy included certain exceptions, was job-related, and was a matter of business necessity. For any chapters interested in adopting a similar policy, he added, the staff at headquarters were ready and able to support them.

As MS finished and began to turn the floor over to his programming director, he was interrupted by one of the chapter directors, JJ. JJ was a long-time staff member for one of the organization's oldest chapters and had recently assumed the director role after the founder had stepped down. MS had had a fairly contentious relationship with JJ's predecessor, and so far, from MS's perspective, JJ was cut from the same cloth. "Does this mean B-Kind will make the chapters get vaccinated, too? I gotta tell you, if that's what you all are up to, I'm outta here—and I'm taking my chapter with me. You're infringing on my personal freedoms here."

MS felt his blood pressure rise. He'd just about had it with this chapter; they were always stirring up trouble. And he certainly did not agree with their politics—they were right-wingers, in his opinion. He bit his tongue, took a deep breath, and responded as calmly as he could: "No, JJ, we will not be requiring chapters to vaccinate their staff or their volunteers. We are leaving that decision up to each of you to make in the best interests of your organization and your staff. We are ready and willing to help you, however, should you decide to adopt that policy."

The meeting moved on, and MS relaxed. About 15 minutes later, he noticed that there was a long chat message from JJ to all meeting attendees. In it, JJ accused the organization of discrimination based on vaccination status, which he claimed was a private medical issue. He could not, he went on, support such a policy, and he was concerned about the long-term viability of B-Kind if policies like this became the norm.

At first, MS kept his silence and tried to pay attention to the material that LM, one of the staff members, was presenting. He kept glancing back at the message and could feel his fury rising a little more every time he re-read it. He thought to himself, "He just doesn't get it, does he? And why is he trying to stir things up? He is always doing stuff like this!" Finally, as LM finished her presentation, he broke in.

"I want to be really clear that it is YOU, JJ, that is infringing on MY freedoms. This is a public health and safety issue, and you are preventing me from being able to feel safe in my job—." JJ cut him off, and the conversation quickly turned into a shouting match which lasted for more than 5 minutes. Finally, another chapter director asked the two of them to take it offline. At that point, the call ended.

CASE STUDY QUESTIONS

1. Using Goleman's model of EI, describe where MS displayed EI and where he did not.
2. What do you think MS should do now? How would you advise him to handle future, similar situations? (Please frame your answers using Goleman's model.)
3. Have you ever had an interaction with a coworker or group that you later regretted? What would you do differently now, based on what you have learned about EI?

CASE STUDY: HANDLING COVID-19 WITH EMOTIONAL INTELLIGENCE

Jacinda Ardern, the prime minister of New Zealand, has been praised for her leadership during the COVID-19 crisis. On March 23, 2020, she announced a minimum 4-week national lockdown to fight the COVID-19 outbreak, the first of any country. Here is a partial transcript of her speech; you may also wish to view her speech online.

Good afternoon.

The cabinet met this morning to discuss our next actions in the fight against COVID-19.

Like the rest of the world, we are facing the potential for devastating impacts from this virus. But, through decisive action, and through working together, we do have a small window to get ahead of it.

On Saturday I announced a COVID-19 alert level system and placed New Zealand at Alert Level 2.

I also said we should all be prepared to move quickly. Now is the time to put our plans into action.

We are fortunate to still be some way behind the majority of overseas countries in terms of cases, but the trajectory is clear. Act now or risk the virus taking hold as it has elsewhere.

We currently have 102 cases. But so did Italy once. Now the virus has overwhelmed their health system and hundreds of people are dying every day.

The situation here is moving at pace, and so must we.

We have always said we would act early. Today 36 new cases were announced. While the majority of these cases continue to be linked to overseas travel in some way, I can also confirm, as did the director general of health, that we have two cases where public health officials have been unable to find how they came in contact with COVID-19. On that basis, we now consider that there is transmission within our communities.

If community transmission takes off in New Zealand the number of cases will double every 5 days. If that happens unchecked, our health system will be inundated, and tens of thousands [of] New Zealanders will die.

...Right now we have a window of opportunity to break the chain of community transmission—to contain the virus—to stop it multiplying and to protect New Zealanders from the worst.

Our plan is simple. We can stop the spread by staying at home and reducing contact. Now is the time to act.

That's why [the] cabinet met today and agreed that effective immediately, we will move to Alert Level 3 nationwide.

After 48 hours, the time required to ensure essential services are in place, we will move to Level 4.

These decisions will place the most significant restriction on New Zealanders' movements in modern history. This is not a decision taken lightly. But this is our best chance to slow the virus and to save lives.

Let me set out what these changes will mean for everyone...

...Now I want to share with you what will happen while we are all in Alert Level 4 to get ahead of COVID-19.

We will continue to vigorously contact trace every single case. Testing will continue at pace to help us understand the current number of cases in New Zealand and where they are based. If we flush out the cases we already have and see transmission slow, we will potentially be able to move areas out of Level 4 over time.

But for the next while, things will look worse before they look better. In the short term the number of cases will likely rise because the virus is already in our community. But these new measures can slow the virus down and prevent our health system from being overwhelmed and ultimately save lives.

To be successful though, to stop community transmission which has a lag time, these measures will need to be in place for 4 weeks. Again, I want to reiterate, you will be able to make regular visits to essential services in that time.

If ... after those 4 weeks we have been successful, we I hope will be able to ease up on restrictions. If we haven't, we'll find ourselves living with them for longer. That's why sticking to the rules matters. If we don't—if you hang out with that friend at a park or see that family member for lunch, you risk spreading COVID -19 and extending everyone's time in Level 4...

New medical modelling considered by the cabinet today suggests that without the measures I have just announced up to tens of thousands of New Zealanders could die from COVID-19.

Everything you will all give up for the next few weeks, all of the lost contact with others, all of the isolation, and difficult time entertaining children—it will literally save lives. Thousands of lives.

The worst-case scenario is simply intolerable. It would represent the greatest loss of New Zealanders' lives in our country's history. I will not take that chance.

I would rather make this decision now, and save those lives, and be in lockdown for a shorter period, than delay, [and] see New Zealanders lose loved ones and their contact with each other for an even longer period. I hope you are all with me on that.

Together we have an opportunity to contain the spread and prevent the worst.

I cannot stress enough the need for every New Zealander to follow the advice I have laid out today.

The government will do all it can to protect you. Now I'm asking you to do everything you can to protect us all. None of us can do this alone.

Your actions will be critical to our collective ability to stop the spread of COVID-19.

Failure to play your part in the coming days will put the lives of others at risk. There will be no tolerance for that and we will not hesitate in using enforcement powers if needed.

We're in this together and must unite against COVID-19.

I am in no doubt that the measures I have announced today will cause unprecedented economic and social disruption. But they are necessary.

I have one final message. Be kind. I know people will want to act as enforcers. And I understand that, people are afraid and anxious. We will play that role for you. What we need from you, is support one another. Go home tonight and check in on your neighbours. Start a phone tree with your street. Plan how you'll keep in touch with one another. We will get through this together, but only if we stick together. Be strong and be kind.[43]

CASE STUDY QUESTIONS

1. Identify three examples where Prime Minister Ardern exhibited EI in her speech. You may use any model outlined in the chapter, but please refer specifically to the constructs and tie your example(s) to each.

2. Do you think her use of EI contributed positively to New Zealand's response to COVID-19? Why or why not? (You may wish to conduct additional research to support your answer.)

3. Choose another world leader who you think did not do an effective job in responding to the pandemic. Provide a short analysis, from an EI standpoint, of the deficiencies in that person's actions.

ADDITIONAL RESOURCES

LEADERSHIP MEASUREMENT TOOLS/EXERCISES

Emotional Intelligence 2.0

■ Travis Bradberry and Jean Greaves have developed a highly popular and accessible model and self-assessment of EI, *Emotional Intelligence 2.0*. The model, which is similar to Goleman's in its emphasis on the influence of personal and social competencies on leadership, also incorporates constructs such as organizational justice, character, and development. The book and the assessment are affordable and available online; the book and the authors' website, TalentSmartEQ, offer resources such as individual reports, suggestions for improvement strategies, and the ability to set goals and track progress.[44]

BOOKS

The Basics

- *Emotional Intelligence: Why It Can Matter More Than EQ*, by Daniel Goleman
- *Emotional Intelligence 2.0*, by Travis Bradberry and Jean Greaves
- *HBR Guide to Emotional Intelligence*

For Leaders

- *Working With Emotional Intelligence*, by Daniel Goleman
- *Primal Leadership: Unleashing the Power of Emotional Intelligence*, by Daniel Goleman, Richard Boyatzis, and Annie McKee
- *The Emotionally Intelligent Manager: How to Develop and Use the Four Key Emotional Skills of Leadership*, by David R. Caruso and Peter Salovey

VIDEOS

- *Daniel Goleman Introduces Emotional Intelligence* (www.youtube.com/watch?v=Y7m9eNoB3NU)
- *The Power of Emotional Intelligence*—a TEDx talk by Travis Bradberry (www.youtube.com/watch?v=auXNnTmhHsk)
- *Emotional Intelligence: From Theory to Everyday Practice*—by Mark Brackett at the Yale Center for Emotional Intelligence (www.youtube.com/watch?v=e8JMWtwdLQ4)
- *Emotional Intelligence: How Good Leaders Become Great*—from the UC Davis Executive Leadership Program (www.youtube.com/watch?v=HA15YZlF_kM)

WEBSITES

- American College of Healthcare Executives (www.ache.org)—The ACHE offers several EI webinars and workshops, including an online EQ assessment (EQ-I).
- TalentSmartEQ (www.talentsmarteq.com)—This is the companion website to Travis Bradberry and Jean Greaves' best-selling *Emotional Intelligence 2.0* (see Leadership Measurement Tools/Exercises below). The site offers self-assessment, multi-rater and 360-degree EI appraisals, in-person and virtual training programs, and coaching services.
- Consortium for Research on Emotional Intelligence in Organizations (www.eiconsortium.org)—The EI Consortium's mission is to "advance research and practice of emotional and social intelligence in organizations through the generation and exchange of knowledge." The site offers research reports, describes the various EI assessment tools, highlights model EI programs, contains interviews and podcasts from EI experts and scholars, and includes a calendar of events.

REFERENCES

1. MacCann C, Jiang Y, Brown LER, Double KS, Bucich M, Minbashian A. Emotional intelligence predicts academic performance: a meta-analysis. *Psychol Bull*. 2020;146(2):150–186. doi:10.1037/bul0000219

2. Fernandez-Berrocal P, Alcaide R, Extremera N, Pizarro D. The role of emotional intelligence in anxiety and depression among adolescents. *Individ Differ Res*. 2006;4(1):16–27.

3. Lopes PN, Grewal D, Kadis J, et al. Evidence that emotional intelligence is related to job performance and affect and attitudes at work. *Psicothema*. 2006;18(suppl):132–138. https://www.psicothema.com/pi?pii=3288

4. Karakurt G, Silver KE. Emotional abuse in intimate relationships: the role of gender and age. *Violence Vict*. 2013;28(5):804–821. doi:10.1891/0886-6708.vv-d-12-00041

5. Bar-On R. A broad definition of emotional intelligence according to the Bar-On Model. https://www.reuvenbaron.com/e-emotional-intelligence-glossary/

6. Goleman D. *Emotional Intelligence: Why It Can Matter More Than IQ*. Bantam Books; 1995.

7. Sternberg RJ. Images of mindfulness. *J Soc Issues*. 2000;56(1):11–26. doi:10.1111/0022-4537.00149

8. Spearman C. General intelligence, objectively determined and measured. *Am J Psychol*. 1904;15:92. doi:10.2307/1412107

9. Thurstone L. The vectors of mind. *Psychol Rev*. 1934;41:32. doi:10.1037/h0075959

10. Guilford JP. *The Nature of Human Intelligence*. McGraw-Hill; 1967.

11. Sternberg RJ. *Beyond IQ: A Triarchic Theory of Human Intelligence*. CUP Archive; 1985.

12. Gardner H, Hatch T. Educational implications of the theory of multiple intelligences. *Educ Res*. 1989;18:6. doi:10.3102/0013189X018008004

13. Gardner H. Frames of Mind: The Theory of Multiple Intelligences. Basic Books, Inc.; 1983.

14. Thorndike EL. Intelligence and its uses. *Harper's Magazine*. 1920:140, 227–235.

15. Salovey P, Mayer JD. Emotional intelligence. *Imagin Cogn Pers*. 1990;9(3):27. doi:10.2190/DUGG-P24E-52WK-6CDG

16. The Mayer–Salovey–Caruso Emotional Intelligence Test (MSCEIT). Consortium for Research on Emotional Intelligence in Organizations. http://eiconsortium.org/measures/msceit.html

17. O'Connor PJ, Hill A, Kaya M, Martin B. The measurement of emotional intelligence: a critical review of the literature and recommendations for researchers and practitioners. *Front Psychol*. 2019;10:1116. doi:10.3389/fpsyg.2019.01116

18. Brackett MA, Rivers SE, Salovey P. Emotional intelligence: implications for personal, social, academic, and workplace success. *Soc Personal Psychol Compass*. 2011;5(1):88–103. doi:10.1111/j.1751-9004.2010.00334.x

19. Petrides KV, Furnham A. Trait emotional intelligence: psychometric investigation with reference to established trait taxonomies. *Eur J Pers*. 2001;15(6):425–448. doi:10.1002/per.416

20. Petrides KV. Ability and trait emotional intelligence. In: Chamorro-Premuzic T, von Stumm S, Furnham A, eds. *The Wiley-Blackwell Handbook of Individual Differences*. Wiley Blackwell; 2011:656–678.

21. Wolff S. *Emotional Competence Inventory: Technical Manual*. Hay Group; 2005. https://www.eiconsortium.org/pdf/ECI_2_0_Technical_Manual_v2.pdf

22. Goleman D. *Working With Emotional Intelligence*. Bantam Books; 1998.

23. Plus M. Limbic system. https://medlineplus.gov/ency/imagepages/19244.htm

24. *The Emotional and Social Competency Inventory Research Guide and Technical Manual*. Vol. 17.1a. 2017. https://www.readkong.com/page/emotional-and-social-competency-inventory-research-guide-1210527

25. The Emotional Quotient Inventory (EQ-i 2.0). Consortium for Research on Emotional Intelligence in Organizations. http://www.eiconsortium.org/measures/eqi.html

26. Nelis D, Quoidbach J, Mikolajczak M, Hansenne M. Increasing emotional intelligence: (how) is it possible? *Pers Individ Differ*. 2009;47(1):36–41. doi:10.1016/j.paid.2009.01.046

27. Alkozei A, Smith R, Demers LA, Weber M, Berryhill SM, Killgore WDS. Increases in emotional intelligence after an online training program are associated with better decision-making on the Iowa gambling task. *Psychol Rep*. 2019;122(3):853–879. doi:10.1177/0033294118771705

28. Persich MA-O, Smith RA-OX, Cloonan SA-O, et al. Emotional intelligence training as a protective factor for mental health during the COVID-19 pandemic. *Depress Anxiety*. 2021;38(10):1018–1025. doi:10.1002/da.23202

29. Lim MD, Lau MC. Can we "Brain-Train" emotional intelligence? A narrative review on the features and approaches used in ability EI training studies. *Front Psychol*. 2021;12:569749. doi:10.3389/fpsyg.2021.569749

30. Cherniss C, Goleman D, Emmerling R, Cowan K, Adler M. Bringing emotional intelligence to the workplace: a technical report issued by the Consortium for Research on Emotional Intelligence in Organizations. 1998. https://www.eiconsortium.org/reports/technical_report.html

31. Ackley D. Emotional intelligence: a practical review of models, measures, and applications. *Consult Psychol J Pract Res*. 2016;68(4):17. doi:10.1037/cpb0000070

32. Rosete D, Ciarrochi J. Emotional intelligence and its relationship to workplace performance outcomes of leadership effectiveness. *Leadersh Organ Dev J*. 26(5):388–399. doi:10.1108/01437730510607871

33. Northouse P. *Leadership: Theory and Practice*. SAGE Publications; 2021.

34. Kumar S. Establishing linkages between emotional intelligence and transformational leadership. *Ind Psychiatry J*. 2014;23(1):1–3. doi:10.4103/0972-6748.144934

35. George B. *True North: Discover Your Authentic Leadership*. Jossey-Bass; 2007.

36. Miao C, Humphrey RH, Qian S. Emotional intelligence and authentic leadership: a meta-analysis. *Leadersh Organ Dev J*. 2018;39:679–690. doi:10.1108/LODJ-02-2018-0066

37. Dulewicz V, Higgs M. Can emotional intelligence be measured and developed? *Leadersh Organ Dev J*. 1999;20(5):242–253. doi:10.1108/01437739910287117

38. Goleman D. *What Makes a Leader?* Harvard Business Review; 2004.

39. Côté S, Lopes PN, Salovey P, Miners CTH. Emotional intelligence and leadership emergence in small groups. *Leadersh Q*. 2010;21(3):496–508. doi:10.1016/j.leaqua.2010.03.012

40. Melita Prati L, Douglas C, Ferris GR, Ammeter AP, Buckley MR. Emotional intelligence, leadership effectiveness, and team outcomes. *Int J Organ Anal*. 2003;11(1):21–40. doi:10.1108/eb028961

41. Detels R, Gulliford M, Karim QA, Tan CC. *Oxford Textbook of Global Public Health*. 6th ed. Oxford University Press; 2015.

42. Barry-Jester AM, Recht H, Smith MR. Pandemic backlash jeopardizes public health powers, leaders. https://khn.org/news/article/pandemic-backlash-jeopardizes-public-health-powers-leaders/

43. PM Jacinda Ardern's Full Lockdown Speech. https://www.newsroom.co.nz/2020/03/23/1096999/pm-jacinda-arderns-full-lockdown-speech

44. TalentSmartEQ. https://www.talentsmarteq.com

Chapter 6

The Situational Approach
to Leadership

Eduardo Sanchez and John Wiesman*

INTRODUCTION

The situational approach to leadership requires that an effective leader adapt their style to the demands of different situations and to meet the changing competencies, confidences, and needs of individual team members.

The situational leadership framework (sometimes referred to as a theory or model in the literature) centers on the interpersonal relationship between a leader and their "followers" to address a situation. Followers can be team or group members or subordinates. The framework depicts leadership as the interplay of interactions between a leader and follower or followers as they respond to and resolve a particular problem or challenge. This chapter explores the origins of the situational leadership framework, its evolution, and its application. The chapter includes published examples of situational leadership applications, including public health applications, and it concludes with case studies of personal leadership experiences and relates them to situational leadership.

As described in other chapters, leadership has been admired, described, defined, and studied for decades[1-7] if not centuries. The business sector, academic and applied, has long been interested in studying leadership as a process of influence and as a discipline in the workplace.[8] Leadership in public health, specifically, has also been the focus of numerous texts, peer-reviewed articles, and of popular media.[9-12]

Some have considered leadership as primarily a reflection of intrinsic characteristics of extraordinary individuals, so-called "born leaders." Others have suggested that leadership primarily derives from extrinsic factors. Leadership is arguably a mix of both intrinsic characteristics and extrinsic influences. Nevertheless, the study of leadership is driven, in part, by the desire to learn to be a better leader by learning from others but also to teach leaders and those interested in being leaders how to be better leaders. The study of leadership has included categorization of leadership styles—think autocratic (individual control by the leader over all decisions) versus democratic (involvement of team members in decision-making). Kellerman has written about bad leadership and has posited that bad leadership must also be carefully studied and understood.[5] The study of leadership has led to the development and evolution of different leadership theories, concepts, models, and frameworks. The historic evolution of the different conceptualizations and characterizations of leadership by periods of time has been described.[7,13] One of those frameworks, situational leadership, is covered in this chapter.

---

* John Wiesman contributed the Case Study on "Situational Leadership in the COVID-19 Response: Washington State," which appears at the end of this chapter.

By the end of this chapter, the reader will be able to:

■ Define and understand situational leadership as one of several leadership theories/frameworks/concepts/approaches/models.
■ Describe examples of situational leadership applications in public health.
■ Give several original personal/professional examples of situational leadership.
■ Discuss case studies applying situational leadership.

DEFINITIONS AND CONCEPTS

The situational leadership framework can be described as a leadership concept and approach in which leaders adapt their behavior—specifically, their leadership style—to both the demands of a particular challenge and the person or persons identified or assigned to address that challenge. The situational leadership framework is contingent on the interplay of a leader and the situation at hand as well as the interactions between a leader and follower or followers in three interrelated domains: task-oriented direction and leadership, relational-oriented direction and leadership, and the "readiness" or development level exhibited by followers or subordinates. See Figure 6.1 for a general representation of the situational leadership framework.

In the initial version of the situational leadership framework, the interaction between a leader and an individual follower can take one of four forms of interaction that are determined by the readiness of followers.[14] Readiness, as defined in situational leadership, describes the degree to which a follower is equipped to take on an assignment or role to address a situation and has two dimensions: ability and willingness. The least evolved stage of readiness (R1) is exhibited by a person in the early stages of ability and willingness: untested or low competence and low confidence. This is a person who can be part of a response to a situation with a leadership style that is more task-oriented and directive (i.e., "do this, do that, and then do that"). The most mature state of readiness (R4) is that level of readiness exhibited by a person with tested or demonstrated ability—that is, skill and competence—and

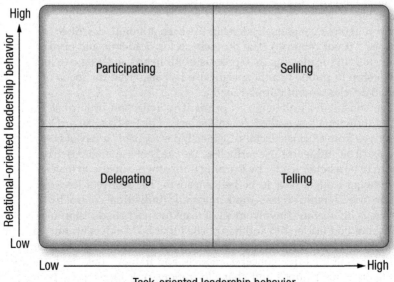

FIGURE 6.1: General Framework for Situational Leadership.

a high degree of "willingness," or confidence. This is a person who, apprised of a situation and the desired outcome or outcomes, requires very little task-direction or relationship-orientation. Between least evolved or low readiness and most evolved or high readiness are two intermediate stages (R2 and R3). Low readiness evolves to a low-intermediate stage (R2) in which the person is still at the early stages of ability and low competence, but willing and confident. The leader will still provide task-oriented or task-based direction and supportive communication to reinforce willingness, whereas in the next stage of readiness (R3), high-intermediate, which then evolves to high readiness (R4), the follower can be characterized as having the ability or skill to accomplish the task (without direction) but may lack confidence or not be willing. The R3 follower can be interacted with using a supportive relational-oriented leadership style ("You've got this"). The leadership style categories that correspond with levels of readiness R1, R2, R3, and R4 are telling, selling, participating, and delegating, respectively.

HISTORY AND EVOLUTION OF SITUATIONAL LEADERSHIP

The theory of situational leadership was first introduced in 1969 by Paul Hersey and Ken Blanchard in their book *Management of Organizational Behavior: Utilizing Human Resources*.[14] Hersey and Blanchard's work came from a business/management orientation with a primary focus on developing human resources, that is, people. The consideration of a relationship between leadership and situation has been explored by others, but Hersey and Blanchard's theory of situational leadership has stood the test of time as evidenced by the 10th edition of their book published more than 40 years after the introduction of the situational leadership theory.[15,16]

In 1997, almost three decades after situational leadership was introduced, Hersey observed that there is no single all-purpose leadership style but that successful leaders are those who can adapt to their unique situations.[17] In addition, he commented that 30 years after the introduction of situational leadership, he considered it as an applicable model rather than an academic theory. Theories are plausible explanatory propositions conceptualized to link causes to effects, whereas models are schematic representations constructed to improve one's understanding about the world and/or to predict outcomes.[18] Hersey shared his thought that the situational leadership "model" provides a construct that makes leadership as objective as the practice of medicine or law and that, through training, individuals can be better leaders in a variety of situations. He stated that leadership is about being effective as a leader.[17]

The situational leadership model is operationalized based on the situation; on the leader's recognition of the situation; on the stage of readiness of followers; on the interplay between the leader and a follower or followers from needing, primarily, concrete directives, tasks, to having the capacity, competence, and confidence to assume more, and even full, delegated responsibility and authority for actions taken; and on the evolution of the amount of concrete task-oriented direction a leader gives and the amount of "socio-emotional" support a leader provides a follower or followers as competence and confidence evolve, and presumably grow, over time. The leader matches their leadership behaviors (the behaviors used to influence or guide a follower) with the needs or with the skills and competence of the individual the leader is working with. Situational leadership is effective when the right mix of directive behaviors and supportive behaviors is used based on the "readiness" of the follower for the performance of required tasks or functions. Hersey has said that it is the amount of ability being used that counts, not how much there is.[17]

In the situational leadership model, the amount and manner of task-specific direction a leader gives an individual follower are characterized as task behaviors (specific, concrete direction); the amount and manner of socio-emotional support a leader provides are characterized as relationship behaviors and the readiness of followers, which informs the leader's behavior approach, evolves from needing and receiving specific direction to assuming responsibility with less concrete direction because of acquired competence and confidence.

Not only has the situational leadership model endured, but it has evolved. In a 25-year retrospective review of situational leadership, Blanchard, the other developer of the original situational leadership model, and two coauthors included an overview of the description of the situational leadership theory published in 1969 and modifications made to the theory in the early 1980s.[19] According to the authors, the situational leadership theory was informed by, and builds on, the leader and leadership analysis starting in the early 1960s that includes the contingency leadership model. The Contingency Theory of Leadership Effectiveness is described as an influence process contingent on three factors: (1) a leader's relations with followers (using the term from the situational leadership model); (2) the amount of structure in the task to be performed; and (3) the leader's power and authority.[15]

The Blanchard article also describes revisions made to the original situational leadership model by Blanchard and others (not including Hersey) to fashion the revised Situational Leadership II.[19] The four original leadership style categories—telling, selling, participating, and delegating—were renamed to directing, coaching, supporting, and delegating, respectively, corresponding to leadership behaviors that are highly directive and less interactive for the directing style ("do this"); highly directive and highly interactive for the coaching style ("let's talk and do mostly what I think"); less directive and highly supportive for the supporting style ("let's talk and do mostly what you think"); and less directive and less interactive ("you got this") for the delegating style.

The term "development" is adopted in the Situational Leadership II model to replace "readiness" and maturity regarding the mastery of skills required for the task or tasks to address a situation.[19] The revised model characterizes the development of the mastery of skills using the terms "competence" and "commitment" to replace the original terms, "ability" and "willingness," respectively. The four development levels, which correspond to R1, R2, R3, and R4, are described as: level 1(low competence, high commitment); level 2 (some competence, less commitment); level 3 (high competence, variable commitment); and level 4 (high competence, high commitment). It might be easier to think of the four levels of development or readiness in terms of competence and confidence with a progression from level 1 (low competence and little to low confidence); level 2 (low competence, high confidence); level 3 (high competence, little to low confidence); and level 4 (high competence and much confidence).

The authors reported that, between 1983 and 1993, over 50 dissertations, masters' theses, and research papers related to Situational Leadership II and leadership analysis had been published. They concluded that use of the model had benefits for understanding, describing, and guiding leadership but that additional research and investigation would help refine the model and its usability.[19]

Please note that for the remainder of the chapter, the original situational leadership model is the primary point of reference.

THE STUDY OF SITUATIONAL LEADERSHIP

One important area of situational leadership analysis describes the utility of the situational leadership framework for the study and teaching of leadership in general. The investigators of a 2018 study, in which 620 military managers with leadership roles but a wide range of experience as managers attending an advanced military leadership program, completed a leadership style self-assessment, and found that the selling leadership style and the participating leadership style merged as dominant.[20] These styles correspond to the moderate levels of development in the situational leadership model (R2 and R3). The authors concluded that situational leadership self-assessment might be an important tool to help managers identify their primary leadership style but also to be aware of deficits and develop the skills and ability to lead followers who fall into the lowest and highest levels of development (R1 and R4, respectively).[20]

In a subsequent study, 129 experienced managers attending a project management educational program completed leadership self-assessments and participated in a project simulation.[21] The managers found the self-assessment helped them understand how their leadership style fit project management. Another observation of the study was that a leader's primary leadership style evolved from task-oriented at the beginning of the simulated project to primarily a relationship-oriented style as the project progressed. The authors conclude that project management teaching should include attention to leadership approaches and leadership behavioral styles but also attention to self-assessment to further develop leadership skills and practice.[21]

A different set of investigators compared and contrasted assessment of followers' ability and commitment with followers' self-assessment. They concluded that the situational leadership model works best (optimal leadership style and a good outcome) when there is congruence between leader and follower assessment of ability and commitment.[22] Leadership self-assessment, leadership assessment of followers, and followers' self-assessment may each play a role in best addressing a situation. One 2008 article describes a light-hearted and innovative approach to teach leadership to college students using *Grey's Anatomy*, a popular U.S. television series, to apply vicarious "real world experience" to understand the situational leadership model.[23]

An online search in Medline for references between 1990 and 2021 on situational leadership in health or healthcare demonstrates interest in situational leadership applications in health and healthcare and resulted in a yield of 75 articles, a small number of which are described in this section.

The Person-Centered Situational Leadership (PCSL) Framework, an adaptation of the Situational Leadership Theory, was implemented and evaluated to improve patient-centered care in nursing homes in the United Kingdom.[24] The "situation" in the nursing home was to meet the changing needs of individual residents throughout the day. The interplay of leaders (clinical leads) and followers (nursing home staff) was described, and the authors concluded that the PCSL Framework has applicability in other care settings and contexts globally. The situational leadership model was analyzed while observing physicians in residency-training engaged in simulated hospital-based scenarios.[25] Video recordings of teams of residents in simulated clinical care scenarios were observed and assessed. The authors concluded that the situational leadership framework could be used as a tool to assess leadership performance in the context of evolving clinical care situations.

Chatalalsingh and Reeves applied the situational leadership theory to explore leadership and team learning in healthcare.[26] They analyzed two interdisciplinary nephrology teams made up of 15 members and 20 members with leadership from 12 individuals representing medicine and nursing. This study identified formal leaders, those with organizationally designated leadership responsibilities, and informal leaders by virtue of expertise. Each of the four leadership styles—directing, coaching, supporting, and delegating, which correspond to telling, selling, participating, and delegating, respectively—was observed and described. The authors contend that using the situational leadership model can be helpful in understanding how leaders use a range of leadership styles that are dependent on clinical context and advance interprofessional team learning.

Situational leadership has also been applied to public health contexts.[27–29] In one 2015 study, four local health department directors were interviewed and 33 staff from the four agencies participated in focus groups relating to public health leadership to explore answers to questions about most appropriate leadership style or styles for effective leadership in local health departments.[27] The top factors identified for good public health leadership from the interviews and focus groups were leading by example, the ability to provide followers with individualized consideration, and to approach leadership experiences "situationally." The authors concluded that the situational leadership model should be used by public health leaders to develop and guide their leadership.

A local public health agency case study related to the organization's pursuit of Public Health Accreditation Board (PHAB) accreditation describes the agency's experience with the accreditation process through the lens of the situational leadership model.[28] The local public health agency's experience with the public health accreditation process closely matched progression through the four stages of "follower" readiness and, as a result, the corresponding situational leadership styles. Early in the process, agency staff were at a low level of competence and confidence (R1) and advanced to an R2 level of readiness by the time of document submission for accreditation. The agency was at R3 by the next important milestone, a site visit by PHAB, and by the time site visit feedback was received, the agency staff members were at an R4 level of readiness. At the same time, the director's (the leader's) style of engagement with staff evolved from task-direction initially to almost complete delegation of authority and decision-making to a coordinator. The authors conclude that the situational leadership model can be useful for a local public health agency as an approach to guide the organization in seeking accreditation, specifically, but in meeting its public health mission, more broadly.

One pre-COVID-19 pandemic analysis of public health leadership to effectively address public health crises or emergencies posits that understanding and applying situational leadership are critical in public health emergency and crisis situations.[29] The authors cite the 2008 report, "World at Risk: The Report of the Commission on the Prevention of WMD Proliferation and Terrorism," which includes a recommendation to enhance the U.S. capability for rapid response to prevent mass morbidity and mortality in the event of a bioterrorism attack to make their case.[30] Burrell and coauthors believe that while the public will look to public health authorities, health scientists, and clinicians for leadership and management during times of any public health crisis, there is a lack of formal academic or "clinical" training that teaches situational leadership. They argue that public health leaders need to understand and properly execute situational leadership in crisis management situations. The authors conclude that acquiring sound leadership skills based on the situational leadership framework is critical for public health, health administration, and clinical professionals.[29]

SITUATIONAL ASSESSMENT

Situational leadership has been described as an approach in which the stage of readiness of a person or persons, so-called followers, assigned to address a situation or respond to a challenge informs the leadership style of the leader in relation to the followers. The leader assigns duties and provides direction to team members or followers based on the team member's skills (specifically competence and confidence) to fit the situation. The determination of readiness depends on the individuals and, again, the competence and confidence they bring to a particular situation. The same person can be at an R3 or R4 readiness stage for one situation or assignment and at R1 or R2 for others. Therefore, optimal situational leadership might be complemented by adopting an approach to assess situations and make informed decisions using a tool like the Josephson Institute's Seven-Step Path to Better Decisions.[31]

Each of the seven steps from the Seven-Step Path is accompanied by questions for leaders to ask related to situational leadership:

1. **Stop and Think:** Wait. What's going on? What is the situation? And how might I/we thoughtfully and effectively address it?
2. **Clarify Goals:** What is the end game? What am/are I/we trying to accomplish?
3. **Determine Facts:** What exactly is going on? What's the background and context of this situation?
4. **Develop Options:** How can I/we best address this situation? And who on the team has the competency and/or confidence to take on tasks or responsibilities? Are there alternative options, approaches, or persons to assign to tasks?
5. **Consider Consequences:** What might be unintended consequences?
6. **Choose**: How can I/we execute the best plan possible with team members assigned tasks and/or responsibilities using the situational leadership model to guide leadership behaviors?
7. **Monitor and Modify:** How are things going? How will we know we are making progress? And how can we do better?

Many of the references in this chapter highlight that readiness and leadership styles can evolve in the course of addressing a situation. Others highlight that situations are not static and can change over time. The situational leadership model and use of the Seven-Step Path for situational assessment are complementary approaches to inform decision-making in public health and healthcare in emergency situations but also in their day-to-day routine functions.

SITUATIONAL LEADERSHIP IN TEXAS

The situational leadership model will be used to describe three experiences in Texas, all related to building Texas' preparedness capacity for bioterrorism emergencies. The first experience is the rationale and work of the Texas Department of Health (TDH) 2001 bioterrorism working group. Second is with the formulation of the Texas Preparedness Coordinating Council (PCC). And the third is a description of the preparation for an August 2005 Strategic National Stockpile (SNS) exercise in North Texas.

One clear and statutorily defined responsibility of the TDH and the Commissioner of TDH is to respond to public health emergencies. Chapter 81 of the Texas Health and Safety codes starts with a statement that the state has a duty to protect the public health.[32] Two challenges were evident to the new commissioner of health starting his tenure in November 2001 in the aftermath of the September 11 attack and the anthrax attacks of 2001. Despite a request for preparedness funding from TDH during the 77th Texas Legislative Session, which met from January 9, 2001, to May 28, 2001, no funding was appropriated. The proposed preparedness plan was put on the shelf. Secondly, although TDH and its commissioner had the responsibility and authority to determine and respond to public health emergencies, the necessary assets (personnel, equipment, and facilities) were largely under the control of local government and local health departments and in private, nongovernmental health system hands (healthcare workforce, hospitals, pharmaceutical products).

THE TEXAS DEPARTMENT OF HEALTH 2001 BIOTERRORISM WORKING GROUP

In response to the first challenge, or situation, TDH created the Bioterrorism Preparedness Working Group (BTWG) and dusted off the bioterrorism preparedness plan that had been shelved when no funding was appropriated, nor explicit authority granted by the Texas legislature. Every single operational unit of TDH, from the vaccine program to vital statistics, procurement, hospital certification, and obesity programs, was asked to review the bioterrorism plan and find their most appropriate role or roles in the plan or make the compelling case for why that particular operational unit should not be a part of the new operational TDH unit that would oversee the state's response in the event of a bioterrorism event. The BTWG approach was a variation of how situational leadership is generally characterized in which the focus is on the interaction between the leader and a follower's (or subordinate's or team member's) readiness to step into a management or contributing role. The BTWG situation challenge was to build TDH's capacity and ability to "protect Texas" from the effects of a bioterrorism incident. The TDH BTWG process focused on the capacity (readiness) of operational units to be part of the TDH BT unit. The organizational units that ended up being included in the BTWG and in the creation of a BT operational unit ran the situational leadership development (readiness and maturity) continuum and included units that could be at all four levels of development: level 1 (low competence, low confidence); level 2 (low competence, more confidence); level 3 (high competence, variable confidence); and level 4 (high competence, high confidence). For example, the TDH infectious disease surveillance and investigations unit, which was already regularly monitoring reportable communicable diseases, conducting epidemiologic investigations, and responding to control disease outbreaks, was very competent and very confident (level 4), whereas the TDH-administered Women, Infants and Children (WIC) program, funded by the U.S. Department of Agriculture (USDA) for supplemental foods, healthcare referrals, and nutrition education for low-income pregnant, breastfeeding, and nonbreastfeeding postpartum women, and to infants and children up to age 5, did not see itself as able, at first, but confident and willing (level 2).

THE TEXAS PREPAREDNESS COORDINATING COUNCIL

The responsibility and authority to respond to public health emergencies is written in Texas law, but the resources that may be needed to appropriately respond in 2001 were largely in the hands of non-state-governmental entities. In response, TDH created the PCC. The PCC was conceptualized as an advisory body and a planning body, initially informal for both functions. The PCC was meant to afford TDH and its commissioner the perspectives and guidance of relevant stakeholders related to emergency response. The PCC included the state's medical association (Texas Medical Association), nursing association, hospital association, and civil liberties organization (The American Civil Liberties Union [ACLU]), to list a few. One of the first activities of the PCC was to review Texas state statutes related to public health emergency response, become aware of the legal authority and the limitations of state law, and to recognize that an optimal response might best be realized with a commitment to a systems, coordinated response to a bioterrorism incident or other public health emergency that, based on size, severity, and time, might necessitate the engagement and participation of non-state-governmental players. The PCC met quarterly. Trust, respect, transparency, humility, and familiarity among members and member organizations were engendered. Many months after inception, the U.S. Congress authorized funding for preparedness that was put to work in Texas with full view from, and engagement of, the PCC stakeholders. In September 2004, the recently created Texas Department of State Services (DSHS), which included the former TDH, was launched. The work of the PCC continued. The PCC set the stage for a better prepared TDH and then DSHS on behalf of the state of Texas.

The creation of the PCC is, again, a variation of how situational leadership is generally considered. With regard to the PCC, the situation was to build TDH's capacity and ability to more effectively stage a state-level response to a public health emergency with pre-coordination and communication to better coordinate a response. The PCC process started with an understanding of a potential situation with the evolution of most members from no situational awareness and a low level of readiness (low competence and low confidence) to a higher level of readiness. The Texas Hospital Association (THA) started at a higher level of readiness than other members of the PCC. THA had some degree of competence (individual hospitals prepared to respond to local mass trauma events, for example) but less confidence in a state-coordinated response (level 2). By the time, in 2005, that Hurricane Rita was projected to make landfall on the Texas gulf coast, just weeks after Hurricane Katrina had hit Louisiana and resulted in hundreds of thousands of Louisiana evacuees in Texas, THA had moved to a level of readiness between levels 3 and 4—with regards to a response to a state public health emergency. THA had the capacity to inventory and manage hospital bed supply and utilization in areas away from the coast and was willing to be more self-directed in doing so. During the response to Hurricane Rita and early recovery, DSHS and THA connected daily at the end of each day to assess the day's work and anticipate the next day, rather than meet more frequently throughout the day.

THE STRATEGIC NATIONAL STOCKPILE (SNS) EXERCISE

The third example of an application of the situational leadership model is related to a North Texas Strategic National Stockpile Exercise (SNS) conducted in North Texas in 2005. The SNS is part of the U.S. Department of Health and Human Services emergency medical response infrastructure that can supplement medical countermeasures needed by states, tribal nations, territories, and the largest metropolitan areas during public health emergencies.[33]

Lifesaving supplies, medications (including antibiotics, vaccines, chemical antidotes, and antitoxins), and devices contained in the stockpile can be secured when, during an incident, needed materials may not be otherwise available or sufficient. The federal SNS team supports states and local preparedness activities. The SNS exercise conducted in North Texas in August 2005 was to be the largest such exercise to date (larger than any single state-level exercise). Texas had been informed of the upcoming exercise weeks in advance of the event. The specifics of the incident—the incident scenario—would be revealed on the day of the exercise. It was revealed in advance that the exercise would involve the need for mass distribution of mock vaccines or antibiotics or both at multiple sites across a multi-county region.

After considering the readiness (competency) and willingness (confidence) of several senior team members to oversee this high priority, high visibility operation, the choice was narrowed to two individuals—the deputy commissioner of public health (DCPH) and the chief operations officer (COO). The two were equal in organizational rank and both had considerable organizational leadership experience, competence, and confidence. Considering that the COO had been an elected county executive in Texas, which was public-facing and necessitated negotiating and compromising skills; that he had successfully worked for a private firm to introduce and institute the children's health improvement plan (CHIP) in another state against tight timelines; and that he was the person who had overseen the successful transition to a paper-less vital statistics records system for Texas on time and under budget, it was clear that the COO was best suited to assure attention to detail and had the highest likelihood of successful execution. The commissioner made the decision to put the COO in charge of the SNS exercise preparation. Operational oversight, once the exercise was initiated, would be largely in the hands of the incident command team, which included the DCPH.

The decision was not without rancor and controversy, but in this case, the situation called for a manager to whom the task could be fully delegated with little need for the commissioner to provide much, if any, task-oriented direction. The exercise and the review that followed positioned Texas and DSHS to apply learnings to the response to the influx of the approximately 500,000 persons from Louisiana because of Hurricane Katrina over Labor Day weekend, just weeks after the SNS exercise. Texas' responses to Hurricanes Katrina and Rita were better because of the BTWG work, the PCC work, and the insights gained from them and applied to the preparation and execution of the SNS exercise.

One unintended but positive consequence of engaging the COO was his innovative approach to arrange to get hundreds of people to several mock mass distribution locations to stand in line to get mock medications or vaccines and then return to the line to simulate thousands of persons needing prophylaxis and/or treatment. After exploring options to simulate a mobilization of the masses, one obvious choice was to work through a staffing agency or staffing agencies to get "boots on the ground" where they were needed; however, the COO also explored working with social services agencies and other nonprofit organizations whereby the organization or organizations under contract would make arrangements to have individuals (ostensibly their staff, volunteers, or supporters) show up at the staging locations. The organizations would be "paid" for delivering persons to be the mock public and could use the funds to do the mission-driven work of the nonprofit. To conclude, the SNS exercise was scored an A-, a very big win for the agency. The DSHS's own review of the exercise revealed opportunities for improvement that were addressed almost immediately, and the formal review of the SNS exercise also revealed opportunities for improvement that resulted in changes. In this example, the more traditional situational leadership was utilized in which the best person for the situation was based on the interaction between the leader and the followers' readiness to step into a management role. The situation was to prepare for a large-scale buildup of TDH's capacity and ability to "protect Texas" from a bioterrorism incident. The process of assessment and determination of best fit for the situation resulted in a choice between two persons at the highest level of readiness or development, level 4—high competence, high confidence.

SUMMARY

The situational approach to leadership requires that an effective leader adapt their style to the demands of different situations and to meet the changing competencies, levels of commitment, and needs of individual team members. The situational leadership framework focuses on the interplay between a leader and their "followers" as they respond to and resolve a particular problem or challenge. Successful application of this leadership approach requires a leader to effectively modulate the degree of direction or support they provide. This approach to leadership has been popularized by the publication and application of the SLII® model, and is noted for its usefulness, practicality, prescriptive value, and emphasis on leader flexibility.[7] The peer-reviewed literature provides numerous examples of the evidence-base for situational leadership, including the use of situational leadership self-assessment; the use of PCSL Framework in long-term care facilities; the value of situational leadership in public health practice; and the use of situational leadership in public health accreditation.

DISCUSSION QUESTIONS

1. According to the situational leadership framework, why does being an effective leader require adaptation?
2. Compare the interactions between a leader and an individual who is confident and competent with that of a leader and an individual who is untested and new.
3. One of the foundations upon which the situational leadership model is operationalized is the leader's recognition of the situation. Explain why this is true.
4. Contrast direction with support provided by a leader in the situational leadership model.
5. How can situational leaders assess a situation and determine which leadership style to use?

PERSONAL REFLECTIONS: CHANCE FAVORS THE PREPARED MIND

I am going to start this section with a full and, in my opinion, important disclosure. My name is Eduardo Sanchez. I am a first-generation U.S. citizen. My parents are from the Dominican Republic. I am a Latino male living in the United States. And I had the great honor and privilege of serving as the first and, up to now, only Latino commissioner of health for the state of Texas.

"Chance favors the prepared mind," a quote attributed to Louis Pasteur, has been a guiding principle and prophetic reality for most of my professional life. The statement speaks to me and spoke to me as a promise—from early in my career, and early in my life, to graduating from medical school, to completing residency and public health training. And it has informed my continuous search for knowledge, for new information, for new ways of understanding. I have benefitted from leadership training throughout my career, among them chief resident leadership training in residency, the Centers for Disease Control and Prevention (CDC)-supported Public Health Leadership Institute early in my career, and the Association of State and Territorial Health Officers (ASTHO) training for new state health officers.

Among the myriad opportunities for optimized public health leadership, I believe that good public health leadership in times of public health emergencies or crises is critical, if not most important. I began my tenure as Texas commissioner of health 8 weeks after 9/11 and in the aftermath of the anthrax attacks of 2001. One thing was certain, and that was that preparedness, a state of readiness (FEMA definition), for public health emergencies or crises would have to be a top priority for the TDH. I was serving in the commissioner role in the not-yet-1-year-old DSHS during Labor Day weekend 2005. One half-million Louisianans traveled or were brought to Texas because of Hurricane Katrina's destruction. And several weeks later, the challenge in Texas was compounded by Hurricane Rita, which necessitated the evacuation of hundreds of thousands of Texas residents from coastal counties to safety inland. That exacerbated an already challenging response to about 250,000 Louisianans being housed in public shelters throughout the state.

Years of training to be a public health and family medicine physician, a few years of trying to sort out how best to more effectively prepare for and respond to a Texas public health emergency, and the opportunity afforded the state of Texas because of available federal bioterrorism preparedness funding converged to result in the chance to be prepared to more competently and more confidently attend to the displacement of and accommodations for hundreds of thousands of Louisianans and Texans who had been displaced from their homes, who needed shelter, food, public health services in shelters, and medical care and prescription drugs for some.

The previous section described three examples of situational leadership in Texas in the context of preparedness. What follows are two additional and personal examples associated with the state's response to Hurricanes Katrina and Rita.

CASE STUDY: HURRICANE KATRINA AND HURRICANE RITA

HURRICANE KATRINA

Over Labor Day weekend in 2005 and in the days that followed, several public shelters were stood up across Texas including large scale operations in Houston, Dallas, Austin, and San Antonio. The shelters were staffed by local emergency response personnel, local health department personnel, state health department personnel, and volunteer medical care staff. On the Sunday after Labor Day, I received a call from the U.S. Department of Health and Human Services Region 6 administrator to inform me that a team of 20 or so employees of the New Orleans local health department, including the department director and a second senior physician, had been evacuated and were "sheltered" in the Dallas Convention Center shelter along with thousands of others from New Orleans and other parts of Louisiana. Days earlier, I had been contacted by the leadership of the CDC Foundation to inform me of funds available from the CDC Foundation to cover unanticipated costs or costs not covered by other mechanisms that were Katrina response costs. Very quickly, following the massive accommodation of so many persons from Louisiana, it became clear that staffing to optimally respond to and meet the demands of persons, particularly persons with limited resources but with medical or other immediate needs, who had come to Texas from Louisiana would be a challenge. This situation was intriguing. On the one hand, public health colleagues from Louisiana were in a Texas shelter. On the other hand, we, in Texas, were shorthanded. In this situation, the situational leadership approach was one where the followers were persons (or really an organizational unit) outside of DSHS.

The initial assessment of the situation and discussions that included all affected parties led to a plan to hire the New Orleans health department team as DSHS employees. I was convinced of the readiness and eagerness of the New Orleans health department staff to get to work. The DSHS chief financial officer was asked to find the fastest way to hire the New Orleans health department staff. We requested funds from the CDC Foundation to immediately put the New Orleans health department staff into hotels with a per diem to feed themselves and to purchase laptop computers for the New Orleans health department staff. The staff was on the DSHS payroll in a few days. I recall traveling to Dallas and seeing the pride and joy of the New Orleans health department staff as I was apprised by the team of the situation in the shelter and more importantly seeing the pride and joy of persons who were in the shelter when they saw the New Orleans health department staff wearing New Orleans health department fluorescent vests on the floor of the shelter.

Applying the situational leadership model to this particular situation, the followers were three individuals, who were the DSHS CFO, the New Orleans health department director, and CDC Foundation CEO, and an organizational unit—the 20 staff of the New Orleans health department. The DSHS CFO had, time and again, demonstrated competence and confidence in the only 1-year-old DSHS; she was at a high state of readiness to do the due diligence to hire the New Orleans staff, and the leadership style for this was the delegating approach. The New Orleans health department director had made initial contact with the DHHS regional administrator and in subsequent discussions exhibited competence and confidence; he was at a high state of readiness to lead the New Orleans health department team, and the leadership style for this was also the delegating approach. The CDC Foundation CEO was fully engaged and demonstrated that they would need very little direction to support the immediate but temporary per diem needs and the computer purchases described earlier. The leadership style for this relationship was a supporting/delegating approach.

HURRICANE RITA

By the time Hurricane Rita made landfall in Western Louisiana near the Texas-Louisiana state line, hundreds of thousands of persons had evacuated from threatened coastal counties including thousands from Louisiana who had evacuated once already because of Hurricane Katrina and were staying in public shelters. As the emergency response team at DSHS considered the situation, the options included using already staffed public shelters, opening new shelters, and exploring creative opportunities. The situation was daunting and, as suggested in the description of the inception of the PCC, response to public health emergencies in Texas depends on a multisectoral, comprehensive, coordinated approach with multiple willing participants. In this situation, the situational leadership approach was one where followers were persons outside of DSHS.

In the days that Hurricane Rita was forming and clearly heading into the Gulf of Mexico and threatening the Texas coast, I was contacted by Dr. P. K. Carlton with an interesting proposition in anticipation of the possibility of needing to evacuate persons from coastal counties. Dr. Carlton, faculty at Texas A&M University and a former U.S. Air Force Surgeon General, with whom I had had an ongoing relationship, reached out to me and DSHS to propose using the not-yet-open-for-patients large animal veterinary hospital at Texas A&M University in the Texas Brazos Valley to accommodate several hundred persons who needed medical supervision in addition to needing to be evacuated. We learned that much of the medical equipment used in large-animal hospitals is equipment designed and approved for use in humans.

The facility had not yet been used, had state-of-the-art technology and infection control capability, and would be staffed by volunteer healthcare personnel from Brazos County. DSHS staff quickly arranged and conducted a site visit; and although the DSDS staff expressed concern with the optics and messaging, they conveyed full confidence in the capacity and competence of the hospital, the oversight of the proposed operation, and the local, volunteer workforce.

Applying the situational leadership model to this particular situation, the followers were an individual, P. K. Carlton, and an organizational unit, both outside of DSHS. The individual was at a high state of readiness—competent and confident—and the leadership style to the situation could be characterized as the delegating approach. The organizational unit—the hospital and the workforce, also competent and quite confident to accommodate and take care of persons with medical needs—would be led with a supporting/delegating leadership style.

DISCUSSION

In each of the situational leadership situations described in the case studies, previously unknown "followers" entered the situational stage at just the right time. In the first situation, an unanticipated need for personnel and services—an influx of persons from Louisiana needing food, housing, and personal hygiene services, and social and medical services—could be addressed, at least for one location, the Dallas Convention Center, with a highly ready (competent, willing, and committed) group from outside of the usual pools of staff (DSHS, local health departments, volunteers). Chance favored the prepared organization or leader. In the second situation, a predictable and anticipated increase in need for facilities and personnel who could care for persons needing a higher level of care than that which could be provided in a general public shelter could be addressed in one part of the state with a highly ready (competent, willing, and committed) group with a state-of-the-art facility that had not been considered in the preparedness work that had been conducted to date; however, the resources (facility and people) could be readily accommodated in the response infrastructure and capacity. Again, chance favored the prepared mind.

CASE STUDY QUESTIONS

1. Compare and contrast the situational leadership situations in each case. How is each similar to and distinct from the traditional situational leadership model? How is each similar to and distinct from the other?
2. How would the situation and the approach have changed had the New Orleans Health Department staff been deemed willing (confident) but not competent to be employed by Texas DSHS and deployed in the Dallas Convention Center shelter?
3. How would the situation and the approach have changed had the New Orleans Health Department staff been deemed competent and willing but the ability to hire them as DSHS staff been deemed not administratively possible?
4. How would the situation and the approach have changed had the veterinary hospital been deemed unfit and unsafe to provide human medical services yet the competent and willing volunteers in that community expressed an interest in helping anyway?

CASE STUDY: SITUATIONAL LEADERSHIP IN THE COVID-19 RESPONSE: WASHINGTON STATE

On the afternoon of Monday, January 20, 2020, while most Americans were celebrating the Martin Luther King, Jr. holiday, public health officials at the CDC and Washington state learned of a blood test result that would soon disrupt every American's daily life, on a scale that last happened 102 years prior. Ahead would be long-term school closures; complete closure of "non-essential" businesses; overwhelmed public health staff, nursing home staff, healthcare workers and medical examiners; job losses in the millions; a torn-apart economy that would require massive amounts of emergency government funding; over 47.3 million cases, 3.3 million new hospitalizations, and 764,000 American deaths in 23 months;[34] and the rapid development and deployment of a new vaccine. The following morning, the CDC along with Governor Jay Inslee from Washington state, his secretary of health, John Wiesman, and the Snohomish County health officer, Dr. Christopher Spitters, announced in two press conferences the United States' first known case of 2019 novel coronavirus, now known as COVID-19 or SARS-CoV-2.[35–38]

In those initial hours and days, public health incident management teams were mobilized, press conferences were held, public health disease investigators interviewed the initial case to understand his movements and who may have been exposed to this new virus, and contact tracing began for those who were potentially exposed. Critical questions requiring urgent decisions had to be made in the absence of complete knowledge.

- During what time frame did public health officials think the patient was infectious? With past coronaviruses, one wasn't infectious until symptoms developed. Was that the case with this one?
- Who was going to be considered a close contact and notified they were at risk for this new disease? That depended upon how one believed the virus was transmitted (direct contact? droplet? airborne?).
- Should the patient be hospitalized even though he was medically stable at the time and in isolation alone at home?[39] If he was to be hospitalized, who would pay the hospital and medical bills, since it didn't appear he needed that level of medical care?
- What would the public need to know about this new disease? How concerned would they need to be for their own health and safety? How should they protect themselves? Should they change their behavior?

The Washington state secretary of health, John Wiesman, had a highly trained, competent, experienced, and deeply committed team. Drs. Kathy Lofy and Scott Lindquist were top-notch health officers and infectious disease epidemiologists; Nathan Weed was exceptionally trained with vast experience as an incident commander; and all were well supported by a cadre of experts from the CDC, some of whom were on the ground with them in Washington state within 20 hours of the positive test result. Key to the core team was the well-trained Washington state Department of Health incident management team that had been mobilized over two dozen times in the last 7 years responding to measles outbreaks, a massive mudslide wiping out a whole hillside neighborhood killing 43 people, a radiation leak at a major research facility, and the immediate health crisis of over 8,000 pain patients who suddenly lost their medical care.

This situation, however, presented unique circumstances. This was a new virus and there wasn't much known about it, so *everyone's* competency in addressing it was lower than usual. John and his team had been watching the case counts climb rapidly in China and were extremely concerned with the rapid spread and wondered if China was forthright with all it knew about the outbreak. Having the first case in the nation was going to put every communication, every action, and every misstep into the spotlight, and John's colleagues all over the nation were going to be eager to learn from him how to best handle the response should they get a case. There had been limited advanced warning and, if this was going to get big, John knew all systems were going to be quickly overwhelmed. He understood far too well that leaders and workers across all sectors were not fully prepared—operationally, financially, mentally, or emotionally. And it was an election year. John's boss, Governor Inslee, was running for a third term as governor. How well public health and the governor's team responded would reflect directly on the governor's leadership and could affect his re-election. So, John had to stop and think about how to best lead in this environment.

The initial goals were clear: (1) identify any contacts and control the spread, (2) learn as much about the virus and how it affected someone who was infected and how it behaved in populations as quickly as possible, and (3) communicate frequently with the public, being the first out with the information, being right with the information shared, and being credible with the communication. The facts were less clear given this was a new virus with much uncertainty, and he knew their knowledge would grow as they gained more experience with the situation, and thus their advice to the public would be refined and even changed as time progressed.

John's options were to proceed as usual or take a different path. Proceeding as usual would mean delegating the entire response to the department's incident management team and John would serve as a high-level policy decision-maker "over to the side". His customary role was responding to the team's needs for resources; providing decisions on key policy questions the team needed answered; linking to the elected officials such as the governor, house, and senate members as well as with the governor's executive team and cabinet officials; and serving as a key spokesperson at crucial moments. This would "keep John in his usual lane" and allow the team to do as they were trained. The risk with this approach was that in this fast-moving environment with a new virus, key decisions might be slowed, John's situational awareness might be outdated too quickly, and the state's and nation's confidence in the team could erode with an early misstep, causing panic.

John took a different path. He immediately activated the department's incident management team. He gave them their charge to investigate the case and control the outbreak, keep the workers safe, and communicate frequently and timely with the media and public. He delegated authority to Nathan and the department's incident command team to lead the overall response as the team was highly competent in this foundational public health work and highly committed to leading public health responses.

However, unlike previous responses, John relocated himself for months from the department's headquarters in Olympia, WA, to the state's public health laboratory in Shoreline, WA, where Kathy, Scott, the department's epidemiologists and laboratory staff, and the CDC field team were located. He focused 100% of his time on the response. He engaged in real-time discussions at the operational level, sometimes engaging in a "Let's talk and do what I think" and "Do this" mode. He coached decisions on criteria for defining a close contact, a key issue so the public health case and contact investigators could do their job, but also a critical one as getting this "wrong" might miss cases, cause panic, and undermine confidence in the response. John supported the idea that the initial case should be hospitalized and directed that the state would "somehow" pay for the hospitalization if the patient's insurance or the federal government wouldn't pay. He felt this was no time to risk the patient deteriorating quickly or for the public to fear his presence in the community, and frankly, this was an unknown disease—they had to learn what they could as quickly as possible about the disease progression. The team found John's presence reassuring and assisted them in making faster decisions, allowing the response to proceed at the pace it needed.

Following this first case, Washington had the nation's first known death, and first nursing home outbreak. As the outbreak grew in Washington state and across the country and as testing became more available, health departments reported daily the number of new COVID tests conducted, the percent positive, and, as best they could, the demographics of those persons being testing.

Most public health data systems around the country were inadequate for the large volumes of tests coming in 24/7. Some were electronically delivered into the automatic data processing systems, others forwarded in spreadsheets that needed to be manually processed, and still others sent data via fax and telephone that had to be entered into data systems.[40] Epidemiology and Information Technology (IT) staff were stretched way beyond any reasonable limits with the on-boarding of hundreds of new inexperienced case and contact investigation staff, reporting out the data at a set time every single day of the week as policy-makers immediately used the data for their decision-making while the media promptly reported on it. Another challenge was maintaining and fixing data systems that were operating 24/7 with no maintenance time and with slow processing speeds that couldn't keep up with the incoming volume of data. Like the testing data systems, the case and contact investigation data systems were not designed to handle a full pandemic response. The data systems were not sufficient to handle the number of investigators entering data, the scripts needed to assist inexperienced staff in conducting the interviews, and the full extent of information needed in this response.

John, Kathy, and Scott regularly found themselves in a place of having to let the governor and his team know that the data systems were down or that errors in data processing had given questionable information that had to be problem-solved before data could be released. They also had to explain the challenges to the skeptical media.[41] While their teams of epidemiologists and IT staff were competent and capable of complex problem-solving under "routine" infectious disease outbreaks, they were greatly challenged in the pandemic due to cognitive and physical exhaustion, the sheer volume of work, and their reluctance at times to accept outside help.

Their staff was tremendously committed and totally exhausted. John and Kathy found themselves "managing up" to the governor, his team, and the media to give staff the time and space they needed to solve the many data processing and system issues that were occurring almost daily. And while doing that, they were personally meeting with staff to understand the problems, ask questions to help problem-solve, offer additional resources, and both relieve and keep the pressure on regarding the urgency of getting the systems fixed. The private technology sector assisted the teams, and that took staff time away from their own efforts to solve problems as they got others up to speed on the systems. John and Kathy moved from delegating to coaching the staff into solutions for help as they were committed but their ability was declining due to cognitive exhaustion and being overwhelmed. There were times when data could not be reported out for a few days and up to a week or more.[42] Most times, the policy-makers were able to make sound decisions despite the delay in data; however, there was a time when the data systems were down so long it was threatening that ability. John found himself having to switch from coaching to directing the team to accept help, and he questioned himself about whether he had waited too long to make that switch in his leadership style.

CASE STUDY QUESTIONS

1. In the first days of the response, John delegated, coached, supported, and directed parts of the response to *highly competent and highly committed staff*. He veered away from the situational leadership model that says you focus on assessing the follower's competency and commitment and then adjust your leadership style. What made him focus on assessing the situation and then deciding his leadership style? Was there another way he might have done this? When using the situational leadership style based on analyzing the situation rather than the follower, how do you decide when to switch to analyzing the followers for determining your leadership style?

2. The data system challenges described here were not unique to Washington state, and some health leaders lost their jobs due to data system problems.[43] The public health IT infrastructure across the United States contains many legacy systems that have needed urgent replacement for years. How do you suppose John and Kathy were balancing their supporting, coaching, and directing styles as they worked with their staff, the governor, and the media regarding COVID-19 data system challenges? How would you know when you need to switch from the supporting and coaching role to directing? Is that switch something you do suddenly or with preparation? If you do it suddenly, what do you suppose are the risks and what do you gain? How do you mitigate the risks? If you do it with preparation, what do you suppose you risk and what do you gain? How do you mitigate those risks?

A robust set of instructor resources designed to supplement this text is located at http://connect.springerpub.com/content/book/978-0-8261-4924-4. Qualifying instructors may request access by emailing textbook@springerpub.com.

REFERENCES

1. Blanchard KH, Johnson S. *The One Minute Manager*. The Berkley Publishing Group; 2001.
2. Carnegie D. *How to Win Friends & Influence People*. Simon and Schuster; 1998.
3. Collins J. *Good to Great: Why Some Companies Make the Leap and Others Don't*. HarperBusiness; 2001.
4. Covey S. *The 7 Habits of Highly Effective People*. Free Press; 1989.
5. Kellerman B. *Bad Leadership: What It Is, How It Happens, Why It Matters*. Harvard Business Review Press; 2004.
6. Kotter JP. *Leading Change*. Harvard Business School Press; 1995.
7. Northouse P. *Introduction to Leadership*. Sage; 2021.
8. T. B. Leadership Theories and Studies. 2011. https://www.referenceforbusiness.com/management/Int-Loc/Leadership-Theories-and-Studies.html
9. Callahan R, Bhattacharya D. *Public Health Leadership: Strategies for Innovation in Population Health and Social Determinants*. Routledge; 2017.
10. Capper SA, Ginter PM, Swayne LE. *Public Health Leadership and Management: Cases and Context*. Sage Publications; 2001.
11. Rowitz L. *Public Health Leadership: Putting Principles Into Practice*. Jones & Bartlett Learning; 2013.
12. Sharfstein JM. *The Public Health Crisis Survival Guide: Leadership and Management in Trying Times*. Oxford Press; 2018.
13. McCleskey JA. Situational, transformational, and transactional leadership and leadership development. *J Business Stud Q*. 2014;5(4):117–130.
14. Hersey P, Blanchard KH. *Management of Organizational Behavior: Utilizing Human Resources*. Prentice-Hall; 1969.
15. Hill W. A situational approach to leadership effectiveness. *J Appl Psychol*. 1969;53(6):513–517. doi:10.1037/h0028667
16. Hersey P, Blanchard KH, Johnson DE. *Management of Organizational Behavior: Utilizing Human Resources*. Prentice-Hall; 2013.
17. Schermerhorn JR. Situational leadership: conversations with Paul Hersey. *Mid-American J Bus*. 1997;12(2):5–11.
18. Wunsch G. Theories, models, and data. *Demografie*. 1994;36(1):20–29. https://www.jstor.org/stable/29788398
19. Blanchard KH, Zigarmi D, Nelson RB. Situational leadership® after 25 years: a retrospective. *J Leadersh Organ Stud*. 1993;1(1):21–36. doi:10.1177/107179199300100104
20. Henkel T, Bordeau D. A field study: an examination of manager's situational leadership style. *J Divers Manag*. 2018;13(2):7–14. doi:10.19030/jdm.v13i2.10218
21. Henkel TG, Marion JW, Bordeau DT. Project manager leadership behavior: task-oriented versus relationship-oriented. *J Leadersh Edu*. 2019;18(2). doi:10.12806/V18/I2/R8
22. Thompson G, Glasø L. Situational leadership theory: a test from three perspectives. *Leadersh Organ Dev J*. 2015;36(5):527–544. doi:10.1108/LODJ-10-2013-0130
23. Torock JL. Bringing the emergency room to the classroom: using "Grey's Anatomy" to simplify situational leadership. *J Leadersh Edu*. 2008;7(2):69–78. doi:10.12806/V7/I2/AB5
24. Lynch BM, McCance T, McCormack B, Brown D. The development of the person-centred situational leadership framework: revealing the being of person-centredness in nursing homes. *J Clin Nurs*. 2018;27(1–2):427–440. doi:10.1111/jocn.13949
25. Skog A, Peyre SE, Pozner CN, Thorndike M, Hicks G, Dellaripa PF. Assessing physician leadership styles: application of the situational leadership model to transitions in patient acuity. *Teach Learn Med*. 2012;24(3):225–230. doi:10.1080/10401334.2012.692269
26. Chatalalsingh C, Reeves S. Leading team learning: what makes interprofessional teams learn to work well? *J Interprof Care*. 2014;28(6):513–518. doi:10.3109/13561820.2014.900001
27. Carlton EL, Holsinger JW Jr, Riddell MC, Bush H. Full-range public health leadership, part 2: qualitative analysis and synthesis. *Front Public Health*. 2015;3:174. doi:10.3389/fpubh.2015.00174
28. Rabarison K, Ingram RC, Holsinger JW Jr. Application of situational leadership to the national voluntary public health accreditation process. *Front Public Health*. 2013;1:26. doi:10.3389/fpubh.2013.00026
29. Burrell DN, Rahim E, Omar-Abdul M, Huff A, Finklea K. *An Analysis of the Application of Situational Leadership in the Post 9/11 Evolving Public Health Managerial Environments*. A.T. Still University; 2018.

30. Commission on the Prevention of Weapons of Mass Destruction Proliferation and Terrorism. *World at Risk the Report of the Commission on the Prevention of WMD Proliferation and Terrorism.* Library of Congress; 2008.

31. Institute J. *The seven-step path to better decisions.* 2017. https://josephsoninstitute.org/med-4sevenstep-path

32. Communicable Disease Prevention and Control Act, 71st Texas Leg., ch. 678, Sec. 1, §Chapter 81. 1989.

33. Office of the Assistant Secretary for Preparedness and Response. Strategic national stockpile. U.S. Department of Health and Human Services. https://www.phe.gov/about/sns/Pages/default.aspx

34. Centers for Disease Control and Prevention. COVID data tracker weekly review. Centers for Disease Control and Prevention. November 19, 2021. https://www.cdc.gov/coronavirus/2019-ncov/covid-data/covidview/index.html

35. Transcript of update on 2019 Novel Coronavirus (2019-nCoV). Centers for Disease Control and Prevention. January 21, 2020. https://www.cdc.gov/media/releases/2020/t0121-Telebriefing-Coronavirus.html

36. Case of 2019 novel coronavirus confirmed in Washington state resident. Washington State Department of Health. January 21, 2020. https://www.doh.wa.gov/Newsroom/Articles/ID/1068/Case-of-2019-novel-coronavirus-confirmed-in-Washington-state-resident-20-006

37. Brown A, Hutton C, Sanders J-G. Snohomish county man is first U.S. case of new coronavirus. *HeraldNet.* January 21, 2020. https://www.heraldnet.com/news/snohomish-county-man-is-first-us-case-of-new-coronavirus/

38. First travel-related case of 2019 novel coronavirus detected in United States. Centers for Disease Control and Prevention. January 21, 2020. https://www.cdc.gov/media/releases/2020/p0121-novel-coronavirus-travel-case.html

39. Holshue ML, DeBolt C, Lindquist S, et al. First case of 2019 novel coronavirus in the United States. *N Engl J Med.* 2020;382:929–936. doi:10.1056/NEJMoa2001191

40. Banco E. Inside America's COVID-reporting breakdown: crashing computers, three-week delays tracking infections, lab results delivered by snail mail: state officials detail a vast failure to identify hotspots quickly enough to prevent outbreaks. *Politico.* August 15, 2021. https://www.politico.com/news/2021/08/15/inside-americas-covid-data-gap-502565

41. Hudetz M, Kamb L. Six months into pandemic, Washington state still struggles with COVID-19 data. *The Seattle Times.* August 14, 2020. https://www.seattletimes.com/seattle-news/six-months-into-pandemic-washington-still-struggles-with-covid-19-data/

42. O'Sullivan J. 'We should have been better prepared': COVID-19 draws attention to Washington state's underfunded public health programs. *The Seattle Times.* March 1, 2021. https://www.seattletimes.com/seattle-news/politics/we-should-have-been-better-prepared-covid-19-draws-attention-to-washington-states-underfunded-public-health-programs/

43. Myers J. California's public health director resigns in wake of coronavirus data errors. *Los Angeles Times.* Updated August 10, 2020. https://www.latimes.com/california/story/2020-08-09/california-public-health-director-resigns-in-wake-of-questions-about-coronavirus-test-data

Chapter 7

Transformational Leadership

Donna J. Petersen

INTRODUCTION

Effective leadership is critical to the success of any organization though it remains in short supply. Persons placed in leadership positions often lack leadership skills or are distracted by managerial responsibilities that take precedence because of their perceived urgency. Our healthcare and public health systems face complex challenges that demand leadership approaches that engage diverse communities in difficult work that may involve years of perseverance. A lack of leadership at the top of an organization is often compounded by the lack of leadership inside an organization, and often created by the lack of opportunity to demonstrate and contribute leadership to organizational efforts from within. Among the many theories of leadership, the transformational leadership approach seeks to address this challenge by cultivating a leadership culture within organizations, giving individuals and groups opportunities to shape and contribute to a shared and inspiring vision. This chapter will present transformational leadership as an important construct in the evolution of thought on the concept of leadership, particularly within the health fields. This approach has the added benefit of being highly applicable to the diversity, equity, and inclusion imperative essential in the promotion of human and community health. Definitions, discussions, and examples will be supported by case studies.

OBJECTIVES

By the end of this chapter, the reader will be able to:

- Distinguish transformational leadership from other leadership styles.
- Describe the four behaviors of transformational leadership.
- Appreciate the attributes of transformational leaders.
- Discuss the importance of transformational leadership in public health and in health systems.
- Relate transformational leadership styles to leadership tasks.
- Describe examples of transformational leadership and their impact relative to other styles.

TERMINOLOGY AND BACKGROUND

The concept of transformational leadership is relatively new in the pantheon of leadership theories. In the mid-1800s, Thomas Carlyle popularized the "great man theory," promoting the idea that leaders were born, not made, though critics noted that leaders were only tasked to lead because of the circumstances in which they found themselves.[1] The "trait theory," promoted by Ralph Stogdill in the 1930s, expanded on the great man theory by identifying select personality traits that were necessary for successful leadership, though once again, critics argued that these did not necessarily have to be innate but could be acquired depending on the leadership situation.[1]

This debate led to the "behavioral theories" of the 1940s that focused more on the roles and tasks of leaders and less on intrinsic traits. These theories examined differences between leadership tasks and management tasks and led to the "contingency" theories of the 1960s that suggested that all leadership was situational. Later scholars proposed "transactional" theories of leadership which were quickly discredited and led to the emergence of what we currently espouse: "transformational" theories. **Transformational theories** focus on the relationships that leaders develop with others, the intrinsic personality characteristics and traits of leaders, various leadership roles, and the central importance of team motivation.[1]

The concept was introduced by James V. Downton and later advanced by James MacGregor Burns.[2] What Burns called "transforming leadership" was characterized by "leaders and followers helping each other to advance to a higher level of morale and motivation."[2(p16)] He distinguished leaders, who transform, from managers, who transact, noting that a key distinction between leaders and managers was the extent to which they sought to change culture versus simply working within an existing culture. A common axiom about this difference posits that managers do things right while leaders do the right things, suggesting that managers are concerned with immediate transactions, operations, and products while leaders have a higher-level responsibility to look to the future, anticipate trends, and seek to optimize outcomes through changes in the organizational culture. The word "transforming" was replaced by the word "transformational" by Bernard Bass in his work describing the impact of transformational leaders on the motivation and performance of the leader's followers.[3] Harkening in some ways back to the trait theory of leadership, Bass believed that transformational leaders provided "idealized influence" (earlier referred to as "charisma"), as well as intellectual stimulation and individual consideration. Transformational leaders offer an inspiring vision and create an environment based on trust, loyalty, and respect that recognizes and cultivates the contributions of individuals and gives them room to be innovative, often altering the environment to enable creative ideas to flourish and contribute to immediate and lasting success. This is in direct contrast to transactional leadership approaches that are typically based on give-and-take arrangements and contingent rewards within a more typical hierarchical structure.[4,5]

The focus of the transformational leader on the performance of the group is manifested in what are considered the four behaviors of transformational leaders, all beginning with the letter "I": inspirational motivation, idealized influence, intellectual stimulation, and individualized consideration.[6] Note the emphasis on the individuals within the organization, those who actually perform the work. An effective transformational leader, so the theory goes, gets more out of their followers because of this focus, enabling those working with them to achieve unexpected or remarkable results (Figure 7.1).[7]

- Inspirational motivation refers to the ability of the leader to communicate a vision that is clear and compelling to others, engendering commitment to the vision and loyalty to the leader.

- Idealized influence is reflected in the leader's power as an authentic role model, someone others wish to emulate.

- Intellectual stimulation is manifest in the way leaders empower others to challenge themselves and the status quo, to imagine and to innovate, and to take risks.

- Individualized consideration is grounded in a high degree of emotional intelligence (see Chapter 5, "Emotional Intelligence") and empathy through which the leader expresses care and concern for each member of the team and provides opportunities for growth and higher-level contributions to the overall vision.

Much of the success of this approach is predicated on the ability of the transformational leader to build relationships. Relationships are central to transformational leadership as they are necessary in building trust within groups and organizations. Trust supports a sense of collective opportunity and responsibility, builds morale and motivation, and results in positive performance outcomes at the individual, group, and organizational levels.[8]

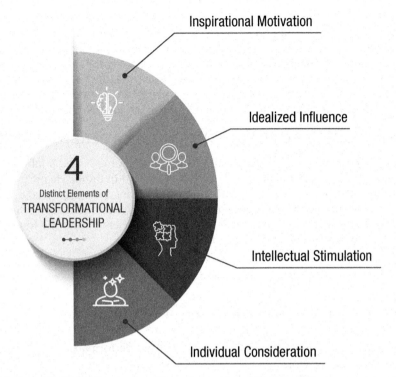

FIGURE 7.1: Four Distinct Elements of Transformational Leadership.
Source: Reproduced with permission from Bass BM, Avolio BJ. *Improving Organizational Effectiveness Through Transformational Leadership*. Sage; 1994.

A sign of how popular this approach to leadership has become is that it was featured in an article in the Business section of the *Cape Cod Times* on Sunday July 4, 2021, in response to a question about how one can become a better leader. Of note, the writer, Marc L. Goldberg, stated that "leadership is not something you do to people but do with people" and later, when describing the reciprocal form of leadership that is characteristic of transformational leadership, ". . . this works especially well in workplaces where the organization is launching innovative practices and approaches to solving age-old problems."[9(pC1)] One of the "age-old" problems in public health is the ultimate upstream determinant of health: systemic and structural racism. The importance of transformational leadership in the dismantling of racist systems will be addressed later in this chapter.

IMPORTANCE OF TRANSFORMATIONAL LEADERSHIP IN PUBLIC HEALTH

Public health is what societies do collectively to create conditions in which people can be healthy.[10] The importance of the collective cannot be overstated and sets up an important premise: that leadership in public health is more important than leaders. The three core functions of public health, also articulated in the Future of Public Health report—assessment, policy development, and assurance—further imply engagement and inclusivity among professionals, sectors, and communities.[10] Leadership that guides these efforts to be engaged and inclusive is essential at all levels of an organization and the system. It is posited that leadership in public health exists and must be nurtured at three levels: the positional leadership level, the individual leadership level, and the community leadership level. As an integral part of a functioning public health system, the healthcare system has struggled for decades to promote equitable access and high quality while trying to control costs. These challenges are formidable and require all the constituent stakeholders to work together to consider implementable solutions. This includes government, insurance companies, employers, healthcare institutions and organizations, providers, and patients. Autocratic leadership styles will not effect change in a system as complex and consequential as this one. Transformational leadership in positional leaders, individuals, and the organizations themselves is required.

TRANSFORMATIONAL LEADERSHIP AND LEADERSHIP TASKS

In 2014, the National Board of Public Health Examiners commissioned a Job Task Analysis as part of a review and revision of the items on the Certified in Public Health examination.[11] Thousands of public health professionals, including clinicians, were surveyed to understand the tasks they perform while doing their jobs. The tasks were then sorted into common themes using factor analysis. Leadership was one of the themes, and the following list of tasks associated with leadership were identified:

Tasks in the Leadership Domain:

- Utilize critical analysis to prioritize and justify actions and allocation of resources.
- Apply team building skills.
- Apply organizational change management concepts and skills.
- Apply conflict management skills.
- Implement strategies to support and improve team performance.
- Apply negotiation skills.
- Establish and model standards of performance and accountability.
- Guide organizational decision-making and planning based on internal and external assessments.
- Prepare professional development plans for self or others.
- Develop strategies to motivate others for collaborative problem-solving, decision-making, and evaluation.
- Develop capacity-building strategies at the individual, organizational, or community level.
- Communicate an organization's mission, goals, values, and shared vision to stakeholders.
- Create teams for implementing health initiatives.
- Develop a mission, goals, values, and shared vision for an organization or the community in conjunction with key stakeholders.
- Develop a continuous quality improvement plan.
- Implement a continuous quality improvement plan.
- Evaluate organizational performance in relation to strategic and defined goals.
- Implement organizational strategic planning processes.
- Assess organizational policies and procedures regarding working across multiple organizations.
- Align organizational policies and procedures with regulatory and statutory requirements.
- Maximize efficiency of programs.
- Ensure that informatics principles and methods are used in the design and implementation of systems.

In reviewing this list, one may wonder if some of these are not more managerial, or transactional, types of tasks. Some may seem to be directed at individuals or small teams, rather than large organizations or systems. The reader should pick any one of these and think about a situation that illustrates this task being performed. Think about how such a task would lend itself to a leadership role. Finally, imagine a leader engaging in this task *not* utilizing the principles of transformational leadership. Recall these principles of behaviors include inspirational vision, idealized influence, intellectual stimulation, and individual consideration.

Here is an example of inspirational vision: *Communicate an organization's mission, goals, values, and shared vision to stakeholders.* At first glance, this seems two-dimensional and uni-directional (i.e., "I have a message and I communicate it"). But thinking about this more deeply, why is a leader communicating the organization's mission, goals, values, and shared vision? Might not such a communication be delivered in a way that invites a response? How were the mission, goals, values, and shared vision developed in the first place? Did the leader make them up on their own? How effective will their delivery of the communication be if they are the sole author of the message? More importantly, how impactful will the mission, values, goals, and shared vision be if they were not developed through an inclusive, inspiring process? These are the questions a transformational leader will ask themselves. Warren Bennis and Burt Nanus, in their book *Leaders: Strategies for Taking Charge,* speak about the critical importance of creating and communicating a vision.[12] They posit that this is a unique leadership task, and the essence of the difference between leadership and management, stating that "by focusing attention on a vision, the leader operates on the emotional and spiritual resources of the organization, on its values, commitments and aspirations. The manager, by contrast, operates on the physical resources of the organization, on its capital, human skills, raw materials, and technology."[12(p85)]

Here is an example of intellectual stimulation from the author's own experience: *align organizational policies and procedures with regulatory and statutory requirements.* Not only does this sound obvious, but it also sounds deadly boring; of course, any organization, especially a governmental organization, is going to follow the rules. But read this again. This task speaks to *alignment*, and to a transformational leader, that says opportunity. Following rules takes effort; it requires procedures, documentation, and clearly defined mechanisms for accountability, often manifested in required signatures from many different individuals. Much "work" in public health and in healthcare is taken up serving the unrelenting and unforgiving master of regulations and statutory requirements. A transformational leader, who, by definition, is anticipating and managing change, will want to assure the rules line up with the policies and procedures, not just the other way around. As a consultant, as a state health public leader, and as a public health academic leader, the author has encouraged this type of thought experiment, and it can be a lot of fun. Ask the question: to what regulation or statutory requirement is this policy or procedure linked? In other words, why are we doing this? Why are we gathering this information? Why are we having multiple people sign this form? Where do the forms go? What would happen if we no longer completed these forms? Forcing yourself and your team to seriously ask these questions may reveal effort that can be redirected to more creative ventures. It is likely that when one asks these questions, they will find that the law no longer exists or never actually existed; that the regulation has been changed; that the "regulation" was an internal policy that is no longer enforced; or that there is a much simpler way to comply with the rules than the cumbersome way it has been done. Rules really can set people free if they let them.

One more example of individualized consideration and a nice segue to the next section on the levels of leadership: *prepare professional development plans for self and others.* This seems very specific and transactional. But again, looking more deeply and considering how important professional development is to oneself, to team members, to the organization, and to the community at large, one can see the possibilities for professional development plans to become a powerful tool in the hands of a transformational leader. Why have professional development plans? Ostensibly because of the desire to have oneself, and one's colleagues and organizations, maintain current knowledge and learn new tools and skills. Having professional development plans is also about achieving goals, using resources most efficiently and effectively, and engaging the most precious resource—people—in pursuit of something bigger than themselves. Professional development plans can become the individualized blueprints of one's overall master plan and ensure that the motivations of individuals are reflected in that plan, and that the vision of the plan is reinforced in the individual opportunities for growth.

TRANSFORMATIONAL LEADERSHIP AT ALL LEVELS

As noted earlier, leadership in public health operates at least at three levels. The first is typically thought of as the roles and responsibilities of the person in a leadership position. Within public health and healthcare, this is typically the state or local health officer, or the CEO of a hospital or health system. When asking students to think of a leader, they typically note President Barack Obama or Reverend Dr. Martin Luther King, Jr. If they are older, they may remember former Surgeon General C. Everett Koop and in present times they would likely say Dr. Anthony Fauci. Today, the list of leaders could also include Jacinda Ardern, prime minister of New Zealand or the minister of health of Canada, Dr. Patty Hadju (for whom the John Fluevog shoe company in 2020 named a limited-edition designer shoe). All these individuals were visionaries; they inspired others, they took risks to achieve what they believed to be important goals, and they motivated others to be bold in tackling pressing social problems. They each embody the essential characteristics of transformational leaders: honesty, integrity, humility, and empathy. They are good communicators; they listen well and are open to new ideas. They motivate, delegate, congratulate, share credit, and champion their colleagues. They are good partners, capable of building coalitions, and are experts at resolving conflicts. They all exemplify idealized influence.

The second level is the leadership that is provided as a field to the larger community. If the public's health is a goal, then public health as a system must champion societies' interest in enjoying good health and doing what is necessary to realize that interest. This speaks to the notion that the field itself provides leadership in the public's interest and that, therefore, everyone working in it must embrace this leadership responsibility. As healthcare organizations embrace their role in promoting population health, they too become active change agents in improving community health. The *fields themselves* provide leadership in the global effort to attain a higher quality of life for everyone.

The third level is leadership demonstrated by individuals. Anyone can emerge as a leader in service to a public health cause (even when the cause is not identified as "public health" per se). The story of the hero-leader who single-handedly takes on a cause and prevails is a popular subject of books and movies. Everyday people engage in similarly courageous work, whether it be around environmental issues or improving access to care for vulnerable populations. This type of local advocacy requires a leader or leaders to emerge to maintain the momentum needed to address the issue. This level also includes public health professionals or persons in related organizations who accept responsibility for a particular task and provide the leadership necessary to see it through, regardless of what title they hold.

At every level, it should be obvious that the same characteristics that make people in leadership positions successful also contribute to success of the field and of individuals within the field or the community. Communicating effectively, authentically engaging others, motivating and inspiring, supporting and adapting. These traits and skills are essential if we are going to achieve long-term sustainable health goals.

CHANGE LEADERSHIP

It should be apparent that this style of leadership may be best suited to longer term change management, to culture change, or to a shift in the focus of investments (see also Chapter 11, "Leading Change"). Above all else, effective transformational leadership requires time, which means the leader must have abundant amounts of patience. The faculty and staff of the author's current institution, a school of public health, spent over 3 years deliberating a change in its structure. They began with an analysis of the external environment and a deep examination of how the current college structure was not aligned with the external reality. Following a full faculty retreat, which generated more questions than answers, several months were devoted to open conversations about each question, one per month. The summaries of those conversations were shared with the full faculty at monthly meetings to allow for further engagement. At the end of that period, the faculty voted to adopt several of the resulting recommendations and then formed six workgroups to address outstanding issues on which consensus could not be achieved. These were also reported to the faculty at monthly meetings. While the departmental structure was being debated, faculty took it upon themselves to re-examine the faculty assembly structure and asked the dean's office to do the same for the college administrative offices. Over the years that it took for these conversations to take place, all policies and procedures were intentionally scrutinized, seeking every way possible to maximize faculty time for creative pursuits. When the final vote was taken, over 3 years after the conversation was begun, the college had eliminated departments, streamlined the dean's office, consolidated faculty assembly committees from seven to three, dramatically changed the composition of the College Executive Committee, changed the staffing structure, and eliminated many unnecessary processes that took up time but added no value.[13] While not perfect, criticisms have been few, and the college continues to recruit outstanding faculty, staff, and students to the College. Contrast that with the experience of coming to work one day to be presented with a new organization chart that eliminates your division or has you reporting to a completely different person. The time it takes to engage not only provides a better product but enlists the community in owning the process and the result.

COLLECTIVE IMPACT

This style of leadership is also essential in working toward collective impact.[14] The concept of collective impact arose in the nonprofit community as an approach that seeks to bring all the available resources to bear on a problem, rather than relying on individual organizations to address the problem independently. Such an approach can be effective, bringing together like-focused organizations—for instance, multiple food banks—to devise a plan to gather more available food and distribute it to more people through an organized effort. But it can also be helpful in addressing multiple factors that each contribute to a problem. The Hillsborough County Health Care Plan (HCHCP),[15] a sales-tax funded health insurance program for low-income adults in Tampa, Florida, has as its primary goal to provide access to quality healthcare for persons who have no other access to health insurance coverage. But the program has achieved greater success by partnering with other governmental and nongovernmental organizations to address the factors that make accessing care difficult, such as transportation, and the factors that contribute to poor health, like housing, paying utility bills, job training, and childcare. "Collective impact" increases the overall yield of individual efforts by magnifying their singular contribution and linking their contributions in a comprehensive approach to solving challenging problems.

TRANSFORMATIONAL LEADERSHIP AND ANTIRACISM

Deeply embedded systems, structures, and policies based on racism are challenging to identify, much less root out. Dismantling these pernicious barriers to health equity will take decades and, of necessity, must involve coalitions working in concert toward shared goals. Leaders with conviction and patience who can sustain the energy it will take to do this work must be able to inspire and motivate others, must trust those with lived experience to chart the course forward, and must build sustainable platforms that support the work and cement the accomplishments so that there is no back-sliding. A quote attributed to Audre Lorde says, "The master's tools will never dismantle the master's house."[16(p2)] If the jobs in public health and in healthcare are to assure full health for all, opportunities to enjoy the conditions that can make everyone healthy, full access to the goods and services that support a high quality of life, and the elimination of negative social, economic, cultural, political, and moral determinants of health, then there is no choice but to remove the obstacles to health equity, which at their roots were sown in racism. Imagine the effort this work demands.[17–19] Transformation of this magnitude will only be achieved if leaders and leadership organizations come together and actively employ the four behaviors that characterize transformational leadership: inspirational motivation, idealized influence, intellectual stimulation, and individualized consideration. One can also draw a parallel to the levels of leadership discussed earlier. Racism manifests itself at three important levels: individual, institutional, and structural. Positional leaders within institutions have a particular responsibility to authentically and intentionally seek out and address racist policies, procedures, and practices within their institutions. Public health as a leading field must employ its transformational leadership talents in pursuit of structural and systemic racism that perpetuates institutional and societal behavior. And individuals, seeking to lead from wherever they are, must actively educate themselves, reflect on, and modify where necessary their own beliefs, attitudes, and behaviors that may hinder their efforts to address institutional and structural racism.

TRANSFORMATIONAL LEADERSHIP AND VALUES

Are leaders born? Some are, certainly. But they can also be made, by learning the underlying behaviors that lead to success and avoiding those tactics that demoralize a team and stifle creative, committed action. As a final note, though transformational leaders must have conviction, tenacity, and patience, they must also exhibit a high degree of humility and act always within an ethical framework. Every health profession has an established code of ethics, and as the work of public health is in increasingly interprofessional environments, it is important to be well-versed in one's own code of conduct, as well as that of others in the workplace. The values of public health, focused as they are on the quality of life of the entire population, provide an umbrella within which professional standards can be applied. These essential values include social justice and health equity; evidence-based decision-making; accountability and stewardship of the public's trust; transparency; and the personal values of honesty, integrity, and humility. Transformational leaders embody and express these values in everything they do but the most important attribute may be trust. To be effective in fully engaging, motivating, and inspiring others, especially over the long-haul that public health and health system reform demand, transformational leaders must trust and be trustworthy.[5,12]

ASSESSMENT INSTRUMENTS

Perhaps the best-known instrument to assess capacity for transformational leadership is the Multifactor Leadership Questionnaire™ developed by Bernard Bass and Bruce Avolio (copyright 1995).[20] The tool has been extensively validated and used by researchers and those working in leadership development; it is designed to assess various leadership styles, including transformational, transactional, and passive/avoidant styles. A short version (MLQ 5X) helps identify leadership behaviors that have been demonstrated through prior research to be strongly linked to both individual and organizational success. If the reader is interested in this instrument, it can be purchased on the www.mindgarden.com site.

The self-assessment that appears as Appendix 7.1 was developed by Don Clark, who maintains a website (http://nwlink.com/~donclark/index.html) on various topics related to leadership. He offers this tool to help aspiring leaders gauge their general level of preference or comfort with transformational leadership.[21]

SUMMARY

Transformational leadership, as its name implies, requires individuals with the ability to change beliefs, motivations, and what Bennis and Nanus call the "social architecture" of organizations toward systemic change in people, institutions, and systems.[12] Threats to health abound and demand courageous leadership willing to commit to altering upstream social, environmental, political, and moral structures, including racism, that far too often determine the fate of people and communities long before healthcare and public health professionals have a chance to introduce their downstream interventions. Motivation, influence, stimulation, and consideration of everyone working to make the changes necessary to secure better futures for all are the essential roles that leaders in public health and healthcare must embrace. Leaders must devote the time and energy to leading that it requires and leave the management to others. Leaders must connect and build sustainable relationships and partnerships. Leaders must nurture trust and patience within learning organizations. Leaders must seek collective impact and champion collective celebration. Leaders must create agents of social change in order to achieve social justice.

DISCUSSION QUESTIONS

1. Transformational leadership is typically linked to successful long-term change processes. How important is trust in managing and achieving change? Why?

2. Many leaders emphasize strategy and minimize the impact of culture when leading change. Transformational leadership suggests an emphasis on culture is paramount to achieving lasting change. Do you believe one is more important than the other? Can either one be ignored? If you believe both are important, how would you achieve a balance between the two? What attributes of successful transformational leaders might prove most effective?

3. In much of the world, a ministry of health oversees the entire health system, including public health and clinical care strategies to improve population health. In the United States, these two spheres are not so directly connected. Given the clear and compelling evidence in support of addressing social determinants of health, including racism, to achieve population health goals, what advice might you give a healthcare leader regarding their role in transformational leadership at the larger societal level? What advice would you give a public health leader regarding their role in transformational leadership within the healthcare system?

CASE STUDIES

The following two case studies illustrate transformational leadership in action first within a large complex organization and second within a diverse community.

CASE STUDY: AN EPIC TRANSFORMATION

The following case study is derived from the author's interviews with Charles Lockwood, Sidney Fernandes, and Patrick Gall.

The Morsani College of Medicine (MCOM) at the University of South Florida does not own its own hospital, but partners with hospitals and healthcare systems in the

Tampa Bay Region. It's 600+ member University of South Florida Physician's Group (USFPG) works most closely with Tampa General Hospital (TGH), MCOM's primary teaching hospital. In the mid-2000s, USFPG and TGH chose different electronic medical record (EMR) platforms. Changes in the healthcare market that signaled an opportunity for these two entities to clinically integrate highlighted this incompatibility. At the same time, the USFPG was facing a looming deadline to upgrade the existing EMR to accommodate revisions to the International Classification of Diseases (ICD) codes and needed to modernize the system to fully transition to electronic billing. Looking to the future, Dr. Charles Lockwood, dean of MCOM and director of the USFPG, determined that the time was right for USF to transition to Epic, the EMR system used by TGH.

Dr. Lockwood crafted an inspiring vision to guide this work, which needed to be accomplished in record time (7 months versus the recommended 18 months). He placed his trust in his chief information systems officer (CIO) and his chief technology officer (CTO). They in turn encouraged him to form a senior leadership team to guide the effort and, very importantly, to define what "success" would look like. "Tears are not the metric," Sidney Fernandes, CIO, recalls saying. "We need clear metrics of success," and not surprising, the senior leadership team emphasized revenue cycle performance metrics. Patrick Gall, CTO, built a timeline backing into the deadline to adopt ICD-10 codes for billing, and began to form teams working through the various levels of the organization, such that the ultimate decision-makers guiding the work would be those persons closest to it. Each group was given clear guidance on the scope of their decision-making authority, their responsibilities, and the tight timelines they were working under. Each group was afforded trust from the other groups; full transparency and open communications encouraged people to disclose concerns as well as to share ideas.

Provider champions representing every clinical department were motivated by their desire to create a better experience for the patients and their fellow providers. Positive experiences in these areas would lead to better documentation, which would support a transition to a successful electronic billing system. This group was instrumental in guiding the development of the system and then evangelizing it to their peers. A group of "super users," individuals who best understand clinical workflows, was engaged to make sure each aspect of the system would function as intended while achieving desired outcomes and avoiding audit criticisms. This group was trained on the new system first, before the providers were trained, so that there would be built-in back up—"at the elbow support"—when the system went live.

Communication across constituent groups was essential. In addition to several layers of working groups, who enjoyed frequent opportunities to discuss the transition, a series of open lunch and learn sessions was held to engage stakeholders, further inform the system design, and to begin to prepare for the launch.

Knowing the launch had to go as smoothly as possible, a central command center was formed with a unique phone number and additional response capabilities. IT staff were on hand in the clinics, very visible in special colored polo shirts. This not only made them easy to identify when a problem arose but provided tangible visible evidence that the commitment to provide support was being fully honored. Finally, the team advocated that resources be set aside to support what they called "provider workflow optimization," or adjustments after the launch, based on lived experience. Rather than invest only in the development and the launch, senior leadership recognized the need to continue to invest to make sure the performance metrics were achieved, the system worked as intended, and that the ultimate users were comfortable with and confident in the new system.

This case study highlights the importance of the four distinct behaviors of transformational leadership. First, Dr. Charles J. Lockwood, MCOM dean and chief of USFPG, made the case for change through departmental, departmental chair and faculty council meetings, town halls, and the USFPG executive council. He repeatedly pointed out that while this change would be difficult, failure to change would be far worse. He noted that the existing EMR system was an ambulatory-only product that did not cover impatient services at TGH, thus limiting providers' ability to provide seamless care and follow-up. It did not allow for electronic charge capture or integrated billing, driving up accounts receivable (AR) and driving down USFPG's net collection rate. The Epic EMR would allow USF to capture federal funding from the federal HITECH act's meaningful use provisions and would facilitate the imminent transition to ICD-10 coding. Epic would also provide a much richer dataset (electronic data warehouse) for clinical research, quality improvement, and patient safety efforts. Finally, this transition was strongly supported by TGH, which could provide financial support under the "safe harbor" provisions of the HITECH act. Thus, the transition would result in receiving a world class EMR at bargain pricing and significant cost-savings.

Second, Dr. Lockwood possesses a high degree of both passion and integrity, which gives him authenticity. As a practicing physician himself, he could empathize with his colleagues but also set the behavioral expectation. He remained engaged, meeting regularly with constituent groups to "cheer them on." The USF CIO partnered with the TGH CIO to make sure everyone in their various roles within each organization understood the transition, had input into its design, and could voice any concerns or ideas at any time. They had social capital that they could expend within their organizations, but also supported each other, not only facilitating the transition but further solidifying the working relationship between the two entities.

Third, the amount of latitude Dr. Lockwood afforded the working groups and the IT experts may have seemed risky but it paid off. He understood that it was his job to clearly articulate the vision and to be focused on the outcome, not on the process. He trusted the process and those leading it, and never wavered in providing his full support to either, even when the going got rough (which it will in a transition of this magnitude).

Fourth, though the effort was being undertaken at the level of the system, the change impacted individuals across job categories. From physicians, to nurses, to pharmacists, to medical records clerks, coders and billers, everyone had a stake in this process and in assuring an optimal outcome. A great deal of thought and effort went into building steering committees and identifying the "champions" who actively promoted awareness, engagement, and morale. By creating a shared leadership model that encouraged transparent communication, every individual had an opportunity to be heard and to support the effort. "All of us are smarter than any one of us at any given point in time," says Patrick Gall, CTO. "This effort succeeded because everyone checked their egos at the door and worked within a culture of trust to get this job done in record time."

For more information: https://health.usf.edu

CASE STUDY QUESTIONS

1. The change to a new EMR system was complex and significant. Can you identify how the four behaviors of transformational leadership were operationalized?
2. Given the strict timeline imposed for this effort, wouldn't a more traditional transactional leadership approach have made more sense? Can you think of any unintended consequences of a transactional approach?
3. Which aspects of transformational leadership were most important in completing the project in record time?
4. How important was the element of trust in this project? Who trusted? Who earned trust?

CASE STUDY: TRANSFORMING COMMUNITY-DRIVEN COVID MITIGATION THROUGH A RACE EQUITY FRAMEWORK

The following case study is derived from the author's interviews with Randall Russell and Carl R. Lavender.

The Foundation for a Healthy St. Petersburg was formed as a health conversion foundation in 2013 upon the sale of nonprofit Bayfront Hospital to a for-profit corporation. The assets were sizable for a community the size of St. Petersburg, Florida, and the visionaries that shaped the Foundation saw an opportunity to address population health on a grand scale with the luxury of being able to commit to a long-term strategy to address the systemic contributors to poor health, including systemic racism. The mission of the Foundation, simply put, is to achieve health equity through race equity.

With a mission that significant and that bold, the Foundation has thoughtfully and intentionally created opportunities to promote success through a social change approach that depends on a transformational leadership style, not just in the CEO but in the entire organization. Listening with intention; engaging with authenticity; building relationships with grassroots, grass-tops, and systems-level leaders; leveraging the power of social institutions including government, the media, the business community, and the faith community; nurturing trust; creating data dashboards to promote accountability; and communicating an inspiring vision have been the hallmarks of the Foundation and its work.

Having established the Foundation as an activist philanthropy with a race equity mission, embedded in and responsive to the community, it was well-positioned to apply the principles of transformational leadership in guiding a COVID-19 mitigation strategy to the benefit of the local BIPOC (Black, Indigenous, and Persons of Color) community. One element of this strategy forms the basis of this case study.

When the availability of federal Coronavirus Aid, Relief and Economic Security (CARES) Act money was announced, Foundation staff immediately contacted the county administrator to suggest that because of the disproportionate impact of COVID-19 on the BIPOC community, the county needed to adopt a new strategy to deploy these resources to best use. In the past, the county would have issued a request for proposal (RFP) and the funds would have gone to the usual suspect agencies, the ones with seasoned grant-writing teams. Instead, the county allowed the Foundation to form a coalition to direct where and to what efforts the money would be allocated and agreed to set aside

$33 million of the $137 million available exclusively for nonprofit organizations. The coalition included government leaders, faith leaders, community advocates, healthcare providers, other philanthropies, and charitable organizations. They developed the criteria and reviewed the requests, many of which came from small nonprofits that served vulnerable communities but were unfamiliar to county leaders; all monies were distributed by the Pinellas County Community Foundation, which was reimbursed by the county from the CARES fund. Also, for the first time, a revolving loan fund was established to advance capital to the deep-rooted smaller nonprofits to make sure they had equal opportunity to access funds. All of this required a high degree of trust among people and entities with already established relationships and a willingness to work cooperatively.

This same level of trust was evident when the county office of the Florida Department of Health called to ask for advice on where to locate vaccination sites and the Foundation was able to offer its Center for Health Equity, located in a predominantly BIPOC community, for the purpose. This same relationship allowed the Foundation to share data and information publicly through its Equity Atlas dashboard and to be a voice not just for the BIPOC community, but for the entire county on public health policy matters including mask mandates, school openings, and the distribution of resources. Relationships with the faith-based community based on a shared understanding of how BIPOC communities learn, engage, and galvanize enabled the Foundation to persuade many churches to stop meeting in person, even on Easter Sunday, despite huge pressure on these same churches to provide succor and places for human connection.

The patience and persistence demonstrated by the Foundation since its founding created the building blocks on which a new kind of response could be implemented in real-time to assure typically marginalized populations, also at higher risk, would not be left behind in the pandemic. Key transformational leadership tools including the effective communication of a motivating vision, the engagement of those who do the work to create the success, and the ability to rely on relationships built on trust and mutual accountability allowed the Foundation for a Healthy St. Petersburg to provide critical leadership in a time of crisis. Going forward, the Foundation intends to codify these learnings in new systems and structures that reflect the power of transformation in saving lives and building communities.

For more information: https://healthystpete.foundation

CASE STUDY QUESTIONS

1. What would you say was the inspirational motivation of the Foundation that enabled this opportunity to be realized?

2. Can you identify or surmise how the other three behaviors of transformational leadership were employed in this effort?

3. The need to act quickly when these funds became available required a high degree of cooperation among a variety of players. How important were relationships in achieving the aims of this effort, that is, in securing dedicated funds for BIPOC communities?

4. Although the securing of these dedicated funds happened relatively quickly, what about this case illustrates the importance of patience in transformational leadership?

A robust set of instructor resources designed to supplement this text is located at http://connect.springerpub.com/content/book/978-0-8261-4924-4. Qualifying instructors may request access by emailing **textbook@springerpub.com.**

REFERENCES

1. Leadership-central.com. Leadership theories. www.leadership-central.com/leadership-theories .html#axzz4oysDbIEs

2. Burns JM. *Leadership*. Harper Collins; 1978.

3. Bass B. *Leadership and Performance*. Free Press; 1985.

4. Odumeru JA, Ogbonna IG. Transformational vs. transactional leadership theories: evidence in literature. *Int Rev Manag Business Res*. 2013;2(2):355–361. https://www.irmbrjournal.com/papers/1371451049. pdf

5. Podsakoff PM, MacKenzie SB, Moorman RH, Fetter R. Transformational leader behaviors and their effect on followers' trust in leaders, satisfaction, and organizational citizenship behaviors. *Leadersh Q*. 1990;1(2):107–142. doi:10.1016/1048-9843(90)90009-7

6. Warrilow S. Transformational leadership theory–the 4 key components in leading change and managing change. https://ezinearticles.com/?Transformational-Leadership-Theory---The-4-Key -Components-in-Leading-Change-and-Managing-Change&id=2755277

7. Bass BM, Avolio BJ. *Improving Organizational Effectiveness Through Transformational Leadership*. Sage; 1994.

8. Bass B. *The Handbook of Leadership: Theory, Research, and Managerial Applications*. 4th ed. Free Press; 2008.

9. Goldberg MC. Reciprocal leaders get what they give. *Cape Cod Times*. July 4, 2021.

10. Institute of Medicine. *The Future of Public Health*. National Academy of Sciences; 1998.

11. Kurz RS, Yager C, Yager JD, Foster A, Breidenbach D, Irwin Z. Advancing the certified in public health examination: a job task analysis. *Public Health Rep*. 2017;132(4):518–523. doi:10.1177/0033354917710015

12. Bennis W, Nanus B. *Leaders: Strategies for Taking Charge*. 2nd ed. Collins Business Essentials; 2007.

13. Petersen DJ. Form follows function: a new structure for a school of public health in the 21st century. *J Public Health Manag Pract*. 2021;28(2):E324–E332. doi:10.1097/PHH.0000000000001350

14. Collective Impact Forum. 2014. https://www.collectiveimpactforum.org/what-collective-impact

15. Hillsborough County Health Care Plan. 2021. https://www.hillsboroughcounty.org/residents/ social-services/health-care-plan

16. Lorde A. The masters tools will never dismantle the master's house. 1984. https://collectiveliberation .org/wp-content/uploads/2013/01/Lorde_The_Masters_Tools.pdf

17. WHO Commission on Social Determinants of Health. Closing the gap in a generation: health equi- ty through action on the social determinants of health [Internet]. World Health Organization; 2008. https://apps.who.int/iris/bitstream/handle/10665/43943/9789241563703_eng.pdf

18. Galea S. *Well: What We Need to Talk About When We Talk About Health*. Oxford University Press; 2019.

19. Berwick DM. The moral determinants of health. *JAMA*. 2020;324(3):225–226. doi:10.1001/ jama.2020.11129

20. Bass BM, Avolio BJ. Multifactor Leadership Questionnaire (MLQ). *APA PsycTests*. doi:10.1037/t03624-000

21. Clark DR. Transformational leadership survey. 2011. http://www.nwlink.com/~donclark/leader/ transformational_survey.html

APPENDIX 7.1: TRANSFORMATIONAL LEADERSHIP SURVEY

Using the following scale, check the box to the right of each statement that you believe comes closest to your level of proficiency and comfort.

Scale: 1 = rarely; 2 = sometimes; 3 = often; 4 = almost always

ITEM #	ITEM	1	2	3	4
1	I go out of the way to make others feel good around me.				
2	I help others with their self-development.				
3	I help others to understand my vision through the use of tools, such as images, stories, and models.				
4	I ensure others get recognition and/or rewards when they achieve difficult or complex goals.				
5	I let others work in the manner they want.				
6	I get things done.				
7	I have an ever-expanding network of people who trust and rely upon me.				
8	I provide challenges for my team members to help them grow.				
9	I use simple words, images, and symbols to convey to others what we should or could be doing.				
10	I manage others by setting standards that we all agree with.				
11	I rarely give direction or guidance to others if I sense they can achieve their goals.				
12	I consistently provide coaching and feedback so that my team members know how they are doing.				
13	People listen to my ideas and concerns not out of fear, but because of my skills, knowledge, and personality.				
14	I provide an empathetic shoulder when others need help.				
15	I help others with new ways of looking at new and complex ideas or concepts.				
16	I ensure poor performance is corrected.				
17	As long as things are going smoothly, I am satisfied.				
18	I monitor all projects that I am in charge of to ensure the team meets its goals.				

Scoring

This survey measures your leadership skills on six factors: Charisma, Social, Vision, Transactional, Delegation, and Execution. Each factor is measured by three questions as shown in the text that follows. Your score is determined by adding your three scores together for each factor in the following chart. Note that the lowest score you can get for each factor is 3, while the highest score is 12.

Strength and Weakness Chart for Transformational Leadership Factors
Charisma (questions 1, 7, 13) Total_____
Social (questions 2, 8, 14) Total_____
Vision (questions 3, 9, 15) Total_____
Transactional (questions 4, 10, 16) Total_____
Delegation (questions 5, 11, 17) Total_____
Execution (questions 6, 12, 18) Total_____
Total the scores and enter the number here _____. The highest score possible is 72, while the lowest possible score is 18.

As noted earlier, there are no correct answers. However, this survey gives you an idea of what transactional leadership factors you might be more comfortable with and the ones you might be less comfortable with. Generally, a score of about 54 or higher means that you are well on your way to becoming a transformational leader.

The highest scoring factors in the previous chart are your stronger leadership factors, while the lower scoring factors are your weaker ones. You should spend some time reflecting and then taking action on the factors you score 9 or less on. To help you, look for opportunities to increase your knowledge and skills with the following factors:

■ **Charisma** (questions 1, 7, 13): You are a role model that shows true dedication, trust, and respect to others, who in turn do the same to you.

■ **Social** (questions 2, 8, 14): You help others to learn by coaching and mentoring them. You create challenging environments to help them reach their full potential. When others have difficulties, you are not afraid to empathize with them and help guide them.

■ **Vision** (questions 3, 9, 15): You provide challenging visions and help people to understand them so that they are motivated to join in.

■ **Transactional** (questions 4, 10, 16): You ensure others understand what you expect from them by using mutual agreement. In addition, you ensure that if poor performance does occur, you take action to ensure it does not affect the moral of the team.

■ **Delegation** (questions 5, 11, 17): You delegate both the task and the authority to get things accomplished.

■ **Execution** (questions 6, 12, 18): While you should delegate as many tasks as possible with the authority to accomplish them, as a good steward of the organization's resources, you should also follow-up to ensure things are going as planned.

(*Source*: Don Clarke, http://nwlink.com/~donclark/index.html)

Chapter 8

Authentic Leadership

Paul C. Erwin, Stephanie B. C. Bailey, and Susan C. Helm-Murtagh

INTRODUCTION

This above all: to thine own self be true,
And it must follow, as the night the day,
Thou canst not then be false to any man.

   Hamlet. Act 1 Scene 3. William Shakespeare.

Authentic leadership centers on the genuineness of the leader being true to themselves and to their followers through self-awareness, transparency, and self-regulation. First formally described in the academic literature by Henderson and Hoy in 1983, authentic leadership was popularized by former Medtronic CEO Bill George in his 2003 book, *Authentic Leadership: Rediscovering the Secrets to Creating Lasting Value.*[1,2] Its popularity was propelled in part by several corporate scandals (e.g., Enron and WorldCom) because such experiences were seen as the antithesis of authenticity—the opposite of authentic leadership is leadership that is spurious, a sham, or a counterfeit. In that light, authentic leadership has also taken on a moral or ethical quality. It is the leadership approach most frequently chosen by students in a graduate-level public health leadership course at the Gillings School of Global Public Health at the University of North Carolina as the foundation for their leadership practice, in part because of its simplicity, its attractiveness at face value, and its applicability across a range of work settings (see Chapter 21, "Creating Your Leadership Framework").

OBJECTIVES

By the end of this chapter, the reader will be able to:

- Understand the definition of authentic leadership.
- Describe the conceptual framework of authentic leadership.
- Relate the development of authentic leadership theories and models with its popular treatment in leadership books.
- Describe the use of authentic leadership in public health and healthcare settings.
- Utilize instruments and tools to assess one's own capacity for authentic leadership.

TERMINOLOGY AND BACKGROUND

"Authenticity" refers to the quality or state of being authentic, reliable, and genuine, with synonyms of true, actual, and original.[3] "Authentic" is derived from the Greek *"authentikos,"* which has its own origin in the ancient Greek *"authentes,"* for "one acting on its own authority," a joining of two words: *"autos"* (self) and *"hentes"* (doer, being).[4] Early writers on authenticity connected it to the Greek aphorism "Know Thyself," which is one of three maxims inscribed in the forecourt of the Temple of Apollo at Delphi.[5] As a philosophical construct, the processes related to authenticity have attempted to show "how people discover and construct a core sense of self, and how this core self is maintained across situations and over time."[6(p1121)] According to Kernis and Goldman, "authentic functioning is characterized in terms of people's (1) self-understanding, (2) openness to objectively recognizing their ontological realities (e.g., evaluating their desirable and undesirable self-aspects), (3) actions, and (4) orientation towards interpersonal relationships."[7(p284)] Avolio et al. defined authentic leaders as "those individuals who are deeply aware of how they think and behave and are perceived by others as being aware of their own and others' values/moral perspective, knowledge, and strengths; aware of the context in which they operate; and who are confident, hopeful, optimistic, resilient, and high on moral character."[8(pp802-804)]

The academic and popular development of authentic leadership takes these philosophical constructs of authenticity and attempts to build theories and models within the context of leadership. Work that pre-dated Henderson and Hoy's 1983 article on authentic leadership focused first on how an organization's authenticity manifested in its leadership.[9] Henderson and Hoy's initial definition of authentic leadership contained elements of both the leader and the organization: the authentic leader is one who (a) accepts personal and organizational responsibility for actions, outcomes, and mistakes; (b) does not manipulate subordinates; and (c) manifests the prominence of the self (as in being true to oneself).[1] Luthans and Avolio defined authentic leadership "as a process that draws from both positive psychological capacities and a highly developed organizational context, which results in both greater self-awareness and self-regulated positive behaviors on the part of leaders and associates, fostering positive self-development."[10(p243)] Gardner et al. build further on this definition by describing authentic leadership first as a leader achieving authenticity through self-awareness, self-acceptance, and authentic actions and relationships.[11] Furthermore, "authentic leadership extends beyond the authenticity of the leader as a person to encompass authentic relations with followers and associates. These relationships are characterized by (a) transparency, openness, and trust; (b) guidance toward worthy objectives, and (c) an emphasis on follower development."[11(p345)] In subsequent work involving Gardner, Avolio, and others, Walumbwa et al. have defined authentic leadership as "a pattern of leader behavior that draws upon and promotes both positive psychological capacities and a positive ethical climate, to foster greater self-awareness, an internalized moral perspective, balanced processing of information, and relational transparency on the part of leaders working with followers, fostering positive self-development."[12(p94)]

Bill George's popular book, *Authentic Leadership: Rediscovering the Secrets to Creating Lasting Value,* is less concerned with presenting formal definitions of authentic leadership and instead focuses on what authentic leaders *are* and what they *do*: authentic leaders are people of highest integrity, committed to building enduring organizations; they have a deep sense of purpose and are true to their core values; they have the courage to build their organizations in ways that meet the needs of all stakeholders; and they recognize the importance of their service to society.[2]

In the following sections, authentic leadership will be explored first through theories and models most prevalent in the academic literature, and second through the popular writings of Bill George and others.

THEORIES AND MODELS

THE ACADEMIC PERSPECTIVE

According to Luthans and Avolio, the theoretical foundations of authentic leadership can be located within Positive Organization Behavior (POB) and Transformational/Full-Range Leadership (FRL).[10] POB stems from the positive psychology movement of the late 1990s and early 2000s, which focuses more on what is right with people and organizations and building on those strengths, rather than being preoccupied with what is wrong and focusing on weaknesses.[10] Germane to public health, the positive psychology movement also influenced the development of community assessment and planning approaches that focus more on identifying and maximizing a community's assets, rather than focusing (exclusively) on their needs (i.e., what they lack). POB draws directly from the field of positive psychology and can be defined as "the study and application of positively oriented human resource strengths and psychological capacities that can be measured, developed, and effectively managed for performance improvement in today's workplace."[13(p59)] The POB capacities (as opposed to inherent traits) of confidence, hope, optimism, and resiliency become the antecedents in the model of authentic leadership shown in Figure 8.1.

While POB serves as the basis for antecedents, FRL "provides the context, leader characteristics, and ethical/moral theoretical foundation" for authentic leadersip.[10(p246)] In the FRL model, as developed by Bass and Avolio,[14] transformational leadership comprises the highest degree of leadership engagement and efficiency across the three leadership elements, with the other two being Laissez-Faire leadership and Transactional Leadership. Authentic leadership builds on but goes beyond FRL: authentic leaders "transcend their self-interest because they are guided by something more important than self-interest, which is to be consistent with their high-end values, which were shaped and developed across a leader's lifespan. Such development centers in part on building the moral capacity of leaders to be able to make 'selfless' judgments."[10(p247-8)] Merging POB and FRL, Luthans and Avolio proposed an initial model of authentic leadership as shown in Figure 8.1.

In the model, life experiences give rise to, or create, the milieu for the positive psychological capacities of confidence, hope, optimism, and resiliency. A highly developed organization is the positive organizational corollary to the individual leader's positive psychological capacities. Trigger events and challenges can be positively promoted through a highly developed

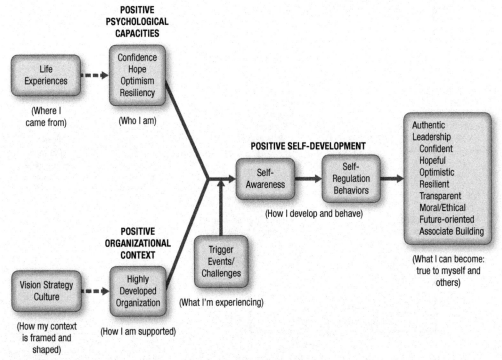

FIGURE 8.1: Authentic Leadership Development Model.
Source: Reproduced with permission from Luthans F, Avolio BJ. Authentic leadership development. In: Cameron KS, Dutton JE, Quinn RE, eds. *Positive Organizational Scholarship*. Berrett-Koehler; 2003;241–258.

organizational context and culture for leadership development. These antecedents set the stage for positive self-development through self-awareness and self-regulation. Self-awareness is critical in the context of change—"if the target leader for development is not aware of areas [they] can self-reinforce and strengthen, then little or no energy will be allocated to the task of development."[10(p257)]

Gardner et al. subsequently proposed a "self-based model of authentic leader and follower development" (Figure 8.2).[11] The central concept is that through increased self-awareness, self-regulation, and positive modeling, authentic leaders foster the development of authenticity in followers. In turn, followers' authenticity contributes to their well-being and the attainment of sustainable and veritable performance.[15]

In its most recent formulation by Gardner et al., drawing on the work of Kernis, authentic leadership comprises (a) self-awareness; (b) relational transparency; (c) balanced processing; and (d) internalized moral perspective.[16,17] The theoretical foundations for the Gardner et al. model are in the literature on the self and identity, which is reflected in the fundamental notion of authenticity as being true to oneself. Personal history comprises the unique life experiences that are described in the model, and may include family influences, early role models, and educational and work experiences.[11] Trigger events are the "catalysts for heightened levels of leader self-awareness and can be either perceived positively or negatively";[11(p347)] these can be subtle or dramatic changes in the leader's circumstances that (in a positivist context) allow for personal growth and development. By continuously asking the question "Who am I?" authentic leaders develop a high level of self-awareness that allows them to be in sync with their core values, identity, emotions, motives, and goals. Self-awareness is one of two critical factors in the development of authentic leadership, with the other one being self-regulation.

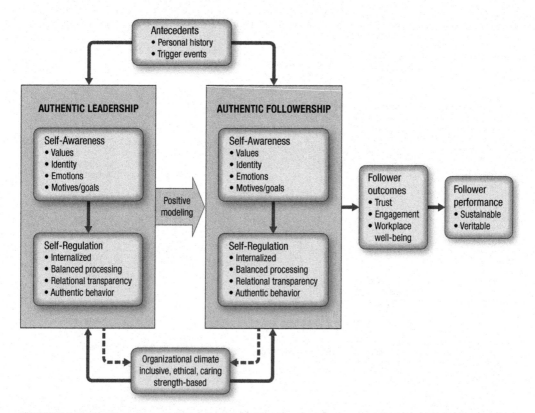

FIGURE 8.2: The Conceptual Framework for Authentic Leader and Follower Development.
Source: Reproduced with permission from Gardner WL, Avolio BJ, Luthans F, May DR, Walumbwa F. "Can you see the real me?" A self-based model of authentic leader and follower development. *Leadersh Q.* 2005;16(3):343–372. doi:10.1016/j.leaqua.2005.03.003

The "internalized" aspect of self-regulation is meant to reflect the leader's internal drive that shapes regulation, as opposed to responding to external forces. Balanced processing is the act of collecting and interpreting self-related information in as unbiased a process as possible. Originally labeled "unbiased processing," this aspect of self-regulation requires a fair and objective collection and interpretation of information, while realizing that no one is completely free of bias. Relational transparency reflects openness and honesty in relationships, especially in conveying one's true self to others. This may include both positive and negative attributes of the leader. Finally, authentic behavior "refers to the actions that are guided by the leader's true self as reflected by core values, beliefs, thoughts and feelings, as opposed to environmental contingencies or pressures from others."[11(p347)] For Gardner, "authenticity and authentic leadership are aspirational endeavors whereby one strives to be one's best self at work."[16(p5)]

While the models presented in Figures 8.1 and 8.2 are focused on authentic leadership *development*, a slightly earlier (2004) model from Avolio et al. proposed the relationship between authentic leaders and follower attitudes and behaviors.[8] In other words, the former models focus on *how* a person develops and becomes an authentic leader, whereas the latter is about *what* authentic leaders do and the impact they have. This model is presented in Figure 8.3.

Followers must first resonate with the authentic leader on a personal level, as authentic leaders lead by example. By creating a deeper sense of high moral values, honesty, and integrity, authentic leaders increase followers' social identification. The three constructs that are most important for developing lasting relationships and influencing followers' behaviors are hope, trust, and positive emotions. Followers must be able to see *their* hopes reflected in the authentic leader's goals. Trust is established when the authentic leader is able to be transparent in conveying their attitudes, values, aspirations, and weaknesses to followers. Authentic leaders are able to connect with followers' emotions in ways that can alter followers' behaviors and attitudes. Through instilling hope, trust, and positive emotions, authentic leaders create a sense of optimism in followers. Such optimism influences the followers' levels of commitment, job satisfaction, meaningfulness, and engagement. A follower with higher levels of these attitudes is more likely to be a higher performer, willing to extend extra efforts, and less likely to exhibit the "withdrawal" behaviors of turnover, tardiness, and absenteeism.[8]

Subsequent scholarship on authentic leadership focused on both authentic leadership development and how authentic leaders actually influence followers' behaviors and attitudes and the impact this has on personal and organizational performance. The advances in scholarship since these theories and models were proposed are presented in a later section of this chapter.

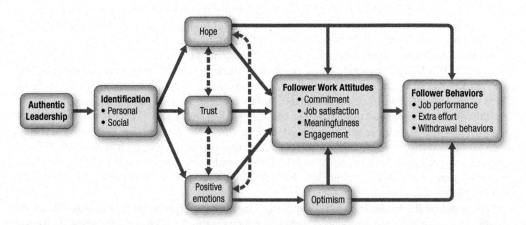

FIGURE 8.3: A Proposed Framework Linking Authentic Leadership to Followers' Attitudes and Behaviors.

Source: Reproduced with permission from Avolio BJ, Gardner WL, Walumbwa FO, Luthans F, May DR. Unlocking the mask: a look at the process by which authentic leaders impact follower attitudes and behaviors. *Leadersh Q.* 2004;15(6):801–823. doi:10.1016/j.leaqua.2004.09.003

THE POPULAR PERSPECTIVE: BILL GEORGE

Bill George, CEO of Medtronic (a Minnesota-based medical technology company) from 1991 to 2003, is credited with popularizing the concept of authentic leadership in practice. His 2003 book, *Authentic Leadership: Rediscovering the Secrets to Creating Lasting Value*, came out in the wake of several high visibility corporate scandals (including Enron) and was largely viewed as the antidote to the leader as scam artist. George pushed to have leaders (current and aspiring) critically evaluate their roles in business and in life, noting that a moral/ethical standard is of utmost importance to leadership. In his observation, corporate leaders were giving in to power and greed. George observed that examples of corruption, including corporate bailouts, abuse of power, financial mishaps, and fraud, captured in media and various publications, were indeed reflective of both the character of the leadership and of the corporate values. Such examples of corporate and political corruption created a groundswell from the public for increased integrity, transparency, accountability, and authenticity in leadership as well as an insertion of a moral compass in order to restore trust.

George is less concerned with definitions of authentic leadership, preferring to describe the characteristics of authentic leaders and what they do. This is also captured in his 2008 interview with the *Harvard Business Review*:

> *Authentic leaders have a deep sense of purpose for their leadership and are true to their core values. They are people of the highest integrity who are committed to building enduring organizations. Authentic leaders see themselves as stewards of the assets they inherit and servants of all their stakeholders. They lead with their hearts, not just their heads, yet they have the self-discipline to produce consistently strong results.*[18]

George's conceptualization of authentic leadership comprises five dimensions, or qualities, that authentic leaders demonstrate, as he has determined through his many experiences in leading others:[2]

1. Understanding their (i.e., the leader's own) purpose
2. Practicing solid values
3. Leading with heart
4. Establishing connected relationships
5. Demonstrating self-discipline

For each of these dimensions, George describes a developmental quality that is necessary for authentic leaders to be effective. These dimensions and developmental qualities are shown in Figure 8.4, George's model for authentic leadership. The five dimensions are located in the inner circle, while the authentic leader's developmental qualities, or characteristics, associated with each of these dimensions are located in the outer circle.

For George, leadership begins with asking a fundamental question: "Leadership for what purpose?"[2] If a leader does not know their own purpose for leading, why would anyone want to follow? The authenticity aspect of this dimension is that the purpose must truly be one's own, not a borrowed or even aspirational purpose that belongs to someone else. Without this genuine, *understanding their (i.e., the leader's own) purpose*, "leaders are at the mercy of their egos and are vulnerable to narcissistic impulses."[2(p19)] Passion for the purpose comes from being "highly motivated by your work because you believe in its intrinsic worth, and you can use your abilities to maximum effect."[2(p37)] Understanding oneself is the prerequisite to knowing one's purpose – this is akin to the self-awareness in the Gardner model described earlier (Figure 8.2).

Values define the leader's moral compass in George's experience, the deep sense of knowing the difference between wrong and right *and* acting on this. It is the act—the actual behavior of the authentic leader—when tested in the "crucibles of life's experiences" that distinguishes this type of leader. It is being true to one's values in practice that matters most. The one value that is required above all others for the authentic leader is integrity—"not just the absence of lying, but telling the whole truth."[2(p20)] Without values, without integrity, there is no trust,

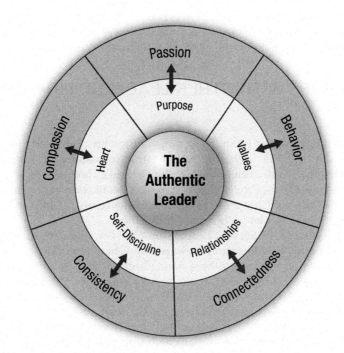

FIGURE 8.4: Bill George's Authentic Leadership Dimensions and Characteristics.
Source: Reproduced with permission from George B. *Authentic Leadership: Rediscovering the Secrets to Creating Lasting Value.* Jossey-Bass; 2003.

and, as with the absence of purpose, without trust why would anyone ever follow the leader? *Practicing solid values* resonates with both the moral/ethical elements of the Luthans and Avolio model (see Figure 8.1) as well as the internalized moral perspective of Gardner et al. (see Figure 8.2).

Authentic leaders truly care about their employees—*leading with the heart* is leading with empathy and compassion. This dimension, perhaps above the others, is one that must be visibly genuine—employees can detect fake or empty expressions of caring and empathy before the "leader" finishes the sentence. The "proof is in the pudding": leading with the heart is an act of doing, it is truly "walking the talk." Passion in the purpose, without *com*passion, does not build followership. In the model of Gardner et al., caring is both a positivist aspect of relational transparency for the authentic leader and a positive attribution of the organization (organizational caring) in which an authentic leader thrives.

George quotes the Indian philosopher Jiddu Krishnamurti in describing the importance of *establishing enduring relationships*: "Relationship is the mirror in which we see ourselves."[2(p23)] For George, employees in today's organizations demand a more personal relationship with their leader, not a detached one, and the authentic leader is one who has the capacity to develop enduring, trusted, caring relationships. Through such deeply connected relationships, Krishnamurti's mirror reflects the "true self I can become" in the Luthans and Avolio model. This dimension of authentic leadership is also a part of the relational transparency in the Gardner et al. model.

Although George includes *demonstrating self-discipline* as the fifth dimension of authentic leadership, its importance is viewed only on a grand scale: "authentic leaders must have the self-discipline to do everything they can to demonstrate their values through their actions."[2(p24)] This self-discipline must be manifested consistently, across time, place, and context. George attains that self-discipline through consistent practices of meditation and regular exercise—keeping both the mind and body fit—as well as balanced nutrition and adequate sleep. Teaching the body and mind through these consistent practices allows the authentic leader to build the self-discipline that is necessary to function across a plethora of challenges. Self-discipline equates to the self-regulation that is present in both of the academia models of authentic leaders described earlier (see Figures 8.1 and 8.2).

RELATIONSHIPS WITH OTHER LEADERSHIP THEORIES AND MODELS

Authentic leadership has most often been compared to and contrasted with several other positivist leadership theories, including servant, transformational, charismatic, spiritual, and ethical leadership, as well as emotional intelligence (EI). Three are discussed briefly here; however, each of these theories are explored in greater detail elsewhere in this textbook. For additional information, see Chapter 5, "Emotional Intelligence," Chapter 7, "Transformational Leadership," and Chapter 9, "Servant Leadership."

As described in Chapter 9, "Servant Leadership," the key characteristics of servant leadership include empathy, listening, and stewardship. The hallmark of servant leadership is putting followers first—serving others—and through this, followers in turn become servant-leaders. Authentic leaders also focus on followers; Avolio and Gardner go so far as to state that "one of the central premises of authentic leadership development is that both leaders and followers are developed over time as the relationship between them becomes more authentic."[15(p327)] Follower outcomes and performance are both important constructs in the Gardner et al. model. In both servant and authentic leadership there is the recognition, either implicitly or explicitly, of leader self-awareness and regulation.[15] The two leadership theories are also similar in having an explicit moral dimension.[19] Avolio and Gardner contend, however, that leader awareness, empathy, and vision in authentic leadership have a stronger grounding in theoretical constructs compared to servant leadership, and are supported through empirical research.[15]

In the academic leadership literature, authentic leadership was initially described as a subtype of transformational leadership.[20] Avolio et al. "consider authentic leadership as a root construct that can incorporate transformational and ethical leadership."[8(pp805–806)] As noted earlier, the theoretical foundations of authentic leadership are in the FRL model, where transformational leadership comprises the highest degree of leadership engagement and efficiency.[14] The four components of transformational leadership, as described in Chapter 7, "Transofrmational Leadership," are:

- charisma or idealized influence
- inspirational motivation
- intellectual stimulation
- personal and individual attention

Transformational leaders have several characteristics in common with authentic leaders, including being optimistic, hopeful, developmentally oriented, and of high moral character.[15] According to Avolio and Gardner, in order to be viewed as a transformational leader, the leader must be authentic; however, being an authentic leader does not necessarily define one as being transformational.[15] As Avolio and Gardner further contend,

> We believe the key distinction is that authentic leaders are anchored by their own deep sense of self; they know where they stand on important issues, values, and beliefs. With that base they stay their course and convey to others, oftentimes through actions, not just words, what they represent in terms of principles, values, and ethics. Transformational leaders may also have this deep sense of self... or they may be able to transform others and organizations, through a powerful, positive vision, an intellectually stimulating idea, attention to uplifting the needs of followers and by having a clear sense of purpose.[15(p329)]

Although Banks et al. found a strong overlap between authentic and transformational leadership in their meta-analysis (see later), it is curious that in a more recent article on authentic leadership, Gardner (one of the co-authors of the Banks paper) and Karam state that there is very little relationship between transformational and authentic leadership, as the two theoretical constructs were developed independently.[16,21]

As described in Chapter 5, EI is commonly understood as the ability to understand, regulate, and use emotions positively, both one's own and those of others. Among the four main models of EI—the Ability EI Model, the Trait EI Model, the Goleman EI Model, and the Emotional-Social Intelligence Model—the closest resemblance to authentic leadership can be found in Goleman's model. Goleman and his co-authors' model of EI emphasizes five dimensions: self-awareness, self-regulation, motivation, empathy, and social skills.[22] These are similar in nomenclature to the four domains of authentic leadership: self-awareness, balanced processing, relational transparency, and internalized moral perspective. In a recent meta-analysis on EI and authentic leadership, Miao et al. examined three constructs of EI: ability EI, self-report EI, and mixed EI.[23] Ability EI measures are based on the theory that EI is a type of intelligence; self-report EI considers EI as a type of personality trait that should be assessed via self-report; and mixed EI includes self-report measurement items as well as behaviors, skills, and competencies.[23] The meta-analysis found a strong positive correlation between the four dimensions of self-awareness, self-management, social awareness, and so-cial/relationship management in the Goleman EI Model with the dimensions of authentic leadership (self-awareness, balanced processing, relational transparency, and internalized moral perspective). The authors found a stronger relationship between authentic leadership and self-report EI and mixed EI, compared to ability EI, stating that such findings provide stronger support for the trait perspective of EI.[23] In their view, Miao et al. believe that with authentic leadership's influence on workplace outcomes, "organizations should recruit and/or promote emotionally intelligent individuals as leaders because these individuals are capable of using effective leadership styles, such as authentic leadership, to influence their followers and achieve desirable outcomes across individual, group, and organization levels."[23(p687)]

To summarize, Covelli and Mason note that the key differentiating feature of authentic leadership from other forms of (positivist) leadership styles is that a leader may be more or less authentic, while still possessing various characteristics of the other leadership styles. "In other words, a leader may be charismatic but inauthentic or authentic but not charismatic. Nevertheless, the most important element of authentic leadership is not the leader's style and whether he or she is transformational or charismatic or not but rather the extent of their authenticity."[24(p3)]

ADVANCES IN ACADEMIC AND PRACTICE-BASED PERSPECTIVES

THE ACADEMIC PERSPECTIVE

Following a special issue of *The Leadership Quarterly* in 2005 that included several foundational articles, the academic exploration of authentic leadership expanded rapidly. Gardner et al. provided a 2011 review of the literature and research agenda on authentic leadership, identifying 91 publications that focused on authentic leadership.[6] Gardner et al. credit Luthans and Avolio's 2003 conceptualization of authentic leadership (the source of Figure 8.1) for reigniting scholarly interest in authentic leadership. The challenges in understanding the literature are apparent from having no less than 13 definitions of authentic leadership, with nine of those proposed since 2003. Noting only seven publications before 2003, by 2010, the authors included a total of 59 theoretically focused publications, 25 empirical, and seven focused on practitioners. Of the 203 total authors of these 91 publications, 152 (75%) were from the United States, with Canada a distant second at 7.9%. Authors were chiefly affiliated academically with management (65%), business (8.9%), or education (8.4%). The primary purpose of the publications, when clearly stated, was more often on extending and linking authentic leadership theory (75.7%) and less about developing a new theory (9.8%).

Among the small number of articles that focused on antecedents to authentic leadership, the POB states of optimism, resiliency, and hope, and an aggregate measure of psychological capacity were positively related to authentic leadership.[6] There was a much greater focus in the literature reviewed on the outcomes of authentic leadership, ranging from personal and social/organizational identification, to trust in leadership, to follower job satisfaction. Several mediating relationships that were posited by authentic leadership theory were supported empirically, including how the relationship between the follower and the supervisor mediates the outcome of actual work engagement. To further build the evidence-base for authentic leadership, Gardner et al. called for stronger theory building, an expansion of the "nomological network" of authentic leadership (i.e., closing the gaps between the theoretical and empirical frameworks), the use of more rigorous and diverse research methods, attention to authentic followership, and a greater focus on authentic leadership development.

In a 2016 meta-analysis that examined the antecedents, correlates, and consequences of authentic leadership, and compared authentic and transformational leadership, Banks et al. utilized 100 samples from published and unpublished work, involving 24,452 individuals.[21] Key findings of this study included (a) statistically strong and significant relations among the four dimensions of authentic leadership (self-awareness, relational transparency, balanced processing, and internalized moral perspective); (b) strong correlations between authentic leadership and both attitudinal and behavioral outcomes predicted in the models, including job satisfaction, follower satisfaction with the leader, group or organization performance, leader-rated effectiveness, task performance, organizational citizenship behaviors of followers, and organizational commitment; and (c) a statistically strong overlap between authentic and transformational leadership, raising concerns that these are not independent constructs.

While other reviews and meta-analyses have followed (e.g., Hoch et al. and Sidani and Rowe), perhaps the most interesting and enlightening academic examination of authentic leadership appeared as an exchange of letters in *The Leadership Quarterly* between Gardner and Karam with Alvesson and Einola.[16,25,26] This exchange was prompted by an Alvesson and Einola article in 2019, entitled "Warning for Excessive Positivity: Authentic Leadership and Other Traps in Leadership Studies."[27] The gist of this article was to find mainstream authentic leadership theory fundamentally flawed, with "shaky philosophical and theoretical foundations, tautological reasoning, weak empirical studies, nonsensical measurement tools, unsupported knowledge claims, and a generally simplistic and out of date view of corporate life."[27(p383)] The two pairs of authors exchanged a total of four letters, all published as a single article. While there were areas of agreement on both authentic leadership theory as well as measured attributes, ultimately there was more "agree to disagree" in the exchange.

Alvesson and Einola have a fundamental disagreement with the concept of "authentic leadership" as *authentic* and *leadership* are, for them, two distinct phenomena. In the end, in their view, people may act authentically, and may be more or less authentic at work, but not primarily as leaders and followers. To reiterate, this is a terrifically enlightening exchange that goes far beyond academic ivory tower arguments over words, but rather appears to be a valid attempt to probe the true meaning and nature of authentic leadership. The reader can learn much about both authentic leadership as well as the fair and free exchange of ideas, both in agreement and disagreement—how refreshing in the current climate of the politicization of COVID-19.

THE PRACTICE/POPULAR PERSPECTIVE

Bill George followed his highly popular successful book, *Authentic Leadership: Rediscovering the Secrets to Creating Lasting Value* with additional books on authentic leadership, including *True North: Discover Your Authentic Leadership, Finding Your True North: A Personal Guide*, and, most recently, *Discover Your True North*.[2,28–30] The last of these will be the focus of this section.

In *Discover Your True North*, George provided an expanded version of his earlier "True North" books, where he not only circled back to many of the 125 authentic leaders he identified in earlier works, but also included 47 new leaders. George provides no methodological explanation for selecting the leaders that are included in this book. In part one of the book, George examines three topics:

1. Framing one's life story
2. The risk of losing one's way
3. The roles that "crucibles" play in one's leadership

For George, understanding one's life story is the key to being an authentic leader; it is the way to discover one's "true north" (i.e., their moral compass). It is less about the facts of one's life and more about how one understands themselves. This is similar to the most basic dimension of self-awareness in the academic models. The life story evolves as the leader ages into leadership, from preparing for leadership, to leading as leadership experiences accumulate, to *generativity*—actively sharing knowledge and wisdom with the generation of leaders that will follow. Leaders who do not ground themselves in their life stories risk losing their way, by being imposters (lacking self-awareness), rationalizers (deviating from personal values), glory seekers (motivated by acclaim), loners (failing to develop support structure), and shooting stars (rapidly rising and descending).[30] His example of Lance Armstrong's "ruthless quest for glory" may be one of the most recognizable examples of losing one's way. One can surmise that those who "lose their way" have a lack of the self-regulation that is such a prominent feature of the academic models.

In George's experience, most of the leaders interviewed and included in his book were shaped by one or more significant personal trials he terms "crucibles." These can be triggered by negative work experiences such as the loss of a job, or by painful life experiences such as divorce, death of a loved one, or severe personal illness. Such experiences can lead to a re-framing of one's life story.

George's five elements of authentic leadership development in *Discover Your True North* build on his earlier description of the five dimensions of authentic leadership, as shown in Table 8.1. The two descriptions of authentic leadership are mostly similar in George's presentations.

The first two dimensions/elements are identical. The third in the later book—sweet spot—is described by George as "the intersection of your motivations and your greatest strengths."[30(p123)] Whereas "leading with heart" was more about caring and compassion—an external expression of leaders to followers—the sweet spot is more about the internal drive, when what the leader loves doing most is actually what they are best doing. The fourth element—support team—is what one develops through establishing connected relationships. An "integrated life" is mostly about work–life balance, but it is equally concerned with being the same person at home as at work—the authentic self. This requires the fifth dimension from the earlier book—demonstrating self-discipline.

In the final section of the book, George builds on moving the authentic leader from the internally focused dimensions (self-awareness, knowing one's values) to being externally engaged: going from "I" to "We." This transformation allows the authentic leader to fully realize and actualize their purpose: "For you as a leader, your purpose is the way you translate your True North

TABLE 8.1: Dimensions and Elements of Authentic Leadership, Bill George

BOOK	AUTHENTIC LEADERSHIP: REDISCOVERING THE SECRETS TO CREATING LASTING VALUE[2]	DISCOVER YOUR TRUE NORTH[30]
Dimensions	Understanding their (i.e., one's own) purpose	Self-awareness
	Practicing solid values	Values
	Leading with heart	Sweet spot
	Establishing connected relationships	Support team
	Demonstrating self-discipline	Integrated life

Source: Data from George B. *Authentic Leadership: Rediscovering the Secrets to Creating Lasting Value*. Jossey-Bass; 2003; George B. *Discover Your True North*. Jossey-Bass; 2015.

into making a difference in the world."[30(p199)] While George's book does not advance the scholarship on authentic leadership, that is not *his* purpose; the book is more about inspiring the authentic leader (or the authentic leader-to be) as they evolve in their leadership journey. Reading the stories of the likes of Hank Paulson, Oprah Winfrey, Warren Buffet, Tim Cook, and Arianna Huffington and many more leaders who may be less widely known gives impetus to the reader to hold the mirror up and ask, *Do I know who I am? Do I know my purpose? Am I moving from "I" to "We" and staying balanced and disciplined on this path?* In any context or setting, at any point in the evolution of a leader, George reminds us of the fundamental importance of these questions.

Robert Goffee and Gareth Jones have also popularized the concept of authentic leadership in a series of articles and books, beginning with a 2000 *Harvard Business Review* article entitled "Why Should Anyone Be Led by You?"[31] A book with the same title followed in 2006, with an updated version released in 2015.[32,33] Their most recent book, *Why Should Anyone Work Here?*, views authentic leadership from an organizational level.[34] The two authors provide both an academic and practice perspective on authentic leadership, but in a different setting from George: The authors are both British and use many examples unique to that setting. It is notable how much of their earliest work mentioned previously, from 2000, resonates with George's practice perspective on authentic leadership, as well as the early academic models and theories. Leadership behaviors such as being genuine, being willing to show vulnerabilities, and empathizing with employees are all consistent with others' conceptualization of authentic leadership. Goffee and Jones also stress the importance of both context and relationships—authentic leadership requires followers, and in their view leadership is something that is done *with* followers, not *to* followers. When people deeply care about their work and their employees, "they're more likely to show their true selves. They will not only communicate authenticity, which is the precondition for leadership, but they will show that they are doing more than just playing the role."[31(para22)] In *Why Should Anyone Work Here?*, Goffee and Jones outline six elements they believe are necessary for creating an "authentic organization," using the acronym "DREAMS"[34–36]:

- **Difference:** By "difference," the authors mean diversity, but also the differences that a diverse workforce (e.g., diversity of race, gender) brings in terms of perspectives, ideas, and workplace behaviors, all of which can increase organizational creativity.

- **Radical honesty:** Openness and transparency are critical for organizational reputation. In Goffee's words, "Tell the truth before someone else does."[36(para13)]

- **Extra value:** An authentic organization adds value to employees (e.g., training of low-skilled workers), who then may have better employment opportunities, including within the organization—this in turn can benefit customers/clients of the organization.

- **Authenticity:** Authentic organizations require leaders (and followers) who are authentic as people.

- **Meaning:** Everyone in the organization must understand the organization's purpose and their purpose, and how their individual contributions to the work plays a part in the ultimate product(s).

- **Simple rules:** The rules that work best for the business also work best for individuals when they are kept simple (see Chapter 20, "Leadership Intangibles," and "Touch" with Peter Ginter).

AUTHENTIC LEADERSHIP IN PUBLIC HEALTH AND HEALTHCARE

Authentic leadership has been a focus within healthcare since the early 2000s, with many references in the academic literature. It has most frequently been applied to, or viewed from, the nursing profession, but one can find articles across numerous healthcare disciplines and topics, from chief executive officers in healthcare organizations, to authentic leadership in nuclear medicine, leadership in organizations providing services to people with disabilities, and to authentic leadership in healthcare teams.[37–40]

In one sense, authentic leadership seems to be a natural fit in public health and health-care—*caring* is one of the fundamental tenets of these dimensions of health, whether one is caring for a community or an individual, and *caring* about work and employees is at the core of authentic leadership. Providing empathetic care and communicating with courage are as necessary in responding to individual patient needs as they are in addressing issues of concern at a community level. It is easy to imagine that if asked to elaborate by a healthcare provider or public health practitioner, the response to every one of the dimensions and attributes in the George model would be, "Yes, this is what I do."

Authentic leadership in nursing will be the primary focus of this section because nursing has been the most frequently written-about discipline. In searching the literature, few public health-focused articles on authentic leadership can be readily identified, with an article by Altman et al. anchoring this part of the section that follows.[41]

Shirey is largely credited with being among the first to describe the need and potential for authentic leadership in nursing, beginning with her 2006 article "Authentic Leaders Creating Healthy Work Environments for Nursing Practice."[42,43] In this seminal work, Shirey first acknowledges the forward-thinking document on establishing healthy work environments by the American Association of Critical-Care Nurses (AACN), published in 2005.[44] Understanding the critical importance of healthy work environments for recruiting and retaining nurses *and* for patient safety, AACN proposed six standards for establishing and sustaining healthy work environments: skilled communication, true collaboration, effective decision-making, appropriate staffing, meaningful recognition, and authentic leadership.[44] As Shirey notes, the inclusion of authentic leadership was not accompanied by much in the way of defining the term, nor what it comprised, or how to achieve it.[43] This is not surprising, as there was very little in either the popular or academic literature on authentic leadership at that time. Shirey adapted both the 2004 model from Avolio et al.[8] (Figure 8.3, linking authentic leadership to followers' attitudes and behaviors) and George's 2003 model[2] (Figure 8.4) to create a model that proposed the mechanisms whereby authentic leaders create healthy work environments (Figure 8.5). In her model, authentic leadership is the input, or antecedent, with the proximal outcome being followers' attitudes and behaviors through employee psychological engagement, and the distal outcome is a healthy work environment.[43] Shirey also proposed a research agenda to further develop the empirical and theoretical base to

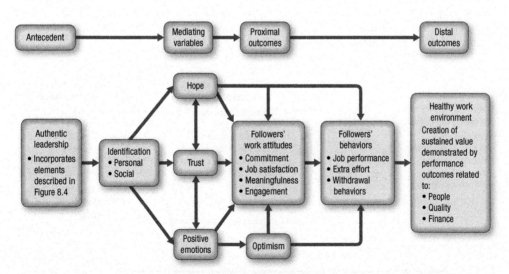

FIGURE 8.5: Shirey's Proposed Model by Which Authentic Leaders Create a Healthy Work Environment.

Source: Reproduced with permission from Avolio BJ, Gardner WL, Walumbwa FO, Luthans F, May DR. Unlocking the mask: a look at the process by which authentic leaders impact follower attitudes and behaviors. *Leadersh Q.* 2004;15(6):801–823. doi:10.1016/j.leaqua.2004.09.003

support the link between authentic leadership and a healthy work environment—it is likely that this research agenda served as the impetus for much of the subsequent scholarly work on authentic leadership and nursing.

Over the ensuing decade and a half, the literature on authentic leadership and nursing has expanded significantly—a cursory check on published articles through PubMed, with authentic leadership and nursing in the article title or abstract, revealed 64 articles since Shirey's 2005 article. Empirical evidence has accumulated that validates much of Shirey's model of antecedents, as well as proximal and distal outcomes, described earlier.[45,46] Most recently, researchers have explored the influence of authentic leadership in nursing in the setting of the COVID-19 pandemic.[47] Raso et al. repeated an earlier study on the empirical relationship between authentic leadership in nursing and healthy work environments, but this time in the context of the pandemic.[45,47] This study also confirmed this relationship in part, although the effects of the pandemic were apparent: four of the six healthy work environment standards were reported as not being present (collaboration, decision-making, staffing, and recognition), while the strongest correlation between a healthy work environment was with the authentic leadership domain of the healthy work environment standards.[47]

Alilyyani et al. have conducted the most comprehensive literature review to date on authentic leadership in healthcare (i.e., not limited to nursing).[42] Their systematic review sought to identify the antecedents, mediators, and outcomes associated with authentic leadership in healthcare.

The findings of this systematic review are best summarized in the model the authors provide, adapting the 2004 model from Avolio et al. (see Figure 8.3), and including the signficant associations between authentic leadership, mediators, and outcomes. As decribed by the authors, in Figure 8.6, "the solid lines indicate that findings from the review support demonstrated relationships. Double lined boxes indicate additions to the original theory."[42(p59)]

Saxe-Braithwaite and Gautreau provide the most recent study on authentic leadership in healthcare executives.[48] Their study examined 14 chief executives and 70 direct reports in healthcare organizations in Ontario, Canada. The authors sought to document the authentic leadership qualities evident in and important to healthcare executives and the degree of congruence between these executives' self-rated assessment of authentic leadership and their direct reports' ratings. Not surprisingly, the healthcare executives rated themselves higher on authentic leadership than did their direct reports. Across the four domains of the authentic leadership (self-awareness, relational transparency, balanced processing, and internalized moral perspective), the most significant difference between the executives' self-rating and the rating of their direct reports was on self-awareness.

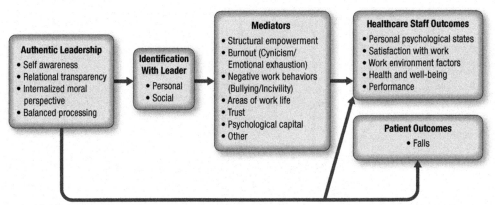

FIGURE 8.6: Adapted Authentic Leadership Model Based on Findings of Systematic Review of Authentic Leadership in Healthcare.

Source: Reproduced with permission from Alilyyani B, Wong CA, Cummings G. Antecedents, mediators, and outcomes of authentic leadership in healthcare: a systematic review. *International Journal of Nursing Studies.* 2018;83:34–64. doi:10.1016/j.ijnurstu.2018.04.001

Finally, one publication clearly in the public health domain is an article featured in the "Management Moment" section of the *Journal of Public Health Management and Practice*, which has been led for more than 15 years by Dr. Ed Baker, a contributor to this textbook. This brief commentary by Altman, Taylor, and Baker[41] provided a public health lens to the qualities of authentic leadership. To be authentic means to "say what you mean and mean what you say," but balancing authentic communications with empathy. Similar to George's "leading from the heart," the public health leader who is authentic "relates to individuals first as who they are, not just for what they can accomplish."[41(p90)] Written at a time when many public health jobs were being eliminated because of state and local budget cuts, Altman stressed the importance of authentic leaders delivering difficult messages in ways that simultaneously exhibited courage on the part of the leader, and doing so with empathy. Such behaviors build trust; the opposite approach would damage both trust in the leader and organizational cohesion. Similar to relational transparency in the academic models and establishing enduring relationships in George's model, the authentic leader must avoid "masking"—hiding their real emotions or vulnerabilities so severely that both individual and organizational authenticity are eroded—while followers experience anger and resentment. Authentic leaders in public health must develop the capacity to balance opposing behaviors—being "tough while being empathetic; courageous and vulnerable; passionate and compassionate; pillars of strength and regular folks; self-reliant and trusting of others; and change advocates and conservers of the past."[41(p91)]

Given the experiences during the COVID-19 pandemic, authentic leadership in public health and healthcare is needed now more than ever. Being true to oneself for those in public health and healthcare has meant leading with evidence and allowing the science to inform policy and procedures. Yet, because of significant pushback from many who either do not accept or understand the science, communicating messages with empathy has been critical to implementing strategies to mitigate the spread of the virus. If not for the passion, heart, and self-discipline for the work and the care for their communities and patients, many more public health practitioners and healthcare providers would have left the field.

Finally, as the nation recovers from the COVID-19 pandemic, and as vacant positions in public health and healthcare get filled, leaders will need to be mindful that their newer, younger employees bring different values, attitudes, and expectations to the workplace, compared to the older workforce. In a thoughtful article that explored millennials' (defined as those born between 1982–1999) work-related attitudes and behaviors, Anderson et al. caution that leadership styles that have resonated with prior generations may be less relevant for millennials.[49] With specific regard to authentic leadership, the authors posited that:

- because millennials are more individualistic, it may be difficult to achieve the value congruence that is fundamental to authentic leader–follower relationships;
- because millennials place a greater value on work–life balance, they may be less inclined to follow their leaders' stronger work ethic; and,
- because millennials place a higher value on extrinsic rewards—salary, promotions—they may not identify with the intrinsic rewards of work that their leaders espouse.

Conversely, millennials also bring new strengths to the workplace—they tend to be more technologically savvy, perhaps less biased in hiring and performance decisions, and part of a more diverse workforce than the baby boomer generation.

AUTHENTIC LEADERSHIP AND STRUCTURAL RACISM

While the authors could not identify articles or books that specifically addressed authentic leadership in the context of structural racism, a recent review on racism in nursing by Iheduru-Anderson et al. provides an opportunity for meaningful discourse.[50] By taking the findings of this review and placing them in the Shirey model (see Figure 8.5) for how authentic leaders influence follower behaviors and attitudes and thus impact the work environment, the impacts of racism vis-à-vis authentic leadership are clearly apparent. Refer back to Figure 8.5 to more clearly visualize where and how structural racism can destroy the antecedents, mediators, and outcomes of authentic leadership.

In the example of nursing, it can be challenging for followers of color to identify with leaders, when the largest nursing organization in the United States, the American Nurses Association, has had only three presidents of color since its inception in 1911. Iheduru-Anderson et al. reference the work of Waite and Nardi, who had identified two presidents of color as of 2017; in 2018, Ernest Grant became the third president of color and the first male president.[51,52] Social identification is further hindered when leaders fail to understand the meaning of intersectionality and the lived experiences of nurses of color. According to Iheduru-Anderson, experiences of racism destroy trust and lead to deeply negative emotions between leader and follower. Such negative emotions can result in a hostile work environment, which impacts retention of nurses of color. This can in turn negatively impact patient care and lead to worsening health inequities when there is racial discordance between providers and patients. With its negative impact on retention, there are fewer opportunities for nurses of color to attain positions of leadership, and thus the overall effect of structural racism is to create a vicious cycle. For Iheduru-Anderson et al., critical self-reflection, with the development of awareness and sensitivity—actually the fundamental tenets of authentic leadership—can be the basis for change.

AUTHENTIC LEADERSHIP METRICS

A commonly used instrument for assessing authentic leadership is the Authentic Leadership Questionnaire (ALQ).[19] Based on the models of Avolio et al. and the conceptualizations of Ilies et al., the ALQ was operationalized and validated by Walumbwa et al. in 2008.[12,15,53] The ALQ consists of four components: relational transparency (five items), internalized moral perspective (four items), balanced processing (three items), and self-awareness (four items). The ALQ has been most widely used in the United States, but it has also been tested and used in many other countries, including China, Kenya, Portugal, Belgium, Canada, New Zealand, Germany, and India.[54]

The ALQ is a proprietary instrument, copyrighted by Bruce J. Avolio, William L. Gardner, and Fred O. Walumbwa, and available through Mind Garden at www.mindgarden.com/69-authentic-leadership-questionnaire. The ALQ may be used as a self-assessment or as an assessment of others' authentic leadership qualities.

In 2011, Neider and Schriesheim proposed a new measure of authentic leadership, the Authentic Leadership Inventory (ALI).[55] Based on the theoretical foundation established by Walumbwa et al. in developing the ALQ, Neider and Schriesheim first proposed a 16-item instrument, using the four constructs in the ALQ—self-awareness, relational transparency, balanced processing, and internalized moral perspective. After further psychometric testing, the ALI was reduced to a final 14-item instrument (see Appendix 8.1). In practice, the ALI has been used by applying a five-point Likert type scale, ranging from 1 being "disagree strongly" to 5 being "agree strongly" for each item. Scores have been summed across the 14 items and averaged across the four constructs, but there is no scoring rubric (for interpretation) currently in use.

We suggest that a potential use of the ALI, even without a scoring rubric, is as a self-assessment mechanism and as part of a 360-degree evaluation. This will allow the leader to gain insights about their strengths and weaknesses as an authentic leader, and to serve as a basis for leadership growth. The instrument can then be used on a recurring basis to assess changes in authentic leadership development. The suggested questionnaire, with instructions and interpretation guidance, is shown as Appendix 8.1.

SUMMARY

Authentic leadership is leading while being true to oneself and to followers through self-awareness, transparency, and self-regulation. The authentic leader is genuine and lives their values in all settings. Authentic leadership has both a scholarly foundation in theories and models as well as popular appeal, especially through several books by Bill George. The development of authentic leaders is rooted in one's life experiences, which give rise to confidence, hope, optimism, and resiliency. Influenced by organizational context, certain trigger events and challenges can lead to positive self-development through self-awareness and self-regulation. This development is fulfilled in the authentic leader who is then confident, hopeful, optimistic, resilient, transparent, moral and ethical, and future and follower oriented. Authentic leaders influence followers' work attitudes and behaviors through personal and social identification and the building of hope, trust, and positive emotions. Authentic leadership is similar to several other positivist leadership theories, including servant leadership and transformational leadership, and it also reflects many elements of EI. Across a number of healthcare settings, but most commonly studied in the nursing profession, when authentic leadership flourishes, a healthy work environment is created. Bill George, who has done so much to popularize authentic leadership in practice, sums it succinctly:

> Authentic leaders genuinely desire to serve others through their leadership. They are more interested in empowering the people they lead to make a difference than they are in power, money, or prestige for themselves. They are as guided by qualities of the heart, by passion and compassion, as they are by qualities of the mind.[2(p12)]

DISCUSSION QUESTIONS

1. How do you know whether or not you are an authentic leader?
2. When all is said and done, who or what will validate you as an authentic leader?
3. Think about the basis for your leadership development and the path you need to follow to become an authentic leader. What life stories have defined you?
4. Think of a current leader you are familiar with (work with, know through other people, have come in contact with) and identify the traits that would lend themselves to authenticity and those that would not. In your response, provide your own definition of authentic leadership.

CASE STUDY: IDENTIFYING AUTHENTIC LEADERSHIP CHARACTERISTICS—AN INFORMAL SURVEY

Stephanie B. C. Bailey, MD, MSHSA

As you read in this chapter, *authentic leadership* is grounded in a leader's ability to be true to themselves and their followers through self-awareness, transparency, and self-regulation; *authentic behavior*, according to Bill George, is guided from one's core values and beliefs.[2] Those core values and beliefs, in turn, are shaped through our life experiences. It would stand to reason, then, that leaders may have different ideas of the characteristics critical to authentic leadership.

To help illustrate this point, I conducted an informal survey of colleagues and friends, many of whom work in traditional leadership roles (as well as some who do not). The persons surveyed operate in a wide variety of industries and professions: healthcare, public health, academia, technology, religion, insurance, financial institutions, government, national/state associations (public health and healthcare), and pharmaceutical. The question posed to them was simply: *When you think of the phrase "authentic leadership," what three characteristics come immediately to mind?*

TABLE 8.2: Authentic Leadership Characteristics Most Frequently Identified by Survey Respondents

CHARACTERISTIC	MENTIONS	CHARACTERISTIC	MENTIONS
Integrity	13	Self-awareness	4
Honesty	10	Compassion	4
Vision	9	Competency	3
Empathy	8	Passion	3
Transparency	7	Trustworthiness	3
Communicator	7	Strategic	3
Listener	6	Emotional intelligence	3
Humility	6	Ethical	3
Courage	5	Vulnerability	3
Purpose	4	Decisive	3
Grounded in truth	4	Results driven	3

Invitations were sent to 102 people, with nine emails returning as undeliverable. This resulted in a final total number of 93 invitations sent. I received 62 responses, for a response rate of 67%. This group supplied 181 characteristics overall; some submitted only one, and a few submitted more than three. All responses were included in Table 8.2 to provide a sampling of current day perspectives on the characteristics of authentic leadership from 62 thoughtful people.

Other characteristics that the literature identifies with authentic leadership, such as *true to self, genuine, lead from the heart, morally strong, shows values/leads by example, consistent, authenticity, and sensitive/respectful of flock*, were mentioned by one or two respondents.

The results were as nuanced as the literature. While there was not one characteristic which was a clear winner, *integrity* and *honesty*, traits commonly associated with authentic leadership, garnered 23 mentions from the 62 respondents (37%). Further, if we were to combine responses arguably related to *integrity*, we could also add *genuine, trustworthy, grounded in truth*, and *transparent* to that category, bringing the total number of mentions for the characteristics related to *integrity* to 37 (60%).

CASE STUDY QUESTIONS

1. How do you interpret these results? Where do you see consistency or inconsistency between these results and the material from the chapter? Please provide support for your answer.

2. If you were participating in the survey, what three characteristics would you choose? Why?

3. In your opinion, are there any characteristics listed in Table 8.2 that do NOT belong on this list? Which one(s), and why?

CASE STUDY: RUTH BADER GINSBURG

Supreme Court Justice Ruth Bader Ginsburg was born on March 15, 1933, in the low-income, working-class Flatbush neighborhood of Brooklyn, NY. She was the second of two daughters of Celia and Amster Bader; her father was a Jewish emigrant from Ukraine and her mother's parents were from Krakow, Poland.[56] Ruth's older sister died of meningitis when Ruth was still an infant.

Ruth's mother Celia, an avid reader and excellent student, graduated from high school at age 15. She did not attend college, however; instead, she worked in a garment factory to help pay for her brother's college education.[57] Celia, who played an active role in Ruth's early education and encouraged her to be both a lady and independent, died of cancer while Ruth was still in high school.

Ruth went on to graduate first in her class from Cornell in 1954, where she met her future husband, Martin D. Ginsburg (Marty). After giving birth to their first child in 1955, Ginsburg enrolled in Harvard Law School in 1956. She was one of nine female students in a class of 500.

When her husband landed a job in New York in 1958, Ginsburg transferred to Columbia Law School to complete her degree. That same year, Marty was diagnosed with testicular cancer; she cared for him and their daughter while attending law school, taking notes for him in classes.[57]

After graduating from Columbia in 1959 at the top of her class, Ginsburg clerked for United States District Judge Edmund L. Palmieri. In 1971, she co-founded and directed the Women's Rights Project of the ACLU. From 1962–1973, she taught law at Rutgers University and at Columbia, where she became that university's first female tenured professor. In 1980, Ginsburg was appointed to the United States Court of Appeals for the District of Columbia Circuit by President Jimmy Carter. In 1993, she was nominated as an Associate Justice of the Supreme Court by President Bill Clinton, taking her seat as Supreme Court Justice on August 10, 1993. She was the Court's second female justice (after Sandra Day O'Connor); she was the only female justice between 2006 and 2009.

During her tenure on the Supreme Court, Justice Ginsburg advocated for gender equality, civil rights, voting rights, the rights of workers, and separation of church and state. She was considered a brilliant legal strategist; her early approach to combating sexism included arguing cases where men were being treated unfairly, correctly surmising that arguing for equal rights for men would likely resonate with male judges.[58] And despite her reputation as a liberal justice, she strongly believed in judicial restraint on issues of social change and she favored states' autonomy, notably siding with conservatives in several such instances.[59] And she famously enjoyed a close, long-term friendship with Justice Antonin Scalia, her conservative judicial counterweight.

Throughout her life, Ginsburg continuously encountered gender barriers: she was not permitted to celebrate bat mitzvah, since Jewish Orthodox law prohibited women from reading from the Torah[60]; she and her fellow female classmates at Harvard were asked by the dean why they were there, taking the place of a man; she was demoted at the Social Security Administration when she became pregnant with her first child;[61] and she had difficulty finding employment at the beginning of her law career, later reflecting, "In the fifties, the traditional law firms were just beginning to turn around on hiring Jews. . . . But to be a woman, a Jew, and a mother to boot, that combination was a bit much."[62]

After battling cancer for two decades, Justice Ginsburg died from complications of pancreatic cancer on September 18, 2020, at age 87, leaving an indelible mark on the law, civil rights, abortion rights, and even pop culture (see "Notorious RBG"). To get a sense of how she led, perhaps it is best to hear from her in her own words:

"You can disagree without being disagreeable."

"Reacting in anger or annoyance will not advance one's ability to persuade."

"For both men and women the first step in getting power is to become visible to others, and then to put on an impressive show. . . . As women achieve power, the barriers will fall. As society sees what women can do, as women see what women can do, there will be more women out there doing things, and we'll all be better off for it."

"Don't be distracted by emotions like anger, envy, resentment. These just zap energy and waste time."

"Fight for the things that you care about but do it in a way that will lead others to join you."

"I would like to be remembered as someone who used whatever talent she had to do her work to the very best of her ability."

"I'm a very strong believer in listening and learning from others."

"Some of my favorite opinions are dissenting opinions. I will not live to see what becomes of them, but I remain hopeful."

"Whatever you choose to do, leave tracks. That means don't do it just for yourself. You will want to leave the world a little better place for having lived."

CASE STUDY QUESTIONS

1. What do you think were Justice Ginsburg's values? How did her life experience shape her values?

2. Using Bill George's five dimensions of authentic leadership, discuss Ruth Bader Ginsburg's authentic leadership style:

    a. Understanding her purpose

    b. Practicing solid values

    c. Leading with heart

    d. Establishing connected relationships

    e. Demonstrating self-discipline

3. What leadership lessons can you learn from the late Justice Ginsburg?

ADDITIONAL RESOURCES

■ The Authentic Leadership Questionnaire (ALG) is a proprietary instrument, copyrighted by Bruce J. Avolio, William L. Gardner, and Fred O. Walumbwa (2007), and available through Mind Garden at www.mindgarden.com/69-authentic-leadership-questionnaire. The ALQ may be used as a self-assessment or as an assessment of others' authentic leadership qualities.

Several institutions offer a certificate and/or executive education in authentic leadership. Inclusion here is meant to provide examples only, not an endorsement by the authors or publishers.

- Harvard Business School: www.exed.hbs.edu/authentic-leader-development/
- Harvard University: https://pll.harvard.edu/course/authentic-leader-development%E2%80%94virtual?delta=0
- Wake Forest University: https://business.wfu.edu/executive-education/open-enrollment/short-courses/authentic-and-effective-leadership/
- Northwestern University: www.kellogg.northwestern.edu/executive-education/individual-programs/executive-programs/lsphere.aspx

In addition, Bill George has published several videos on authentic leadership that are publicly available on YouTube.

 SPRINGER PUBLISHING CONNECT™ A robust set of instructor resources designed to supplement this text is located at http://connect.springerpub.com/content/book/978-0-8261-4924-4. Qualifying instructors may request access by emailing textbook@springerpub.com.

REFERENCES

1. Henderson J, Hoy W. Leader authenticity: the development and test of an operational measure. *Educ Psychol Rec*. 1983;3(2):63–75.
2. George B. *Authentic Leadership: Rediscovering the Secrets to Creating Lasting Value*. Jossey-Bass; 2003.
3. Merriam-Webster Dictionary. 2022. https://www.merriam-webster.com/dictionary/authentic
4. LinkedIn. What does authenticity mean? 2022. https://www.linkedin.com/pulse/what-does-authenticity-mean-caroline-claeys/
5. Parke HW, Wormell DEW. *The Delphic Oracle/1 the History*. Blackwell; 1956.
6. Gardner WL, Cogliser CC, Davis KM, Dickens MP. Authentic leadership: a review of the literature and research agenda. *Leadersh Q*. 2011;22(6):1120–1145. doi:10.1016/j.leaqua.2011.09.007
7. Kernis MH, Goldman BM. A multicomponent conceptualization of authenticity: theory and research. In: Zanna MP, ed. *Advances in Experimental Social Psychology*. Vol 38. Academic Press; 2006:283–357.
8. Avolio BJ, Gardner WL, Walumbwa FO, Luthans F, May DR. Unlocking the mask: a look at the process by which authentic leaders impact follower attitudes and behaviors. *Leadersh Q*. 2004;15(6):801–823. doi:10.1016/j.leaqua.2004.09.003
9. Novicevic MM, Harvey MG, Ronald M, Brown-Radford JA. Authentic leadership: a historical perspective. *J Leadersh Organ Stud*. 2006;13(1):64–76. doi:10.1177/10717919070130010901
10. Luthans F, Avolio BJ. Authentic leadership development. In: Cameron KS, Dutton JE, Quinn RE, eds. *Positive Organizational Scholarship*. Berrett-Koehler; 2003;241–258.
11. Gardner WL, Avolio BJ, Luthans F, May DR, Walumbwa F. "Can you see the real me?" A self-based model of authentic leader and follower development. *Leadersh Q*. 2005;16(3):343–372. doi:10.1016/j.leaqua.2005.03.003
12. Walumbwa FO, Avolio BJ, Gardner WL, Wernsing TS, Peterson SJ. Authentic leadership: development and validation of a theory-based measure. *J Manag*. 2008;34(1):89–126. doi:10.1177/0149206307308913
13. Luthans F. Positive organizational behavior: developing and managing psychological strengths. *Acad Manag Perspect*. 2002;16(1):57–72. doi:10.5465/ame.2002.6640181
14. Bass BM, Avolio BJ. *Improving Organizational Effectiveness Through Transformational Leadership*. Sage; 1994.
15. Avolio BJ, Gardner WL. Authentic leadership development: getting to the root of positive forms of leadership. *Leadersh Q*. 2005;16(3):315–338. doi:10.1016/j.leaqua.2005.03.001
16. Gardner WL, Karam EP, Alvesson M, Einola K. Authentic leadership theory: the case for and against. *Leadersh Q*. 2021;32(6):101495. doi:10.1016/j.leaqua.2021.101495
17. Kernis MH. Toward a conceptualization of optimal self-esteem. *Psychol Inq*. 2003;14(1):1–26. doi:10.1207/S15327965PLI1401_01
18. Harvard Management Update. The call for authentic leadership. *Harvard Business Review*. February 28, 2008. https://hbr.org/2008/02/the-call-for-authentic-leaders-1

19. Northouse PG. *Leadership: Theory and Practice.* 7th ed. Sage; 2016.

20. Avolio BJ. Pursuing authentic leadership development. In: Nohria N, Khurana R, eds. *Handbook of Leadership Theory and Practice.* Harvard Business Press; 2010:739–765.

21. Banks GC, McCauley KD, Gardner WL, Guler CE. A meta-analytic review of authentic and transformational leadership: a test for redundancy. *Leadersh Q.* 2016;27(4):634–652. doi:10.1016/j.leaqua.2016.02.006

22. Goleman D. *Emotional Intelligence: Why It Can Matter More Than IQ.* Bantam; 2012.

23. Miao C, Humphrey RH, Qian S. Emotional intelligence and authentic leadership: a meta-analysis. *Leadersh Organ Dev J.* 2018;39(5):679–690. doi:10.1108/LODJ-02-2018-0066

24. Covelli BJ, Mason I. Linking theory to practice: authentic leadership. *Acad Strateg Manag J.* 2017;16(3):1–10. https://www.abacademies.org/articles/Linking-theory-to-practice-authentic-leadership-1939-6104-16-3-124.pdf

25. Hoch JE, Bommer WH, Dulebohn JH, Wu D. Do ethical, authentic, and servant leadership explain variance above and beyond transformational leadership? A meta-analysis. *J Manag.* 2018;44(2):501–529. doi:10.1177/0149206316665461

26. Sidani YM, Rowe WG. A reconceptualization of authentic leadership: leader legitimation via follower-centered assessment of the moral dimension. *Leadersh Q.* 2018;29(6):623–636. doi:10.1016/j.leaqua.2018.04.005

27. Alvesson M, Einola K. Warning for excessive positivity: Authentic leadership and other traps in leadership studies. *Leadersh Q.* 2019;30(4):383–395. doi:10.1016/j.leaqua.2019.04.001

28. George B. *True North: Discover Your Authentic Leadership.* Jossey-Bass; 2007.

29. George B. *Finding Your True North: A Personal Guide.* Jossey-Bass; 2008.

30. George B. *Discover Your True North.* Jossey-Bass; 2015.

31. Goffee R, Jones G. Why should anyone be led by you? *Harv Bus Rev.* 2000;78(5):62–70. https://hbr.org/2000/09/why-should-anyone-be-led-by-you

32. Goffee R, Jones G. *Why Should Anyone Be Led by You? What It Takes to Be an Authentic Leader.* Harvard Business Review Press; 2006.

33. Goffee R, Jones G. *Why Should Anyone Be Led by You? With a New Preface by the Authors: What It Takes to Be an Authentic Leader.* Harvard Business Review Press; 2015.

34. Goffee R, Jones G. *Why Should Anyone Work Here?: What It Takes to Create an Authentic Organization.* Harvard Business Review Press; 2015.

35. Clayton M. Rob Goffee and Gareth Jones: authentic leadership. 2017. https://www.pocketbook.co.uk/blog/2017/09/05/rob-goffee-and-gareth-jones-authentic-leadership/

36. Jacobs K. Goffee and Jones: why should anyone work here? *HR.* 2016. https://www.hrmagazine.co.uk/content/features/goffee-and-jones-why-should-anyone-work-here

37. Saxe-Braithwaite M, Gautreau S. Authentic leadership in healthcare organizations: a study of 14 chief executive officers and 70 direct reports. *Healthc Manag Forum.* 2020;33(3):140–144. doi:10.1177/0840470419890634

38. Johnson SL. Authentic leadership theory and practical applications in nuclear medicine. *J Nucl Med Technol.* 2019;47(3):181–188. doi:10.2967/jnmt.118.222851

39. Brady LT, Fong L, Waninger KN, Eidelman S. Perspectives on leadership in organizations providing services to people with disabilities: an exploratory study. *Intellect Dev Disabil.* 2009;47(5):358–372. doi:10.1352/1934-9556-47.5.358

40. Marques-Quinteiro P, Graça AM, Coelho FA Jr, Martins D. On the relationship between authentic leadership, flourishing, and performance in healthcare teams: a job demands-resources perspective. *Front Psychol.* 2021;12:692433. doi:10.3389/fpsyg.2021.692433

41. Altman D, Taylor S, Baker E. Leading with authenticity in challenging times. *J Public Health Manag Pract.* 2011;17(1):90–91. doi:10.1097/PHH.0b013e31820425c0

42. Alilyyani B, Wong CA, Cummings G. Antecedents, mediators, and outcomes of authentic leadership in healthcare: a systematic review. *Int J Nurs Stud.* 2018;83:34–64. doi:10.1016/j.ijnurstu.2018.04.001

43. Shirey MR. Authentic leaders creating healthy work environments for nursing practice. *Am J Crit Care.* 2006;15(3):256–267. doi:10.4037/ajcc2006.15.3.256

44. American Association of Critical-Care Nurses. AACN standards for establishing and sustaining healthy work environments: a journey to excellence. *Am J Crit Care.* 2005;14(3):187–197. doi:10.4037/ajcc2005.14.3.187

45. Raso R, Fitzpatrick JJ, Masick K. Clinical nurses' perceptions of authentic nurse leadership and healthy work environment. *J Nurs Adm*. 2020;50(9):489–494. doi:10.1097/NNA.0000000000000921

46. Labrague LJ, Al Sabei S, Al Rawajfah O, AbuAlRub R, Burney I. Authentic leadership and nurses' motivation to engage in leadership roles: the mediating effects of nurse work environment and leadership self-efficacy. *J Nurs Manag*. 2021;29(8):2444–2452. doi:10.1111/jonm.13448

47. Raso R, Fitzpatrick JJ, Masick K, Giordano-Mulligan M, Sweeney CD. Perceptions of authentic nurse leadership and work environment and the pandemic impact for nurse leaders and clinical nurses. *J Nurs Adm*. 2021;51(5):257–263. doi:10.1097/NNA.0000000000001010

48. Saxe-Braithwaite M, Gautreau S. Authentic leadership in healthcare organizations: A study of 14 chief executive officers and 70 direct reports. *Healthc Manage Forum*. 2020 May; 33(3):140–144. doi: 10.1177/0840470419890634. Epub 2019 Dec 11.

49. Anderson HJ, Baur JE, Griffith JA, Buckley MR. What works for you may not work for (Gen) Me: limitations of present leadership theories for the new generation. *Leadersh Q*. 2017;28(1):245–260. doi:10.1016/j.leaqua.2016.08.001

50. Iheduru-Anderson K, Shingles RR, Akanegbu C. Discourse of race and racism in nursing: an integrative review of literature. *Public Health Nurs*. 2021;38(1):115–130. doi:10.1111/phn.12828

51. Waite R, Nardi D. Nursing colonialism in America: implications for nursing leadership. *J Prof Nurs*. 2019;35(1):18–25. doi:10.1016/j.profnurs.2017.12.013

52. American Nursing Association. The first black male ANA president: a milestone in nursing. 2021. https://onlinenursing.duq.edu/blog/the-first-black-male-ana-president-a-milestone-in-nursing/

53. Ilies R, Morgeson FP, Nahrgang JD. Authentic leadership and eudaemonic well-being: understanding leader–follower outcomes. *Leadersh Q*. 2005;16(3):373–394. doi:10.1016/j.leaqua.2005.03.002

54. Datta B. Assessing the effectiveness of authentic leadership. *Int J Leadersh Educ Stud*. 2015;9(1):62–75.

55. Neider LL, Schriesheim CA. The Authentic Leadership Inventory (ALI): development and empirical tests. *Leadersh Q*. 2011;22(6):1146–1164. doi:10.1016/j.leaqua.2011.09.008

56. Godin B. Women of interest: Ruth Bader Ginsburg. The Voice website. https://www.voicemagazine.org/2020/10/21/women-of-interest-ruth-bader-ginsburg/

57. Ruth Bader Ginsburg. A&E television networks. Women's History website. March 24, 2021. https://www.history.com/topics/womens-history/ruth-bader-ginsburg

58. Donvito T. 15 ways Justice Ruth Bader Ginsburg has made history. *Reader's Digest*. November 23, 2021. https://www.rd.com/article/ruth-bader-ginsburg/

59. Wehle K. Opinion: the surprising conservatism of Ruth Bader Ginsburg. Politico website. 2020. https://www.politico.com/news/magazine/2020/09/20/ruth-bader-ginsburg-conservatism-418821

60. Kaplan Sommer A. Why Ruth Bader Ginsburg had an intimate, yet ambivalent relationship with Judaism and Israel. Haaretz. December 15, 2020. https://www.haaretz.com/us-news/.premium-bader-ginsburg-had-an-intimate-yet-ambivalent-relationship-with-judaism-and-israel-1.9169497

61. Justice Ruth Bader Ginsburg passes the torch. https://www.icrw.org/news/justice-ruth-bader-ginsburg-passes-the-torch/

62. Alexander KL. Ruth Bader Ginsburg. October 2, 2020. https://csub.libguides.com/RBG

APPENDIX 8.1. AUTHENTIC LEADERSHIP INVENTORY (ALI)

Abbreviations used in the chart that follows are for the four authentic leader constructs: (S) = self-awareness (three questions); (R) = relational transparency (three questions); (M) = internalized moral perspective (four questions); and (B) = balanced processing (four questions).

Instructions:					
This questionnaire is designed to provide insights into your authentic leadership by assessing the four constructs of authentic leadership: relational transparency, internalized moral perspective, balanced processing, and self-awareness. Using the 5-point scale, respond to each statement by selecting the number that best represents your response to the item. **Scale:** 1 = Strongly Disagree; 2 = Disagree; 3 = Neither Agree Nor Disagree; 4 = Agree; 5 = Strongly Agree					
1. My leader clearly states what he/she means. (R)	1	2	3	4	5
2. My leader shows consistency between his/her beliefs and actions. (M)	1	2	3	4	5
3. My leader asks for ideas that challenge his/her core beliefs. (B)	1	2	3	4	5
4. My leader describes accurately the way that others view his/her abilities. (S)	1	2	3	4	5
5. My leader uses his/her core beliefs to make decisions. (M)	1	2	3	4	5
6. My leader carefully listens to alternative perspectives before reaching a conclusion. (B)	1	2	3	4	5
7. My leader shows that he/she understands his/her strengths and weaknesses. (S)	1	2	3	4	5
8. My leader openly shares information with others. (R)	1	2	3	4	5
9. My leader resists pressures on him/her to do things contrary to his/her beliefs. (M)	1	2	3	4	5
10. My leader objectively analyzes relevant data before making a decision. (B)	1	2	3	4	5
11. My leader is clearly aware of the impact he/she has on others. (S)	1	2	3	4	5
12. My leader expresses his/her ideas and thoughts clearly to others. (R)	1	2	3	4	5
13. My leader is guided in his/her actions by internal moral standards. (M)	1	2	3	4	5
14. My leader encourages other to voice opposing points of view. (B)	1	2	3	4	5
Scoring:					
1. Add your responses to statements 1, 8, and 12; divide by 3. This is your relational transparency score. 2. Add your responses to statements 2, 5, 9, and 13; divide by 4. This is your internalized moral perspective score. 3. Add your responses to statements 3, 6, 10, and 14; divide by 4. This is your balanced processing score. 4. Add your responses to statements 4, 7, and 11; divide by 3. This is your self-awareness score.					

Source: Neider LL, Schriesheim CA. The Authentic Leadership Inventory (ALI): development and empirical tests. *Leadersh Q.* 2011;22(6):1146–1164. doi:10.1016/j.leaqua.2011.09.008

Chapter 9

Servant Leadership

Paul C. Erwin

INTRODUCTION

Servant leadership centers on empathy for, attentiveness to, and nurturing of followers. Servant-leaders are ethical; they empower their followers, and help them realize their full development potential. The hallmark of servant leadership is putting followers first—serving others—and through this, followers in turn become servant-leaders. Key characteristics of servant leadership include empathy, listening, and stewardship. First developed by Robert Greenleaf in a 1970 essay entitled, *The Servant as Leader*, servant leadership has grown in its fields of use, from business, to higher education, to health and medical care, and to public health. Through both popular media as well as workshops and trainings available from several organizations, including The Greenleaf Center for Servant Leadership at Seton Hall, servant leadership has become increasingly accessible to potential adherents. Scholarship on servant leadership has been expanding in the past 20 years, with a recent review including 285 published articles. With its emphasis on social justice, and a practice perspective that leans into equity, the field of public health is particularly fertile for servant leadership to thrive. And, in an even larger sense, the whole notion of healthcare—serving others—is the perfect pallet for a portrait of servant leadership.

OBJECTIVES

By the end of this chapter, the reader will be able to:

- Understand the history and development of servant leadership.
- Describe the key characteristics of servant leadership.
- Understand the current state of research on servant leadership.
- Recognize servant leadership in practice, from business, to nonprofit organizations, to health and medical care.
- Identify resources and instruments for assessing servant leadership.
- Apply concepts of servant leadership through case studies.

HISTORY AND DEVELOPMENT OF SERVANT LEADERSHIP

THE SERVANT AS LEADER—ROBERT GREENLEAF

Robert Greenleaf created the term "servant leadership" in a seminal 1970 essay entitled *The Servant as Leader*.[1] At that time a retired executive who had worked for AT&T for 38 years, Greenleaf took his inspiration for servant leadership from a book by Hermann Hesse,

Journey to the East. On a presumably mythical journey in search of the "League," a group of travelers is accompanied by the servant Leo, who goes about serving others through daily chores, often with singing and levity. The journey goes smoothly until Leo suddenly disappears, and the travelers become disenchanted as they lose their way and wander about. After many years of aimless travel, the narrator finds Leo, who turns out to have been the leader of the League, which had sponsored the original journey. In Greenleaf's own words, this story ". . . clearly says that *the great leader is seen as servant first.*"[1(p2)] From that singular moment of inspiration, Greenleaf wrote his 27-page essay that has served as the foundation of servant leadership, and later expanded this into his best-selling book, *Servant Leadership: A Journey Into the Nature of Legitimate Power and Greatness.*[2]

For Greenleaf, the servant-leader is servant-first, not leader-first:

> *The difference manifests itself in the care taken by the servant-first to make sure that other people's highest priority needs are being served. The best test, and difficult to administer, is: Do those served grow as persons? Do they, while being served, become healthier, wiser, freer, more autonomous, more likely themselves to become servants?*[1(p6)]

Greenleaf describes the importance of the leader's ability to listen and understand, and the primacy of this for the servant-leader: ". . . only a true natural servant automatically responds to any problem by listening first . . . because true listening builds strength in other people."[1(p8)] Through listening, Greenleaf's servant-leader accepts and empathizes, which allows followers to "grow taller" and more trusting of the servant-leader. Although Greenleaf acknowledges the need for the servant-leader to have intellectual capacity, he proposes two intellectual abilities that "are not formally assessed in an academic way: [the servant-leader] needs to have *a sense for the unknowable* and be able to *foresee the unforeseeable.*"[1(p11)] The servant-leader must be able to bridge the information gap between these two poles, by intuition. This leads to another key characteristic of Greenleaf's servant-leader: foresight, or prescience for "*what* is going to happen *when* in the future."[1(p12)] Awareness, perception, persuasion, conceptualizing, and healing are additional attributes of Greenleaf's servant-leader, some of which may bring wholeness to the servant-leader themselves.

Finally, in his 1970 essay, Greenleaf describes *institutions as servants*, and builds on this in his book: "An institution starts on a course toward people-building with leadership that has a firmly established context of *people first.*"[1(p22)] As goes the servant-leader, so goes the institution of the servant-leader.

Eva et al., in their comprehensive review of the research on servant leadership, provide this new definition of servant leadership:

> *Servant leadership is an (1) other-oriented approach to leadership (2) manifested through one-on-one prioritizing of follower individual needs and interests, (3) and outward reorienting of their concern for self towards concern for others within the organization and the larger community.*[3(p114)]

This new definition comports to the current models of servant leadership that include Antecedent Conditions, Servant-Leader Behaviors, and Outcomes. These models and Eva's review are presented in more detail in the sections that follow.

EVOLUTION OF SERVANT LEADERSHIP

Following Greenleaf's 1970 essay and 1977 book, few publications referenced servant leadership à la Greenleaf until the early 1990s, and most of these were of a religious nature or affiliation (e.g., as in Jesus being the first and greatest example of the servant-leader). Graham's 1991 article entitled "Servant Leadership in Organizations: Inspirational and Moral,"[4] is one of the first to appear in a scholarly publication. Graham was exploring the boundaries of *charismatic leadership*, noting the challenges to morality in considering that, for example, both Gandhi and Hitler could be described as charismatic leaders in their followers' views. As an alternative to charismatic leadership, servant leadership provided the model for Graham

---

Box 9.1: Spears' 10 Characteristics of Servant Leadership

1. Listening
2. Empathy
3. Healing
4. Awareness
5. Persuasion
6. Conceptualization
7. Foresight
8. Stewardship
9. Commitment to the growth of people
10. Building community

---

that was inspirational, but also contained moral safeguards. Servant leadership "encourages in followers not only intellectual and skill development but enhanced moral reasoning capacity as well. Followers become autonomous moral agents, i.e., they are not bound within the context of the leader's goals."[4(p116)]

In 1995, Larry Spears published the first book beyond Greenleaf on servant leadership, *Reflections on Leadership*,[5] an edited book with contributions from popular leadership writers including M. Scott Peck and Peter Senge. In his own contribution, Spears identified 10 characteristics of servant leadership (Box 9.1), reproduced in the list that follows with permission:

1. **Listening:** Servant-leaders are not only present for communication and decision-making skills, but also to make a deep commitment to listening intently to others.
2. **Empathy:** Servant-leaders understand and empathize with others, accept them, and value them for their special unique spirits.
3. **Healing:** Servant leadership has a tremendous potential for healing oneself and others of broken spirits and emotional hurts and scars.
4. **Awareness:** The servant-leader, by fostering self-awareness and general awareness, can aid in the understanding issues of ethics and values.
5. **Persuasion:** Servant-leaders usually rely on persuasion rather than positional authority and convince rather than coerce. This characteristic highlights the differences between a traditional authoritarian leadership model and servant leadership.
6. **Conceptualization:** Instead of the traditional manager approach and concern toward short-term operational goals, a servant-leader goes beyond the day-to-day realities and dreams great dreams.
7. **Foresight:** This is probably the only servant-leader characteristic with which one may be born, while all others can be consciously developed—foresight enables servant-leaders to learn from the past, accept the present, and be in tune with the future.
8. **Stewardship:** CEOs, staff, directors, and trustees of all institutions play significant roles in holding their institutions in trust for the greater good and benefit of society.
9. **Commitment to the growth of people:** Instead of people being valued only at their level of external or tangible contributions, servant-leaders are committed to "seeing" the intrinsic value—personal, professional, and spiritual—of each individual.
10. **Building community:** Because of the shift from local communities to large institutions through the industrialization of America, there is a sense of loss of community spirit. Servant-leaders pursue building community back into the workplace environment at the lowest level possible.[5]

Spears' book included essays from several leadership writers and scholars, showing that the field on servant leadership was growing.[5] That same year (1995), Melrose[6] published a book on servant leadership as the CEO of Toro Motor Company, and since then, books by

Hunter,[7,8] Autry,[9] Keith,[10] Blanchard and Miller,[11] Jennings and Stahl-Wert,[12] Blanchard,[13] and most recently Burkhart and Joslin,[14] as well as others, have expanded popular access to servant leadership as a distinct leadership type. Research on servant leadership evolved more slowly than did popular books on the subject and will be reviewed in a section to follow.

THE POPULARITY OF SERVANT LEADERSHIP

In addition to a recent plethora of best-selling books, servant leadership has grown in popularity over the past two decades through the establishment of several servant leadership-focused organizations, some of which are highlighted in the text that follows.

Greenleaf Center for Servant Leadership

There are now several education and training organizations focused on servant leadership, but Greenleaf initiated the first, where the early ideas about servant leadership began to incubate. In 1964, he established the Center for Applied Ethics, renamed the Robert K. Greenleaf Center for Servant Leadership in 1985.[15] In 2019 the Greenleaf Center moved from Atlanta to Seton Hall University, one of the country's leading Catholic universities.[15] The Greenleaf Center offers a certificate program of three courses for individuals at varying levels of servant leadership learning; annually selects several Greenleaf Scholars, providing financial support for servant leadership–related scholarly work; and hosts an annual International Servant-Leader Summit.[16]

Servant Leadership Institute

The Servant Leadership Institute was founded in 2008 by Art Barter, former CEO of Datron World Communications.[17] Barter, who was introduced to servant leadership through the author Ken Blanchard, credits the replacement of a traditional power-led management style with servant leadership in growing Datron from a $10 million company to a $200 million company in 6 years. Barter's approach, and the spirit of the Servant Leadership Institute, is one of application: "We didn't start the Servant Leadership Institute to become a consultant company or a leadership training company. We started it to share our knowledge of what we learned in implementing servant leadership."[18(para6)] Barter hired Tony Baron to serve as president of SLI, who later authored *The Art of Servant Leadership*,[19] largely based on interviews with Barter about his application of servant leadership. Today, the Servant Leadership Institute offers hands-on training and coaching, interactive workshops, keynote speakers, and leadership consulting.

The Spears Center for Servant Leadership

Larry Spears became president and CEO of the Greenleaf Center for Servant Leadership shortly before Robert Greenleaf's death in 1990, and he served in that capacity until 2007. In 2008, he established the Larry C. Spears Center for Servant Leadership with a mission to "create a more caring and serving world through the understanding and practice of servant leadership, and with a primary emphasis upon the books and related publications by Robert K. Greenleaf and Larry C. Spears."[20(para2)] In its early years, the Spears Center provided a mechanism for speaking engagements and workshops on servant leadership. Spears also became faculty at Gonzaga University, which publishes *The International Journal of Servant Leadership* in collaboration with the Spears Center.

CHARACTERIZING SERVANT LEADERSHIP

MODELS

Based on the Spears characteristics noted in Box 9.1 and additional characteristics described by others, leadership scholars have attempted to construct both a theory about, and models of, servant leadership. This is challenging, given that scholars are not in agreement with ei-

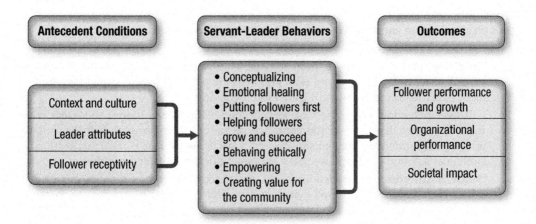

FIGURE 9.1: A Model of Servant Leadership.
Source: Reproduced with permission from Northouse PG. *Leadership: Theory and Practice*, 7th ed. SAGE Publications, Incorporated; 2016; Adapted from Liden RC, Panaccio A, Meuser JD, Hu J, Wayne SJ. Servant leadership: antecedents, processes, and outcomes. In: Day DV, ed. *The Oxford Handbook of Leadership and Organizations*. Oxford Library of Psychology; 2014:357–379.

ther the characteristics of servant leadership or whether it is a trait or a behavioral process.[21] Liden and colleagues have produced some of the most extensive scholarly work on servant leadership, and in 2014 published a model that included three main components, each with several subcomponents: Antecedent Conditions, Servant Leader Behaviors, and Outcomes.[22] While a more detailed and comprehensive model is available in Xu, Zhong, and Liden's recent systematic review of research on servant leadership, a simplified version adapted by Northouse suffices for ease of explanation and application (Figure 9.1).[23]

RESEARCH

Following Graham's 1991 article mentioned earlier, as described in Liden et al., a handful of articles explored various taxonomies of servant leadership, including Page and Wong, Spears and Lawrence, and Barbuto and Wheeler.[24-27] Liden and colleagues' publications, beginning with the 2008 article that presented a multidimensional measure and multi-level assessment of servant leadership, have been among the most cited scholarly works on servant leadership.[24] As described in a comprehensive review by Eva et al. in 2018 (with Liden as the senior author), research on servant leadership can be characterized in three phases: (1) conceptual—based on the early writings of Greenleaf and Spears; (2) cross sectional measurement—developing measures of servant leadership and testing associations between servant leadership attributes and performance outcomes; and, (3) causal model development—understanding the relationship between the antecedents and outcomes, and the mediating mechanisms and boundary conditions between these.[3]

The review by Eva et al. spanned 1998 to 2018, identifying 285 published articles on servant leadership. In this review, the authors attempted to provide conceptual clarity of servant leadership, in particular how it could be differentiated from other leadership approaches such as transformational leadership, authentic leadership, and ethical leadership. The authors credit van Dierendonck for differentiating servant leadership from transformational leadership in that servant leadership is more focused on the psychological needs of followers as a goal in itself, while transformational leadership places the leader at the center of the leadership process and puts followers' needs secondary to the organization's goals.[28] While servant leadership is similar to authentic leadership in the recognition of the role of leader self-awareness and regulation, Eva postulates that the source of this self-awareness and regulation in servant-leaders comes from either a spiritual or altruistic motive to serve others.[29]

Finally, Eva delineates servant leadership from ethical leadership by the servant-leader's focus on stewardship and the long-term perspective that such a focus requires.

Eva summarizes these studies as follows:

- **Antecedents:** Leaders who are more agreeable, less extraverted, with a strong sense of confidence in themselves and who identify strongly with their organization are more likely to exemplify servant leadership behaviors.

- **Follower behavior:** The impact of servant leadership is to produce followers who will likely serve their organization and people around them, through helping, collaboration, corporate social responsibility, and proactiveness. This is the actualization of Greenleaf's notion of the follower of a servant-leader in turn serving others.

- **Follower attitudes:** Servant leadership is associated with employee engagement, job satisfaction, psychological well-being, and positively linked to employees' perceptions of work–life balance and family support.

- **Performance:** Servant leadership is positively associated with employee and team performance, being linked to an innovation orientation, and to knowledge sharing among employees.

- **Leader-related outcomes:** The servant-leader has higher perceived trust, effectiveness, integrity, and a better quality relationship with followers.

- **Team and organizational outcomes:** Servant leadership is associated with team effectiveness, psychological safety, creativity, and innovation. At the organizational level, servant leadership is positively related to firm performance through service climate and to organizational commitment and operational performance.

SERVANT LEADERSHIP IN PRACTICE

The application of servant leadership has been widespread, beginning in the business and industry sectors, then extending to use in nonprofit and governmental organizations, and health and medical care. The Modern Servant-Leader blog currently lists 115 companies or organizations that use servant leadership, including for-profit, nonprofit, and governmental entities, but not including primary religious organizations.[30] "Use of servant leadership" is defined as: "There must be at least one publicly documented reference to the organization and its view of, support for, or belief in servant leadership principles. This may be in job descriptions, news articles, employee posts or other publicly available sources."[30(para5)] While noting several examples of servant leadership in various categories in the text that follows, more emphasis will be given to those in health and medical care.

INDUSTRY AND BUSINESS

An internet search query of "companies that use servant leadership" will return all manner of lists, including:

1. Five Companies That Embrace Servant Leadership, from book publisher Berrett-Koehler[31]
   - Balfour Beatty
   - The Container Store
   - Marriott International
   - Starbucks
   - Nordstrom's
2. Five Real-Life Brands That Embody Servant Leadership, from the HR Daily Advisor[32]
   - Starbucks
   - Southwest Airlines

- Synovus Financial
- Popeye's Louisiana Kitchen
- The Container Store

And, as noted in Eva et al., the list of companies adopting servant leadership also includes Ritz-Carlton, ServiceMaster, TDIndustries, SAS, and Zappos.com.[3] Perhaps the best described is that of Datron World Communications, as former CEO Art Barter used his experience of implementing servant leadership at Datron to establish the Servant Leadership Institute.[18] In an essay in Blanchard and Broadwell's *Servant Leadership in Action*, Barter described taking over ownership of Datron in the wake of a Department of Justice investigation that had left the company in turmoil, despite no illegal findings.[33] Having learned about servant leadership from Ken Blanchard, Barter began to implement elements of servant leadership throughout the company, putting employees first (throwing out the traditional organizational chart) and building trust through listening. For Barter, servant leadership is "a life-giving, life-freeing mindset that releases people."[33(p221)] Its one overarching ideal is simple: caring about people, and "when you treat individuals with dignity and respect, you unlock their vast potential."[33(p221)] From a $10 million company to $200 million in 6 years, followed by a record contract of $495 million in 2016, Barter credits his company's extraordinary performance with staying true to servant leadership.

GOVERNMENTAL

In the Modern Servant-Leader's list of entities that use servant leadership, you will find the United States Air Force, Army, Marine Corps, and Navy. U.S. Army Brigadier General Jeffrey Foley also contributed an essay to Blanchard and Broadwell's book, entitled *Five Army-Tested Lessons of Servant Leadership*.[33] Despite its hierarchical command and control structure, General Foley indicates that, for the vast majority of time, when lives are not on the line, "In the Army, true leadership is not about being a master – it's about being a servant."[33(p122)] His five lessons are:

- Commit to lead by oaths, values, and creeds.
- Listen by squinting with your ears.
- Be relentless in the development of leaders.
- Communicate your purpose and intent.
- Build trusted relationships.

Servant leadership, for General Foley, is at the core of what makes the Army the Army: "Sergeants are the leaders of the enlisted branch of the Army. The origin of the term *sergeant* is from the Latin *serviens*, which means *one who serves*."[33(p124)]

In a second essay on servant leadership and the military in Blanchard and Broadwell, Robin Blanchard bases her lessons learned in the application of servant leadership on 29 years of active duty in the National Guard: (1) People need to feel valuable—"Remember that no matter how senior or junior you are in the workplace, praise releases the recipient's creative genius—and organizations reap the benefits."[33(p190)]; and (2) People need to be equipped for success—". . .a servant-leader must ensure that people know what is expected of them, understand policies and procedures, and receive whatever training is needed."[33(p193)]

HEALTH AND MEDICAL CARE

Servant leadership is featured in a wide array of health-related and medical fields, including nursing, physicians and residents, dentistry, occupational therapy, physician assistants, interprofessional, public health, nurse practitioners, pharmacy, and healthcare organizations.[34-53] A brief summary of three of these categories—nursing, public health, and healthcare organizations—follows. This is not meant to be an exhaustive review of the literature on servant leadership in these sectors; rather, the examples provided will give the reader a general sense of the range of settings in which servant leadership is being applied.

Nursing

The peer-reviewed literature includes numerous nursing and servant leadership–related citations. The heart and soul of the nursing profession is to care for others; thus, it is an environment that is conducive to having leaders care for followers through servant leadership. As Fahlberg and Toomey describe in a 2016 essay, "This idea of serving first and the ability to foster relationships are common characteristics of some of the best nursing leaders. We lead, speak up, volunteer, and advocate because it's the right thing to do. . . . Many of us have become leaders, not because we want power or prestige, but because we care. We want to help. We want to make something better. We see a wrong, and we want to make it right, so we do something. Soon, others join in, becoming leaders as they learn and grow through their own service."[54(p50)] Two articles in particular serve to represent the published work on nursing and servant leadership—one addressing workforce shortages in nursing and the other focusing on quality of care and staff satisfaction. Although their 2004 article may seem dated, Swearingen and Liberman address a nursing challenge that remains present to this day: how to contend with the nursing workforce shortages.[34] To begin with, they recognize that servant leadership and nursing share a common pursuit—that of healing. Servant-leaders heal both themselves and their relationships with others through serving first. This search for wholeness in relationships is a perfect fit with nursing: "What better place to practice healing of relationships than in an industry that heals the bodies of others?"[34(p103)] Nurse leaders who adopt servant leadership can help recruit and retain nurses because their organizations will:

- Emphasize mentoring and modeling.
- Focus on customer service and excellence.
- Hire people who will be flexible and do whatever it takes to get the job done.
- Listen to others, including new hires.
- Look for ways to empower new hires.
- "Put their money where their mouth is" through nurse leaders at the top who desire to serve.

Neill and Saunders provide a case example of the application of servant leadership in a Medical Intensive Care Unit (MICU) of a Veterans Administration hospital to enhance quality of care and staff satisfaction.[35] Servant leadership in this setting was an opportunity to blend idealism and pragmatism: idealism in that servant-leaders care about the dignity and self-worth of others, recognizing that "a leader's power is generated from those who are led,"[35(p396)] and practical in that "only a leader who is competent and committed to the well-being of others can truly lead in the most difficult situations."[35(p396)] Neill and Saunders provide examples of Spears' 10 principles of servant leadership as applied to the MICU setting, including:

- **Empathy:** The nurse leader would never ask a nurse to do something that the nurse leader would personally be unwilling to do.
- **Awareness:** Recognizing the critical life events in employees that impact workplace performance
- **Commitment to the growth of people:** A conscious effort to recognize the unique talents of each nurse and channel their development
- **Building community:** Engaging other providers and patients in the MICU to enhance accountability and generate continuous quality improvement of nursing care

Public Health

A previous commissioner of the Tennessee Department of Health, Dr. Freida Wadley, would often describe the work of public health practice as "doing the Lord's work." While she meant this symbolically, many public health practitioners would likely agree with her. With its bend toward social justice and an internal ethic of identifying and serving those most in need, one might assume that the literature is full of examples of servant leadership in this domain; however, a search in PubMed of abstracts and titles that use the terms "servant leadership" AND "public health" yields only two references, and only one of these actually describes servant leadership: Koh, in 2009.[47] At the time of the article, Howard Koh was serving as the assistant secretary for health in the U.S. Department of Health and Human Services. Koh describes public health as having egalitarian roots, and being much less hierarchical than business and the military: "public health leadership starts with a foundation of science but ultimately requires social strategy, political will, and interpersonal skill."[47(pS12)]. In searching for a model of leadership that fits public health, Koh wrote that "in contrast, then, to some classic leadership models portraying bold leaders directing passive followers, the public health culture favors a more collaborative, facilitative leadership that recognizes the value of complementary and synergistic leadership functions among multiple contributors. Such servant-leaders motivate and inspire individual and organizational commitment for change in a manner that is [and then quoting Greenleaf[2]] 'insistent yet not domineering . . . credible rather than powerful . . . concerned with process as much as content.'"[47(pS14)] For Koh, it is the public health leader as servant-leader who can bring together disparate voices for a common mission, and that by "working between and above the levels of leadership of self, others and organizations, these transcendent leaders can ultimately shift the paradigm from 'no hope' to 'new hope' and create a renewed sense of community."[47(pS17)]

Public health practice is about doing and acting, not theorizing, so in one sense it stands to reason why there is a paucity of published material that connects servant leadership and public health. A scan of the websites of two major public health representative organizations—the National Association of County and City Health Officials (NACCHO) and the Association of State and Territorial Health Officials (ASTHO)—yields little information on servant leadership. One may conjecture, then, that leaders in public health may often be practicing servant leadership as "public servants" without recognizing it.

Healthcare Organizations

There are many references to servant leadership in the healthcare/medical care sectors, to cite just a few.[49–53] In communications with Larry Spears during the writing of this chapter (June 11, 2021), he indicates that "I am in the third and final day of the online servant leadership conference, and I see that there are a number of healthcare presenters and sessions (7), including people talking about servant leadership at the VHA [Veterans Health Administration], at Cleveland Clinic, Devereaux Health, and others" (personal communication, used with permission). The central mission of most healthcare organizations is to provide for people who are ill, that is, to serve the sick. It is therefore no surprise that many leaders of healthcare organizations adopt a servant leadership approach for themselves and their organizations. Change is an ever-present force in the healthcare sector, as powerful today as it was 20 years ago when Schwartz and Tumblin encouraged physician leadership within healthcare organizations to adopt servant leadership as the model for addressing both internal and external demands within that sector.[53] In the ideal setting, the healthcare leader will blend aspects of situational leadership (see Chapter 6, "The Situational Approach to Leadership"), transformational leadership (see Chapter 7, "Transformational Leadership"), and servant leadership in order to create a learning organization. Without this approach to leadership, they contend, transformation—that is, adapting to change—cannot occur, and without such transformation a healthcare organization cannot compete successfully in a market economy. Referencing the work of Kanter,[55] Schwartz and Tumblin identify five characteristics of adaptable organizations that can easily fit within Spears' 10 characteristics of servant leadership:

- great flexibility
- commitment to the individual
- superior use of teams
- strong core competencies
- a taste for diversity

In order to achieve and sustain a transformational and adaptable environment, healthcare organizations must recognize the strategic advantage of the "social transformation" of the organization, away from the traditional individualistic, hierarchical, and commodity-based transactional environment. Referencing the work of Nahapiet and Ghoshal, those healthcare organizations that "generate the highest degree of social capital will be most successful at creation of new intellectual capital and eventually will capture market share."[53,56(p1425)] In their view, servant leadership is the path to such transformation.

Trastek, Hamilton, and Niles take a somewhat different approach in applying servant leadership to the healthcare setting: here the focus is on serving the patient first.[57] "The ethical and moral aspects of servant leadership require a health-care provider to put the physical, emotional, and financial needs of the patient first."[57(p380)] Such leadership is necessary in order to build trust between providers and patients, the fundamental ingredient that will ultimately result in improved quality of care and lower costs. Trust will allow providers to effectively provide patients with the skills, tools, and feedback that is necessary for self-determination, and it is that empowerment of patients that will change the value equation in the healthcare setting. Furthermore, by organizing teams of healthcare providers to produce high-value patient care, the servant-leader will help other providers achieve their own goals and inspire high performance and innovation throughout the organization.

SERVANT LEADERSHIP AND STRUCTURAL RACISM

Structural racism, with synonyms of institutional racism and systemic racism, can be defined as "a system in which public policies, institutional practices, cultural representations, and other norms work in various, often reinforcing ways to perpetuate racial group inequity."[58] Policies and institutions, though, are made by people or made up of people. If the focus of servant leadership is to serve others that they may "while being served, become healthier, wiser, freer, more autonomous, more likely themselves to become servants,"[1(p6)] then it stands to reason that servant leadership, if universally adopted, could bring about change in addressing structural racism. The egalitarian nature of servant leadership and the sense of building community that it evokes provide further support for this assertion. Writing in the *Journal of the American Heart Association*, Mezu-Ndubuisi makes a strong argument for the potential of servant leadership to unmask systemic racism through servant-leaders holding one another accountable for promoting equity and diversity.[59] Mezu-Ndubuisi's call for addressing systemic racism and unconscious bias in medical workplaces resonates with many of the characteristics and attributes that Greenleaf and Spears have described for servant leadership: structural racism can be eradicated only "when staff and leadership collaboratively renew individual commitments to serve, learn, love, heal, and teach—not just with words but by compassionate example, striving to become servant-leaders."[59(p4)]

SERVANT LEADERSHIP MEASUREMENT TOOLS

LIDEN'S SL-28 AND SL-7

While Eva et al. describe several servant leadership measurement instruments, those of Robert Liden and colleagues are featured most prominently.[3] Liden et al. developed and validated a 28-item servant leadership assessment instrument (SL-28), and later created a more concise 7-item version (SL-7).[24,60] Both of these instruments can be used as objective assessments of the servant-leader, as well as for self-assessment (Appendices 9.1 and 9.2). Robert Liden generously provided these measurement tools and his permission to use them here. To interpret results, Dr. Liden states, "The scale anchors provide a guide. We always add each respondent's responses to the questions and then divide by the number of questions. That way, the mean corresponds to the response scale" (personal communication, Dr. Robert Liden, June 3, 2021).

PERSONAL REFLECTIONS ON SERVANT LEADERSHIP

In searching and reading the peer-reviewed and popular publications on servant leadership in writing this chapter, two individuals—Dr. Jill Graham and Mr. Larry Spears—generously provided personal stories about their own journeys into servant leadership. Responding to "cold calls" from a stranger, they have given their time and thoughtfulness in the true spirit of servant leadership.

DR. JILL GRAHAM: EARLY SCHOLARSHIP ON SERVANT LEADERSHIP

Jill Graham, PhD, is professor emerita at the Quinlan School of Business, Loyola University in Chicago. Graham's 1991 article on servant leadership, "Servant Leadership in Organizations: Inspirational and Moral"[4] was one of the earliest scholarly assessments of servant leadership. Reflecting on her original interest in servant leadership and what drew her to do some of the early scholarship on the topic, Dr. Graham offered the following observations:

> My interest in leadership as a topic of study began when I was in graduate school at Northwestern back in the early 1980s. As one who had been a high school and undergraduate student activist in the 1960s and continued to be active in my local community through my early adult years, I have long been sensitive to (and suspicious about) authoritarian leaders who desire blind loyalty from unquestioning followers. Learning about the Asch and Milgram experiments (and, later, the Stanford prison study) primed me to care deeply about the development of independent critical thinking and resistance both to groupthink and autocratic leadership, even when the latter has the attractive appearance of charisma. So, when my graduate studies included the various theories of leadership prominent back then, the only one that offered any promise in my view was that form of transformational leadership that included intellectual stimulation of followers as one of its possible outcomes. I gave my first paper entitled 'Leadership: A Critical Analysis' at the Academy of Management annual meeting in 1982, and another in 1985 entitled 'Transformational Leadership: Fostering Followers' Autonomy, **Not** Automatic Followership' at the 8th Biennial Leadership Symposium, later published in James G. Hunt, B. Rajaram Baliga, H. Peter Dachler, & Chester A. Schreisheim (eds.), Emerging Leadership Vistas, Lexington Books, 1988, 73–79.
>
> In addition to academic study, I've long loved Bible study. Because of my fear of the potential dark side leaders described as charismatic, together with the fact that many authors include Jesus as an example of a charismatic leader, I decided to try using scripture as a source for models of positive leadership theory. Two that came first to mind (other than the authoritarian rule of the Egyptian pharaohs and Roman imperialists) were the Good Shepherd and the Servant-leader. I happen to have friends who had a small sheep farm on Washington Island, Wisconsin (in Lake Michigan), and they agreed to let me camp on their land and observe both their sheep and their shepherding. (I called this my 'field research.') I took only my Bible and a notebook along with my camping gear. While that experience taught me quite a lot about sheep and shepherding, I concluded that being a Good Shepherd, by itself, is not a good model for leading human followers. Sheep are incredibly stupid animals and need to be led even to a fresh field of grass when the field they are in has been thoroughly grazed; they resist leaving the familiar, now barren ground, even for a lush new field. Even when thirsty, they won't drink from a newly

filled tank until the water has stopped moving and is still. (This gave me new insight into the 23rd Psalm's reference to 'still waters.') Sheep sometimes stumble and have difficulty righting themselves; a shepherd's crook is then used to help lift them back on all four legs. And there is no way even the most caring and devoted shepherd can somehow train or develop sheep into becoming more independent animals, willing to take some initiative. I concluded the Good Shepherd model of leadership is equivalent to a form of leader consideration and benevolence, even of love. It is beautiful and admirable, but appropriate only when leaders and followers are essentially of irrevocably different natures, when followers can never be trained or developed into leaders themselves. No sheep ever becomes a shepherd.

So that left servant leadership as a possible Biblical model for human leadership of followers who could be developed as independent critical thinkers and leaders themselves. Didn't Jesus do exactly that? He taught his disciples, but he also empowered them to be teachers and healers of others. Jesus served them and instructed them to serve one another. Yes, Jesus was also a considerate and loving leader, but he was more than that, more than a Good Shepherd. He was a servant-leader and called others and modeled for others how to be a servant-leader. So that is my answer to your question, Paul. I first learned about servant leadership from the Bible. It was only when I was drafting the paper that eventually was published in The Leadership Quarterly *in 1991, that I happened to hear a talk by the president of Loyola University Chicago, Father Raymond Baumhart, S.J., where I was a relatively new member faculty. Fr. Baumhart mentioned 'servant leadership' in his address. Afterwards I was bold enough to mention to Fr. Baumhart that I was working on a paper that concerned servant leadership and he asked to see it. (Earlier in his career, Fr. Baumhart had taught in the business school, and even chaired the Management Department, where I was then teaching.) In our subsequent conversation about my draft paper, Fr. Baumhart introduced me to the work of Robert Greenleaf and the Greenleaf Center on Servant Leadership. While that first paper already was done, I subsequently became well acquainted with the Greenleaf Center and attended several events there.*

LARRY SPEARS, AND A DIRECT CONNECTION TO ROBERT GREENLEAF, CARRYING ON HIS LEGACY

Larry Spears served as president and CEO of the Greenleaf Center for Servant Leadership from 1990 to 2007, then established the Larry C. Spears Center for Servant Leadership in 2008, which continues today. While reviewing the early history of the Greenleaf Center and Spears' own work in servant leadership, the author corresponded with Mr. Spears to learn more about his connections to Robert Greenleaf and his ongoing work at the Spears Center. True to the nature of servant leadership, Mr. Spears was generous and immensely helpful in providing information, links to interviews that he had done, and guidance on the contents of this chapter. Here is a sample of some of our correspondence, used with his permission.

Here is a link to the NBC Dateline interview that I did back in 2004: http://www.spear scenter.org/about-larry/interviews/dateline?id=65. And here is a longer interview that Ben Lichtenwalner of Modern Servant-leader did with me about 5 years ago: https://www.modern servantleader.com/servant leadership/an-interview-with-larry-spears-a-servant leadership-leg end/. Perhaps these interviews can provide you with something that might be useful by way of information, or even quotes for your chapter.

Also, I spent just a single day with Robert Greenleaf, 8 days before he died in September of 1990. So, at that point, I did not know him well. However, I felt like I eventually came to know him in a deeply personal way through going through his archival papers, discovering many previously unknown writings by him, and in editing or co-editing all five of his available books. I am attaching a short remembrance of my one visit with Greenleaf, which I wrote shortly after his death in 1990. It also appears as a chapter in Fortuitous Encounters.

Remembering Bob Greenleaf, by Larry Spears

Note: The remembrance that follows has been edited for this book; the full version is available at Fortuitous Encounters[61]

On September 20, 1990, I had my one-and-only encounter with Bob Greenleaf, which occurred just nine days before his death. I had been appointed as the new director of The Greenleaf Center in February of 1990. Several scheduled trips were planned and postponed during the Spring and into the Summer, due to Bob's strokes and related health issues.

At that time, the future of servant leadership, and of The Greenleaf Center, seemed not nearly as strong as they are today. Awareness of Greenleaf's writings was still mostly word-of-mouth, and there were a few people who had voiced doubts to me as to the likelihood of The Greenleaf Center continuing after his passing. I was also aware of Bob Greenleaf's own concerns as to his legacy, and so as I planned for what turned out to be our one-and-only morning together, I sought to share with him my vision and insights into what I believed was a brighter future still to come for the organization that carried his name. I felt in my bones that servant leadership was about to blossom all over the world as a result of the many seeds that he had sown in the preceding 20 years, and I shared ideas with him as to how I thought The Greenleaf Center could be of greater help in nurturing those seeds and many more in the future.

Immediately prior to visiting with Bob, I spent a half hour talking with Lisa Sweeney, the social worker who frequently read to him. Ms. Sweeney mentioned that he was one of the least assuming people she had ever met, and she recounted a story that seemed illustrative of his modest nature: Bob Greenleaf had supposedly once been asked by a new resident at Crosslands what kind of work he had done in the past. Greenleaf, who had retired as Director of Management Research at AT&T, and who went on to become a noted author, lecturer, and consultant to corporations, universities, and foundations, had simply responded, "I worked in an office."

Greenleaf tenderly examined photocopies of a series of ten display advertisements that I had recently put together and which had been placed in various magazines. As Bob heard about the significance of this project—and particularly when he was told that his work and ideas would be reaching a new audience of over a half-million readers through the advertisements in these publications—he chuckled and said, "Good work."

I then read to Bob some heartfelt and laudatory letters that I had received from a dozen different people.

As I finished, a look of amazement swept across his face. Bob seemed profoundly touched by hearing these expressions of appreciation from others who had, in turn, been touched by him and his writings. As Quakers, Bob and I found great meaning and comfort in silence, and so we sat quietly together for quite some time.

There was, of course, nothing that he needed to say. It was I who had come to do the saying on behalf of many of us—to remind him of the legacy that he has left each of us—and to thank him for his life's work. I told him of my own appreciation of the opportunity to serve as the Greenleaf Center's own servant-leader. Bob listened as I also told him of the hundreds of people whom I had already met by that time who had been profoundly influenced by the servant-leader concept. I said to him that I believed that his ideas were likely to become increasingly influential in the coming years. He stared intently for a few moments, and then gave a relaxing sigh.

I stood up and took Bob's hand in mine, and I thanked him for our time together. He stared thoughtfully at me and slowly said, "Thank you, Larry." As I walked out of his room, I turned around for one final look.

Bob had picked up the [Greenleaf] Center's newsletter and was slowly turning the page.

A CODA AND ACKNOWLEDGMENT

I want to express my appreciation to Larry Spears for reviewing an earlier draft of this chapter and correcting several errors I had made. In addition, where I had used the term "servant leader" rather than "servant-leader" in the earlier version, Larry offered this comment: "Paul, I also noted that you have not included a hyphen when using the word(s) servant leader (servant-leader). While there are many who do not do so, I can tell you that it was important to Robert Greenleaf that the hyphen be included in servant-leader. I am including (below) a brief article that I included as a chapter in *The Spirit of Servant Leadership*, and which I use as an instructor's announcement in my Gonzaga graduate courses. This article, by David Wallace, is titled, "The Power of a Hyphen: The Primacy of Servanthood in Servant Leadership."[62] I invite you to read it, in case you may be persuaded to also include the hyphen in your chapter/book."

SUMMARY

Servant leadership is serving others first, which allows those who are served to grow as persons and become healthier and more likely themselves to become servants. Servant leadership has grown in popularity over the past two decades, with the establishment of several servant leadership–focused organizations and through numerous best-selling books. At the same time, scholarly publications on servant leadership have provided evidence of its value and impact. The very nature of public health *practice* and health*care* is serving others, thus it is the ideal setting for servant leadership to thrive. Servant leadership is similar to, yet can still be distinguished from, other forms of leadership, particularly transformational, authentic, and ethical leadership. A model of servant leadership includes three primary domains: Antecedent Condition, Servant Leader Behaviors, and Outcomes. Using these domains as a template, servant leadership measurement tools can facilitate both the objective assessment of servant leadership attributes as well as a subjective assessment (i.e., a self-assessment).

DISCUSSION QUESTIONS

1. In what ways is servant leadership similar to, but distinct from, other forms of leadership, particularly transformational, authentic, and ethical leadership?
2. In the popular literature, as well as in the scholarly work, why might there be more written about servant leadership in business than in the nonprofit and public health sectors?
3. What might be the potential harms of servant leadership? (Hint: Read Xu, Zhong, and Liden.[23])

CASE STUDY: SERVANT LEADERSHIP IN PUBLIC HEALTH PRACTICE

[Note: This case study is based on the published case study, "Intentional Paradigm Change: A Case Study on Implementation of Mobilizing for Action Through Planning and Partnerships (MAPP)" in the Journal of Public Health Management and Practice, *and exerted and adapted with permission.[63]]*

In mid-2006, while Dr. Martha Buchanan (a.k.a., Dr B.), then medical director and health officer for the Knox County Health Department (KCHD), Tennessee, contemplated the changes taking place in her work environment, she came to this existential moment: "What have I become medical director of?" The shifts in personal and professional roles and responsibilities since joining the KCHD as assistant health officer in 2004 felt, as she imagined, like propagating waves in an earthquake. With a background in clinical medicine, and in the setting of a health department rigidly structured on personal healthcare services for low-income persons, the changing landscape underfoot was indeed seismic: the long-standing comprehensive prenatal care program had ended, and there was already discussion about outsourcing the $5.25 million indigent primary care program and the pediatric primary care clinic. Jobs were being lost, including those of highly skilled nurse practitioners with years of experience. Anxiety among remaining KCHD staff members created palpable tension in every corner, as purpose and focus dissolved. "Will I be next?" A combination of internal and external drivers of change was at play, and there was no certainty whether the eventual outcome would be toxic or lead to a new beginning. One thing, though, was certain for Dr B.: this was the proverbial "paradigm shift" she had been reading about in perusing the online material about MAPP (Mobilizing for Action Through Planning and Partnerships), a community based strategic planning process. She could walk away from local public health and return to a safer, more comfortable world of clinical medicine, or she could try to understand and help guide this paradigm shift. She chose the latter.

Dr. B. was committed to serving the community, but in order to serve the community best, she needed to do two things first: (1) serve her employees by leading an organizational strategic planning process that established a new vision, mission, values, and strategic priorities, and (2) empower her employees with knowledge about MAPP. This work on the organizational strategic plan did not proceed unchallenged. Internally, there was early pushback from some leaders within the KCHD, challenging the KCHD director because of their realm of influence and undermining the efforts to involve all staff members. Dr. B. was trying to break down silos, and this required a special, direct appeal to some because of the influence they wielded. Several one-on-one meetings between Dr. B. and these leaders were necessary to work through their concerns, both during the process of developing the strategic plan and after the strategic issues were identified.

CASE STUDY QUESTIONS

1. Of the 10 characteristics of servant leadership identified by Spears, which are most apparent in Dr. B.'s case?
2. How does *choice* figure in the practice of servant leadership?

CASE STUDY: BECOMING A SERVANT-LEADER

My first significant leadership position after all the academic preparation was as the regional health officer for the Tennessee Department of Health, for a region of 22 county health departments in east Tennessee. For context, this was mostly in a rural Appalachia setting. The culture of the organization that I came into was very hierarchical, and very top down in its management style, with the "boss" being the regional director, an administrator to whom I reported directly. Those in supervisory positions directed employees, and the culture of listening to and following the directions of your supervisor was deeply rooted. I was 33 years old, just back from a 2-year International

Health Fellowship in Karachi, Pakistan, with a freshly minted MPH degree. Directly reporting to me were county health officers, communicable disease control staff, and a few isolated employees, some of whom (as they told me) "had been doing public health practice all your life." The leader attributes I brought to this work included a sense of fairness, that everyone's voice mattered, respect, and a willingness to learn. But it was clear to me at the outset: before I could do any directing, any talking, I had a great amount of listening to do. I did not realize it at the time, but this was putting into action Greenleaf's view of the servant-leader described earlier: "only a true natural servant automatically responds to any problem by listening first . . . because true listening builds strength in other people."[1(p8)] I found my direct reports receptive to my listening approach, as they found it quite refreshing. Through listening, I was putting followers first, and the listening allowed my direct reports to better formulate their own solutions to challenges, helping followers to grow and succeed. This had the effect of empowering employees who previously felt that they had no voice. Although not measured in any formal way, the general sense of an improved organizational performance was pervasive.

CASE STUDY QUESTION

1. Identify the following elements of servant leadership (refer to Figure 9.1):
   a. Antecedent Condition
   b. Servant-Leader Behaviors
   c. Outcomes

A robust set of instructor resources designed to supplement this text is located at **http://connect.springerpub.com/content/book/978-0-8261-4924-4**. Qualifying instructors may request access by emailing **textbook@springerpub.com**.

REFERENCES

1. Greenleaf R. The servant as leader. http://www.ediguys.net/Robert_K_Greenleaf_The_Servant_as_Leader.pdf
2. Greenleaf RK. *Servant Leadership: A Journey Into the Nature of Legitimate Power and Greatness.* Paulist Press; 1977.
3. Eva N, Robin M, Sendjaya S, van Dierendonck D, Liden RC. Servant leadership: a systematic review and call for future research. *Leadersh Q.* 2019;30(1):111–132. doi:10.1016/j.leaqua.2018.07.004
4. Graham JW. Servant-leadership in organizations: inspirational and moral. *Leadersh Q.* 1991;2(2):105–119. doi:10.1016/1048-9843(91)90025-W
5. Spears LC. *Reflections on Leadership: How Robert K. Greenleaf's Theory of Servant-Leadership Influenced Today's Top Management Thinkers.* Wiley; 1995.
6. Melrose K. *Making the Grass Greener on Your Side: A CEO's Journey to Leading by Serving.* Berrett-Koehler Publishers; 1995.
7. Hunter JC. *The Servant: A Simple Story About the True Essence of Leadership.* Currency; 2008.
8. Hunter JC. *The World's Most Powerful Leadership Principle: How to Become a Servant Leader.* Currency; 2004.
9. Autry JA. *The Servant Leader: How to Build a Creative Team, Develop Great Morale, and Improve Bottom-Line Performance.* Currency; 2007.
10. Keith KM. *The Case for Servant Leadership.* Greenleaf Center for Servant Leadership; 2015.
11. Blanchard KH, Miller M. *Great Leaders Grow: Becoming a Leader for Life.* Berrett-Koehler Publishers; 2012.
12. Jennings K, Stahl-Wert J. *The Serving Leader: Five Powerful Actions to Transform Your Team, Business, and Community.* Berrett-Koehler Publishers; 2016.

13. Blanchard K. *Servant Leadership in Action: How You Can Achieve Great Relationships and Results*. Berrett-Koehler Publishers; 2018.

14. Burkhardt J, Joslin J, eds. *Inspiration for Servant-Leaders: Lessons From Fifty Years of Research and Practice*. The Greenleaf Center; 2020.

15. Pine L. Seton Hall selected as new home for Robert K. Greenleaf Center for Servant Leadership. https://www.shu.edu/news/seton-hall-selected-as-new-home-for-greenleaf-center.cfm

16. Greenleaf Center for Servant Leadership. https://www.greenleaf.org/

17. Servant Leadership Institute. Welcome to the Servant Leadership Institute. https://www.servantleadershipinstitute.com/

18. Servant Leadership Institute. About the institute. https://www.servantleadershipinstitute.com/about-the-institute

19. Baron T. *The Art of Servant Leadership: Designing Your Organization for the Sake of Others*. Wheatmark, Inc.; 2010.

20. Larry C. Spears Center for Servant-Leadership. The Spears Center mission and key initiatives. http://www.spearscenter.org/spearscenter/missioninitiatives

21. Northouse PG. *Leadership: Theory and Practice*. 7th ed. SAGE Publications, Incorporated; 2016.

22. Liden RC, Panaccio A, Meuser JD, et al. Servant leadership: antecedents, processes, and outcomes. In: Day DV, ed. *The Oxford Handbook of Leadership and Organizations*. Oxford Library of Psychology; 2014:357–379.

23. Xu H, Zhong M, Liden R. The state of the art in academic servant leadership research: a systematic review. In: Burkhardt J, Joslin J, eds. *Inspiration for Servant-Leaders: Lessons From Fifty Years of Research and Practice*. The Greenleaf Center; 2020:46–102.

24. Liden RC, Wayne SJ, Zhao H, Henderson D. Servant leadership: development of a multidimensional measure and multi-level assessment. *Leadersh Q*. 2008;19(2):161–177. doi:10.1016/j.leaqua.2008.01.006

25. Page D, Wong TP. A conceptual framework for measuring servant leadership. In: Adjibolooso S, ed. *The Human Factor in Shaping the Course of History and Development*. American University Press; 2000:110.

26. Spears LC, Lawrence M. *Focus on Leadership: Servant-Leadership for the Twenty-First Century*. John Wiley & Sons; 2002.

27. Barbuto Jr JE, Wheeler DW. Scale development and construct clarification of servant leadership. *Group Organ Manag*. 2006;31(3):300–326. doi:10.1177/1059601106287091

28. van Dierendonck D, Stam D, Boersma P, de Windt N, Alkema J. Same difference? Exploring the differential mechanisms linking servant leadership and transformational leadership to follower outcomes. *Leadersh Q*. 2014;25(3):544–562. doi:10.1016/j.leaqua.2013.11.014

29. Avolio BJ, Gardner WL. Authentic leadership development: getting to the root of positive forms of leadership. *Leadersh Q*. 2005;16(3):315–338. doi:10.1016/j.leaqua.2005.03.001

30. Servant Leadership Companies List. *Modern Servant Leader* blog. https://www.modernservantleader.com/featured/servant-leadership-companies-list

31. Berrett-Koehler. 5 companies that embrace servant leadership. https://medium.com/@BKpub/5-companies-that-embrace-servant-leadership-cf18114ee891

32. Creighton K. 5 real-life brands that embody servant leadership. *HR Daily Advisor*. https://hrdailyadvisor.blr.com/2018/06/01/5-real-life-brands-embody-servant-leadership/

33. Blanchard K, Broadwell R. *Servant Leadership in Action: How You Can Achieve Great Relationships and Results*. Berrett-Koehler Publishers; 2018.

34. Swearingen S, Liberman A. Nursing leadership. Serving those who serve others. *Health Care Manag (Frederick)*. 2004;23(2):100–109. doi:10.1097/00126450-200404000-00002

35. Neill MW, Saunders NS. Servant leadership: enhancing quality of care and staff satisfaction. *J Nurs Adm*. 2008;38(9):395–400. doi:10.1097/01.NNA.0000323958.52415.cf

36. Hanse JJ, Harlin U, Jarebrant C, Ulin K, Winkel J. The impact of servant leadership dimensions on leader–member exchange among health care professionals. *J Nurs Manag*. 2016;24(2):228–234. doi:10.1111/jonm.12304

37. Yancer DA. Betrayed trust: healing a broken hospital through servant leadership. *Nurs Adm Q*. 2012;36(1):63–80. doi:10.1097/NAQ.0b013e31823b458b

38. Anderson D. Servant leadership, emotional intelligence: essential for baccalaureate nursing students. *Creat Nurs*. 2016;22(3):176–180. doi:10.1891/1078-4535.22.3.176

39. Thomas CM, Allen R, Edwards J. Strategies for successful nurse-student preceptorships. *J Christ Nurs*. 2018;35(3):174–179. doi:10.1097/cnj.0000000000000506

40. Anselmo-Witzel S, Heitner KL, Dimitroff LJ. Retaining generation y nurses: preferred characteristics of their nurse managers. *J Nurs Adm.* 2020;50(10):508–514. doi:10.1097/nna.0000000000000926

41. Specchia ML, Cozzolino MR, Carini E, et al. Leadership styles and nurses' job satisfaction. Results of a systematic review. *Int J Environ Res Public Health.* 2021;18(4):1552. doi:10.3390/ijerph18041552

42. Garber JS, Madigan EA, Click ER, Fitzpatrick JJ. Attitudes towards collaboration and servant leadership among nurses, physicians and residents. *J Interprof Care.* 2009;23(4):331–340. doi:10.1080/13561820902886253

43. Oostra RD. Physician leadership: a central strategy to transforming healthcare. *Front Health Serv Manag.* 2016;32(3):15–26.

44. Certosimo F. The servant leader: a higher calling for dental professionals. *J Dent Educ.* 2009;73(9): 1065–1068. doi:10.1002/j.0022-0337.2009.73.9.tb04793.x

45. Dillon TH. Authenticity in occupational therapy leadership: a case study of a servant leader. *Am J Occup Ther.* 2001;55(4):441–448. doi:10.5014/ajot.55.4.441

46. Huckabee MJ, Wheeler DW. Physician assistants as servant leaders: meeting the needs of the underserved. *J Physician Assist Educ.* 2011;22(4):6–14. doi:10.1097/01367895-201122040-00002

47. Koh HK. Leadership in public health. *J Cancer Educ.* 2009;24(2 suppl):S11–S18. doi:10.1007/bf03182303

48. Diggins K. NP collaborative practice and servant leadership. *J Christ Nurs.* 2015;32(3):144. doi:10.1097/cnj.0000000000000184

49. Aij KH, Rapsaniotis S. Leadership requirements for Lean versus servant leadership in health care: a systematic review of the literature. *J Healthc Leadersh.* 2017;9:1–14. doi:10.2147/jhl.S120166

50. Cottey L, McKimm J. Putting service back into health care through servant leadership. *Br J Hosp Med (Lond).* 2019;80(4):220–224. doi:10.12968/hmed.2019.80.4.220

51. der Kinderen S, Valk A, Khapova SN, Tims M. Facilitating eudaimonic well-being in mental health care organizations: the role of servant leadership and workplace civility climate. *Int J Environ Res Public Health.* 2020;17(4):1173. doi:10.3390/ijerph17041173

52. Ahmad N, Scholz M, Arshad MZ, et al. The inter-relation of corporate social responsibility at employee level, servant leadership, and innovative work behavior in the time of crisis from the healthcare sector of Pakistan. *Int J Environ Res Public Health.* 2021;18(9):4608. doi:10.3390/ijerph18094608

53. Schwartz RW, Tumblin TF. The power of servant leadership to transform health care organizations for the 21st-century economy. *Arch Surg.* 2002;137(12):1419–1427; discussion 1427. doi:10.1001/archsurg.137.12.1419

54. Fahlberg B, Toomey R. Servant leadership: a model for emerging nurse leaders. *Nursing 2021.* 2016;46(10):49–52. doi:10.1097/01.NURSE.0000494644.77680.2a

55. Kanter RM. *The Change Masters: Innovation for Productivity in the American Corporation.* ERIC; 1983.

56. Nahapiet J, Ghoshal S. Social capital, intellectual capital, and the organizational advantage. *Acad Manag Rev.* 1998;23(2):242–266. doi:10.2307/259373

57. Trastek VF, Hamilton NW, Niles EE. Leadership models in health care–a case for servant leadership. *Mayo Clin Proc.* 2014;89(3):374–381. doi:10.1016/j.mayocp.2013.10.012

58. The Aspen Institute. Structural racism and community building. https://www.aspeninstitute.org/wp-content/uploads/files/content/docs/rcc/aspen_structural_racism2.pdf

59. Mezu-Ndubuisi OJ. Unmasking systemic racism and unconscious bias in medical workplaces: a call to servant leadership. *J Am Heart Assoc.* 2021;10(7):e018845. doi:10.1161/jaha.120.018845

60. Liden RC, Wayne SJ, Meuser JD, Hu J, Wu J, Liao C. Servant leadership: validation of a short form of the SL-28. *Leadersh Q.* 2015;26(2):254–269. doi:10.1016/j.leaqua.2014.12.002

61. Davis P, Spears LC. *Fortuitous Encounters: Wisdom Stories for Learning and Growth.* Paulist Press; 2012.

62. Wallace D. The power of a hyphen: the primacy of servanthood in servant-leadership. https://fliphtml5.com/uhie/uyha/basic

63. Erwin PC, Buchanan M, Read E, Meschke LL. Intentional paradigm change: a case study on implementation of Mobilizing for Action through Planning and Partnerships (MAPP). *J Public Health Manag Pract.* 2017;23(6):627–637. doi:10.1097/PHH.0000000000000584

APPENDIX 9.1: SERVANT LEADERSHIP MEASURES (SL-28 AND SL-7)[24]

Section A. In the following set of questions, think of _____
_____, your immediate supervisor or manager (or team leader); that is, the person to whom
you report directly and who rates your performance.
Please select your response from Strongly Disagree = 1 to Strongly Agree = 7 presented in the table
that follows and enter the corresponding number in the space to the left of each question.
****
****

Strongly Disagree	Disagree	Slightly Disagree	Neutral	Slightly Agree	Agree	Strongly Agree
1	2	3	4	5	6	7

____1. My manager can tell if something work-related is going wrong.

____2. My manager gives me the responsibility to make important decisions about my job.

____3. My manager makes my career development a priority.

____4. My manager seems to care more about my success than his/her own.

____5. My manager holds high ethical standards.

____6. I would seek help from my manager if I had a personal problem.

____7. My manager emphasizes the importance of giving back to the community.

____8. My manager is able to effectively think through complex problems.

____9. My manager encourages me to handle important work decisions on my own.

____10. My manager is interested in making sure that I achieve my career goals.

____11. My manager puts my best interests ahead of his/her own.

____12. My manager is always honest.

____13. My manager cares about my personal well-being.

____14. My manager is always interested in helping people in our community.

____15. My manager has a thorough understanding of our organization and its goals.

____16. My manager gives me the freedom to handle difficult situations in the way that I feel is best.

____17. My manager provides me with work experiences that enable me to develop new skills.

____18. My manager sacrifices his/her own interests to meet my needs.

____19. My manager would **not** compromise ethical principles in order to achieve success.

____20. My manager takes time to talk to me on a personal level.

____21. My manager is involved in community activities.

____22. My manager can solve work problems with new or creative ideas.

____23. When I have to make an important decision at work, I do **not** have to consult my manager first.

____24. My manager wants to know about my career goals.

____25. My manager does whatever she/he can to make my job easier.

____26. My manager values honesty more than profits.

____27. My manager can recognize when I'm disappointed without asking me.

____28. I am encouraged by my manager to volunteer in the community.

SERVANT LEADERSHIP SHORT FORM (SL-7)[60]

____1.   My manager can tell if something work-related is going wrong.

____2.   My manager makes my career development a priority.

____3.   I would seek help from my manager if I had a personal problem.

____4.   My manager emphasizes the importance of giving back to the community.

____5.   My manager puts my best interests ahead of his/her own.

____6.   My manager gives me the freedom to handle difficult situations in the way that I feel is best.

____7.   My manager would **not** compromise ethical principles in order to achieve success.

APPENDIX 9.2: SERVANT LEADERSHIP SELF-REPORT[24]

In the following set of questions, think of your own leadership style. Please select a response indicating the extent to which you agree or disagree with the following questions using the following seven-point rating scale:

Strongly Disagree	Disagree	Slightly Disagree	Neutral	Slightly Agree	Agree	Strongly Agree
1	2	3	4	5	6	7

____1.   I can tell if something work related is going wrong.

____2.   I give my subordinates the responsibility to make important decisions about their jobs.

____3.   I make the career development of my subordinates a priority.

____4.   I care more about my subordinates' success than my own.

____5.   I hold high ethical standards.

____6.   My subordinates would seek help from me if they had a personal problem.

____7.   I emphasize the importance of giving back to the community.

____8.   I am able to effectively think through complex problems.

____9.   I encourage my subordinates to handle important work decisions on their own.

____10. I am interested in making sure that my subordinates achieve their career goals.

____11. I put my subordinates' best interests ahead of my own.

____12. I am always honest.

____13. I care about my subordinates' personal well-being.

____14. I am always interested in helping people in our community.

____15. I have a thorough understanding of our organization and its goals.

____16. I give my subordinates the freedom to handle difficult situations in the way that they feel is best.

____17. I provide my subordinates with work experiences that enable them to develop new skills.

____18. I sacrifice my own interests to meet my subordinates' needs.

____19. I would **not** compromise ethical principles in order to achieve success.

____20. I take time to talk to my subordinates on a personal level.

____21. I am involved in community activities.

_____22. I can solve work problems with new or creative ideas.

_____23. When one of my subordinates has to make an important decision at work, I do **not** expect him/her to consult me first.

_____24. I want to know about my subordinates' career goals.

_____25. I do whatever I can to make my subordinates' jobs go more smoothly.

_____26. I value honesty more than achieving organizational goals.

_____27. I can recognize when my subordinates are disappointed without asking them.

_____28. I encourage my subordinates to volunteer in the community.

Chapter 10

Adaptive Leadership

Laura Magaña-Valladares, Sandro Galea, and Angelina Casazza

INTRODUCTION

Adaptive leaders anticipate, react to, and navigate change, mobilize people to tackle evolving challenges, and help teams and organizations thrive in new realities. This chapter builds on the concept of adaptive leadership first developed by Heifetz in 1994 and subsequently refined by others.[1] The concept is further developed using the authors' own leadership experiences to propose seven guiding pillars that can help advance adaptive leadership in healthcare and public health settings.

To illustrate these seven guiding pillars, the authors examined contributions from the world of academic public health about adaptive leadership in the face of the COVID-19 pandemic as well as their institutions' responses to other changes. The pandemic was a crisis to which healthcare and public health were forced to rapidly respond with no clear roadmap. This, for better or for worse, tested organizations' and leaders' adaptive capabilities. Case examples in this chapter will demonstrate how public health academia adapted to shifts in the environment and shifting priorities during the pandemic as well as through other organizational and environmental shifts, illustrating the principles of adaptive leadership along the way.

OBJECTIVES

By the end of this chapter, the reader will be able to:

- Discuss the importance of adaptive leadership.
- Demonstrate the value of adaptive leadership as an approach to lead in public health and healthcare settings.
- Introduce and analyze seven foundational pillars of adaptive leadership.
- Examine illustrative leadership case studies from academic public health including examples from the COVID-19 pandemic.
- Apply adaptive leadership concepts in different scenarios.

BACKGROUND

The authors are indebted to the foundational works of Heifetz et al. that formally introduced the concept of adaptive leadership to the literature, as summarized in Figure 10.1. Although many of their findings and arguments now may seem obvious to seasoned change agents, their framework was fundamental in informing how the authors discuss adaptation as a particular opportunity for strong leaders.

Adaptive leaders must observe and diagnose the situation, the organization, and the context—the *what*. They then must interpret those data to find meaning and strategy—the *why*. And then they must intervene and design action to drive and sustain change—the *what next*.[2]

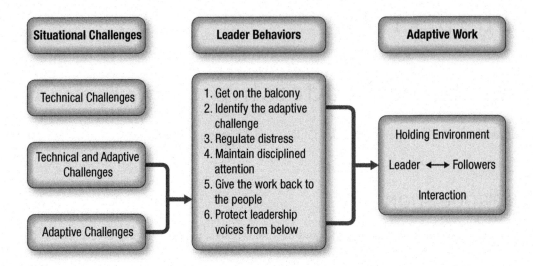

FIGURE 10.1: Model of Adaptive Leadership. The figure presents a visual representation of Heifetz's 1994 adaptive leadership model.

Source: Reproduced with permission from Northouse P. *Leadership: Theory and Practice*. 7th ed. SAGE Publications; 2016:261. Copyright © 2016 by SAGE Publications, Inc.

In working on this diagnosis all the way through to action, adaptive leaders must take a step back to strategically see the big picture, which Heifetz et al. refer to as "getting on the balcony" to look down at the "dance floor." This helps the leader identify the challenge at hand. In brainstorming ways forward, adaptive leaders should look to blend conservative and progressive approaches by also identifying what is working in the current environment that they want to maintain and build up. According to Heifetz et al., it is important to diagnose a system through the "getting on the balcony" above the "dance floor" to depict how things really are from a distance and find the accurate perspective. When adaptive leaders use the balcony perspective, they might have a totally new and very different picture of the people on the dance floor, because they can see the segmented groups that make up the great picture. When moving back and forth between the balcony and the dance floor, they can assess what is happening in the organization and make corrective decisions, make a list of what they see, look for indicators, focus on diagnosis while taking actions, develop more than one interpretation of facts, and share their perspectives with others before taking the next step.

In designing interventions, adaptive leaders should be committed to embracing an experimental mindset, being flexible and open when determining success criteria, redirecting when they miss the mark, and continuously engaging a diversity of perspectives. In this designing action stage, Heifetz et al. quote F. Scott Fitzgerald, who said "The test of a first-rate intelligence is the ability to hold two opposing ideas in mind at the same time and still retain the ability to function."[2(p37)]

Concepts can often be best understood in relation to the ideas that they are not. One such useful contrast is the difference between an adaptive leadership approach and a technical solutions approach (Figure 10.2). A technical solutions approach may very well be complex and mission-critical, but it differs from adaptive approaches in that it leans on traditional authority-driven leadership expertise and existing knowledge, procedures, and parameters. Adaptive approaches require learning beyond what currently exists to both identify and solve the problem and must be executed as a partnership among diverse stakeholders. Heifetz et al. acknowledge that many organizational challenges are in fact a blend between technical and adaptive, but that the adaptive elements are what drive the learning and need for stakeholder participation. In addition, adaptive leadership should not be confused with what is commonly referred to as simply leadership—having a hierarchical position of power, often (hopefully) paired with doing the job well and employing informal power (e.g., trust,

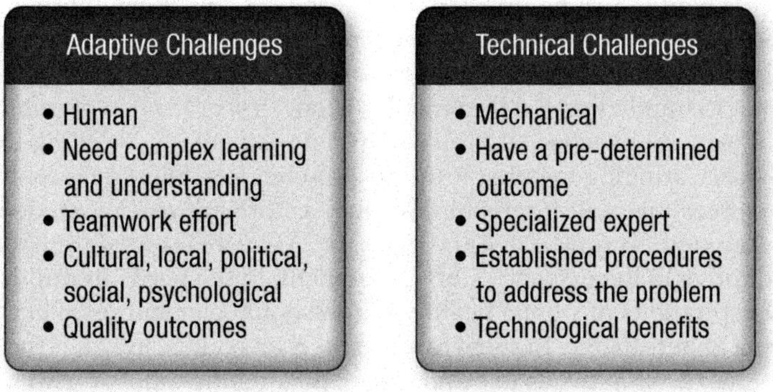

Adaptive Challenges	Technical Challenges
• Human • Need complex learning and understanding • Teamwork effort • Cultural, local, political, social, psychological • Quality outcomes	• Mechanical • Have a pre-determined outcome • Specialized expert • Established procedures to address the problem • Technological benefits

FIGURE 10.2: Differences Between Adaptive and Technical Challenges.

credibility). Adaptive leaders are those who, on behalf of a cause or mission they care deeply about, challenge expectations, dance on the edge of current accepted practices and priorities, and point out contradictions. This can be a dangerous and unpopular position but is the space one has to inhabit in order to drive and lead teams through adaptive changes.[2]

Useem interprets the adaptive leadership framework in the context of the United States Armed Forces and explains how central tenets of military leadership are aligned with key adaptive skills.[3] He explains that a strong leader must meet the troops and create personal connections, which become key when leading through challenges. The leader must make sound and timely decisions; must focus on the mission by establishing common ground, building up allies, and putting personal needs aside; and must always put their strategic objectives clear and in front, while avoiding the temptation to micromanage their execution.

Ramalingam et al. take lessons from Heifetz et al. and apply it to their own list of five principles and use the COVID-19 pandemic as an illustrative example.[4] They explain that adaptive leadership requires 4 A's:

> *Anticipation of likely future needs, trends and options; **Articulation** of these needs to build collective understanding and support for action; **Adaptation** so that there is continuous learning and the adjustment of responses as necessary; and **Accountability**, including maximum transparency in decision making processes and openness to challenges and feedback.*[4(para3)]

They outline their own five principles: learning and adapting based on evidence; continuously stress-testing underlying theories; streamlining the process of making deliberative decisions; emphasizing transparency, inclusion, and accountability; and mobilizing collective action. The authors provide strong examples of why the COVID-19 pandemic necessitates these five principles, which are used to help build the seven pillars that follow as well.

WHY PUBLIC HEALTH NEEDS AND LENDS ITSELF TO ADAPTIVE LEADERSHIP

Public health is concerned with creating the conditions for people to be healthy. A modern conception of public health considers transportation, urban environments, and economic policies all within the remit of public health, and as nondiscretionary foci of public health attention.[5,6] Such an expansive definition of public health calls for the engagement of a broad range of actors to coordinate action that can address large-scale, "upstream" drivers of health. The upside of this approach is substantial. Shifting large-scale population drivers of health has the potential to affect shifts in the health of whole populations, improving substantially on individual-based approaches that aim to change individual behavior by achieving person-by-person change. The downside of this approach is that it is far harder to achieve success while working on a larger canvas, and any effort to bring about desired changes will be undoubtedly complicated and require the engagement of multiple stakeholders, aligning them toward achieving shared ends. This makes effective leadership—and management to implement the leadership vision—a *sine qua non* of public health. This makes adaptive leadership especially important. Fundamentally, working toward achieving large-scale goals, bringing together multiple stakeholders, aligning incentives, and minimizing disincentives that will fragment coalitions is difficult and must, definitionally, be responsive to changing circumstances and contexts. As such, leadership that is responsive, flexible, and adaptive to the exigencies of the moment, to the needs of multiple stakeholders, and to the aspirations of public health is an essential element of public health action that aims to bring about change. In some respects, perhaps public health is the paradigmatic enterprise where leadership needs to be adaptive, making the topic of this chapter particularly apposite to the field.

CONTEXT OF COVID FOR ADAPTIVE LEADERSHIP

There has perhaps been no more marked illustration of the need for adaptive leadership in public health and healthcare than during the COVID-19 pandemic. COVID-19 swept the world throughout 2020 and is continuing through 2021 and well into 2022. As of May 2022, more than 6 million people worldwide have died of COVID-19, including more than 1 million people in the United States. The pandemic was the worst global pandemic since the 1918 influenza pandemic, more than a hundred years previously. COVID-19 upended lives worldwide, with countries adopting different degrees of restrictive control measures to halt the spread of disease, shuttering economies, and changing the normal course of operations for the private and public sector alike for more than 2 years.

Public health was at the center of this upheaval. COVID-19 was clearly a public health crisis, a novel infectious disease that defied early efforts at testing, isolation, and containment. The response to COVID-19 had enormous implications for health in both the short and long term. For example, as routine preventive health efforts shut down as a result of COVID-19, mortality from non-COVID-19 related causes, such as cardiovascular disease and cancer, rose in 2020.[7] Actions taken to stem the spread of COVID-19 are also likely to have public health implications in the long term. For example, many jurisdictions shut down schools during the pandemic. This is likely to be associated with delayed educational and social-developmental attainment, limiting economic prospects, and affecting health through the lifecourse.[8] In addition, as the COVID-19 pandemic evolved, the actions of public health, or actions aiming to protect the health of the public, were often politicized both in the United States and globally. Public health therefore found itself often in the eye of the storm, literally working to save millions of lives in the short term, balancing actions in the present with their long-term consequences, while dealing with political pressures that often challenged the work of public health and that threatened to undermine confidence in the field for years to come.

These challenges were felt throughout the field of public health, from local public health departments to federal agencies working on the COVID-19 response, from university-based schools of public health to organizations like the Association of Schools and Programs of Public Health (ASPPH) that serves to amplify the voice of academic public health and work with partners throughout the world on creating the conditions for better health. It was a moment that called for leadership in public health at all levels, and, in particular, leadership that was adaptive, that quickly recognized new realities and mobilized people—both inside and outside the profession—to flexibly act as conditions around us were changing. It is probably fair to say that this moment was a defining moment for public health professionals, one that challenged the field but also one that pushed the field to rise to the occasion, where the mission of public health has never been more important. Recognizing the salience that the COVID-19 moment has had for the field and the world, and how adaptive leadership in the field was inextricably linked to the moment, the coming section weaves COVID-19 as an example throughout, illustrating how responding to COVID-19 led to instances of adaptive leadership both in ASPPH and in various schools and programs of public health. Other non-COVID-19 examples will be used to illustrate the pillars of a public health adaptive leadership framework to show both how generalizable this approach is, and also how relevant it is to the particular challenge the field faced in 2020.

Schools and programs of public health had two distinct roles during COVID-19. First, they had a responsibility to advance their mission, to advance the health of the public, engaging with the world around them, communicating around the pandemic, and in many cases working directly with partners in public health practice and in government on containment of the pandemic. Second, however, the schools and programs were also themselves institutions, many of them with thousands of direct constituents—faculty, staff, students—on premises that also needed protecting from the pandemic. This put the schools and programs in an unusual position, one where they were engaging with the broader world about a crisis of import for the public's health and also having to focus on how that crisis was affecting them "at home." The heterogeneity of approaches to the latter across schools and programs of public health well illustrates the challenges that society at large faced during the COVID-19 moment. While many schools shut their doors throughout 2020 and into 2021, moving all their operations to a digital format including education, others chose to implement measures to contain COVID-19 and continue to teach in a hybrid format—using digital technologies but also allowing the possibility of in-person teaching for those who could not avail themselves of digital technologies—throughout the year.

A PUBLIC HEALTH ADAPTIVE LEADERSHIP FRAMEWORK—SEVEN PILLARS

In reviewing the literature about adaptive leadership frameworks and applying and reflecting on the authors' own experiences in leadership in public health, academia, and healthcare, a seven-pillar structure was developed through which to explain how best to practice adaptive leadership (Figure 10.3). Examples are drawn from public health academia—both related to COVID-19 and not—to illustrate the application of each pillar.

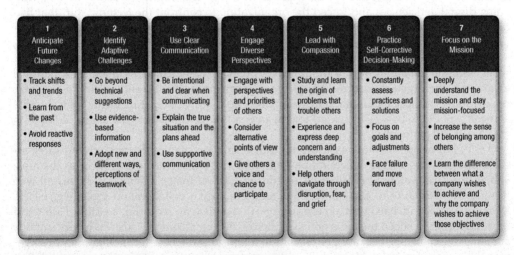

1 Anticipate Future Changes	2 Identify Adaptive Challenges	3 Use Clear Communication	4 Engage Diverse Perspectives	5 Lead with Compassion	6 Practice Self-Corrective Decision-Making	7 Focus on the Mission
• Track shifts and trends • Learn from the past • Avoid reactive responses	• Go beyond technical suggestions • Use evidence-based information • Adopt new and different ways, perceptions of teamwork	• Be intentional and clear when communicating • Explain the true situation and the plans ahead • Use suppportive communication	• Engage with perspectives and priorities of others • Consider alternative points of view • Give others a voice and chance to participate	• Study and learn the origin of problems that trouble others • Experience and express deep concern and understanding • Help others navigate through disruption, fear, and grief	• Constantly assess practices and solutions • Focus on goals and adjustments • Face failure and move forward	• Deeply understand the mission and stay mission-focused • Increase the sense of belonging among others • Learn the difference between what a company wishes to achieve and why the company wishes to achieve those objectives

FIGURE 10.3: Seven Pillars for Adaptive Leadership.

PILLAR 1: ANTICIPATE FUTURE CHANGES

The starting point for leading successful change is anticipation. Adaptive leaders need to be organized and always looking toward what may be coming next. A focus on anticipation protects the leader and the organization from being cornered into a reactive and defensive response when the need for change materializes. Sometimes anticipating a specific change is possible if the leader carefully tracks shifts and trends; however, leaders can also help their teams anticipate general disruptions by creating frameworks and strategies that can flex to tackle new challenges, like considering learning from mistakes and failures to be opportunities, acknowledging the past and the future, relying on analytical procedures and determinism (cause-and-effect sequences), and picturing the outcome of leading actions.[9]

Anticipating what may happen if the rules or environment suddenly change depends on knowing the context in which one operates, as well as learning from what has happened in the past. This awareness of the past and present must also be rooted in clear metrics; without grounding anticipation in facts, leaders run the risk of visualizing an illusion which can make them prepare incorrectly.

Without proper preparation and brainstorming about what potential changes could be coming, leaders only have the option to produce reactive remedies rather than preventive or adaptive solutions. Anticipation in the changing world requires the understanding of new and past options, and adaptive leaders should envision that future while constantly considering the present and sharing their vision; anticipation in adaptive leadership means sharing knowledge with and receiving feedback from all involved.

How Academic Public Health Modeled This Pillar

The digital transformation that enabled ASPPH to flourish during the pandemic had its anticipatory genesis 8 years earlier when public health schools and programs decided to join together under the umbrella of a new association. While expanded membership provided opportunities to strengthen the organization and create greater collective impact, it threatened to overwhelm existing technology capacity. Anticipating the changing IT challenges actually allowed the association to anticipate COVID-19. More problematically, digital platforms and processes were outdated and mired by old-school enterprise IT management theory. The trends disrupting the technology landscape—cloud computing, open-source, agile, and DevOps (the combination of cultural philosophies, practices, and tools that increases an organization's ability to deliver applications and services at high velocity)—had largely gone ignored. As a result, innovation lagged, skills grew stale, and business-as-usual ruled. But the new demands imposed by the expansion of ASPPH brought into sharp focus its widening digital deficiencies and forced the organization to confront the tectonic shift that had taken place. By short-circuiting the status quo, the association's decision to expand had catalyzed the need for fast and dramatic technological change. Learning from past experiences, ASPPH leadership started paying attention to digital trends, perceiving the current environment, and understanding where and how ASPPH had fallen behind. With better situational awareness, the organization could begin to discern future threats and, more importantly, opportunities to close the digital transformation gap. Thus, anticipating technological needs allowed ASPPH to be well prepared for the new adaptive challenges that came along with the COVID-19 pandemic.

ASPPH developed a multi-year digital transformation plan coalescing around three areas: cloud services, digital collaboration tools, and video conferencing. Cloud was the most straightforward if ambitious initiative, migrating 100% of the on-premises servers and web hosting infrastructure to the cloud. Implementing digital collaboration tools (e.g., Slack, Monday.com, Lucidchart) was a more complicated endeavor, requiring a cultural shift and breaking down of siloed business processes across the organization. This was a very important adaptive challenge because people had to adapt to these new technologies and reorganize their everyday tasks. Meanwhile, video conferencing efforts focused on consolidating to a single platform—in a stroke of lucky anticipation, Zoom—instead of the haphazard mix used by various teams. Individually, the three initiatives achieved specific goals as the digital transformation progressed over the years. Due to practicing anticipation, other synergistic benefits soon emerged. IT could manage cloud systems from anywhere and facilitated asynchronous communication across time and space while maintaining team cohesion through frequent face-to-face video interactions. Leadership realized that cloud, digital tools, and video conferencing had converged to remove shared location as a prerequisite for collaboration and innovation. The idea of a distributed workforce began to percolate as an opportunity to attract and retain talent, reduce expensive office space, and build operational resilience. While no one could have predicted the unprecedented work-from-home experiment about to unfold during COVID-19, anticipation for the future of work was well underway. By the time the pandemic lockdowns started, the Association had already implemented comprehensive telework policies and procedures and equipped all employees to work remotely. With all the elements in place and confidence in the vision, adaptation to full-time remote was swift and seamless. The power to anticipate came from situational awareness and connecting concepts to imagine the possible—a new way of working from anywhere, anytime.

PILLAR 2: IDENTIFY ADAPTIVE CHALLENGES (BE QUICKLY ALERT TO WHAT NEEDS THE CHALLENGE BRINGS ABOUT)

Adaptive leaders must convince others about the need for change while engaging them in the process. These changes must go beyond mere technical suggestions. Adaptive challenges involve new and different perceptions of teamwork, communication, beliefs, and values, and often entirely new ways of doing things.

Adaptive challenges are usually long-term issues and require complex learning and involve different types of approaches (human, political, social, behavioral, cultural, perceptional, multidisciplinary) in all types of environments.[10] It is incumbent on the adaptive leader to be alert to when a challenge being faced requires an adaptive leadership approach, instead of a technical solution. A technical solution "fixes" the problem so that the leadership team can continue forward with their predetermined plan. A problem that calls on an adaptive leadership approach requires the leader to think about the difference between aspirations and reality, and to ask themselves if a problem can simply be solved or instead should serve as a catalyst for meaningful change.

In order for adaptive leaders to approach adaptive challenges, they must recognize the potential of an adaptive challenge, be certain of their goal, include others, learn about the past and anticipate future outcomes, share the need for change using evidence-based arguments, and constantly communicate their ideas and the reasons for change. It requires the embrace of the possibility inherent in any particular challenge, and the requisite reorientation of thinking to adapt to the challenge.

How Academic Public Health Modeled This Pillar

When acting as an advocate, managing the balance between core values and political reality—which can shift over time—is essential to being a successful adaptive leader. These tensions can be illustrated by ASPPH's advocacy activities related to harm reduction strategies in the context of the opioid epidemic in the United States and elsewhere. Although research has repeatedly shown that harm reduction strategies, such as needle exchange programs, can greatly reduce associated infectious diseases linked to injectable drug use, Congress banned the use of federal funds for syringe exchange programs in 1988.

After years of advocacy efforts seeking—unsuccessfully—to have the provision fully repealed, which by definition would have been more of a technical change, ASPPH's advocacy leadership sought to find creative ways to reach the Association's objectives. Working with its advocacy allies, the Association developed a new way of looking at how to tackle the federal ban roadblock; the leadership team proposed maintaining the ban on the federal purchase of the hypodermic needles needed for an exchange, but to then allow federal resources to be used for the infrastructure and operation of exchange sites. Such a policy option was rejected by some as being less than the full repeal many in the public health field felt was the only just position. The Association's leaders helped build support for this new compromise, which was ultimately embraced—grudgingly in many cases—by members of Congress from congressional districts seeing major infectious disease outbreaks due to illicit injectable drug usage. The syringe exchange compromise was enacted in 2015.[11] The results have been positive, with HIV and other infectious disease rates dropping in areas with active exchange programs. ASPPH successfully reframed considerations around harm reduction goals and political restrictions to get the necessary funding to do the most good possible, which highlights how adaptive leaders must remain open to innovative solutions, even if they involve unsatisfying intermediate solutions.[12]

ASPPH's creative problem-solving in the face of federal restrictions required a devotion to transparency in decision-making processes, as well as the open discussion of uncertainty and evolving knowledge—both with their public health allies who sought a full repeal and with bureaucratic decision-makers who were hesitant to be seen as supporting drug use. Such openness can contribute to uncertainty and hostility; however, adaptive leaders recognize that such challenges are an essential part of the policy dialogue and provide a continuous learning opportunity, even though the process may be painful.

PILLAR 3: USE CLEAR COMMUNICATION (BOTH ABOUT THE CHALLENGE AND WHAT YOU ARE DOING ABOUT IT)

In order to advance change and help their teams adjust to new goals, adaptive leaders need to be intentional and clear about what they are communicating and how they are doing it. They must dually communicate what truly is going on with the challenge at hand as well as what the plan forward is. That path forward is the formal agenda paired with the guiding vision that sets and drives that agenda. Often, disruption and change cause anxiety and fear within organizations; those heightened emotions can make people look even harder for reassurance and honesty from their leaders. Successful leaders tailor their communications to the environment in which they are operating, including the contexts of emotional intensity. Additionally, supportive communication styles work better than dominant or controlling styles because leaders want to motivate and encourage people rather than force them to follow directions or force them into change without context.

Controlling communication styles, with phrases like "you should," "you must," or "you have to," can frustrate people's need for self-determination or autonomy, reducing the likelihood of people engaging willingly rather than through embarrassment, guilt, or anxiety.[13] Therefore, adaptive leaders are human-oriented leaders who practice interpersonal, realistic, and knowledge-based communication approaches, and thus manage to engage with others due to motivation. Supporting communication styles rely on clarity and promote productive teamwork. When dealing with an adaptive challenge, adaptive leaders use supportive communication styles by concentrating on the challenges and possible solutions while empowering people to help meet the challenges at hand.

Communication, at its core, is the transference of symbols, the assignment of meaning, and the creation of a shared reality.[14] In evaluating if the communications are successful, according to Larson et al., it is important to understand the difference between communication competencies and communication effectiveness. Communication competencies include knowing communication requirements, understanding the environment and needs, and being aware of socially appropriate behaviors, while communication effectiveness relates to the desired outcomes.[15] As they communicate, adaptive leaders should be cognizant of how their messages are interpreted by the entirety of the organization. The old adage of "it's not just what you say, it's what they hear" rings especially true here.

How Academic Public Health Modeled This Pillar

Most schools of public health during COVID-19 converted their teaching to fully online. At Boston University, the School of Public Health (BUSPH) adopted a different approach—choosing to offer in-person classes with an opportunity for virtual engagement. This approach was in many ways the harder of the two approaches. A complete recourse to digital education was more directly in line with the message that COVID-19 was transmitted by person-to-person spread and, as such, limiting person-to-person contact was best achieved by removing such contact. However, the cost of moving all operations to digital was high. Much of the work of public health benefits from in-person collaboration. And, perhaps as or more important than costs, many students, particularly those from more disadvantaged backgrounds, did not have the space to engage in online education and would not have been able to continue their studies if they did not have the opportunity to engage in in-person education. Therefore, BUSPH developed a system of Learn from Anywhere (LfA), affording students the option of learning in person or online. This required faculty to teach in-person (with the exception of faculty with medical reasons for not being on campus) and for an elaborate system of teaching assistants to help with the effort to implement this approach. The university launched a large-scale effort of testing, screening, and isolation of cases, all of which was implemented to keep the community safe as LfA was underway.

This all required an effort at communication to ensure that the entire community was aware of what was being done and why, and of changes that had to be put in place as circumstances changed. The scale of the communication was substantial. By way of example, the dean held 57 virtual events with members of the school community in spring 2020, 10 in summer, 30 in fall 2020, and 35 in spring of 2021. The associate deans held 6 virtual events with members of the school community in spring 2020, 16 in summer, 33 in fall 2020, and 5 in spring of 2021. Therefore, the leadership team held a total of 192 virtual gatherings during the peak pandemic time, from spring 2020 through to the summer of 2021. The dean sent out 15 emailed communications to the school community in spring 2020, 18 in summer, 15 in fall 2020, and 10 in spring of 2021; the associate deans sent out 26 emailed communications to the school community in spring 2020, 24 in summer, 26 in fall 2020, and 26 in spring of 2021. Therefore, the leadership team sent out a total of 160 electronic communications during the peak pandemic time, from spring 2020 through to the summer of 2021. This communication ranged from the mundane—details about protocols for testing, for example—to messages explaining the rationale for particular courses of action. This communication was not, as one might imagine, unequivocally successful. There was resistance in the community to the idea that some of the school's work would continue to be carried out in-person, despite the extensive testing protocols and efforts to make the buildings safe and conducive to in-person learning. The resistance however highlighted how important the communication effort was to ensure that the school could flexibly adapt to the moment and continue its mission.

PILLAR 4: ENGAGE DIVERSE PERSPECTIVES

A truly adaptive leader listens to and engages with the diverse perspectives and priorities of those around them as they diagnose situations and pursue ways to adjust to what comes next. Considering alternative points of view fits squarely into what an adaptive leader is challenged to do—react and adjust to complex and changing situations. While including multiple perspectives, adaptive leaders will increase their awareness of critical context, become more creative, and cultivate the tools to tackle the challenges ahead. Adaptive leaders are constantly learning about different points of view while encouraging their teams to learn alongside them. A stakeholder analysis can be a great framework for inclusion and diversity. Adaptive leadership is dependent on finding and elevating novel ways of thinking. Adaptive leaders must also seek out divergent perspectives—not simply a large number of voices in an echo chamber. By engaging with people who are resistant to the change or who fundamentally disagree with the change strategy, the adaptive leader can continue to utilize the best communication strategies and proposed solutions to bring the organization or group toward the new change. (However, it is important that adaptive leaders not get bogged down by detractors—not everyone will embrace the change.)

By highlighting how people's contributions are indispensable, leaders can encourage them to come forward to collaborate in pursuit of shared adaptive goals. Those whose perspectives are included might not know for sure the outcomes of their efforts in the midst of change, but the fact that their leader gave them a voice and chance to participate is what empowered them to step out of their comfort zone. Adaptive leaders recognize that everyone involved in the change at hand is a stakeholder and how critical it is to build trust with, empower, and constantly communicate with all of them. Intentionally engaging stakeholders in adaptive change efforts has the benefits of capitalizing on local capacity and experience, building a contributor team that has a naturally shared goal, motivating the stakeholders to tackle the challenges ahead, enhancing teamwork, improving the equity of decision-making, and continuously testing the ideas and the reception of those ideas in advance of the adaptive change itself.[16]

How Academic Public Health Modeled This Pillar

Following changes to the Council on Education for Public Health (CEPH) criteria in 2016, the University of North Carolina Gillings School of Global Public Health (UNC) began to create a new approach to core courses for the Master of Public Health (MPH). During the shift from five separate discipline-based courses to integrated courses, the process reached a point where it was obvious that some of the department chairs were not aligned with the process. This meant that the team had to stop, pause forward movement temporarily, listen to and engage a plurality of diverse perspectives, and bring people along.

The process had started with an effort to integrate core courses, partly based on years of feedback from students who were negative about the introductory public health courses. When the revised CEPH criteria were published that no longer required five separate courses, the school decided to integrate the disciplinary content, progressing from simpler to more complex concepts, content, and skill building. Students would have the experience of working across disciplines as they would when they entered or reentered the workforce. Conceptually, it made sense, but it threatened disciplines with a strong sense that if students did not get adequate amounts of their discipline-specific content, they would graduate unprepared.

The school knew the importance of engaging everyone, in particular, the ones who were resistant to the change or disagreed with the change. Sessions were held with department chairs to explain the conceptual model used to design the integrated courses and to have open discussions about the chairs' concerns about losing key disciplinary content in the redesign. School leadership agreed to provide more regular and detailed progress updates. While the school had anticipated future needs in the planning process and articulated them to many stakeholders, clearly, this had not been done sufficiently with the chairs. In pausing, the school adapted the model to the needs of—and based on—the expertise of the chairs, made some refinements in plans, and agreed to be accountable to them and other stakeholders through regular updates. The school committed to collecting and sharing data about student evaluations and performance and assured the department chairs that the school would continue to iterate on the integrated core courses as needed. No set of introductory courses would satisfy everyone, including faculty and students, but the core courses at UNC today are more appropriate, reflective of knowledge needed to be effective in public health, and satisfactory for both students and faculty.

PILLAR 5: LEAD WITH COMPASSION

Leading with compassion is, for many leaders, a developed capability. Everyone has the capacity to do so, but demonstrating it requires intentional action. Adaptive leaders know how to bring out the best in their teams by showing that they care and by giving others a voice.

According to Straus et al., there are five important aspects that define compassion: "recognizing suffering in others; understanding the common humanity of this suffering; feeling emotionally connected with the person who is suffering, tolerating difficult feelings that may arise; and acting or being motivated to help the person."[17(p19)] In this way, adaptive leaders must study and learn the origin of the problem that is troubling others, and then be able to experience and express deep concern and understanding in order to acknowledge others' feelings.

This adaptive leadership pillar can be simply understood when thinking that many times people will not listen to us only because of what we say, but because they know how much we care. A key tenet of Heifetz et al.'s framework is that the failure to adapt is most often attributed to resistance to loss.[2] People resist change when there is real or perceived loss to them or to things that they care about, rather than people simply being stuck or comfortable in their ways. An adaptive leader must show compassion, find out what is at stake (or what people fear is at stake), and continue to provide reassurance and context to bring those people into the new place where they and the organization can thrive. Adaptive leaders must be mindful of what and how they tell people things in order to help navigate through the disruption, fear, and, at times, grief. Admittedly, some of the loss associated with adaptive change may be people themselves—compassion is critical in those situations as well.[2]

Leading with compassion has proven to bring several advantages, such as better outcomes and the promotion of well-being, because compassion motivates others to feel connected to their organization and to act together. When leaders and their teams are connected by common needs and interact in a compassionate way, they are stronger and more prepared to tackle the adaptive changes ahead.

How Academic Public Health Modeled This Pillar

At the University of South Florida, a large and growing academic health center was able to realize an opportunity thanks to a convergence of three situational facts: the opening of a new medical clinic made old clinic space available; budget cuts were forcing consideration of the consolidation of services across four colleges (medicine, nursing, pharmacy, and public health); and a renewed commitment to interprofessional education was encouraging innovative approaches to assuring that each graduate embraced interprofessionalism in practice. After months of deliberations, a group of leaders recommended that the university organize and locate a shared student services operation in the old clinic space reporting to a new vice president and open to students from the four medical professional schools. While there had always been cooperation among the four separate student services offices, each had its own culture, history, and ways of operating and as such, the plan was met with skepticism bordering on hostility.

Adaptive leadership is about managing change and the leadership team understood that change of this magnitude would be more successful if the process authentically engaged those who would be affected. The leaders also appreciated and vocalized that these "operations" were actually "people" and that the professional and personal needs of the people needed to be addressed intentionally. A focus on being compassionate in planning to meet the needs and priorities of the students was paramount. A series of conversations were held within and across each group, culminating in a retreat designed to allow honest expression of fears and concerns but also ideas and opportunities. Using such techniques as active listening, appreciative enquiry, and design thinking, the plan for consolidation was modified and the timeline extended. A vice president was recruited with everyone's input and personnel were relocated to the newly common area, but the consolidation process and timeline were adapted to focus on one functional area at a time, based on student demand, external constraints, and, most importantly, staff readiness. Managing this process with compassion gave the people involved time and space to express their concerns, consider the possibilities, and ultimately come together in what is now a thriving interprofessional service center for all health professions students.

PILLAR 6: PRACTICE ONGOING SELF-CORRECTIVE DECISION-MAKING

As adaptive leaders lead teams and organizations through change, they themselves must often change as well. They must continuously assess their practices and solutions in the face of the changing situations around them. In an ever-changing and complex environment, adaptive leaders must keep their eye on the end goal and be open-minded about how tactics may need adjustment to get to that goal. This chapter has explored how adaptive leaders need to diagnose their environment and what changes are needed as well as how they must coach, communicate, and be compassionate. Leaders also need to apply these lessons to their own mindsets and strategies as well. This openness to self-correction is critical for leading successful adaptation.

In living through change, adaptive leaders must be able to step back to be objective and sometimes critical of their own decisions and strategies and adapt as the situations demand. Adaptive leaders base much of their daily tasks on creative thinking and cognitive competencies that help them visualize, understand, decide, guide, and adapt—all in a continuous loop. Successful leaders know that making quick decisions and prioritizing standing by those decisions may look like strength and confidence; they also know that those actions can in fact block their opportunities to truly assess what is and is not working.

Adaptive leaders must be prepared that their self-reflection may uncover a miscalculation that needs to be corrected moving forward. Failure is uncomfortable but facing it and recalibrating is critical for successful adaptation. Adaptive leaders must constantly question and assess while being open to a need to change their approach to better tackle the overarching changes at hand.

How Academic Public Health Modeled This Pillar

The School of Public Health at the City University of New York was previously structured as a consortial school between four independent entities within the University-Hunter College, Lehman College, Brooklyn College, and the Graduate Center. The first three offered masters degrees and the last offered the doctoral degree. This had several key limitations related to unequal distribution of expertise across public health disciplines, resource control issues, and challenges of four independent decision-making processes. It soon became clear that a unified school would hold much greater promise of cohesiveness, depth, excellence, and success. The school's leadership had to convince faculty, students, and administrators, who had functioned up until that point within the various consortial colleges, of the merits of joining together to establish the new consolidated school—which aspired to be "THE Public School of Public Health."

Faculty and staff had to be shown the tangible benefits in making the transition, united by a core mission. Throughout this process, openness to self-correction was critical to build trust and adjust as necessary. The school's leadership had to embrace adaptive leadership with a particular focus on democratic decision-making. Faculty members were involved in creating the governance plan, and a student governance structure was also established. These governance structures encouraged ongoing reflection and adjustment—the school's leadership certainly did not want to pursue a specific programmatic change if it was no longer resonating with key stakeholders.

This grassroots engagement encouraged faculty, staff, and students to feel a sense of ownership in the school's future. The governance structure facilitated ongoing self-corrective decision-making, and the immediate success was visible to all when 85% of the faculty chose to move to the new entity. The creation of new programs and vehicles of learning allowed for a doubling of the student body, and a vibrant and open interaction among the faculty ensured a rapidly growing research and service portfolio. In receiving ongoing feedback from all key stakeholders, the leadership team was able to reflect and adapt as necessary to produce the best possible end result for the school.

PILLAR 7: FOCUS ON THE MISSION (THE URGENT SHOULD NOT OVERRIDE THE IMPORTANT)

As simple as it may seem, adaptive leaders must be able to deeply understand their mission and push others around them to pursue objectives that support that mission. When people are encouraged to focus on the mission, they often feel an increased sense of belonging. Focusing on and flexing in response to change can have the unintended consequence of overshadowing the overall mission; leaders managing through change must be constantly aware of not letting the urgent—the change or crisis at hand—override the important: the mission. In determining priorities, leaders should keep the Eisenhower Principle in mind "What is important is seldom urgent and what is urgent is seldom important."[18]

Typically, adaptive leaders are working to bring their team or organization safely to the other side of a significant change, and they must stay mission-focused on the journey as well as when they reach that other side. A key motivator of advancing adaptation is to help the organization continue to pursue its mission, regardless of what changes around it. According to Cardona and Rey, there is a very important difference between knowing *what* a company wishes to achieve and *why* the company wishes to achieve those objectives.[19] Leaders must be very clear in stating and restating why they pursue specific objectives to achieve their mission. Keeping that "why" at the center of everything they do and reminding their teams to do the same is a critical strategy for leaders to lead through uncertainty and upheaval. Reminding teams about the mission also helps adaptive leaders reassure people who are anxious about the change or skeptical of the need for adaptation.

How Academic Public Health Modeled This Pillar

The dean of the School of Public Health at Rutgers University assumed the task of growing and redirecting the school after a long period of uncertainty. The goal was to evolve the tenets of the school from a more traditional model of public health based in medicine to a current model based around the concept of health and well-being. Between 2017 and 2019, the School of Public Health at Rutgers University undertook a period of self-reflection, healing, and team-building across its key constituents of students, staff, faculty, and the communities it serves. These efforts were led by an expert in group dynamics whose goal was to assess the school climate, the fear associated with change, and to undertake a team building exercise with the faculty and staff. Toward the end of this process, the school launched a 5-year strategic plan with health equity and social justice front and center. The plan was developed using an interactive consensus building process.

Numerous initiatives have been undertaken to date based on the new mission of the school. These include a diversity post-doctoral program in social justice and health equity designed for underrepresented scholars in academia; the development of a modern urban public health paradigm as one of the university's Big Ideas; the creation of a new Department of Urban-Global Public Health, the conceptualization of an environmental justice concentration; the design and roll out of a diversity, equity, and inclusion assessment for all syllabi and courses; and a collaboration with the New Jersey Department of Health to create the state's COVID-19 contact tracing program. All of these changes in the direction of the school were enacted through open and honest discussion in forums and ongoing messaging about the school's strategic plan. In short, effective leadership requires openness, inclusiveness, and where safe debate can be undertaken in order for such efforts to be moved forward. This work requires leaders to be adaptive in their thinking and for the deliverables and strategies they originally develop as part of the mission to be adaptable also.

THE SEVEN PILLARS: QUESTIONS FOR REFLECTION AND DISCUSSION

PILLAR 1: ANTICIPATE FUTURE CHANGES

Reflection

1. As an adaptive leader, how many times in a work week do you study and analyze changing situations to practice anticipation?
2. Have you developed a scheme that allows you to analyze with others the actions of the past and possible outcomes of the future?

For Discussion

1. Can you think of a situation when you and your team had to react to a situation because of the lack of anticipation? What are some disadvantages you can think of when this happened?

PILLAR 2: IDENTIFY ADAPTIVE CHALLENGES

Reflection

1. As an adaptive leader, have you been able to identify a challenging situation by identifying the root of the problem? What was the most difficult part when diagnosing the situation? Did you include others in the identification process?

For Discussion

1. Describe some differences between adaptive challenges and technical challenges.

PILLAR 3: USE CLEAR COMMUNICATION

Reflection

1. As an adaptive leader, have you ever misused controlling communication styles instead of supportive communication styles? If yes, have you been able to revert that situation?

For Discussion

1. Adaptive leaders effectively communicate the purpose of change. What are the best ways for communicating change outcomes to build understanding, consensus, and collaboration for your team to adapt and embrace change?

PILLAR 4: LISTEN TO AND ENGAGE DIVERSE PERSPECTIVES

Reflection

1. How often do you empower others in your organization to think for themselves and take initiatives for problem-solving?

For Discussion

1. What valuable knowledge or skills have you learned by listening to others' perspectives?

PILLAR 5: LEAD WITH COMPASSION

Reflection

1. When facing an adaptive challenge, have you been able to show your team that you care by giving them a voice?

For Discussion

1. Adaptive leaders must be mindful of what and how they tell people things to help navigate through the disruption, fear, and, at times, grief. Share situations where you as a leader have been successful and unsuccessful practicing this behavior.

PILLAR 6: PRACTICE ONGOING SELF-CORRECTIVE DECISION-MAKING

Reflection

1. Do you consider yourself to be open-minded about adjustments? Why or why not?

For Discussion

1. Describe a situation in which you, as an adaptive leader, learned from self-correction.

PILLAR 7: FOCUS ON THE MISSION

Reflection

1. As an adaptive leader, can you tell the difference between *what* the organization wishes to achieve and *why* the organization wishes to achieve those objectives?

For Discussion

1. In your own words, describe the meaning of the Eisenhower Principle: "What is important is seldom urgent and what is urgent is seldom important."

FINAL CONSIDERATIONS FOR THE ADAPTIVE LEADER

Adaptive leadership is about knowing and managing one's environment but also has a critical self-reflective and self-care element. It is important for adaptive leaders to prioritize their physical, social, and emotional well-being and resilience. Heifetz et al. lay out five elements[20]:

1. Exist in the balance between optimism and realism to avoid being in denial or too cynical.
2. Find sanctuaries (a place or an activity) that allow you to pause, reflect, and recenter your perspective.

3. Find and lean on confidants to debrief with—ideally, external people you trust and who will care more about you than the specific issues you are grappling with.

4. Bring more of your authentic and emotional self to work—when balancing emotion with poise, it reminds the people around you that while change is hard and trying, it is doable.

5. Don't lose yourself in your role or in the change you are managing—you should aim to not be defined by a single issue both because it makes you vulnerable to environmental shifts and because it keeps you from other fulfilling opportunities.

SUMMARY

Leaders in public health and healthcare will best serve their teams and missions by embracing the tenets of adaptive leadership. In following the seven pillars proposed in this chapter, leaders can endeavor to lead through change with a focus on communication and compassion. The worlds of public health and healthcare often present challenges that are time-sensitive and without a clear roadmap—the COVID-19 pandemic is one such example. This chapter explores how academic public health responded to the pandemic as well as other challenges facing the organizations as a means to demonstrate the necessity of truly adapting to shifting environments, rather than proposing technical and formulaic reactionary strategies. By consciously practicing adaptive strategies, health leaders can offer solutions that are contextual and relevant, ensure stakeholder buy-in with compassionate and purposeful communication, and continuously iterate on whether the strategies are best meeting the often-changing needs at hand.

DISCUSSION QUESTIONS

1. Describe some differences between adaptive challenges and technical challenges.

2. Adaptive leaders effectively communicate the purpose of change. What are the best ways for communicating change outcomes to build understanding, consensus, and collaboration for your team to adapt and embrace change?

3. Describe a situation in which you, as an adaptive leader, learned from self-correction.

4. As an adaptive leader, can you tell the difference between *what* the organization wishes to achieve and *why* the organization wishes to achieve those objectives?

5. In your own words, describe the meaning of the Eisenhower Principle: "What is important is seldom urgent and what is urgent is seldom important."

A robust set of instructor resources designed to supplement this text is located at http://connect.springerpub.com/content/book/978-0-8261-4924-4. Qualifying instructors may request access by emailing **textbook@springerpub.com**.

REFERENCES

1. Heifetz RA. *Leadership Without Easy Answers*. Belknap Press of Harvard University Press; 1994.
2. Heifetz RA, Grashow A, Linsky M. *The Practice of Adaptive Leadership: Tools and Tactics for Changing Your Organization and the World*. Harvard Business Press; 2009.
3. Useem M. Four lessons in adaptive leadership. *Harvard Business Review*. November 2010. https://hbr.org/2010/11/four-lessons-in-adaptive-leadership
4. Ramalingam B, Nabarro D, Oqubay A, et al. 5 principles to guide adaptive leadership. *Harvard Business Review*. September 2020. https://hbr.org/2020/09/5-principles-to-guide-adaptive-leadership
5. Galea S, Annas GJ. Aspirations and strategies for public health. *JAMA*. 2016;315(7):655–656. doi:10.1001/jama.2016.0198
6. DeSalvo KB, O'Carroll PW, Koo D, Auerbach JM, Monroe JA. Public health 3.0: time for an upgrade. *Am J Public Health*. 2016;106(4):621–622. doi:10.2105/AJPH.2016.303063
7. Sharpless NE. COVID-19 and cancer. *Science*. 2020;368(6497):1290. doi:10.1126/science.abd3377
8. Christakis DA, Van Cleve W, Zimmerman FJ. Estimation of US children's educational attainment and years of life lost associated with primary school closures during the coronavirus disease 2019 pandemic. *JAMA Netw Open*. 2020;3(11):e2028786. doi:10.1001/jamanetworkopen.2020.28786
9. Nadin MIHAI. How can anticipation inform creative leadership. 2008. https://www.nadin.ws/wp-content/uploads/2010/02/creative-leadership.pdf
10. O'Brien K, Selboe E, eds. *The Adaptive Challenge of Climate Change*. Cambridge University Press; 2015. https://www-cambridge-org.pbidi.unam.mx:2443/core/services/aop-cambridge-core/content/view/DCC65FF4C9422497CBCD50165C41CB90/9781139149389c1_p1-23_CBO.pdf/climate_change_as_an_adaptive_challenge.pdf
11. Public Law No. 105-78, 111 Stat 1515. https://www.gpo.gov/fdsys/pkg/PLAW-105publ78/pdf/PLAW-105publ78.pdf
12. CDC. HIV infection risk, prevention, and testing behaviors among persons who inject drugs–National HIV Behavioral Surveillance: injection drug use – 23 U.S. Cities, 2018. HIV Surveillance Special Report 2020; 24.
13. Vansteenkiste M, Simons J, Lens W, Soenens B, Matos L. Examining the motivational impact of intrinsic versus extrinsic goal framing and internally controlling versus autonomy-supportive communication style upon early adolescents' academic achievement. *Child Dev*. 2005;76(2):483–501. http://citeseerx.ist.psu.edu/viewdoc/download;jsessionid=3F40C2E5A0D79B7FAFFA6A1395BED14C?doi=10.1.1.582.5440&rep=rep1&type=pdf
14. Hackman MZ, Johnson CE. *Leadership: A Communication Perspective*. Waveland Press; 2013. https://books.google.es/books?hl=es&lr=&id=9V4WAAAAQBAJ&oi=fnd&pg=PR1&dq=communication+competencies+in+adaptive+leadership&ots=pA4vosPRJu&sig=jlgIlUWtLJCsQIef8PBpLyJlNcM#v=onepage&q=communication%20competencies%20in%20adaptive%20leadership&f=false
15. Larson C. *Assessing Functional Communication*. 1978. https://files.eric.ed.gov/fulltext/ED153275.pdf
16. Bryson JM, Patton MQ. Analyzing and engaging stakeholders. In: Newcomer KE, Hatry HP, Wholey JS, eds. *Handbook of Practical Program Evaluation*. Jossey-Bass; 2010:3, 30–54. https://www.preventionweb.net/files/7995_APF.pdf#page=52
17. Strauss C, Taylor BL, Gu J, et al. What is compassion and how can we measure it? A review of definitions and measures. *Clin Psychol Rev*. 2016;47:26. https://www.sciencedirect.com/science/article/pii/S0272735816300216#bbb0110
18. Jenkins J. *Urgent Versus Important: Use Your Time Effectively*. Churchill Leadership Group Inc.; 2020. https://churchillleadershipgroup.com/urgent-versus-important-use-time-effectively/
19. Cardona P, Rey C. Management by missions: how to make the mission a part of management. *Probl Perspect Manag*. 2006;4(1):164–174. http://www.dpmc.com.br/wp-content/uploads/sites/5/2020/06/management-by-missions.pdf
20. Heiftez R, Grashow A, Linsky M. Leadership in a (permanent) crisis. *Harvard Business Review*. July–August 2009. https://hbr.org/2009/07/leadership-in-a-permanent-crisis

APPENDIX 10.1: ADAPTIVE LEADERSHIP QUESTIONNAIRE

My Name: _____

Instructions: This questionnaire contains items that assess different dimensions of adaptive leadership and will be completed by you and others who know you (coworkers, friends, members of a group to which you belong).

- ■ Make five copies of this questionnaire.
- ■ Fill out the assessment about yourself; where you see the phrase "this leader," replace it with "I" or "me."
- ■ Have each of five individuals indicate the degree to which they agree with each of the 30 statements that follow regarding your leadership by circling the number from the scale that they believe most accurately characterizes their response to the statement. There are no right or wrong responses.
- ■ Use the following rating scale:
  - ● Strongly Disagree 1
  - ● Disagree 2
  - ● Neutral 3
  - ● Agree 4
  - ● Strongly Agree 5

1. When difficulties emerge in our organization, this leader is good at stepping back and assessing the dynamics of the people involved.
2. When events trigger strong emotional responses among employees, this leader uses his/her authority as a leader to resolve the problem.
3. When people feel uncertain about organizational change, they trust that this leader will help them work through the difficulties.
4. In complex situations, this leader gets people to focus on the issues they are trying to avoid.
5. When employees are struggling with a decision, this leader tells them what he/she thinks they should do.
6. During times of difficult change, this leader welcomes the thoughts of group members with low status.
7. In difficult situations, this leader sometimes loses sight of the "big picture."
8. When people are struggling with a value conflict, this leader uses his/her expertise to tell them what to do.
9. When people begin to be disturbed by unresolved conflicts, this leader encourages them to address the issues.
10. During organizational change, this leader challenges people to concentrate on the "hot" topics.
11. When employees look to this leader for answers, he/she encourages them to think for themselves.
12. Listening to group members with radical ideas is valuable to this leader.
13. When this leader disagrees with someone, he/she has difficulty listening to what the other person is really saying.
14. When others are struggling with intense conflicts, this leader steps in to resolve their differences for them.
15. This leader has the emotional capacity to comfort others as they work through intense issues.
16. When people try to avoid controversial organizational issues, this leader brings these conflicts into the open.

17. This leader encourages his/her employees to take initiative in defining and solving problems.
18. This leader is open to people who bring up unusual ideas that seem to hinder the progress of the group.
19. In challenging situations, this leader likes to observe the parties involved and assess what's really going on.
20. This leader encourages people to discuss the "elephant in the room."
21. People recognize that this leader has confidence to tackle challenging problems.
22. This leader thinks it is reasonable to let people avoid confronting difficult issues.
23. When people look to this leader to solve problems, he/she enjoys providing solutions.
24. This leader has an open ear for people who don't seem to fit in with the rest of the group.
25. In a difficult situation, this leader will step out of the dispute to gain perspective on it.
26. This leader thrives on helping people find new ways of coping with organizational problems.
27. People see this leader as someone who holds steady in the storm.
28. In an effort to keep things moving forward, this leader lets people avoid issues that are troublesome.
29. When people are uncertain about what to do, this leader empowers them to decide for themselves.
30. To restore equilibrium in the organization, this leader tries to neutralize comments of out-group members.

ALQ Scoring Formula

Get on the Balcony: This score represents the degree to which you are able to step back and see the complexities and interrelated dimensions of a situation.

To arrive at this score:

Sum items 1, 19, and 25 and the reversed (R) score values for 7 and 13 (i.e., change 1 to 5, 2 to 4, 4 to 2, and 5 to 1, with 3 remaining unchanged).

1 _____ 7(R) _____ 13(R) _____ 19 _____ 25 _____ Total _____

Identify the Adaptive Challenge: This score represents the degree to which you recognize adaptive challenges and do not respond to these challenges with technical leadership.

To arrive at this score:

Sum items 16 and 20 and the reversed (R) score values for 2, 8, and 14 (i.e., change 1 to 5, 2 to 4, 4 to 2, and 5 to 1, with 3 remaining unchanged).

2(R) _____ 8(R) _____ 14(R) _____ 16 _____ 20 _____ Total _____

Regulate Distress: This score represents the degree to which you provide a safe environment in which others can tackle difficult problems and to which you are seen as confident and calm in conflict situations.

To arrive at this score:

Sum items 3, 9, 15, 21, and 27.

3 ___ 9 _____ 15 _____ 21 _____ 27 _____ Total _____

Maintain Disciplined Attention: This score represents the degree to which you get others to face challenging issues and not let them avoid difficult problems.

To arrive at this score:

Sum items 4, 10, and 26 and the reversed (R) score values for 22 and 28 (i.e., change 1 to 5, 2 to 4, 4 to 2, and 5 to 1, with 3 remaining unchanged).

4 _____ 10 _____ 22(R) _____ 26 _____ 28(R) _____ Total _____

Give the Work Back to the People: This score is the degree to which you empower others to think for themselves and solve their own problems.

To arrive at this score:

Sum items 11, 17, and 29 and the reversed (R) score values for 5 and 23 (i.e., change 1 to 5, 2 to 4, 4 to 2, and 5 to 1, with 3 remaining unchanged).

5(R) _____ 11 _____ 17 _____ 23(R) _____ 29 _____ Total _____

Protect Leadership Voices From Below: This score represents the degree to which you are open and accepting of unusual or radical contributions from low-status group members.

To arrive at this score:

Sum items 6, 12, 18, and 24 and the reversed (R) score value for 30 (i.e., change 1 to 5, 2 to 4, 4 to 2, and 5 to 1, with 3 remaining unchanged).

6 _____ 12 _____ 18 _____ 24 _____ 30(R) _____ Total _____

ALQ Scoring Chart

To complete the scoring chart, enter the raters' scores and your own scores in the appropriate column on the scoring sheet that follows. Find the average score from your five raters, and then calculate the difference between the average and your self-rating.

	RATER 1	RATER 2	RATER 3	RATER 4	RATER 5	AVERAGE RATING	SELF- RATING	DIFFER- ENCE
Get on the Balcony								
Identify the Adaptive Challenge								
Regulate Distress								
Maintain Disciplined Attention								
Give the Work Back to the People								
Protect Leadership Voices From Below								

ALQ Scoring Interpretation

High range: A score between 21 and 25 means you are strongly inclined to exhibit this adaptive leadership behavior.

Moderately high range: A score between 16 and 20 means you moderately exhibit this adaptive leadership behavior.

Moderately low range: A score between 11 and 15 means you at times exhibit this adaptive leadership behavior.

Low range: A score between 5 and 10 means you are seldom inclined to exhibit this adaptive leadership behavior.

This questionnaire measures adaptive leadership by assessing six components of the process: get on the balcony, identify the adaptive challenge, regulate distress, maintain disciplined attention, give the work back to the people, and protect leadership voices from below. By comparing your scores on each of these components, you can determine which are your stronger and which are your weaker components. The scoring chart allows you to see where your perceptions are the same as those of others and where they differ.

There are no "perfect" scores for this questionnaire. While it is confirming when others see you in the same way as you see yourself, it is also beneficial to know when they see you differently. This assessment can help you understand those dimensions of your adaptive leadership that are strong and dimensions of your adaptive leadership you may seek to improve.

(*Source:* Northouse PG. *Leadership: Theory and Practice*. SAGE Publications; 2016. Reproduced with permission of SAGE Publications, Inc.)

Chapter 11

Leading Change

Suzanne M. Babich

INTRODUCTION

There are many possible recipes for effective change leadership. This chapter will explore some of the ingredients that can help change efforts succeed. Key steps include clearly articulating the rationale for change, understanding the environmental context in which the change is to happen, and identifying those with an interest in the change, including understanding the nature of their interests and their potential for assisting or blocking change. This chapter presents strategies that many leaders use to work more effectively with stakeholders, and how those leaders apply lessons gleaned from others, including what has worked in the past, what has not, and why. It also brings together evidence and leadership principles to craft a plan for change that can be effective and sustainable in improving the public's health.

OBJECTIVES

By the end of this chapter, the reader will be able to:

- Identify the underlying problem driving the need for change.
- Describe the environmental conditions that comprise the context for organization or policy level change.
- Assess stakeholders with an interest in influencing the shape, pace, or direction of change.
- Understand key concepts for working effectively with stakeholders to produce change.
- Analyze information about strategic successes, failures, barriers to, and facilitators of change.
- Apply evidence and leadership principles to create a viable vision and plan for change.

PRACTICAL CHANGE LEADERSHIP IN PUBLIC HEALTH AND HEALTHCARE

There is no one right way to lead change. When problems reach the point that the status quo is no longer desirable or possible, there are many potential paths to a solution. Passivity—the "take no action" approach—may leave the future to chance. At times, this may be the strategic choice of some stakeholders, particularly when they have confidence that others will take an active role in advancing their favored agenda. Those who want to actively influence the shape, pace, or direction of change, though, will need to effectively exercise the art and skill of leadership.

In the context of this chapter, public health and healthcare change leadership refers to change at either of two levels:

■ change that increases an organization's ability to improve the public's health; and
■ policy development and implementation at any level—local, state, regional, provincial, national, or international—with the goal of improving the public's health.

The distinction between leading change in *public health* and leading change in *healthcare* merits a brief explanation in relation to the two levels at which this chapter addresses change leadership.

In general, discussion about public health refers to the health of populations in the aggregate. That is, it tends to focus on system-level healthcare in communities of people, whether those people are within local communities, states, provinces, regions, nations, or globally. Public health is often preventive in nature, in that it includes attention to policies, programs, and systems of care that protect the health and well-being of people. Examples include fluoridation of drinking water, governmental policies on immunization, local health department management of infectious disease outbreaks, and monitoring and surveillance of food-borne illness.

In contrast, references to healthcare change leadership often center the change at the level of organizations, often in the context of health services delivery to individuals. Examples include organizational change in hospitals to improve policies to mitigate the incidence of hospital-acquired infections, or improvement of processes at a community health clinic to decrease the wait time for people coming for testing for sexually transmitted infections.

Despite these descriptions, there can be considerable overlap, blurring the distinctions between public health and healthcare. For example, hospital systems that provide care to individual patients may be involved in providing large-scale screening and preventive health services such as education campaigns and screenings for high blood pressure for large groups of people. Public health departments may offer patient-level interventions such as immunizations or well-baby screenings for infants. So, for the purpose of this chapter, policy or organization-level change leadership can be applied in both public health and healthcare settings, as appropriate.

Academic researchers and political scientists have built a body of literature that documents vast knowledge about the process of how organizational or policy change occurs. The details vary depending upon many factors, including the specific governance system in which the change is set; however, the actual leadership of change is more art than evidence. Leadership cannot be learned only didactically; it has to also be learned experientially. For that reason, this chapter—as well as the textbook in which it is embedded—puts the emphasis on practice, including practical advice, tools and insights from leaders who have learned by being actively engaged in broad, diverse communities of practitioners united in a quest to improve the health of people everywhere.

The steps that follow comprise a framework for building an evidence-based plan for change. They describe a sequential, comprehensive approach to assembling information that, when applied with leadership principles, can form the basis of an action plan that has a high likelihood of bringing about effective and sustainable change.

The steps are practical. They involve the systematic collection and analysis of evidence in real-world settings. Given the dynamic conditions of the real-world setting, as well as time and other resource constraints that a leader may face, the evidence base may be incomplete or it may vary in quality. This is a reality for most public health and healthcare leaders, who may have to make decisions and take action despite some level of uncertainty.

Key steps in this approach include:

1) articulating the problem;
2) describing the environmental context for change;
3) identifying the stakeholders or interested parties, and the nature of their interests;
4) investigating what works, what doesn't, and why;

5) applying the art and science of change leadership; and

6) putting it all together in a plan for change . . .

. . . then doing it! Effective change leadership requires not only the knowledge and skill to lead, but also the will to try. Effective leaders may not succeed every time they try, but with a sound evidence base, experience, and commitment, they stand a good chance of making a difference.

STEPS FOR BUILDING AN EVIDENCE-BASED PLAN FOR CHANGE

STEP 1—WHAT IS THE PROBLEM?

Any compelling vision for change has to begin with a clear message about why change is needed. Is there a problem that needs to be fixed? A process that could be improved? A policy that falls short of its intended goal? How significant is the problem? Can it be described in terms of its magnitude and scope? How many people are affected? What is the cost or burden? Can any of this be quantified? What information can be brought to bear to help underscore the urgency of the issue?

If this were translated into an academic exercise, it would be, "Write a problem statement." It sounds like a simple task, but it is not easy. Crafting a strong problem statement can be an effective way, though, for leaders to think through their vision and articulate it in a meaningful way.

Crafting a good problem statement takes practice. It also takes discipline. It requires one to be knowledgeable enough about the issue to be able to describe it in terms that convey its significance and importance. It also requires the skill to focus sharply and distill the statement to its essence. Although it may seem counterintuitive to describe a complex problem in simple terms, the result can give leaders a powerful advantage. Long, complicated problem statements lose their punch. An effective leader needs to be able to communicate their vision in a way that grabs the attention of others and inspires them to follow in the direction of change.

For that reason, a small set of "best practices" has emerged over time. These tips are useful for leaders who want to refine their "calls to action."

Better problem statements often:

- Are concise.
  - Hold the attention of a reader or listener by using shorter statements. Just the exercise of distilling an idea to its essence also forces leaders to focus precisely on what they mean. The discipline of doing this helps to ensure clearer communication.
- Use simple language, free from jargon.
  - Eliminate barriers to understanding, ensuring that the widest audience will get the message.
- Convey a sense of the magnitude, scope, and urgency of a problem.
  - Increase the chances that others will take notice and be motivated to act.
- Pair the problem with a suggested solution.
  - Draw attention to and interest in the direction of support for your preferred action.

There are many other strategies for effectively communicating ideas to the media and other audiences that are beyond the scope of this chapter. Guidance is available in books, multimedia resources, and hands-on workshops that focus on communication training for leaders. Look for support for this type of coaching from professional associations, universities, personal leadership coaches, and other organizations and businesses that specialize in this type of professional development.

It takes time and experience to master strong communications skills. Effective leaders commit themselves to continuous improvement of their communication skills and are constantly seeking to learn and improve over time, with practice.

EFFECTIVE PROBLEM STATEMENTS

Which of the following problem statements do you think are effective? Why? How could they be strengthened?

PROBLEM STATEMENT 1—MICHAEL J. FOX AND PARKINSON'S DISEASE

The following is an excerpt from a 2-minute statement of Canadian actor Michael J. Fox at a September 1999 Senate hearing where he joined other Parkinson's advocates urging Congress to increase research funding for the disease by $75 million.[1]

> [T]he time for quietly soldiering on is through. The war against Parkinson's is a winnable war, and I have resolved to play a part in that victory. . . . 1 million Americans living with Parkinson's want to beat this disease. . . . But with your help, if we all do everything we can to eradicate this disease, in my 50s I will be dancing at my children's weddings. And mine will be just one of millions of happy stories.[1]

In this case, the problem statement, as an advocacy tool, is particularly effective because of its celebrity author, Michael J. Fox, a popular actor who became a "face" of Parkinson's disease when he went public with his own diagnosis. In his statement, he gives a sense of the magnitude and scope of the problem, citing the prevalence of the disease in the United States. A famous name helps to draw attention to a statement such as this, and big figures such as "one million Americans" help to underscore the importance and urgency of the problem. Fox also humanizes his call to action with a sentimental wish to dance at his children's weddings.

Fox, of course, is also pairing his statement with a larger effort to advance a solution—a call for Congress to increase research funding for the disease by $75 million. He uses imagery such as ". . . soldiering on . . ." and ". . . winnable war" to compare efforts to eradicate a disease to those of fighting a military battle. It could be argued that his statement could be even more powerful if he dispensed with this analogy and, instead, simply used clear language to state exactly what he meant: it will take a powerful, cooperative effort, but eradicating Parkinson's disease would relieve the suffering of millions of Americans and those who love them. In writing and speaking, the use of cliches and similar turns of phrase is seldom as powerful as direct, clear language.

What do you think?

PROBLEM STATEMENT 2—DR. RISA LAVIZZO-MOUREY AND YOUR ZIP CODE

The following is an excerpt from a 1.5-minute 2017 video statement from Dr. Risa Lavizzo-Mourey, former president and CEO of the Robert Wood Johnson Foundation, on health inequalities. Risa Lavizzo-Mourey was the first African American to head the foundation.[2]

> Inequality is when your zip code is as important as your genetic code in predicting how long and how well you're going to live. . . . How healthy someone is depends on their whole environment. The zipc code says so much about the immediate environment in which we live. It is often a lens into housing, education, access to healthcare services, access to healthy foods. A zip code is not supposed to be that kind of lens, so we have to change that if we're going to make the zip code about getting mail to people and not about predicting how long they're going to live. Without health, we will not have equity.[2]

Dr. Lavizzo-Mourey introduces the idea that one's zip code is often a proxy for longevity; health researchers can predict the likely length of a person's life based on nothing more than where they live. It may be a surprising concept for some people, and it can be a good stimulus for discussion about the social determinants of health.

(continued)

Zip code is mentioned four times in the short statement, ending with, "A zip code is not supposed to be that kind of lens, so we have to change that if we're going to make the zip code about getting mail to people and not about predicting how long they're going to live."[2] At this point, the statement loses some power, because the main point is cloaked in the ongoing "zip code" frame. The statement could be strengthened by switching to a direct remark, such as, "Everyone has a right to an environment that supports health." Then, it could be further strengthened by pairing the statement with a proposed solution or action. For example, "Commit to eliminating health inequalities." Better yet, be even more specific in defining an actionable solution or step. For example, "Urge your government representatives to vote "yes" on [proposed legislation]."

The very beginning of a statement, as well as the end, are also opportunities to make a lasting impression. The opening is a great opportunity to grab a reader's or listener's attention. The ending is the chance to "stick the landing," or make a point that firmly underscores a point. In this case, the ending reads, "Without health, we will not have equity." A strength of this statement is that it is short and declarative. It could be even stronger if it were even more direct. For example, in the context of the total message, it might be helpful to conclude with, "It's the right thing to do." Another example might be, "Until everyone has an equal opportunity to be healthy, there will be no justice."

What do you think?

PROBLEM STATEMENT 3—AMERICAN SOCIETY OF ADDICTION MEDICINE AND OPIOID USE DISORDER

What follows is the problem statement from the 2020 American Society of Addiction Medicine (ASAM) Public Policy Statement on Treatment of Opioid Use Disorder (OUD) in Correctional Settings.[3]

Individuals who are incarcerated are a vulnerable population and withholding evidence-based opioid use disorder (OUD) treatment increases risk for death during detainment and upon release. ASAM (American Society of Addiction Medicine) recognizes that correctional settings are diverse and that not all resources are universally available. This policy statement describes the standard of care that ASAM believes all detained and incarcerated individuals with OUD should receive. ASAM also advocates for systemic changes to ensure universal access to such care within correctional institutions.[3(p1)]

In this case, the organization ASAM takes a stand and advocates for systemic changes that would result in a higher standard of care for detained and incarcerated individuals with OUD. They do a good job of noting several points that help to explain the complexity of the problem, including the vulnerability of detained and incarcerated individuals with OUD, the diversity of correctional settings, and the variability in access to resources. The statement makes it clear that ASAM supports systemic changes that would make access to quality care possible in correctional facilities. The statement could be strengthened in several ways, however.

The statement starts by remarking that individuals who are incarcerated are vulnerable. It goes on to say that they are at increased risk of death if they do not receive evidence-based OUD treatment. The statement could be improved by attention to the logical progression of the argument for change. It could be more powerful if, for example, it was to begin with a declarative statement that gave a sense of the magnitude or scope of the problem, increasing the sense of importance and urgency of the problem. Opening with a statement such as, "Incarcerated individuals suffering from opioid use disorder are 100 times more likely to die if they don't receive evidence-based OUD care during detainment and after release," is one example of a clearer, more direct approach.

From there, the statement could briefly acknowledge that the vulnerability inherent in being a prisoner, the variations among correctional institutions, and limitations of resources all conspire to make this a challenging problem to solve. It could then move on to briefly

(continued)

summarize a proposed solution, ending with a call to action in support of appropriate standards of care, universal access to that care, and systemic changes to ensure that happens.

Even the last line of the statement could have more impact if it were worded slightly differently. For example, it might be changed from, "ASAM also advocates for systemic changes to ensure universal access to such care within correctional institutions," to "ASAM supports universal access to quality care, regardless of an individual's status as incarcerated." The latter, while perhaps not perfect, is clearer and more concise.

Can you think of a better way to "stick the landing" in this case?

PROBLEM STATEMENT 4—CENTERS FOR DISEASE CONTROL AND PREVENTION AND OBESITY

The following excerpt comes from a statement about the obesity epidemic on the website of the Centers for Disease Control and Prevention.[4]

Obesity is a serious chronic disease, and the prevalence of obesity continues to increase in the United States. Obesity is common, serious, and costly. This epidemic is putting a strain on American families, affecting overall health, health care costs, productivity, and military readiness. Obesity can lead to type 2 diabetes, heart disease, and some cancers. A healthy diet and regular physical activity help people achieve and maintain a healthy weight starting at an early age and continuing throughout life.[4(paras1-2)]

This statement includes some key elements of a strong problem statement, but they are in the wrong order. The statement could be improved by attention to organization and logical progression of the argument, a sharper focus, and a clearer, stronger articulation of the proposed solution.

The second sentence, "Obesity is common, serious, and costly," would be a great start to this problem statement. Move it to the top. The body of the statement could then be reorganized to succinctly emphasize how common, serious, and costly the problem is in America. For example, it might include some facts and figures: "Two-thirds of American children are overweight or obese, sharply raising the risks of diabetes, heart disease, and cancer, degrading their quality of life and shortening lives. The effects of obesity cost us billions of dollars annually in excessive healthcare costs and lost productivity. It's a national disaster needing immediate action."

How could the proposed solution be worded differently? Try: "Health-supporting diet and exercise habits must be supported throughout life. The health and welfare of our nation depend on it." Another option: "We need a national health policy that supports healthful diet and exercise patterns throughout life."

Can you think of other ways to strengthen this problem statement?

STEP 2—CONTEXT FOR CHANGE

Leading change requires the ability to visualize the future and to influence others to follow that vision. Steering others requires an awareness of factors in the environment that must be taken into consideration if they could affect the plan for change in some way.

Just as the pilot of a plane must maintain an awareness of the weather conditions and the level of the fuel supply, public health and healthcare leaders need to be aware of how social, economic, political, and even organizational conditions may affect the path to change. Those conditions are often dynamic, requiring leaders to remain vigilant and to adapt over time. Table 11.1 describes these factors and provides examples of practical questions that can help leaders assess the environmental context for change. Leaders can use this information to conduct an environmental scan, assessing the environmental conditions in terms of opportunities and threats. They can use this information to help inform their approach to change leadership and adapt their strategies and tactics accordingly.

TABLE 11.1: Environmental Conditions Comprising the Context for Change

CONDITION	DESCRIPTION	SAMPLE KEY QUESTIONS
Social	Demographic character of the community or population (e.g., age, gender, political identity, race and ethnicity, socioeconomic status); relevant opinions of consumers, taxpayers, voters, audiences, and the mass media; expectations derived from previous experiences	What are the opinions of the public (consumers, taxpayers, voters, and audiences) about the problem or proposed change? What are the opinions expressed by the mass media about the problem or proposed change? What expectations based on previous experiences may exist during this change process?
Economic	Economy and distribution of resources, including the economic impact of the change on stakeholders	What are the goals (in economic terms)? What tools and resources are available for designing and financing the change? Which interested parties stand to gain or lose financially based upon the change?
Political	Agendas and priorities of those involved; political parties in power (in key governmental or organizational positions, for example)	How public is the debate? What are the media saying? At what level of governance is the change to be initiated?
Organizational	Intra- and inter-organizational relationships and hierarchies	Who are the organizational players? What are their interests? (Control? Financial? Public image? Other?) What are their resource bases? (Size and sources of financing; allocation of staff and/or funds to an issue; expertise; network of organizations in and outside government) What resources are committed to activities pertaining to the proposed change?

The conditions and approach described here are particularly well-suited to understanding the context for policy change at the societal level, whether local, regional, state, or provincial, or even national or international levels. However, the approach can be adapted, in principle, for understanding the context for change within organizations as well, where similar information is just as important. Remember: There is no one correct way to lead change. Leaders need to be able to apply structure and a systematic approach to organizing and understanding a complex and dynamic web of factors. There is room for adaptation and interpretation, to "freestyle," at times. This is the art of leadership, and it improves with experience.

STEP 3—IN WHOSE INTEREST? THE ROLE OF STAKEHOLDERS

By any definition, a leader is someone who influences others to follow along on a vision toward a goal. Doing this requires the ability to identify and engage with a constellation of "interested others"—stakeholders—who may, whether they realize it or not, have a stake in that vision becoming reality. They may have an interest in the shape, pace, direction, and/or outcomes of the change effort. They have the power to support or block change, directly or indirectly, through their actions or inaction.

Interest group theory includes a large body of literature with great practical implications for health leaders. Academic programs in public health leadership, particularly those based in the United States, often use classic texts such as *The Policy Paradox* by Deborah Stone and *Agendas, Alternatives, and Public Policies* by John Kingdon to help teach the importance of and the intricacies of effectively engaging and working with stakeholders to support change actions, especially in the context of governmental policy making, in contrast to organizational policy change.[5,6] These and other resources can be excellent sources of insight to support change leadership planning; however, principles and common behaviors described in such resources are rooted in U.S. cultural norms. Motivations and influences of players, for example, and such dynamics as power and loyalty may not play out the same way in cultures outside the United States. It is vitally important to be aware that strategies for effectively working with stakeholders to advance change may differ in different cultural contexts.

For example, in the United States, current legal frameworks make it relatively easy for interest groups, such as companies that produce pharmaceuticals or medical devices, medical professional associations, hospital systems, and health insurance companies, to wield political influence through campaign donations and other financial levers, such as paying for the services of powerful lobbyists. So, stakeholder groups with substantial financial means often have a disproportionately high level of influence in the U.S. policy making process as compared to stakeholders with lesser means. In contrast, those same stakeholder groups, set in a similarly high-income country setting but within the governance system of the European Union, for example, may have their power greatly reduced by laws that limit their ability to use money to buy influence.

In general, the potential for stakeholders to influence change is highly dependent on the governance system in which the change is being advocated. Stakeholders such as business and industry groups and professional associations may have greater clout in democratically run political systems, for example, than in totalitarian political systems. In other authoritarian systems, for example, stakeholders may have greater influence because of who they know in government than how much money they have to use. In still other countries, corruption and the power of bribes are important factors to consider in understanding the dynamics of change leadership. Public health and healthcare leaders need to take into consideration the total environment for change, including the country, culture, and associated governance systems, as they assess the climate for change and strategize about how best to work with stakeholders.

In this chapter, the discussion of the role of stakeholders pertains primarily to change leadership efforts on the external, or governmental, policy level. For understanding change leadership at the organizational level in the United States, Shortell and Kaluzny's classic text, *Health Care Management: Organization, Design, and Behavior* is used in many schools of public health.[7] Organizational behavior, in contrast to change at the governmental policy level, focuses on the dynamics of primarily internal stakeholders—individuals and groups or teams—in organizational settings. Change leadership in that context centers on the management of those individuals and teams and how best to work with them to meet a desired goal, to get the job done. Like policy level change, organization-level change also requires the ability of leaders to influence others to support the shape, pace, or direction of a desired change, to buy in to a vision. Even within organizations, too, culture matters, and organizational change leadership within U.S. organizations can function very differently than in countries outside the United States. While this chapter focuses primarily on the role of stakeholders in governmental policy level change, those working at the organizational level may find relevance in some of the key concepts described here and apply them in organizational settings.

For example, giving others a voice in important changes that affect them is generally an important consideration in leading change. Regardless of whether change leadership happens in the larger policy context or outside of government within organizations themselves, the importance of a holistic, inclusive, participatory approach, captured in the phrase, "nothing for us without us," is a hallmark of sound change leadership in public health.[8]

While there are many ways to identify stakeholders with an interest in a change action, it is important to think broadly and creatively to ensure the most comprehensive list possible. There is no risk in listing too many. Rather, the risk is in overlooking a key player that may be in a position to support or block change, perhaps one with novel insights that could lead to a better plan.

If the list is long, it can be stratified later to select those stakeholders who are most affected by the proposed change, or who have the greatest power and potential to influence change. Health leaders may want to focus engagement efforts on those primary stakeholders, especially when time or other resources are limited.

One useful approach to creating a stakeholder list is a framework proposed by Kingdon.[6] Six categories serve as prompts for brainstorming stakeholder groups that have an interest in a proposed change (Table 11.2). There may not be many, or even any, stakeholders in every category; however, the prompts help to increase the likelihood that an important stakeholder group has not been overlooked. While the framework is usually applied to change leadership at the policy level, the general approach can be adapted for changes led at the organizational level as well. Any approach that helps to ensure a comprehensive awareness of relevant stakeholders can work.

Regardless of whether change leadership efforts are initiated within an organization or outside, at the policy level, some level of stakeholder analysis is a vital step.

STEP 4—PREPARING FOR CHANGE: CRITICAL QUESTIONS

Engaging stakeholders, whether at the policy or organizational level, involves talking with representatives of those groups to understand their interests and needs. What do stakeholders think about the proposed change? Do they support the proposal? Why or why not? What are stakeholders' views on the short-term and long-term feasibility of the proposed change? How might the proposal be strengthened?

Interviewing key stakeholders individually or in focus groups can reveal valuable information about stakeholders' perceptions about potential barriers or facilitators of a proposed

TABLE 11.2: Kingdon's Stakeholder Categories

CATEGORY	STAKEHOLDER EXAMPLES
Business and Industry	Hospitals, drug and device companies, retail stores, food producers and manufacturers
Professionals	Physician associations, public health associations, allied health associations, nursing associations
Public interest	Consumer groups; counterpoints to self-interested business, industry, labor, and professional groups that place public good ahead of private gain ("people over profits")
Government officials	State and local officials lobbying for or against change
Labor	Organized labor groups
Academic researchers	University faculty and other researchers; think-tank personnel

Source: Data from Kingdon J. *Agendas, Alternatives, and Public Policies.* 2nd ed. Longman; 2011.

Box 11.1: Critical Questions for Stakeholders

1. Do you support the proposed change?
   a. Probe: Why or why not?
2. What are the barriers to implementation of the proposed change?
   a. Probe: Please explain.
3. What might facilitate implementation of the proposed change?
   a. Probe: Please explain.
4. Has anything like this been attempted in the past? What were the results?
   a. Probe: Which strategies succeeded?
      i. Why?
   b. Which strategies failed?
      i. Why?
5. What recommendations would you have for advancing this proposed change?
   a. Probe: Please say more.

---

change, revealing opportunities for leaders to incorporate important modifications to the plan or to mitigate challenges and increase stakeholders' support for change. Stakeholders may also be able to share information about previous or similar change efforts in which they were involved, including which strategies succeeded, which failed, and why. Surveys can be used to gather some of the same information if they are designed with open-ended questions; however, the lack of interactivity through engaged discussion with an interviewer is a potential limitation of surveys.

Integrating ideas, best practices, and recommendations from stakeholders, enabling them to be co-designers of plans for change, greatly increases the likelihood that those change efforts will succeed. Box 11.1 provides some sample questions that may be useful in guiding discussions with key stakeholders. The questions are designed to help leaders better understand stakeholders' motivations and potential to influence the shape, pace, or direction of a proposed change.

STEP 5—APPLYING THE ART AND SCIENCE OF CHANGE LEADERSHIP

Leading change is equal parts art and skill. Within the academic public health community, there is general consensus that successful leadership in public health and healthcare requires a combination of objective and subjective masteries or competencies. This is particularly true of those in mid- to senior-level roles in public health and healthcare settings, where leadership challenges are most often confronted.

In 2009, after a multiyear process that included input and debate among hundreds of stakeholders in a modified Delphi process, members of the Association of Schools and Programs of Public Health (ASPPH) published a competency model for Doctor of Public Health (DrPH) programs in the United States.[9]

This was a set of competencies deemed to be of fundamental importance to being effective in mid- and senior-level positions in public health and healthcare, and it specifically included the ability to lead change. In that context, leadership was defined by ASPPH as: "The ability to create and communicate a shared vision for a positive future; inspire trust and motivate others; and use evidence-based strategies to enhance essential public health services."[9(p13)]

Box 11.2 lists the nine competencies that ASPPH deemed essential to effective leadership in public health and healthcare. It shows how describing the "art and science" of change leadership has been attempted in a systematic way, reconciling and consolidating diverse views into guidance for academic programs developing future public health and healthcare leaders. Anyone who has ever tried to apply metrics to documenting attainment of these

> **Box 11.2: Association of Schools & Programs of Public Health (ASPPH) DrPH Competency Model—Leadership Competencies (2009)**
>
> 1. Communicate an organization's mission, shared vision, and values to stakeholders.
> 2. Develop teams for implementing health initiatives.
> 3. Collaborate with diverse groups.
> 4. Influence others to achieve high standards of performance and accountability.
> 5. Guide organizational decision-making and planning based on internal and external environmental research.
> 6. Prepare professional plans incorporating lifelong learning, mentoring, and continued career progression strategies.
> 7. Create a shared vision.
> 8. Develop capacity-building strategies at the individual, organizational, and community level.
> 9. Demonstrate a commitment to personal and professional values.

Source: Reproduced with permission from ASPPH DrPH Model website. 2009. https://www.aspph.org/teach-research/models/drph-model/ page 13.

competencies by DrPH scholars can attest to the challenge; at some level, demonstration of these competencies reflects "art" in the sense that it may vary according to individual leaders' thoughts, beliefs, attitudes, or ideas, some of which may derive from that individual's unique personal or professional experiences.

Shortly after ASPPH published its DrPH competency model, the Council on Education for Public Health (CEPH), an independent U.S. accreditation agency for schools of public health and public health education programs outside schools of public health, also created its own competencies for the purpose of accreditation of Master of Public Health (MPH) and DrPH programs. Again, through a process similar to that applied earlier by ASPPH, including some of the same stakeholders who participated in the ASPPH competency model project, the agency attempted to define the masteries or competencies needed by successful mid- to senior-level public health and healthcare practitioners, including those competencies necessary for successful change leadership. In this case, the agency defined "D3. DrPH Foundational Competencies."[10] Among the foundational competencies was a subset of 10 leadership, management, and governance competencies, shown in Box 11.3.

> **Box 11.3: Council on Education for Public Health (CEPH) DrPH Foundational Leadership, Management, and Governance Competencies**
>
> 1. Propose strategies for health improvement and elimination of health inequities by organizing stakeholders, including researchers, practitioners, community leaders, and other partners.
> 2. Communicate public health science to diverse stakeholders, including individuals at all levels of health literacy, for purposes of influencing behavior and policies.
> 3. Integrate knowledge, approaches, methods, values, and potential contributions from multiple professions and systems in addressing public health problems.
> 4. Create a strategic plan.
> 5. Facilitate shared decision-making through negotiation and consensus-building methods.
> 6. Create organizational change strategies.
> 7. Propose strategies to promote inclusion and equity within public health programs, policies, and systems.
> 8. Assess one's own strengths and weaknesses in leadership capacities, including cultural proficiency.
> 9. Propose human, fiscal, and other resources to achieve a strategic goal.
> 10. Cultivate new resources and revenue streams to achieve a strategic goal.

Source: Reproduced with permission from Accreditation Criteria: Schools of Public Health and Public Health Programs website. https://media.ceph.org/wp_assets/2016.Criteria.pdf

Although worded differently than the ASPPH leadership competencies for the public health and healthcare workforces, the CEPH leadership competencies reflect a similar range of skills and abilities, based on foundational knowledge and experience. The CEPH competencies are worded in such a way as to be more easily measured objectively for purposes of accountability of educational programs. The CEPH competency set is more prescriptive than the ASPPH competency model in describing the "how to" of leadership, management, and governance. The ASPPH model includes such terms as "collaborate with," "influence others," and "create a shared vision." The CEPH model includes "Communicate . . . for purposes of influencing behavior and policies," "Assess one's own strengths and weaknesses in leadership capacities," and "Cultivate resources" As any DrPH program director can attest, documenting attainment of leadership competencies via objective, quantifiable means can be extremely challenging. These intangible aspects of "influencing others" represent the subjective art of change leadership.

In recognizing that leading change is both an art and a skill, it is then easier to understand why there is no single, correct recipe for effecting change. Leading change is complicated. That is also why preparation and planning is so important. Attention to preparation and planning—using a systematic approach—can increase the potential that the change will be implemented, and that it will be effective and sustainable.

Part of that preparation and planning was discussed earlier in this chapter. It includes assembling a body of evidence that can help to inform a leader's approach to change leadership efforts. That evidence includes background information that can be used to describe the problem, including the magnitude, scope, significance, and urgency of the issue. For example, evidence might include the prevalence of obesity among adults or children in a nation, the impact of tobacco use on the morbidity or mortality rates of a population, the economic cost of delaying treatment for diabetes, and a multitude of other examples. Since there is no end to the amount of evidence a leader could potentially collect, those leaders at some point have to deem themselves sufficiently informed so that they can move on to the next step in a process of deciding how to approach a leadership challenge.

Information about the environmental conditions that comprise the backdrop for change was also discussed earlier in this chapter. Perhaps most importantly, this includes a comprehensive, "360 degree" analysis of the stakeholders—individuals or organizations—with an interest in the proposed change, their position for or against the proposed change, the nature of their interest (a financial stake or their public image, for example), and their rationale for that position. All of this background information is constantly in flux, so leaders need to be able to make reasoned assessments of when they know enough, and when to stop and move on to the next steps in the process. This is part of the "art" of understanding how to lead.

Collectively, this evidence can be brought together to create a cogent, comprehensive, integrated picture of the case for change. The evidence can then be applied to an explicit strategy for addressing the original problem, as well as an action plan—a recipe—for change. Leaders ultimately bring together the evidence, their understanding of the context, as well as those less well-defined, affective "leadership" skills, refined through years of experience, to craft a plan for change. There is no single, correct approach.

The process of synthesizing and making sense of the evidence is shown in Figure 11.1. It can be used as one model for conceptualizing a graphic representation of the evidence and relationships that should be considered in crafting a plan for change.[11] The core elements include:

1) The <u>resources</u> necessary to implement and maintain the organizational change or policy, including people, funds, and other elements of infrastructure

2) The <u>players</u> affecting the change, including key stakeholders (e.g., populations, communities) and key decision-makers

3) The contextual <u>parameters</u> affecting the change including law and policy, organizational or situational authority, ethics, political and public feasibility, and the prevailing social environment and norms

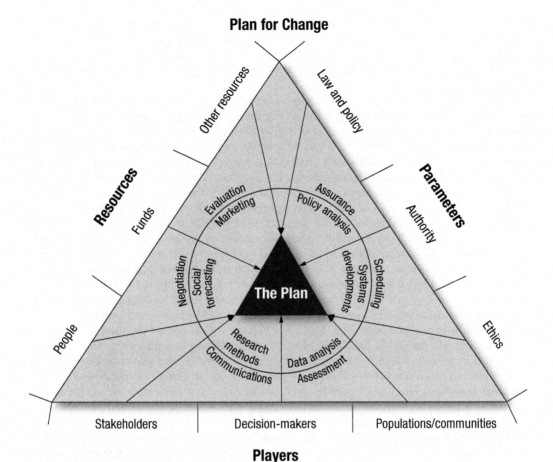

FIGURE 11.1: Crafting a Plan for Change. The core elements of the evidence and relationships that should be considered when crafting a plan for change include the resources necessary to implement and maintain the change, the players affecting the change, and the contextual parameters that affect the change.

Source: Reproduced with permission from the University of North Carolina at Chapel Hill, Gillings School of Global Public Health. Department of Health Policy and Management. Executive Doctoral Program in Health Leadership (DrPH) Program Handbook; 2015.

Other elements, including a range of policy and management tools used by public health leaders (communications, informatics, policy analysis, social forecasting, scheduling, negotiation, assessment, planning, assurance, public relations, marketing, and evaluation), may be incorporated into planning as applicable (see inner circle, Figure 11.1). A plan for change combines these elements in a coherent and comprehensive strategy for making organizational or policy change.

STEP 6—PUTTING IT ALL TOGETHER: A PLAN FOR CHANGE

In crafting a plan for change, skillful, experienced public health and healthcare leaders start with the evidence and bring leadership principles to bear on a strategic approach to influence others to adopt a vision for change. That may sound straightforward, but every plan for change involves a unique mix of elements—problems, solutions, players, resources, and parameters (Figure 11.1)—and leaders with their own, individual personalities and leadership styles.

Other contributors in this book have compared and contrasted varying leadership styles and described best leadership practices and "lessons learned" from leaders in the field who have been effective in creating change. While some common themes or patterns may emerge from interviews with public health leaders, the truth is that there is no foolproof formula for success.

Leaders learn most substantially by doing. Hopefully they learn from their own mistakes, and they improve their own skills by observing the successes and failures of others. While leadership cannot exclusively be taught in a classroom through lectures, readings and other educational resources and programs can help leaders by providing valuable concepts and frameworks that leaders (particularly emerging leaders) can apply to their practices. They learn from experience, tweak the mental models they have developed, and grow as leaders.

Strong leaders continuously develop their skills, and they adapt as the environment changes. One good example of this was brought about by the health inequalities that were accentuated in the United States during the COVID-19 pandemic, and the subsequent attention that was brought to longstanding problems related to systemic racism and inequities. As this text goes to press, many public health and healthcare leaders are working in earnest, with renewed resolve, to reflect on how their own attitudes, beliefs, and practices may contribute to the problem and what actions they need to take to rectify the situation. They are examining ways in which they can improve and do a better job of leading change for health equity and the elimination of systemic racism related to public health and healthcare.

So, what does a "plan for change" look like? What form should it—or could it—take?

It may not be a satisfying answer to hear, but the truth is, plans may vary. There may be an "art and science" to leading change, but there is no single correct way to approach it. Effective leaders glean what they can from others with more or different experience, from the evidence they have found, and from lessons they have learned from their own experiences. Then they attempt to put some structure to what they know, and they create a plan for moving forward.

Though each approach may be different, it can be helpful to organize some best practices into a framework to help guide ideas about a strategic plan for change. One of the best-known change models was developed by John Kotter.[12] The Kotter Model is outlined in Table 11.3.[13]

The Kotter Model has been used widely in the United States since 1995 when the approach was first published in the Harvard Business Review.[12] It has since been updated by its author.[13] It describes an eight-step process that is easy to understand and follow, which is one reason that it is a preferred model for teaching in academic settings. The model is particularly well-suited to traditional, United States-based organizations with a top-down organizational management structure. This approach may be a disadvantage, however, if some stakeholders are left with a sense that they have been left out of key steps, such as setting the initial vision for the change or in other critical junctures in the change creation process. When considering the Kotter Model as a contemporary blueprint for change leadership, it may be a good idea to reflect critically on any ways in which the model may miss opportunities to support or protect the change process. That may be particularly true in the context of change leadership outside the United States or in organizations in which a more collaborative, shared governance is in place as compared to a more traditional, hierarchical management structure.

It is important to underscore that the Kotter Model, while widely used, was developed in the American context, drawing from research and inputs from a largely American pool of cases over a cross section of time. It is one recipe for leadership success, but any application of this framework should be approached with a critical eye to the environmental contexts—including social and cultural—in which it is based. That environment is changing rapidly all over the world, particularly as more people begin to recognize and reconcile the historical impacts of systemic racism and exclusion of women and underrepresented minorities in the leadership of organizations and civil societies.

Despite potential limitations in applying the Kotter Model in public health and healthcare change leadership, however, there is ample evidence in the literature that the tool has been

TABLE 11.3: Kotter's Eight-step Process for Leading Change

STEP	DESCRIPTION
1. Create a sense of urgency	This is achieved by effectively communicating the problem to others, underscoring the magnitude, scope, or other compelling reason that the issue merits immediate action. Link the problem with the proposed vision for a solution—the change that stakeholders will hopefully embrace and help to advance.
2. Build a guiding coalition	Leaders cannot succeed alone. They need others who buy in to their vision for change and can help advance it. In this model, leaders identify a diverse set of champions—perhaps from different areas of an organization—who collectively have the power to create momentum for change.
3. Create a strategic vision and initiatives	Leaders need a clear, strategic vision statement that can be easily communicated to others. It should convey the rationale for the change so that others understand and are more likely to buy in to the change effort. Those who are part of the "guiding coalition" should be able to effectively convey the clear, simple message as well. A series of individual initiatives can then be planned to move the change forward.
4. Enlist a volunteer army	In this step of the change process, emphasis is on growing a contingent of others who have bought in to the change vision and are ready and willing to assist in pushing the change forward. The idea is to create a critical mass of support to help the change effort gain momentum and propel it forward.
5. Enable action by removing barriers	Leaders—and their champions, their guiding coalition—are called on to do what they can to make it possible for others to advance the change. The specific barriers to be removed may vary, but examples could include the need for training, personnel, changes in an organization's structure, funding, and so on. An effective plan for change recognizes impediments to change and includes steps to circumvent, mitigate, or otherwise eliminate them.
6. Generate short-term wins	Better plans include a range of interim goals to provide a sense of accomplishment and forward movement, giving everyone involved a sense of encouragement. It can be helpful to give attention to short-term wins and even reward those who help to achieve them.
7. Sustain acceleration	It is important to ensure that progress toward change is sustained in the long term and that short-term wins do not create complacency. Short-term achievements, while important milestones, do not in themselves constitute success. The concern is that some teams may stop trying once short-term goals are achieved, in the mistaken notion that the ultimate mission is as good as met. So, sustaining acceleration means continuing to push on as short-term wins are identified.
8. Institute change	In this final stage, attention is paid to ensuring that an organization's systems, processes, people, and environment are all aligned to support the change so that the new order becomes the norm. It is institutionalized.

Source: Data from Kotter J. The 8-step process for leading change. n.d. https://www.kotterinc.com/8-steps-process-for-leading-change

broadly effective in helping to conceptualize change efforts, both in the United States and internationally.[14–18] In one study that encompassed nine European countries, a change leadership research question related to polypharmacy management was conceptualized using the Kotter Model, complemented by an implementation model.[19]

LEADING CHANGE TODAY

Much of what is taught all over the world in courses about leadership had its origins in the United States, particularly in American business schools and the self-help publishing market in the context of organizational management and change leadership. In recent years, with increasing recognition of systemic racism and gender bias in the workplace, as well as the impact of globalization and demographic changes, it may be an opportune time to examine how these and other realities should be accounted for and addressed as we consider how best to lead change in the interest of the public's health.

It is the right thing to do, and it is also necessary for change to be effective and sustainable. Principles of cultural competence, for example, discussed in detail in other chapters in this book, explain this rationale well. "Nothing for me without me" means that unless plans for change include consideration of and buy in from stakeholders, they are doomed to fail. Those same stakeholders can block or otherwise fail to implement change that does not reflect and respond to their needs, beliefs, and attitudes.

At this point, there are as many questions as answers about a way forward. Science and technology have advanced to a point that the magnitude, scope, complexity, and urgency of our problems require much more of our leaders than before. Public health and healthcare leaders need to be able to organize and apply massive amounts of data in decision-making. A global perspective is indispensable. Public health and healthcare leaders need to adapt and respond quickly to change. They must be able to respond effectively to advances in technology including informatics, genomics, artificial intelligence, and related ethical issues, such as potential actions to interfere with predictive behaviors, and increasing complexities resulting from globalization and demographic changes, including issues relating to cultural competency, policy and law, public health ethics and human rights, healthy aging, and many others. Leaders need to be equipped to function effectively in multicultural settings and appreciate the ways in which global political, economic, social, and organizational conditions affect health locally.

Public health and healthcare leaders need the necessary skills but also the values, abilities, and intrinsic will to apply these attributes to make a difference, and to push forward, build on the good work that has already been accomplished, and go much further. The massive scale of the COVID-19 public health catastrophe in the United States and worldwide, exposing the magnitude and scope of breakdowns in communication, diplomacy, solidarity, public health preparedness, and trust in government and science, as well as the impacts of persistent socioeconomic inequalities, related health disparities, and systemic racism, highlight the central challenge to public health leadership. What has been done to date to support the public's health has not yet produced the necessary outcome: change on the scale needed to ensure the health and well-being of all people and planet. There is much more work to be done.

SUMMARY

There is no one right way to lead change. In general, better results happen when leaders can clearly articulate a concise and compelling problem and proposed solution, understand the environmental conditions that comprise the backdrop for organization or policy level change, and competently assess stakeholder interests and potential to influence the process. Change leadership requires the ability to make strategic assessments, learn from the past, and apply sound leadership principles for an evidence-based plan for change. Growing awareness of the impacts of systemic racism and gender bias, as well as globalization and demographic changes, have increased the complexity of leading change today. Leading change to improve the public's health demands integrity, an intrinsic motivation to contribute, a global perspective and inclusive attitude, and a commitment to continuous improvement. The need for effective public health leadership has never been more urgent than now.

DISCUSSION QUESTIONS

1. Think of an organizational or policy level change needed to improve the public's health, whether local, national, or international. What is the underlying problem that necessitates this change? Write a short problem statement (2–3 sentences) that succinctly describes the problem and your position on it.
2. In the case you chose in question #1, describe the social, political, economic, and organizational conditions that comprise the environmental context for change at a given point in time. What challenges do these conditions present for change leadership? How should leaders respond?
3. How can leaders gather information that may be helpful in understanding or communicating about change efforts? What are some sources of information about strategies that may have been tried in the past, which succeeded, which failed, and why? How can leaders gain information about potential barriers to or facilitators of change? List some sources and methodologies leaders might use to gain this information.
4. The eight-step Kotter Model for change leadership has been widely applied in the United States and internationally to help conceptualize a plan for accelerating complex change leadership efforts in public health and healthcare. The model was introduced in 1995 and is well-suited to traditional, U.S.-based organizations with a top-down organizational management structure. Consider the Kotter Model in the context of a contemporary blueprint for change leadership in public health and healthcare. Reflect critically on any ways in which the model may miss opportunities to support the change process, with particular emphasis on supporting diversity, equity, and inclusion (DEI) goals. How could the change process be strengthened to support DEI goals?

CASE STUDY: CHANGE LEADERSHIP DURING A CRISIS

During the COVID-19 pandemic, Dr. Anthony Fauci, director of the National Institute of Allergy and Infectious Diseases of the National Institutes of Health, was one of the most publicly visible and respected experts helping to lead the national and international public health responses. In the early days of the pandemic, Dr. Fauci told the public that wearing face masks was unnecessary. Soon thereafter, however, he advised the public that masks were recommended.

Reflect on your own understanding of what transpired during this time of the early unfolding of the pandemic. If you need to refresh your memory or learn more, search online for media accounts or papers describing the early management of the crisis in the United States.

CASE STUDY QUESTIONS

1. How did Dr. Fauci's actions reflect effective change leadership? Discuss factors in Dr. Fauci's approach to advising the public during the pandemic that may have influenced the extent to which people accepted and acted on his advice.

2. Now think about a health leader who played a prominent role in your own local public health response to the pandemic. In what ways did that individual (or organization) demonstrate principles of effective change leadership? Explain. Were there any ways in which the response failed? Why or why not?

CASE STUDY: FORMULATING A CHANGE PLAN

The COVID-19 pandemic exacted a devastating toll on the world. Virtually everybody was affected in some way, either directly or indirectly; however, people around the world were not affected equally. Morbidity and mortality from COVID-19 disproportionately burdened some populations more than others.

Why was the health of some populations affected more adversely than others by COVID-19? How are these outcome differentials linked to change leadership? There is a large and growing body of published studies and commentaries on this topic, including analyses of the varied responses to the pandemic around the world, and the outcomes of those responses.[20–25]

Think about one reason why some people fared worse than others. Now think about the determinants of health of populations.

CASE STUDY QUESTIONS

Imagine that you are writing a post for an influential blog. The title of your post is:

"Why Was the Health of Some People Affected More Adversely Than Others by COVID-19? The Determinants of Health of Populations." Replace the subtitle "The Determinants of Health of Populations" with an alternative subtitle that includes the word "leadership" and includes the need for a structured plan for change in the health system of a specific country, state, or region anywhere in the world.

Next, design that plan in broad terms. The plan you will propose will provide leadership insights into the answer to the question, "Why was the health of some people affected more adversely than others by COVID-19?" and provide guidance on how to change that condition.

"Some people" may be defined differently by different people. Be clear about who "some people" and "other people" are. Formulate a plan that details how a change in policy or practice could address the problem.

At minimum, the plan should include:
- specific set of leadership activities necessary to effect change and timetable for those changes;
- *identification of resources needed (e.g., money, people) and description of how those resources would be applied; and*
- *identification of supporting and opposing stakeholders and how a leader might manage opponents and related political issues.*

REFERENCES

1. United States Senate, One Hundred Sixth Congress, First Session. Hearing before a Subcommittee of the Committee on Appropriations, Special Hearing, Parkinson's Disease Research and Treatment. S. Hrg. 106-373. U.S. Government Printing Office. Pages 12–14. https://www.govinfo.gov/content/pkg/CHRG-106shrg59959/html/CHRG-106shrg59959.htm and https://www.youtube.com/watch?v=fkOkeY0l3Cw

2. Ford Foundation. Risa Lavizzo-Mourey on health inequality. March 29, 2017. https://www.fordfoundation.org/just-matters/ford-forum/inequalityis/risa-lavizzo-mourey-on-health-inequality

3. American Society of Addiction Medicine. Public policy statement on treatment of opioid use disorder in correctional settings. https://www.asam.org/docs/default-source/public-policy-statements/2020-statement-on-treatment-of-oud-in-correctional-settings.pdf

4. Centers for Disease Control and Prevention. https://www.cdc.gov/obesity/about-obesity/index.html

5. Stone D. *Policy Paradox: The Art of Political Decision Making*. 3rd ed. W. W. Norton & Company; 2011.

6. Kingdon, J. *Agendas, Alternatives, and Public Policies*. 2nd ed. Longman; 2011.

7. Burns L, Bradley E, Weiner B. *Shortell and Kaluzny's Health Care Management: Organization, Design, and Behavior*. 6th ed. Delmar Cengage Learning; 2011.

8. Nothing for us, without us. Opportunities for meaningful engagement of people living with NCDs: meeting report. World Health Organization website. 2021. https://www.who.int/publications/i/item/nothing-for-us-without-us-opportunities-for-meaningful-engagement-of-people-living-with-ncds

9. Association of Schools and Programs of Public Health Education Committee. *Doctor of Public Health (DrPH) Core Competency Model*. 2009. https://aspph-wp-production.s3.us-east-1.amazonaws.com/app/uploads/2014/04/DrPHVersion1-3.pdf

10. Council on Education for Public Health. *Accreditation Criteria: Schools of Public Health and Public Health Programs*. Updated October 2016. https://media.ceph.org/wp_assets/2016.Criteria.pdf

11. The University of North Carolina at Chapel Hill, Gillings School of Global Public Health. Department of Health Policy and Management. Executive Doctoral Program in Health Leadership (DrPH) Program Handbook; 2015.

12. Kotter JP. Leading change: why transformation efforts fail. *Harv Bus Rev*. 1995;73:59–67. https://hbr.org/1995/05/leading-change-why-transformation-efforts-fail-2

13. Kotter J. Leading change: why transformation efforts fail. Harvard Business Review website. 1995. https://hbr.org/1995/05/leading-change-why-transformation-efforts-fail-2

14. Aziz AM. A change management approach to improving safety and preventing needle stick injuries. *J Infect Prev*. 2017;18(5):257–262. doi:10.1177/1757177416687829

15. Lv C-M, Zhang L. How can collective leadership influence the implementation of change in health care? *Chin Nurs Res*. 2017;4(4):182–185. doi:10.1016/j.cnre.2017.10.005

16. Chappell S, Pescud M, Waterworth P, et al. Exploring the process of implementing healthy workplace initiatives: mapping to Kotter's leading change model. *J Occup Environ Med*. 2016;58: 1. doi:10.1097/JOM.0000000000000854

17. Carman AL, Vanderpool RC, Stradtman LR, Edmiston EA. A change-management approach to closing care gaps in a federally qualified health center: a rural Kentucky case study. *Prev Chronic Dis*. 2019;16: E105. doi:10.5888/pcd16.180589

18. Small A, Gist D, Souza D, Dalton J, Magny-Normlis C, David D. Using Kotter's change model for implementing bedside handoff: a quality improvement project. *J Nurs Care Qual*. 2016;31:1. doi:10.1097/NCQ.0000000000000212

19. McIntosh J, Alonso A, MacLure K, et al. A case study of polypharmacy management in nine European countries: implications for change management and implementation. *PLoS One*. 2018;13(4):e0195232. doi:10.1371/journal.pone.0195232

20. Adolph C, Amano K, Bang-Jensen B, Fullman N, Wilkerson J. Pandemic politics: timing state-level social distancing responses to COVID-19. *J Health Polit Policy Law*. 2021;46(2):211–233. doi:10.1215/03616878-8802162

21. Treskon M, Docter B. Preemption and its impact on policy responses to COVID-19. 2020. https://www.urban.org/sites/default/files/publication/102879/preemption-and-its-impact-on-policy-responses-to-covid-19.pdf

22. Erwin PC, Mucheck KW, Brownson RC. Different responses to COVID-19 in four US states: Washington, New York, Missouri, and Alabama. *Am J Public Health*. 2021;111(4):647–651. doi:10.2105/AJPH.2020.306111

23. Laffet K, Haboubi F, Elkadri N, Georges Nohra R, Rothan-Tondeur M. The early stage of the COVID-19 outbreak in Tunisia, France, and Germany: a systematic mapping review of the different national strategies. *Int J Environ Res Public Health*. 2021;18(16):8622. doi:10.3390/ijerph18168622

24. Wang D, Mao Z. A comparative study of public health and social measures of COVID-19 advocated in different countries. *Health Policy*. 2021;125(8):957–971. doi:10.1016/j.healthpol.2021.05.016

25. Haider N, Osman AY, Gadzekpo A, et al. Lockdown measures in response to COVID-19 in nine sub-Saharan African countries. *BMJ Glob Health*. 2020;5(10):e003319. doi:10.1136/bmjgh-2020-003319

Chapter 12

Diversity, Equity, Inclusion, and Intercultural Competence in Leadership

Katherine L. Turner

INTRODUCTION

In our increasingly diverse, international, and interconnected world, diversity, equity, and inclusion (DEI), and intercultural competence are essential leadership mindsets, skills, and practices. There is a clear and compelling case for diverse leaders who represent their stakeholders and can understand and deliver on consumer interests and needs. There is an increasingly strong call for inclusive leaders who cherish differences, embrace disruption, adapt with agility, drive innovation, foster a speak-up culture, and can effectively manage a diverse workforce. Public demand for racial, gender, and other forms of justice make an equity mindset and action critical in leaders. DEI and intercultural competence in leadership are vital in public health, given the effects of systemic racism and other forms of oppression on people's health and healthcare systems. This chapter outlines the definitions, evolution, intersections, skills, mindsets, and practices of diversity, equity, inclusion, and intercultural competence in leadership.

OBJECTIVES

By the end of this chapter, the reader will be able to:

- Describe the definitions, evolution, and intersections of DEI and intercultural competence.
- Describe why DEI and intercultural competence in leadership are essential in today's increasingly diverse and dynamic public health and healthcare landscape.
- Describe inclusive leadership traits and practices and their importance.
- Discuss an equity mindset and equity leadership practices and their impact.
- Describe cultural humility and culturally competent leadership.

BACKGROUND ON DIVERSITY, EQUITY, AND INCLUSION AND INTERCULTURAL AND GLOBAL COMPETENCE

DEFINITIONS

Diversity, equity, and inclusion, often referred to by their acronym DEI or EDI, are distinct but interrelated concepts. Leaders must understand their unique meanings and interrelatedness to create strategies, act with clarity and intentionality, and make tangible advances in each.

Accessibility and justice are related concepts that are often included with DEI initiatives. DEI consulting firm Global Citizen, LLC developed and uses the following definitions.[1]

■ **Diversity:** The characteristics that make individuals and groups unique and different from each other, including identity markers, personality types, ways of thinking, ideas, and perspectives.

■ **Inclusion:** Actions to create an environment in which everyone is and feels welcomed, respected, valued, and supported to fully participate.

■ **Equality:** The state of being considered inherently the same worth and accorded the same status, rights, resources, and opportunities, regardless of unique identities and characteristics.

■ **Equity:** Fair treatment, access, opportunity, and advancement for all people, while identifying and shifting power structures, eliminating systemic barriers, and providing needed resources to ensure the full agency, participation, and benefit of people who have experienced discrimination and oppression.

■ **Accessibility:** Giving equitable access to everyone along the continuum of human ability and experience. Accessibility encompasses the broader meanings of compliance and refers to how organizations make space for the unique characteristics that each person brings.

■ **Justice:** Dismantling barriers to resources and opportunities in society so that all individuals and communities can live with dignity and well-being. These barriers include racism, sexism, classism, and other forms of systemic oppression.

EVOLUTION

There has been an evolution in leaders' understanding of and commitment to DEI over recent decades. The field of DEI has its roots in corporate America in the 1960s, sparked by anti-discrimination legislation including the Equal Pay Act of 1963, Title VII of the Civil Rights Act of 1964, and the Age Discrimination in Employment Act of 1967. Throughout that decade, efforts were focused on nondiscrimination and affirmative action. Initially, there was a focus on diversity and representation in the workplace, particularly in large, U.S.-based companies.[2] From the 1970s to the 1990s, many Fortune 500 companies made concerted efforts in diversity hiring, casting a wider net to attract a broader talent pool, with their focus mainly on compliance. Also, as the more diverse Generation X population began entering the workforce, they brought more of a focus on diversity, which influenced organizational cultures.[2]

From the 1990s to the 2000s, organizations began realizing the benefits of a diverse workforce that mirrored their consumer base and that could provide valuable input into their products and services. At the same time, employees were calling for more of a voice in company decisions, which pointed to a need for greater inclusion. More workplace interventions focused on inclusion, and academic research was being conducted on inclusion as well as emotional intelligence, a foundational element of an inclusive culture.[2] When inclusion efforts stalled, and employees felt dissatisfied for these and myriad other reasons, including lack of opportunities for advancement, organizations experienced high turnover, particularly among Black, Indigenous, and people of color (BIPOC); women; and lesbian, gay, bisexual, transgender, queer or questioning (LGBTQ+) employees.[2]

From 2000 to 2015, organizational efforts continued to center on creating a more diverse workforce, particularly on increasing diversity in C-Suites and boards of directors, and they made inclusion more of a focus; however, gains in leadership diversity have been slow.[2] According to McKinsey and Company's data set, among companies that were based in the United States and the United Kingdom, female representation on executive teams rose from 15% in 2014 to 20% in 2019.[3] Across the global data set, for which the data started in 2017, this number moved up just one percentage point, from 14% to 15%, in 2019—and more than a third of companies still had no women on their executive teams. This lack of material progress was evident across all industries and in most countries. Similarly, representation of ethnic minorities on U.S. and U.K executive teams stood at only 13% in 2019, up from just 7% in 2014. For the global data set in 2019, this number was 14%, up from 12% in 2017.[3]

From approximately 2015 onward, more organizations issued commitments to equity in addition to diversity and inclusion; this mainly originated from gender-based equal pay and racial equity initiatives.[2] Some organizations have included accessibility (DEAI or IDEA) and/or justice (DEAIJ or JEDI) as their areas of focus.

In the wake of the murder of George Floyd on May 25, 2020, and the killings of Breonna Taylor, Ahmaud Arbery, and too many other innocent Black people in the United States around the same time—and countless more before then—there was a global surge in the Black Lives Matter and broader antiracism movements. Employees began speaking out more vocally and publicly against workplace microaggressions and discrimination, and leaders made public commitments to advance racial equity and broader DEI in their organizations and beyond. The widespread call for organizational change and social transformation was palpable, urgent, and long overdue and caused a notable increase in organizational DEI activities.[4]

INTERSECTIONS

Intercultural competence (also known as cultural competence), global competence, cultural humility, and DEI are interrelated concepts and practices. Intercultural competence is the process of developing greater appreciation for cultural differences and knowledge, attitudes, and skills that promote effective interaction and communication in diverse cultural contexts. Global competence is the constellation of (a) awareness, (b) understanding, (c) sensitivity, and (d) ethical practice within an individual or a system. This constellation enables effective intercultural and cross-country interactions and partnerships that effect organizational and social transformation and result in mutually beneficial and empowering outcomes for the good of all.[5] Intercultural competence and global competence are important leadership mindsets, skill sets, and processes that enable leaders to advance DEI in service to their organization's mission.[6] They can be practiced and measured at both the individual and organizational levels, while DEI efforts are often more focused on the organizational level.[6] To be effective in international organizations, leaders need to adopt a global mindset and avoid ethnocentrism. There are numerous intercultural and global competence models that comprise interrelated core competencies, including self-awareness, understanding, attitudes, skills, and practices, each with their own components; more recent models have incorporated equity. There are also numerous cultural competence scales and metrics to assess and measure progress in cultural competence in individuals and organizations.[7,8]

Cultural humility is a related concept and an important leadership trait. Cultural humility is expressed through a lifelong commitment to self-evaluation and self-critique, redressing power imbalances, and developing mutually beneficial and nonmaterialistic partnerships with communities on behalf of individual and defined populations.[9] Leaders demonstrate humility by encouraging others to share their constructive feedback; for example, that a leader is showing favoritism, tends to interrupt, or is overlooking important information or perspectives. When leaders demonstrate empathy and consider different perspectives, they offer people hope that the leader cares about them and takes their views into account, rather than barreling on with preconceptions based only on their perspectives. Cultural humility creates a personal connection between leaders and a diverse set of stakeholders, making it easier to develop and implement shared decisions.[10]

WHY DIVERSITY, EQUITY, INCLUSION, AND CULTURAL COMPETENCE IN LEADERSHIP ARE ESSENTIAL

There is both a moral and business imperative for DEI in leadership, and it would be inadequate and shortsighted to focus on the business case alone.[11] There have been criticisms of approaches that focus exclusively on the business case, and many authors argue persuasively for the benefits from a business *and* values perspective.[12]

The workplace is an important site for DEI assessment and interventions because organizational systems and the leaders who operate them are, usually unintentionally, perpetuating inequities against employees and other stakeholders. Leaders also have the ability to revise policies and shift cultural norms more readily than in society at large. "The study of change efforts and the oppositions they engender are often opportunities to observe frequently invisible aspects of the reproduction of inequalities. The concept of inequality regimes may be useful in analyzing organizational change projects to better understand why these projects so often fail and why they succeed when this occurs."[13(p441)]

While much of the research and examples cited in this chapter are from private companies and nonprofit organizations that are not necessarily public health and healthcare related, they are relevant. DEI and intercultural competence are particularly important in public health and healthcare leadership, given the effects of systemic racism and other forms of oppression on people's health and healthcare systems. Social determinants of health are the conditions in the environments where humans live and work that affect our health, functioning, and quality-of-life outcomes and risks. These include the systems and institutions in which people live and work as well as people's relationships and interactions with family, friends, work colleagues, and community members, all of which have an important impact on their health and well-being.[14] These systems and human interactions and their impact can be positive or damaging. Systemic oppression, such as racism, while not easily diagnosable, has a deep, lasting, and intergenerational effect on individual and population health and is therefore a major public health issue.

Building on decades of research on the social determinants of health and the ever-expanding consensus within public health that racism is a public health crisis, the American Public Health Association (APHA), the National Collaborative for Health Equity, and the de Beaumont Foundation created the *Healing Through Policy: Creating Pathways to Racial Justice* initiative. Through this initiative, they are offering a suite of policies and practices that can be implemented at the local level to promote racial healing, advance racial equity, and dramatically improve the conditions in which people live, grow, work, and play.[15]

MORAL IMPERATIVE

There is a strong moral imperative to advance DEI in leadership. Systemic racism, sexism, homophobia, and other forms of oppression are institutionalized and therefore constantly operating. They create structural barriers that serve to advantage people who are part of socially dominant groups and disadvantage those who are not, particularly when it comes to being identified for and pursuing leadership opportunities. BIPOC, women, and LGBTQ+ people may be penalized, often unconsciously, for having certain traits or acting in ways that are not viewed as normative or desirable for leaders from a White, heterosexual, cisgender, Western, male point of view. These male leaders' perceptions and actions are usually unconscious and grounded in implicit biases.[16] People who are not part of the socially dominant groups may engage in "code switching," in which they adjust their speech, and "covering," in which they adjust their behaviors, which can include spotlighting or suppressing aspects of their identities, to gain access to and survive or thrive in leadership. DM, a gay man who worked at a Fortune 500 company with a nondiscrimination policy, said, "I couldn't be fired for being gay, but when partners at the firm invite straight men to squash or drinks, they don't invite the women or gay men. I'm being passed over for opportunities that could lead to being promoted."[17] Unless leaders intentionally work to identify and dismantle these structural inequities, there will be unfair advantages and disadvantages in the allocation of resources, opportunities, and rewards in the workplace that create disparate outcomes.[18]

INCREASINGLY DIVERSE WORKFORCES AND CONSUMERS

In addition to the moral imperative, there is a strong business case for DEI in leadership. Due to rising global migration, populations—and therefore workforces—are becoming increasingly diverse, international, and interconnected.[19] By 2025, the world's middle-class population is expected to reach 3.2 billion, up from 1.8 billion in 2009, with the majority of this increase coming from Africa, Asia, and Latin America. As income levels increase, so does consumer demand.[20] Additionally, consumers are able to use their digital devices to exercise greater choice and therefore expect to exert more of a voice in shaping the products and services they consume.[20] Organizations are increasingly cultivating more consumer-centric mindsets and capabilities by using design thinking, with concepts such as "empathy" and "connectedness," to better understand clients' lives and future needs. Organizations are also increasingly taking a leader-led approach to talent development programs, which puts the responsibility on leaders to teach their teams using practical approaches, reality-based stories and case studies, and teachable moments.[20] Leaders need to be able to relate to their employees to successfully develop their talent. Given the increasingly diverse workforce and consumer base, organizations need leaders who represent diverse constituents, can understand and address their teams' and consumers' unique interests and needs, and are able to inclusively lead diverse teams. All of these dynamics are absolutely playing out in public health and healthcare, in which leaders need to be able to relate to and meets the needs of their diverse communities, employees, and patients.

ATTRACTING TOP TALENT AND CULTIVATING INNOVATION

Organizations that demonstrate a strong commitment to DEI are able to attract top talent, because prospective employees are increasingly prioritizing DEI in their selection criteria. In one study, 80% of respondents indicated that inclusion was important when choosing an employer, 39% reported that they would leave their current organization for a more inclusive one, and 23% (30% of Millennial respondents) indicated that they had already left an organization for a more inclusive one.[21] A more diverse workforce also means diversity of thought, which breeds innovation, a critical leadership and organizational success factor.

There are significant cultural, political, and economic differences in markets, with stiff competition for top talent between local and global companies. The expansion of higher education is creating more highly educated and mobile workers, with a large percentage of the global graduates coming from China and India.[20] However, many companies struggle with successfully attracting, including, and retaining diverse leaders and employees. For example, while their numbers in the workforce are increasing, women hold only 12% of corporate board seats worldwide.[20] In a 2015 survey of 362 executives, only 10% believed that they had the talent needed to win new customers.[20]

In a 2014 survey of 1,500 executives, 75% responded that innovation was among their company's top three priorities; however, 83% rated their companies' innovation capabilities as average (70%) or weak (13%).[20] While many leaders agree that collective intelligence enhances group performance, few understand how to consistently achieve it. A leader's understanding of diversity and inclusion will be critical to their organization's success.[20]

ANTICIPATING AND OVERCOMING RESISTANCE TO DIVERSITY, EQUITY, AND INCLUSION

Despite numerous moral and business reasons to advance DEI, some leaders and employees remain inactive or even resistant. When researchers asked White, heterosexual, cisgender men with white-collar jobs in the United States about their views on DEI in the workplace, only 10% of respondents thought DEI were *not* important at all, but many were not involved in such efforts. The most common reasons they gave was that they were "too busy" or did not feel that advancing DEI would benefit them,[22] which indicates a deeper issue about how company leaders frame the case for and stress the importance of DEI for their employees and organizations. If DEI efforts have not been positioned as mission critical, leadership imperatives, and important for all staff, they may seem to some, particularly those in socially dominant groups, as optional and even extracurricular. Given that White, heterosexual, cis-gender men continue to hold a disproportionate percentage of executive positions, if they see themselves as too busy or not personally implicated in DEI in the workplace, it can be challenging to make significant progress.

Another common reason that people resist embracing and advancing DEI is biases, which, whether implicit or overt, impact the way we see ourselves and others, assess situations, and make decisions. For example, implicit stereotypes cause people to judge others according to unconscious ideas they hold. With similarity-attraction bias, people tend to more easily and deeply connect with people who look and act like them. With in-group favoritism, people favor members of their in-groups, and with attribution error, people use the wrong reason to explain someone's behavior. Coupled with in-group favoritism, this results in a positive attribution for in-group members and a negative attribution for out-group members.[20] These and other biases can cause leaders to recruit and select employees and their replacements who are similar to them, which thwarts diversity efforts, perpetuates existing power structures, and can create a culture of exclusion for those in the out-group.

In the following sections, evidence, traits and characteristics, and strategies for diversity, inclusion, equity, and intercultural competence will be presented.

DIVERSITY AND REPRESENTATION IN LEADERSHIP

Organizations' success depends on their leaders' ability to optimize an increasingly diverse and dispersed talent pool.[23] Additionally, organizations benefit when leaders bring their diverse identities and unique lived experiences to their leadership roles, styles, and approaches, despite overt or subtle pressure to conform to dominant cultural notions of leadership. One research report, based on interviews with leaders in different roles and observation of leadership groups, sought to understand how people identify themselves and their leadership in relation to others, and how individuals assess their inclusive leadership and its impact on their effectiveness.[18] The authors defined diverse leadership as "that which integrates leaders with a wide range of characteristics in a way which cherishes rather than deletes difference and fully utilises the potential benefits of a more heterogeneous leadership."[24(p2)]

CURRENT LACK OF REPRESENTATION

Diversity and representation matter, given that organizations with more diverse leadership teams have better long-term performance.[3] Currently, however, BIPOC, women, and LGBTQ+ people are underrepresented in C-Suites and boards of directors in for-profit companies as well as nonprofit organizations. Around 10% of S&P 500 companies explicitly disclosed their directors' race/ethnicity, and 8 out of 10 of their board members were White.[25] Women comprise half the world's workforce and the majority of college graduates yet hold only about a quarter of leadership roles.[26] Only 4.7% of companies in each of the Russell 3000 and S&P 500 indexes had a female board chair and less than one out of five board committees in the Russell 3000 were led by women.[25] Only 6% of CEOs of S&P 500 companies were women, which equated to merely 30 of 322 companies.[27] Nonprofit organizations in the United States are faring no better. According to BoardSource's 2017 report of nonprofit board practices, 90% of chief executives and 84% of board members reported as White, and 27% of boards identified as entirely White.[28] Since BoardSource began studying diversity data, board diversity has remained largely unchanged, with BIPOC representation never exceeding 18%.[28] Sixty-five percent (65%) of chief executives stated that they were somewhat or extremely dissatisfied with racial and ethnic diversity levels.[28]

According to the Building Movement Project's 2017 *Nonprofits, Leadership, and Race* survey results, respondents, in particular BIPOC respondents, agreed or strongly agreed that executive recruiters do not do enough to identify a diverse pool of qualified candidates for executive nonprofit positions, predominately white boards often do not support the leadership potential of BIPOC staff, and organizations often rule out BIPOC candidates based on the perceived lack of "fit" with the current organizational culture. Additionally, BIPOC respondents reported that it was harder for them to advance because of their smaller professional networks.[29]

The gender leadership gap is also evident at the national and global leadership levels. Women held only 25.2% of parliamentary seats and 21.2% of ministerial positions around the world in 2019, according to the World Economic Forum.[30] Only 68 of the 153 countries covered by the report had a female head of state in the past 50 years.[26]

These patterns are also seen in public health and healthcare leadership. Based on data from the American Hospital Association and American College of Healthcare Executives, 89% of all hospital CEOs in 2019 were White.[33] At local health departments in 2019, 92% of experienced and 90% of new (with less than 3 years of experience) top executives were White.[31] Women, who comprised 66% of top executives, fared better.[31] According to the U.S. Census Bureau, in 2019, 60% of the U.S. population was White.[32] This disparity persists despite two decades of increasing racial and ethnic diversity among graduate students in health administration. Racial or ethnic minority students made up 43.7% of the Association of University Programs in Health Administration graduate programs in the 2018 to 2019 academic year.[33]

There are numerous reasons for the lack of proportionate diversity and representation in leadership. Current organizational leaders must try to understand how their organizational norms might implicitly discourage certain leadership styles or silence certain voices. For example, in companies where most leaders are White men who gain respect by speaking assertively, women of all races and Black men may be perceived negatively for being assertive and subsequently labeled as "aggressive" or "angry." This places leaders of color and women in a double bind. They can conform to the organization's norms, which sometimes means deviating from cultural prescriptions for their group, or they can do the opposite. Either way, they will violate one set of expectations and risk marginalization and diminished opportunities for advancement.[33]

DIVERSITY AS A SUCCESS FACTOR

Increased diversity in C-Suites, boards of directors, and employees overall has been associated with organizational success. Companies that have a disconnect between what they say they are doing and the actual progress they are making in diversity can seriously erode internal and external credibility and further contribute to a lack of inclusion.[3]

In companies that promote two-dimensional (2D) diversity in leadership, in which leaders exhibit at least three inherent and three acquired diversity traits, these leaders are more likely to have their ideas win endorsement from decision-makers, get developed or prototyped, and get deployed in the marketplace.[34] Companies with more than 30% of women on their executive teams are significantly more likely to outperform those with between 10% and 30%, and these companies are more likely to outperform those with fewer or no women executives.[3]

DIVERSITY FOSTERS INNOVATION

Boston Consulting Group found that companies with more diverse management teams had 19% higher revenues due to innovation. An inherently diverse workforce can be a vital source of innovation because individuals with different identities will be more attuned to the unmet needs of consumers who are like them. Organizations with multicultural leaders and workforces in which leaders prize differences, value each employee's voice, and manage rather than suppress disruption have greater means to promote and support innovation.[34] CTI's 2013 report found that when teams had one or more members who represented the gender, ethnicity, culture, generation, or sexual orientation of the end user, the entire team was as much as 158% more likely to understand and innovate effectively for that end user. On the other hand, homogeneity stifles innovation. When leadership lacked innate or acquired diversity, or failed to foster a speak-up culture, fewer ideas with market potential made it to market.[34] STI found that ideas from BIPOC, women, LGBTQ+ people, and Gen-Ys were less likely to win the endorsement they needed to move forward because the predominantly White, male, heterosexual, cisgender leaders who came from similar educational and socioeconomic backgrounds didn't value ideas for which they didn't personally see a need.[34]

LEADERS SPEAK ON DIVERSITY

"There are massive biases and incredible assumptions made about your abilities based on the way you look or on past experiences with others of the same racial and ethnic background,"[50(para1)] states Folasade May, the director of the Melvin and Bren Simon Gastroenterology Quality Improvement Program at University of California Los Angeles Health. She continues, "If the perception is that we are challenging to work with, leadership teams are less likely to take a chance and invite us to the table. This is unlikely to be the case when a white person does not perform well; that person does not reflect poorly on the entire race. It's a heavy burden that we are often responsible for challenging the future perception of our entire race."[50(para1)] Anu Kumar, president and CEO of Ipas, offered, "My advice to women of color who have been overlooked, overworked, or passed over is to recognize that we are part of a system that is rigged against us and to try to make peace with it while continuing the struggle to change it by seizing opportunities when they arrive or creating them."[35(para15)] Her remarks are echoed by Jen Wong, COO of Reddit and the daughter of Chinese immigrants, who stated that although companies are realizing the importance of diversity in the workplace, she has noticed the presence of a "bamboo ceiling" in the United States. She advises women and BIPOC to be "vulnerable and authentic," as there is "nothing more important than being human."[36] Glen Senk, the former CEO of Urban Outfitters, advised other LGBTQ+ leaders and employees to authentically be themselves when leading an organization. He stated, "When you are running an organization and have thousands of people you are trying to align around an objective, there's not time for hidden layers. You need trust, and in order to have trust, you need to be honest. Who wants to live a double life?"[37(para20)] Paul Block, of the U.S. company Merisant, noted, "People with different lifestyles and different backgrounds challenge each other more. Diversity creates dissent, and you need that. Without it, you're not going to get any deep inquiry or breakthroughs."[38(para3)]

STRATEGIES TO INCREASE DIVERSITY AND REPRESENTATION IN LEADERSHIP

There are numerous strategies leaders can employ to increase diversity and representation in senior leadership, which include:

- Create and socialize a strong and customized case for DEI and promote it company wide.
- Strengthen leaders' capability and accountability for DEI.
- Set data-driven goals in workforce plans, taking into account which forms of multivariate diversity to prioritize in addition to race, ethnicity, and gender.
- Ensure equitable promotion opportunities through fair, de-biased, transparent, and monitored processes.
- Promote diverse talent into executive, senior management, and technical roles.
- Enforce a zero-tolerance policy for discriminatory behavior and strengthen managers' capacity to identify and address microaggressions.
- Establish norms for inclusive behaviors and assess leaders and employees against them.

- Build a culture of belonging in which managers tangibly embrace their commitment to multivariate forms of diversity.
- Assess belonging in internal surveys.[3]

To increase diversity in boards of directors, McKinsey and Company recommend:

- Begin planning early, long before a vacancy arises.
- Groom and develop relationships with prospective board members.
- Disrupt the usual search processes that tend to rely on existing board members' networks, which are often composed of people similar to them.
- Conduct a formal search and nomination process with an explicit focus on diversity.
- Widen the search by seeking candidates from different sectors than usual.
- Review and revise board policies, procedures, and practices, especially term limits, to create vacancies that offer opportunities for greater diversity.[39]

Iris Bohnet, a behavioral economist, professor, and director of the Women and Public Policy Program at the Harvard Kennedy School, advocates smart, data-driven, systemic solutions like de-biasing organizations more so than working to change individual leaders' mindsets. Debiasing is a process through which organizational leaders assess and take steps to reduce cognitive biases in organizational policies, procedures, and processes. "I don't think the solution is to fix women or people of color or other underrepresented groups, but eventually we have to move to fixing the system."[40]

INCLUSIVE LEADERSHIP TRAITS AND PRACTICES

The goal of inclusion should be to ensure that everyone in an organization feels welcome, valued, and supported. This is how leaders strengthen employee engagement and retention, and how they create a stage for teams that perform at a high level. On the flip side, organizational cultures that are not inclusive are more likely to experience negative outcomes in terms of employee satisfaction and retention, resulting in higher turnover rates and lower organizational performance.

What makes people feel included in organizations, that they are being treated fairly and respectfully, and that they are valued and belong? There are many components to this. An organization's mission, vision, values, policies, procedures, and practices are all vitally important. Coworker behaviors have a large impact; however, leaders play a pivotal role. What leaders say and do make up to a 70% difference as to whether an individual reports feeling included. This matters because the more people feel included, the more they participate, make an extra effort, and collaborate well, all of which improve organizational performance.[10]

Inclusive leadership is a key differentiating factor to create organizational success.[23] Jim Turley of Ernst & Young drew an important distinction: "Diversity itself is about the mix of people you have, and creating an inclusive culture is about making that mix work."[38(para13)] Inclusive leader behaviors unleash the full potential of a diverse workforce. Leaders who create a speak-up culture position companies to realize greater efficiencies and cut costs.[34] By committing to diversity and inclusion, organizations reap many benefits, including higher employee morale, loyalty, retention, and productivity.[41]

Diversity and inclusion are strongly interrelated, and both are needed to realize organizational success. According to Dr. Stephanie Creary, assistant professor and organizational scholar at the Wharton School, "You think the issue is you need more underrepresented people, but your culture may not be designed to nurture that talent, and that's the problem."[42(p42)]

Inclusion directly enhances performance. Research demonstrated that teams helmed by inclusive leaders were 17% more likely to report that they were high performing, 20% more likely to say they made high-quality decisions, and 29% more likely to report behaving collaboratively. A 10% improvement in perceptions of inclusion increased work attendance by almost one day per year per employee, thereby reducing the cost of absenteeism. However, inclusion in leaders can be challenging to assess. Most leaders in this study were unsure about whether others experienced them as inclusive or not. Only a third (36%) saw their inclusive leadership capabilities as others did, another third (32%) overrated their capabilities, and the final third (33%) underrated their capabilities. Most importantly, leaders were rarely certain about the specific behaviors that impacted their rating as more or less inclusive.[43]

DELOITTE'S SIX SIGNATURE TRAITS OF INCLUSIVE LEADERSHIP

Deloitte surveyed employees about inclusion, interviewed leaders identified as inclusive, and reviewed the academic literature to develop six traits that distinguished inclusive leaders from others and then developed a tool to assess those traits. They outlined the six signature traits of inclusive leadership, asserting that inclusive leadership is about (a) treating people and groups fairly, based on their unique characteristics, rather than on stereotypes; (b) personalizing individuals by seeking to understand and valuing the uniqueness of diverse others while also accepting them as members of the group; and (c) leveraging the thinking of diverse groups for smarter ideation and decision-making that reduces the risk of being blindsided.[20] The six signature traits are:

- **Commitment**: Highly inclusive leaders are committed to diversity and inclusion because they align with their personal values, and they understand the business case for them. Staying the course is hard, but leaders back up their verbal commitments by prioritizing time, energy, and resources to fully address inclusion. Inclusive leaders possess a strong sense of personal responsibility for change and understand that change begins with them.

- **Courage**: Openly acknowledging improvements that are needed means incurring personal risk. Highly inclusive leaders challenge the status quo—beginning with themselves, and then others, and the system. They are courageous to be humble about their strengths and vulnerable about their weaknesses.

- **Cognizance of bias**: Highly inclusive leaders are aware of their own and their organizations' blind spots. They engage in corrective strategies to advance equity. They acknowledge that, despite best intentions, their leaders and organizations have biases, and they institute policies, processes, and structures to mitigate them. They are highly aware of implicit biases, stereotypes, negative attitudes, and process biases, such as confirmation bias and groupthink.[44] They are aware of circumstances, such as fatigue, time pressures, and other stressors, that may cause them to be more susceptible to biases. They understand that humans' natural state, without intervention, leans toward self-interest and replication and that success in a diverse world requires a different approach.

- **Curiosity**: Diverse experiences, ideas, and teams facilitate growth. Highly inclusive leaders have an open mindset, empathy, acceptance of their own limitations, a strong desire to understand how others view and experience the world, and a tolerance for ambiguity. Their followers feel valued, demonstrate loyalty, and therefore provide access to more in-depth information, which enables leaders to engage in more effective decision-making.

- **Cultural intelligence**: Highly inclusive leaders embrace unfamiliar environments and have a desire for learning from diverse others. They understand that people see the world through different cultural frames. They value cultural differences, defy ethnocentric and superior tendencies, build strong connections with people from different backgrounds, and are confident and effective in intercultural communications and interactions.

- **Collaboration**: A diverse-thinking team is greater than the sum of its parts. Highly inclusive leaders create an empowering environment for individuals and teams and effectively leverage the thinking of diverse employees, customers, and other stakeholders.[20]

Commitment is the most critical of these traits; without it, the other five attributes cannot be fully developed.

IDENTIFYING AND DISRUPTING LEADERSHIP BIASES

For those working around a leader, the single most important trait that generates a sense of inclusiveness is a leader's visible awareness of bias. According to comments on a 360-degree Inclusive Leadership Assessment (ILA), participants particularly noticed when a leader "constantly challenged their own biases and encouraged others to be aware of their preconceived leanings." An inclusive leader seeks insight into their biases by, for example, "Asking others to give feedback on whether their thought process is biased."[10]

In addition to awareness and acknowledgment of biases, participants cared about humility, empathy, and perspective-taking.[10] Leadership biases can cause people to overlook great ideas, undermine individual potential, and create a less-than-ideal work experience for colleagues.[45]

Leaders can take the following steps to begin the process of addressing and mitigating biases[45]:

- Accept that biases are operating and commit to learning more about them and how to interrupt them.
- Build a culture where people talk openly about recognizing and mitigating biases and hold each other accountable.
- Assess the current state of biases, work to make improvements, track improvements, and use the data to further hone strategies.

LEADING DIVERSE TALENT AND TEAMS

Future success depends on organizations' and leaders' ability to optimize an increasingly diverse and dispersed talent pool.[23] Inclusive leaders create intentional opportunities for innovation and collaboration. They rely on data, such as diversity of thinking preferences, to design teams that are optimized for creative and innovative thinking, and then they set them up for success. This includes articulating the "why" and giving people frameworks, guidelines, and a toolkit to work together effectively, consider different ideas, and push each other to think in new ways.[46]

In an inclusive culture, employees know that, irrespective of their race, gender, creed, sexual orientation, and physical ability, they can fulfill their personal objectives by aligning them with those of the organization, have a meaningful career, and be valued as an individual. They are valued for how they contribute to the organization's mission.[38]

STRATEGIES AND PRACTICES TO INCREASE INCLUSION

Deloitte determined that inclusive leadership is not about the occasional grand gesture, but rather routine and smaller-scale but genuine comments and actions that leaders practice. Leaders that were determined to be the least inclusive would try to overpower others, display favoritism, and discount alternate views. Verbatim responses from their assessments identified some of the following inclusive leadership behaviors:

- **Shares personal weaknesses**: "[This leader] will openly ask about information that she is not aware of. She demonstrates a humble unpretentious work manner. This puts others at ease, enabling them to speak out and voice their opinions, which she values."
- **Learns about cultural differences:** "[This leader] has taken the time to learn the ropes (common words, idioms, customs, likes/dislikes) and the cultural pillars."
- **Acknowledges team members as individuals:** "[This leader] leads a team of over 100 people and yet addresses every team member by name, knows the work stream that they support and the work that they do."[43(para16–18)]

There are numerous strategies leaders can employ to increase inclusion. These include personal strategies, such as: (a) get to know your blind spots, (b) remain visible and vocal, (c) deliberately seek out differences in thought and approach, and (d) check your impact.[43]

Organizational strategies include[41]:

- Promote your organization's commitment to inclusion.
- Facilitate collaboration across the organization.
- Assess and de-bias your job descriptions:
  - Choose words carefully; select words that do not connote a certain gender, and so on.
  - Use inclusive, gender-neutral pronouns, such as "they."
  - Highlight the organization's investment in employee development and celebrate employees' capacity to grow.

LEADERSHIP TO ADVANCE EQUITY

Public demand for racial, gender, and other forms of justice and equity is clear and urgent. Sixty-one percent of Americans believe the United States needs new civil rights laws to fight discrimination against Black Americans, according to a September 2020 Gallup poll.[47] As much as people in the United States expect their government to increase equity for Black Americans and other vulnerable populations, customers and other stakeholders expect organizational leaders to take even greater action on DEI. In a concurrent Edelman poll,[48] 77% of respondents said companies must respond to injustice in order to earn or keep their trust.[49]

To be able to advance equity, leaders need to develop an equity mindset. United Way Worldwide's Equity Activation Model is a systems-based view for how businesses can activate equity within and outside of their organizations. It is structured around three main spheres of influence: workforce, marketplace, and society. Each sphere, in turn, includes multiple activators—key areas of activity and everyday choices such as talent advancement; products and services; and standards and policies—through which organizations can exert their influence to activate equity. Within each activator, organizations take specific actions in pursuit of equity.[42]

Equity demands systems-level changes, beginning with challenging current policies, procedures, practice, patterns, and cultures and ensuring accountability.[42] Promoting systems-level changes to advance equity needs to occur at different levels and involves many components.

- **Workforce:** access, enablement, and advancement
- **Marketplace:** products and services, marketing and sales, ecosystems and alliances, and supply chain
- **Society:** community impact and partnership, standards, and policy

STRATEGIES TO ADVANCE LEADERSHIP DIVERSITY, EQUITY, AND INCLUSION

Bringing together all three areas, there are numerous key strategies to advance leadership DEI.[20,43,49]

- **Every leader owns and role models DEI:** Every board member and C-suite leader in the organization should own a set of responsibilities for driving DEI in the workplace, marketplace, and society. Every leader needs to see it as their responsibility to role-model inclusive leadership.
- **Strategic alignment:** Executive leaders need to view and promote DEI as core pillars within the organization's strategic plan and workplans. They need to articulate a compelling

narrative as to why inclusive leadership is mission critical and a leadership imperative. They must make meaningful workplace changes to signify the importance of DEI.

- **Recruitment:** HR leaders can ensure that job advertisements emphasize inclusive leadership capabilities and the organization's commitment to DEI. They can incorporate inclusion into their behavioral interview questions.
- **Performance management:** HR leaders can integrate inclusive leadership capabilities into the organization's competency expectations, link key performance indicators (KPIs) to inclusive behaviors and DEI outcomes, ensure that those promoted to senior positions embody inclusive leadership and demonstrate a genuine commitment to DEI, and hold leaders and managers truly accountable for non-inclusive behaviors.
- **Rewards and recognition:** Executive leaders can reward leaders who role-model inclusive behaviors and showcase inclusive leaders and the organizational benefits from their inclusive behaviors.
- **Leadership development:** HR leaders can formally assess inclusive leadership capabilities across senior leaders and managers, identify individual and organizational developmental gaps, and create development plans based on the six signature traits of inclusive leadership. They can require leaders to seek 360-degree feedback on their inclusive leadership practices and incorporate the feedback into their personalized development plans. They can provide inclusive leadership education, coaching, and mentoring to strengthen leaders' capacity. They can integrate inclusive leadership into the organization's talent identification and development strategy to assess readiness and develop current and future leaders.
- **System integration:** Executive leaders can integrate inclusive leadership as well as the broader principles of DEI into the organization's innovation strategy and processes.

SUMMARY

This chapter provides the definitions, evolution, intersections, skills, mindsets, and practices of diversity, equity, inclusion, and intercultural and global competence in leadership. The increasingly diverse, international, and interconnected world calls for inclusive leaders who will commit to advance DEI. Intercultural and global competence are related, essential leadership mindsets, skills, and practices. There is a moral imperative and compelling business case for increased diverse leadership who can represent their stakeholders and deliver services they want and need. The public outcry for justice makes leaders' cultural humility, equity mindset, and action critical. DEI and intercultural and global competence in leadership are vital in public health and health systems, given the effects of systemic racism and other forms of oppression on people's health and healthcare systems.

DISCUSSION QUESTIONS

1. Who are inclusive leadership role models for you, what have you learned from them, and how will you apply what you learned to your leadership practice?
2. Explain and give examples of why DEI and intercultural competence are particularly important in public health and healthcare leadership.
3. What barriers to DEI in leadership have you experienced, and how might you apply some of the strategies outlined in the chapter to address them?
4. Given what you learned about DEI and intercultural competence in leadership in this chapter, what steps will you take to increase your intercultural competence, inclusive leadership, and equity mindset?

CASE STUDY: LEADERSHIP DIVERSITY, EQUITY, AND INCLUSION MISTAKES

INSTRUCTIONS

Read the following case and then respond to the questions that follow. Content warning: This case discusses workplace biases and microaggressions.

CASE

We were only a few minutes into the all-staff meeting, and I, a woman of color who prides herself on her commitment to DEI in the workplace, had just made a terrible mistake. In an effort to start the meeting in an inclusive and welcoming manner, I introduced a new team member to the rest of the employees. I expected the new employee to be impressed and pleased by my efforts to warmly welcome them to our organization; however, I was wrong.

After my warm introduction, I looked at the person, expecting to see their positive reaction. Instead, their face revealed an expression of confusion and hurt, a tense jaw, and eyes that sparkled with tears. I wondered what I had done to cause such a reaction. A few moments later, it clicked. I had not asked for the person's pronouns, and even worse, I had misgendered them by assuming that they used "he/him" pronouns based on my impressions of their physical appearance.

Thoughts rushed into my mind about what I should say to "fix" the situation in the moment, or if I should postpone the rest of the meeting, or if I should address the situation later since I had already caused enough harm. As terrible as I felt, the last thing I wanted to do was exacerbate the situation. I knew that the way I handled this situation in word and deed would be critical. I referred to my new colleague by their name only throughout the rest of the meeting. When the meeting was finished, I asked to speak with the new team member privately, and they agreed.

Once we were alone, I quickly apologized and accepted responsibility for my mistake, but then I stumbled over my words. I fell silent. After a few moments, my colleague generously stated, "I understand that you made an honest mistake, but it's triggering to have to go through this experience over and over again. For most people, starting a new position brings feelings of hope, happiness, and excitement. For me, I always have this sense of anxiety that situations like this will happen, and I'll have to make quick decisions about how to respond, whether to correct the person, or let it go. Simple behaviors that most people do not have to think twice about, such as going to the restroom, cause me extreme anxiety, because at any given moment, I may be subject to the question 'What are you doing here' or 'This isn't the right restroom for you.'"

As I actively listened to their explanation, I was struck by how getting a seemingly small detail wrong could have such a drastic impact on someone's feelings. This "small" detail is actually not small at all. What I learned from these DEI mistakes were that making an assumption and failing to demonstrate gender sensitivity in this situation led to a new employee feeling uncomfortable in their new place of work. This was the complete opposite of my positive intentions. No matter my good intentions, I had still caused harm. In hindsight, I realize the importance of offering my own pronouns and clarifying someone else's pronouns *before* speaking and showing them respect by using their stated pronouns.

CASE STUDY QUESTIONS

1. What critical DEI leadership mistakes did the author make?

2. How did the author take responsibility for her mistakes in the moment?

3. What did the author do to rectify her mistake, and how effective were her actions?

4. Think of a leadership DEI mistake that you have made recently and respond to the following questions:

   ▪ What critical DEI mistake did you make?

   ▪ How did you become aware of your mistake? Was it on your own, or did someone bring it to your attention?

   ▪ How did you take responsibility for your mistake in the moment?

   ▪ What actions have you taken since then to handle similar situations more effectively?

   ▪ What were your most important lessons learned from your mistake?

   ▪ How are you applying your lessons learned to your leadership practice?

   ▪ What are your key lessons learned from this case study activity overall?

CASE STUDY: ORGANIZATIONAL DIVERSITY, EQUITY, AND INCLUSION MISTAKES

INSTRUCTIONS

Read the following case and then answer the questions that follow. Content warning: This case discusses workplace biases, microaggressions, and discrimination complaints. Note the company named is fictitious.

CASE

Santé Corp is a well-known home health agency with over 6,000 employees in 12 regional offices. On trend with many other corporations, Santé Corp's senior leadership team made a public announcement of their company's commitment to DEI; however, they made a series of serious and costly mistakes. In their DEI marketing campaign, they unwittingly portrayed Asian employees as highly professional, logical, and technologically savvy, and the way they depicted Black employees caused them to feel even more alienated. They quickly rolled out a number of DEI activities such as town hall meetings with high-profile BIPOC speakers. They did not conduct an assessment or integrate DEI into their company vision, mission, values, strategic plan, and workplace culture. Several BIPOC, female-identified, and LGBTQ+ employees lodged discrimination complaints. A few former employees publicly shared their complaints on a popular social media business site, with immediate responses from other former employees sharing similar stories about DEI abuses. Santé Corp saw a dramatic spike in resignations, particularly by BIPOC, female-identified people, and LGBTQ+ employees.

Former employee testimonials on social media included:

"My former white, heterosexual, cisgender male boss once told our interview team that he didn't think that a candidate, who was a person of color, was fit for our open position because he was not 'professional' enough. When I asked him to elaborate, he noted the candidate's cultural dress, feminine mannerisms, and speech."

"As a woman of color, I noticed a significant pay gap between me and my male colleagues who were at the same level and career track. When I asked for an explanation from my manager and HR, I was told that it was not an issue of race or gender but assertiveness in the role."

"Although I publicly shared that I was a gay woman, I was frequently asked, 'Is your husband here?' at work social events. Having to constantly correct the assumption that I was heterosexual was draining, demoralizing, and made me feel like I could not be my authentic self in the workplace."

CASE STUDY QUESTIONS

1. What common organizational DEI mistakes did Santé Corp leaders make?
2. How have you made or witnessed similar organizational DEI mistakes, and how would you rectify those mistakes in the future?
3. What lessons have you learned from this case study, and how will you apply them in your leadership practices?

ADDITIONAL RESOURCES

LEADERSHIP MEASUREMENT TOOLS AND EXERCISES

- **Harvard Implicit Association Test (IAT) for Gender-Career and Race** (https://implicit.harvard.edu/implicit/user/agg/blindspot/indexgc.htm).
  - The Gender-Career IAT often reveals a relative link between family and females and between career and males. The Race IAT requires the ability to distinguish faces of European and African origin. It indicates that most people in the United States have an automatic preference for White over Black. Note that the statements can be United States-centric and may or may not be applicable to people from different countries. Once you have completed both IATs, respond to the following reflection questions:
    - How did your results confirm or challenge your understanding of your biases?
    - As a leader, what are the benefits to having a better understanding of your biases?
    - Reflecting back on your life, which of your biases have changed or stayed the same? For those that have changed, what contributed to the changes?
- **The APHA DEI Toolkit** (www.apha.org/-/media/files/pdf/affiliates/equity_toolkit.ashx)
  - Governance Assessment and Tools was created by the APHA and includes five assessments on governance, mission-driven programs, partnerships, communication, and advocacy.
- **The Center for Global Inclusion–DEI Approaches, Insight, and Impact Worksheet** (https://centreforglobalinclusion.org/The-Centre/di-approaches-insight-impact-activity)

- This 20- to 30-minute activity is designed to (a) educate participants on the Five Approaches to DEI that are part of the Global Diversity, Equity, and Inclusion Benchmarks (GDEIB) and (b) help participants gain insight into the impact of the similarities and differences between their personal approach to DEI and their organization's approach to DEI and to determine how those differences or similarities might guide their actions. The one-page worksheet contains activity instructions, a summary of the five approaches, and sections for self-assessment, reflection, and discussion.

ACKNOWLEDGMENTS

I extend my deepest appreciation to: Jennifer Tran, Mariana Rocha-Goldberg, and Priya Shah who provided invaluable assistance with research and formatting for this chapter.

 A robust set of instructor resources designed to supplement this text is located at http://connect.springerpub.com/content/book/978-0-8261-4924-4. Qualifying instructors may request access by emailing **textbook@springerpub.com.**

REFERENCES

1. Global Citizen, LLC. *Equity, Diversity and Inclusion (EDI)*. Global Citizen, LLC.; 2014. https://www.globalcitizenllc.com/equity-diversity-and-inclusion

2. Williams S. Evolution of diversity in the workplace | LinkedIn. *LinkedIn*. February 24, 2020. https://www.linkedin.com/pulse/evolution-diversity-workplace-stacey-williams/

3. McKinsey and Company. *Diversity Wins: How Inclusion Matters*. May 2020. https://www.mckinsey.com/~/media/mckinsey/featured%20insights/diversity%20and%20inclusion/diversity%20wins%20how%20inclusion%20matters/diversity-wins-how-inclusion-matters-vf.pdf

4. Turner KL. Diversity officers unplugged: how to build belonging amidst COVID and racial tensions (panel). Presented at: 2020 Diversity & Inclusion Conference; 2020.

5. Global Citizen, LLC. *Global Competence Training*. Global Citizen, LLC.; 2014. https://www.globalcitizenllc.com/global-competence-training

6. Stubblefield-Tave B, Walker WE. Using cultural competence to advance and sustain DEI efforts. *LinkedIn*. February 17, 2021. https://www.linkedin.com/pulse/using-cultural-competence-advance-sustain-dei-efforts-beau

7. Intercultural Development Inventory. The roadmap to intercultural competence using the IDI. Intercultural development inventory | IDI, LLC. April 10, 2012. https://idiinventory.com

8. Aperian Global. Cultural competence training & consulting. Aperian Global. https://www.aperianglobal.com/solutions/cultural-competence

9. Tervalon M, Murray-García J. Cultural humility versus cultural competence: a critical distinction in defining physician training outcomes in multicultural education. *J Health Care Poor Underserved*. 1998;9(2):117–125. doi:10.1353/hpu.2010.0233

10. Bourke J, Titus A. The key to inclusive leadership. *Harvard Business Review*. March 6, 2020. https://hbr.org/2020/03/the-key-to-inclusive-leadership

11. van Dijk H, van Engen M, Paauwe J. Reframing the business case for diversity: a values and virtues perspective. *J Bus Ethics*. 2012;111(1):73–84. doi:10.1007/s10551-012-1434-z

12. Ely RJ, Thomas DA. Getting serious about diversity: enough already with the business case. *Harvard Business Review*. November 1, 2020. https://hbr.org/2020/11/getting-serious-about-diversity-enough-already-with-the-business-case

13. Acker J. Inequality regimes: gender, class, and race in organizations. *Gender & Society*. 2006;20(4):441-464. doi:10.1177/0891243206289499

14. Healthy People 2030. Social determinants of health. 2021. https://health.gov/healthypeople/objectives-and-data/social-determinants-health

15. American Public Health Association, de Beaumont, National Collaborative for Health Equity. *Healing Through Policy: Creating Pathways to Racial Justice*. Author; October 2021:99. https://apha.org/-/media/Files/PDF/topics/equity/Healing_Through_Policy_Policy_and_Practice_Briefs.ashx

16. García Johnson CP, Otto K. Better together: a model for women and LGBTQ equality in the workplace. *Front Psychol*. 2019;10:272. doi:10.3389/fpsyg.2019.00272

17. Singh S, Durso LE. Widespread discrimination continues to shape LGBT people's lives in both subtle and significant ways. Center for American Progress. May 2, 2017. https://www.americanprogress.org/issues/lgbtq-rights/news/2017/05/02/429529/widespread-discrimination-continues-shape-lgbt-peoples-lives-subtle-significant-ways

18. Morrison M, Lumby J, Maringe F, Bhopal K, Dyke M. *Diversity, Identity and Leadership*; 2007:46. http://citeseerx.ist.psu.edu/viewdoc/download;jsessionid=9C936F466842EF81B4A084EA538C3441?doi=10.1.1.492.651&rep=rep1&type=pdf

19. United Nations, Department of Economic and Social Affairs, Population Division. *International Migration 2019: Report*. UN; 2019.

20. Bourke J. The six signature traits of inclusive leadership. *Deloitte Insights*. April 14, 2016. https://www2.deloitte.com/us/en/insights/topics/talent/six-signature-traits-of-inclusive-leadership.html

21. DeHaas D, Bachus B, Horn E. *Unleashing the Power of Inclusion: Attracting and Engaginc the Evolving Workforce*. Deloitte University Press: The Leadership Center for Inclusion; 2017.

22. Todd S. The number one reason White men give for not getting involved with diversity and inclusion. *Pocket Worthy*. August 10, 2020. https://getpocket.com/explore/item/the-number-one-reason-white-men-give-for-not-getting-involved-with-diversity-and-inclusion?utm_source=pocket-newtab

23. Bourke J, Dillon B. Fast forward: leading in a brave new world of diversity (customers, ideas, talent). *Deloitte Australia*. June 2015. https://www2.deloitte.com/content/dam/Deloitte/au/Documents/human-capital/deloitte-au-hc-trends-forward-diversity-290515.pdf

24. Lumby J, Bhopal K, Dyke M, et al. *Integrating Diversity in Leadership in Further Education Research Report*. March 3, 2007. https://www.researchgate.net/publication/237258453_Integrating_Diversity_in_Leadership_in_Further_Education_Research_Report

25. Tonello M. *Corporate Board Practices in the Russell 3000 and S&P 500: 2020 Edition*. The Conference Board, Inc; 2020. https://conferenceboard.esgauge.org/boardpractices/report

26. Nayyar S. How to support more women in leadership roles. World Economic Forum. March 8, 2020. https://www.weforum.org/agenda/2020/03/international-womens-day-women-leadership-roles

27. Catalyst. Women CEOs of the S&P 500 (List). Catalyst. August 30, 2021. https://www.catalyst.org/research/women-ceos-of-the-sp-500

28. BoardSource. Leading with intent: 2017 National Index of Nonprofit Board Practices; 2017. https://leadingwithintent.org/wp-content/uploads/2017/11/LWI-2017.pdf?hsCtaTracking=8736f801-1e14-427b-adf0-38485b149ac0%7C82ace287-b110-4d8f-9651-2b2c06a43c05

29. Thomas-Breitfeld S, Kunreuther F. *Race to Lead: Confronting the Nonprofit Racial Leadership Gap*. Building Movement Project; 2017. https://buildingmovement.org/wp-content/uploads/2019/08/Race-to-Lead-Confronting-the-Nonprofit-Racial-Leadership-Gap.pdf

30. World Economic Forum. *Global Gender Gap Report 2020*; 2019. https://www.weforum.org/reports/gender-gap-2020-report-100-years-pay-equality

31. National Association of County & City Health Officials. 2019 national profile of local health departments. *NACCHO*. 2020:147. https://www.naccho.org/uploads/downloadable-resources/Programs/Public-Health-Infrastructure/NACCHO_2019_Profile_final.pdf

32. United States Census Bureau. National population by characteristics: 2010–2019. *Census.gov*. October 8, 2021. https://www.census.gov/data/tables/time-series/demo/popest/2010s-national-detail.html

33. American College of Healthcare Executives. Increasing and sustaining racial diversity in healthcare leadership. November 2020. https://www.ache.org/about-ache/our-story/our-commitments/policy-statements/increasing-and-sustaining-racial-diversity-in-healthcare-management

34. Hewlett SA, Marshall M, Sherbin L, Gonsalves T. *Innovation, Diversity, and Market Growth*. Center for Talent Innovation; 2013. https://www.talentinnovation.org/_private/assets/IDMG-ExecSumm FINAL-CTI.pdf

35. Kumar A. *Living Into Leadership as a Woman of Color: Sexism and Subtle Bias*. Forbes Nonporift Council; March 24, 2020.

36. Bahadur N. How C-Suite women of color have powerfully redefined executive presence. *Working Mother*. May 13, 2020. https://www.pressreader.com/usa/working-mother/20200601/page/2

37. Wharton: University of Pennsylvania. When to come out: the challenges facing gay CEOs. July 28, 2014. https://knowledge.wharton.upenn.edu/article/gay-ceos

38. Groysberg B, Connolly K. Great leaders who make the mix work. *Harvard Business Review*. September 1, 2013. https://hbr.org/2013/09/great-leaders-who-make-the-mix-work

39. Wingard J. Diverse boards propel successful companies–three strategies to expand pipelines. *Forbes.* February 21, 2019. https://www.forbes.com/sites/jasonwingard/2019/02/21/diverse-boards-propel-successful-companies-three-strategies-to-expand-pipelines

40. Bohnet I. Talks at Google | What Works; 2016. https://gtalks-gs.appspot.com/talk/what-works

41. Brennan M. 3 ways to make your organization more inclusive. Koya Partners. February 10, 2020. https://koyapartners.com/blog/inclusive-organizations

42. Deloitte. Part III: Act now–the equity imperative. Deloitte United States. February 23, 2021. https://www2.deloitte.com/us/en/pages/about-deloitte/articles/act-now-the-equity-imperative.html

43. Bourke J, Titus A. Why inclusive leaders are good for organizations, and how to become one. *Harvard Business Review.* March 29, 2019. https://hbr.org/2019/03/why-inclusive-leaders-are-good-for-organizations-and-how-to-become-one

44. Deloitte Australia. Inclusive leadership–will a hug do? *Human Capital.* March 2012. http://www2.deloitte.com/content/dam/Deloitte/au/Documents/human-capital/deloitte-au-hc-diversity-inclusive-leadership-hug-0312.pdf

45. Barnett J. The role of leadership in addressing bias in the workplace. *Forbes.* November 8, 2018. https://www.forbes.com/sites/jimbarnett/2018/11/08/the-role-of-leadership-in-addressing-bias-in-the-workplace

46. Lepore M. Why inclusive leadership is essential to innovation. Herrmann Global. 2021. https://blog.thinkherrmann.com/why-inclusive-leadership-is-essential-to-innovation

47. Jones JM. New low in U.S. See progress for black civil rights. *Gallup.com.* September 9, 2020. https://news.gallup.com/poll/319388/new-low-progress-black-civil-rights.aspx

48. Edelman R. Systemic racism: the existential challenge for business. Edelman. September 8, 2020. https://www.edelman.com/research/systemic-racism

49. Deloitte. How business leaders can build a more equitable workforce. *Harvard Business Review.* May 11, 2021. https://hbr.org/sponsored/2021/05/how-business-leaders-can-build-a-more-equitable-workforce

50. Eze N. Driving health equity through diversity in health care leadership. *NEJM Catalyst.* October 20, 2020. https://catalyst.nejm.org/doi/full/10.1056/CAT.20.0521

Chapter 13

Managing and Resolving Conflict

Michael R. Fraser

INTRODUCTION

Workplace conflict is inevitable, but effective leaders can and should manage and resolve conflict. Conflict over ideas has a transformative impact on an organization; however, interpersonal and team relationship conflict erodes trust and creates a toxic workplace culture if not effectively addressed. Some team members thrive in settings where conflict provides the opportunity for creative discussion and development of ideas while others may avoid any kind of conflict entirely. What is most important about managing conflict is that it is dealt with honestly and effectively: avoiding it or accommodating it too often can result in relationship strain and have a negative impact on organizational outcomes. This chapter examines how public health and healthcare managers and leaders can improve team performance by leveraging the opportunities that constructive conflict over ideas presents and providing skills to resolve negative interpersonal conflict.

OBJECTIVES

By the end of this chapter, the reader will be able to:

- Analyze the sources and impact of conflict at work.
- Define five conflict-handling styles.
- Describe how to effectively manage and resolve conflict at work.
- Apply conflict management and resolution skills to two scenarios.

WHAT IS CONFLICT?

Simply put, conflict arises when two or more interests, positions, or concerns appear to be incompatible.[1] Conflict is commonly defined as a disagreement or clash, and many ascribe negative associations to conflict, especially when there is a preference to avoid conflict versus engage in it. In the era of COVID-19, conflict erupts daily between public health leaders, healthcare workers, and different groups in society; for example, conflict between those who support mask mandates and those who do not, or those who support vaccination and those who do not. Conflict has become so intense in many communities that some health officers and elected officials have been physically threatened for decisions they made about COVID-19 prevention and control. Some healthcare workers have threatened to leave or have left their jobs over vaccine mandates in their facilities. National associations of public health officials, including the Association of State and Territorial Health Officials, the National Association of County and City Health Officials, and the Big Cities Health Coalition, have reported almost 250 local and state health officials have left their positions as agency leaders due to the stress and strain of conflict between themselves and their elected leadership, or between their agency and the community it serves.[2,3]

While these conflicts between health professionals and members of their communities play out on a national stage, it is important to remember that disagreements and debate do not have to result in resignations nor an increase in the spread of disease. Thoughtful, intentionally designed, and rational approaches to conflict can allow for better solutions to be reached. Unfortunately, however, this requires both sides to participate in conflict resolution in good faith and with minds open to change, a requirement that many may not be able to abide in an era of hyper-partisanship and political divide. Key to resolving conflict is the will of both parties to do so. Without this will, there is little way for any conflict to be successfully resolved because there is no interest in or room for resolution.

Addressing and managing conflict can lead to healthy and productive conversations about different viewpoints, perspectives, interests, concerns, and needs. It is often through disagreement and debate that new, creative approaches are identified and can be raised up in an organization. Debate and disagreement are also ways to uncover important underlying assumptions and beliefs that would not otherwise be made explicit on a team. Indeed, when opposing and seemingly disparate viewpoints are made known through conflict, managers and leaders can weigh different options and use the interests and information shared to make well informed decisions. The consideration of different options and interests can create new approaches to their team's work, inspire and inform innovation, and result in new approaches to addressing problems. This kind of generative disagreement has been termed "constructive" or "creative" conflict because it leads participants toward positive resolution and creates new thinking and additional value for an organization and its stakeholders.[4]

Understanding the source of conflict is important to managing and resolving it. Conflict over ideas is helpful and transformative. Interpersonal conflict, however, is damaging and toxic to relationships and team performance. As such, it is important to distinguish debate and disagreement over ideas from conflict between individuals that might be the result of personality differences, power differentials, or different work styles and preferences.

In her book *Dealing With Conflict*, Amy Gallo defines four sources of conflict that are helpful to getting to the core reasons that we may experience disagreement and discord with others: relationship, task, process, and status.[5] Relationship conflicts are common in many different settings. Relationship conflicts often focus on subjective observations about how one is being treated or particular personal issues between people. Task conflict is rooted in disagreement on or opposition to a goal or what a group is trying to accomplish, for example when group members disagree with what the outcome of their work should be or have different points of view on a project's objective. Process conflict is centered around differences in how team members may approach the way work is to be accomplished, or how it is to get done. Status conflict arises from disagreement or dispute about who oversees a group or one's position within it. Understanding these sources of conflict allows for more precise resolution. For example, there may be disagreement within a group over how a report is to be written and who is responsible for authoring various sections (process conflict). Conflict over process may be more constructively addressed if the group makes their ideas about their ideal process known and individuals share their assumptions about the authoring process to make expectations and needs clear. It also avoids misattribution of a conflict to another source, such as relationship or status conflict, when that is not actually the cause.

CONFLICT AND EMOTIONAL INTELLIGENCE

Unfortunately, some experiences with disagreement may be associated with damaging or upsetting interpersonal conflict that probably involved hurt feelings and, potentially, other negative experiences. Conflict brings up emotions and feelings that influence individual reactions to it and these emotions can take over the conflict response. These emotional reactions are a natural part of being human and are deeply rooted in biology and psychology. The emotional response is an important survival tactic: the "fight or flight" response to stressors such as an attack kept the species alive and is hardwired in human brains to activate when they feel threatened by others. While this fight response served early humans well when a tribe was attacked by saber-toothed tigers or opposing factions, the fight response does not serve people well in contemporary work settings where there is room for disagreement and debate and perceived attacks are not matters of life or death. The same fight response is certainly not warranted when someone turns in a report late, disagrees with a performance review, makes a mistake, or takes an approach to solving a problem that someone believes does not include what they perceive to be a critical part of the solution.

EMOTIONAL INTELLIGENCE

Because individual responses to conflict can surface emotions, responding to conflict in ways that use the rational/logical parts of the brain instead of the more primal and emotional parts is helpful to regulate each conflict response. Emotional intelligence (EI) is the ability to manage and regulate emotions when interacting with others including how people behave in conflict situations. Work by Goleman[6] and Bradberry and Greaves[7] defines four domains that comprise the core EI approach: self-awareness and self-management make up personal EI competence, and social awareness and relationship management comprise one's social competencies. Self-awareness is being mindful of and understanding the emotions that an individual may experience in a particular situation and why they are experiencing them. Understanding and perceiving one's emotional state while experiencing conflict is critical to then managing the emotional response to it. Self-management is the ability to guide a response to a particular emotion that elicits a constructive outcome, or an outcome that is a rational response to the situation rather than an irrational one. Far too often people jump to a fight-or-flight response in a conflict situation rather than take the time needed to consider different responses to the perceived threat and to manage their emotions to resolve the situation more constructively. Of course, this is difficult to do in the moment itself, but it is critically important to constructive and productive responses to conflict between individuals.

The first two EI domains relate to self: self-awareness and self-management. The other two EI domains relate to how people interact with others. Social awareness is one's ability to sense or pick up on the emotions other people are experiencing. Social awareness has to do with how individuals listen to and observe others, and how aware individuals are of their emotions and the influence they have on the situation about which they are a part. Relationship management is the fourth and last EI domain. Relationship management brings the other three domains together (self-awareness, self-management, social awareness) and has to do with how one maintains connections and strengthens relationships over time.[6,7] Relationship management focuses on the strength of the bonds people have between each other and how these bonds are maintained during and after conflict, difficult conversations, or in times of stress.

A critical insight that EI provides concerning interpersonal conflict is that one can actively and empathetically approach both themselves and others when dealing with disagreement or discord. Far too often, the response to difficult situations may be to avoid them entirely (a flight instinct), or to engage in emotionally driven reactions that may damage relationships (a fight instinct). Assessing one's EI and working to strengthen the requisite skills and abilities in these four domains can help an individual understand their reactions to conflict and consider constructive approaches to resolving it. Another important insight of EI is that there are almost always underlying emotions, needs, interests, expectations, and subjective perceptions at play in any conflict situation. As such, conflicts may not always be about what people are actually arguing over but instead they may be about past issues, unclear or hidden expectations, or different perceptions of the same set of facts. EI provides the capacity to examine the ability of an individual to be aware of and understand those underlying issues, and how they manage their responses to them. (See Chapter 5, "Emotional Intelligence," for more detail.)

THE ICEBERG OF CONFLICT

An adaptation of Cloke and Goldsmith's "iceberg of conflict"[8(p122)] illustrates this point. In Figure 13.1, at the tip of the iceberg is the issue above the surface that is experienced as conflict. Take, for example, a conflict between two coworkers who were asked by their supervisor to present a project update to their health officer but who are actively disagreeing about which one of them should make the presentation. Coworker A wants to present because she believes she contributed the most to the project and coworker B wants to present because she similarly wants to be able to demonstrate what she contributed. What appears to be the issue central in this conflict is disagreement over who gets to present to the health officer, and it may seem that the best resolution is to rationally negotiate between both coworkers about what makes the most sense in this situation; however, under the surface of this conflict may be other factors. These include factors such as individual personalities, feelings of wanting to be seen and appreciated, needs to be recognized by a superior, expectations about the contributions made to the final product and their importance, and perhaps unresolved issues from prior experiences of never having been able to present and watching someone else take credit for work that was not their own.

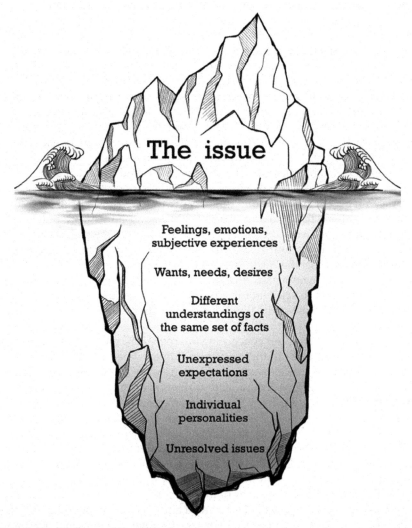

FIGURE 13.1: The Iceberg of Conflict.

Source: Adapted with permission from Cloke K, Goldsmith J. *Resolving Conflicts at Work*. Revised ed. Jossey-Bass; 2005:121–122.

An important part of resolving this conflict between coworkers A and B is to uncover those issues and understand how they influence what might seem like a simple disagreement about who is giving a presentation but in fact are tied to emotions, unmet needs, and hidden expectations. Surfacing and discussing these under the surface factors openly and honestly can lead to resolution of the conflict and deeper understanding between team members. Through that discussion, coworkers can evolve a mutually satisfying resolution or win–win outcome perhaps by agreeing to share the presentation time between them, or to identify a future presentation or update where the other coworker would be able to present individually to the health officer. The dialogue may also strengthen their relationship by providing opportunity for learning and sharing between them. Such an open and honest conversation may uncover the motivations and desires each coworker brings to work, such as the desire to be appreciated or to contribute, and make those desires known so they can be addressed in the future in other situations and opportunities and avoid similar conflict.

WHY CONFLICT MATTERS

As mentioned earlier, one approach to dealing with conflict is to avoid it entirely. In many cultures, especially those where there is a large status or power differential between supervisors and subordinates, disagreement and conflict at work are frowned upon and may even be expressly discouraged. In all cultures, those who are conflict avoidant seek to resolve conflict by not engaging in it at all, while those who seek conflict have little trouble activating their "fight" response in any debate or disagreement. While these cultural norms about conflict and our own personal preferences about avoiding or seeking conflict are important to appreciate, it is also essential to note that there is a tremendous cost to both the individuals and organizations involved.

First, at the personal level, not addressing conflict or reacting to it with anger or emotional outbursts may keep an individual from developing strong personal relationships. As stated earlier, relationship management is a critical part of EI and how bonds of trust are developed between people. If someone avoids sharing ideas and feedback with individuals because they are afraid to upset others, disappoint others, or make others angry, they do not have the chance to hear the individual's perspective, to consider alternatives, and to grow and improve. To feel inspired and engaged at work, people need work that is challenging and personally meaningful but also work that allows them to feel part of a group that is similarly committed to a shared goal or vision. If conflict is avoided, one may not be able to fully commit to a group's course of action or set of ideas, especially if the individual disagrees with or feels differently about the work but is afraid to disclose that disagreement for fear of upset and retribution.

"Groupthink" is a term used to describe what happens when a group prioritizes its desire for harmony over sharing a diversity of ideas.[9] When groupthink is at play, there is little to no disagreement over a group's decision even if members of the group disagree with the decision made or have better ideas to share. Groupthink within a team or organization may arise from conflict avoidance, or from relying upon a group with limited diversity of thought and opinions to make a decision. Rather than suggesting different courses of action or contributing novel ideas to a group's deliberation, members of the group agree on a course of action because it is the expedient thing to do but perhaps not the best thing to do in a given situation. While members of the team may nod their heads and outwardly appear to be agreeing with the group's decision, some may inwardly question the wisdom of the group's decision and actively oppose it in their own minds. Team members may leave the meeting with a false sense of understanding that the group reached agreement when some in the group merely wanted the meeting to end or did not want to be perceived as being contradictory or argumentative.

To help address groupthink, some teams identify a "strategic dissenter" as a way to organizationally support disagreement within a group.[10] The dissenter's job is to question group decisions and direction when or if no one else will, allowing space for debate and consideration of alternatives. This can be a helpful tactic to assuring conflict over ideas is routinized within a group's decision-making process. The dissenter's job is not to disagree with individuals but to raise opposing viewpoints and perspectives as a catalyst to questioning assumptions and to preventing premature consensus. Making it someone's job helps normalize constructive and creative conflict over ideas and can lead a group to consider important alternatives when they may not otherwise.

People often avoid conflict because they do not want to upset or anger someone, or because they fear reprisal or retribution in settings where there are significant power differences between coworkers. One only has to read Hans Christian Andersen's childhood fable "The Emperor's New Clothes" to be reminded of the desire to avoid conflict and disagreement, especially with those in higher positions, even if it means not being honest with each other.[11] In his book *The Five Dysfunctions of a Team*, Patrick Lencioni describes ways that teams can work better together to achieve organizational results and explains what gets in the way of team functioning.[12(p191)] Fear of conflict is a dysfunction that Lencioni describes as the result of lack of trust among coworkers. Because members of a team may not trust each other they are less likely to be vulnerable with each other and share honest feedback, or to take the risks needed to innovate or develop new ideas.

In Lencioni's model, this lack of vulnerability and trust between team members results in conflict avoidance. By avoiding conflict, team members are not fully committed to the team because they do not share their honest ideas or perspectives on the team's work, and if the team's idea fails, they can claim that their team's decision was not their (own) decision in the first place. In short, fear of conflict and lack of trust limit the engagement of team members who then may be less committed to their work, less accountable for results, and ultimately less attentive to successful results or organizational outcomes that matter. Lencioni offers a simple assessment to measure a team's performance on the five dysfunctions model.[12] Three items ranked on the assessment relate specifically to the extent to which fear of conflict is a problem that a team needs to address[12(pp192–193)]:

- team members are passionate and unguarded in their discussion of issues;
- team meetings are compelling, and not boring; and
- during team meetings, the most important—and difficult—issues are put on the table to be resolved.

If members of the team being assessed rank these items as low or uncommon on their teams, there may be an opportunity to address fear of conflict and ways that encourage constructive disagreement within the group. If team members rank these items high or common on their teams, it is a good indication that disagreement and debate over ideas is taking place and should be supported and continued.

Critical to Lencioni's model is the idea that an organization's work may ultimately be less effective when team members lack trust and avoid conflict because they are less committed to the work of their team. Not sharing ideas or perspectives because of a fear of conflict or inability to effectively manage disagreement holds people back both in their personal relationships and their relationships with coworkers. Constructive or creative conflict allows individual contributors to openly share divergent points of view and critique one another's ideas without fear of interpersonal strife. This conflict of ideas, not of individual personalities, is what organizations need so they can change, evolve, innovate, and ultimately thrive.

DIVERSITY AND ADDRESSING CONFLICT

Lack of trust and fear of conflict are especially important to address in contemporary public health practice and healthcare settings where coworkers are multigenerational, come from different backgrounds, have diverse life experiences, and may comprise different racial and ethnic backgrounds. Diversity is a strength of any organization when leveraged appropriately; the different ways in which people think and their lived experiences can help shape successful program growth, policy implementation, and product or service development. Emerging research in the management and organizational development literature suggests that diverse teams are essential to an organization's ability to innovate and create products and services that capture new markets in ways that homogenous teams do not.[13] Health departments may similarly be well served by recruiting and retaining diverse public health professionals and leveraging this diversity to address the population health needs and perspectives from a variety of personal perspectives and professional training. Likewise, healthcare facilities and clinical settings should recruit for diversity so that their workforce represents the community they serve and understands patient and population health needs more clearly.

Diversity, however, must be effectively managed and leveraged within an organization for it to be a significant contributor to an organization's success: it is not enough to recruit and retain diverse teams if that diversity is not leveraged to improve organizational performance. When members of a team do not trust their coworkers to support and help them at work they may disengage from their jobs and may not fully commit to organizational goals and outcomes. Conflict, especially conflict between different racial or ethnic groups, becomes personally damaging and perpetuates organizational and systemic inequities. When conflict is not constructively addressed it creates hostile work environments where individuals feel attacked, marginalized, discriminated against, and disrespected. It can lead to high turnover, hostile work environments, and work experiences that are personally difficult and professionally damaging.

An approach to addressing racial conflict in the workplace involves multiple factors, all of which require the commitment of organizational leaders and group members to obtain measurable and lasting change. Open and honest discussions about both interpersonal relationships and structural or systemic discrimination or inequity need to take place with an eye toward healing, reconciliation, and creating an environment that celebrates difference as a positive aspect of the organization's culture. The Truth, Racial Healing, and Transformation (TRHT) movement provides a guide to this important work.[14] One aspect of TRHT efforts includes creating supportive and helpful individual relationships between coworkers that leverage difference as a value and promotes a common understanding of shared humanity. This includes developing trust and individual appreciation for the positive impact that different experiences have on organizational performance and results. A second aspect of TRHT work involves engaging in organization-wide discussions of institutional policies and procedures that may advantage some groups over others and provides the space for meaningful opportunities to raise issues and then eliminate these disparities through policy change and organizational transformation. This work can bring up conflict between individuals with different experiences at the same organization and needs to be openly and honestly addressed by management with a genuine commitment to equity and improvement.

While some leaders and managers may avoid conversations about disparities and inequities within the workplace because they can be difficult and uncomfortable, avoidance most likely will make the problems on a team even worse. Thoughtful and intentionally designed processes to manage and resolve these conflicts will lead to greater organizational success by allowing coworkers the opportunity to share their experiences, identify potential resolutions, and collaboratively develop a path forward that promotes equity, diversity, and the meaningful participation of everyone in the workplace. A part of TRHT work is to acknowledge that tension or conflict may emerge as part of the TRHT process, and to develop ground rules and processes to discuss and resolve it.[14(p21)] Efforts to advance TRHT have to be authentic, sincere, and supported by organizational leaders. This alone can generate conflict between organizational leaders and/or coworkers who want to avoid conflict by glossing over differences or denying that inequity or discrimination exist in their workplace or on their teams. Leaders have to create an environment of trust before they can initiate these difficult conversations and manage and handle conflicts in a way that encourages growth, learning, and transformation, rather than isolation, retreat, or separation.

CONFLICT MANAGEMENT AND RESOLUTION APPROACHES

The *Thomas-Kilmann Conflict Mode Instrument* or TKI is a widely used approach to measuring and describing the different ways individuals behave when experiencing interpersonal conflict and their preferred conflict management styles.[1] The TKI is based on the work of Kenneth Thomas and Ralph Kilmann who describe five approaches to handling conflict across two main dimensions of conflict behavior: assertiveness and cooperativeness.[1] The assertiveness dimension describes how forcefully an individual emphasizes or attempts to meet their own needs or interests in a conflict, and the cooperativeness dimension describes how forcefully an individual attempts to satisfy the needs of others. While an individual may have a preferred or default mode to handle conflict, effective conflict management involves thoughtfully using each mode in a given situation and understanding the pros and cons of each. These modes include[1(p5)]:

- **Competing:** An approach to conflict is assertive and uncooperative; an individual tries to maximize their own interests or concerns often at the expense of the other person's interests or concerns (high assertiveness, low cooperativeness).
- **Collaborating:** An approach to conflict is assertive and cooperative; an individual seeks to achieve a win–win position that satisfies both individuals' interests and concerns (high assertiveness, high cooperativeness).
- **Compromising:** An approach to conflict that partially resolves the individuals' concerns or issues; is in the middle space or mid-range on the assertiveness and cooperativeness dimensions (medium assertiveness, medium cooperativeness).
- **Avoiding:** An approach to conflict that is unassertive and uncooperative; individuals' concerns are not addressed because conflict is avoided (low assertiveness, low cooperativeness).
- **Accommodating:** An approach to conflict that is unassertive and cooperative; an individual satisfies the concerns of the other without satisfying their own (low assertiveness, high cooperativeness).

Kilmann and Thomas suggest there is no best style for handling interpersonal conflict. Instead, all five modes have a place in how people manage conflict with others. The potential benefits, cautions, and when to potentially employ each mode when managing interpersonal conflict are summarized in Table 13.1.

While no one style is best, the TKI suggests that the most satisfying resolutions to conflict may come from the collaborating approach. This is primarily due to the emphasis on creating a "win–win" position for both parties. While acknowledging that competing, accommodating, and avoiding are sometimes necessary, the cautions with these approaches and their costs to individuals may outweigh their benefits. Compromising, a handling mode used by many to resolve conflicts at work, is also acknowledged as a realistic option but one that can lead to both parties feeling the conflict was not truly resolved to their full satisfaction. This may mean that additional discussion and dialogue are needed in the future and that the conflict is not truly resolved even when a compromise position that is acceptable to both parties is reached.

Assessing team members' conflict management preferences using the TKI can help improve a team's EI by helping team members become more self-aware of their preferred conflict-handling modes and how they influence their behavior in conflict situations. The TKI can be administered through several different leadership development consultants and organizations and then used to consider individual approaches to managing conflict and reactions to it. In their commentary "Building Conflict Competence," Lynn Fick-Cooper and Edward Baker summarize the preferred styles of public health leaders that used the TKI to assess their conflict-handling style preferences as part of the Public Health Leadership Institute.[15] The scholars' results indicated that the most common conflict-handling modes used

TABLE 13.1: Five TKI Conflict-Handling Modes and Their Benefits, Cautions, and When to Use

CONFLICT-HANDLING MODE	BENEFITS	CAUTIONS	WHEN TO USE
Competing	Clearly asserts your interests and concerns; may be expedient to a resolution if you have authority/power	May hurt relationships when the other's concerns are not addressed, or they perceive they "lost"; may avoid a better resolution that could result from collaboration	When collaboration is not feasible; when you have to "win" or have to defend yourself; when an unpopular action needs to be taken or when consensus fails
Collaborating	Creates synergy; allows for learning and communication; may strengthen relationships; may lead to an optimal result through development of new ideas or options	May take time; requires consideration of novel views and ideas; if a resolution is not reached could lead to hurt feelings	When both positions are vital to the organization's success; when new solutions are needed; when you need commitment from all involved
Compromising	Realistic; a way to resolve conflict in a manner that is "good enough" to both parties; may lessen strain on relationships if perceived as neither party getting what they wanted but all parties got something	Sacrifices a potentially more optimal resolution; if not resolved satisfactorily the conflict issue could come back up again; may end up with less innovative solutions than collaboration	When you need a temporary solution to a difficult issue; when you need to reach a quick resolution of a conflict; when competing or collaborating have not been successful
Avoiding	Lowers stress; saves time; may allow for resolution at a later time that might be more appropriate	May increase interpersonal conflict rather than resolve it; when people avoid disagreement or debate the work culture may lack candor needed to build trust; can degrade relationships	When you want to avoid emotional conflict; when issue is unimportant; when issue may be too sensitive; when you need more time to honestly and clearly share your concerns
Accommodating	Restores "harmony"; may be a chance to help the other; can potentially allow for relationship building by ceding self-interest; may save time	Sacrifices one's own interests and could lead to resentments as a result; may acquiesce instead of fully agree	When you are persuaded by the other person's position; when you are overruled or outvoted; when you know you are wrong; when you need to boost others and can sacrifice your own interests to do so

Source: Adapted from Kenneth WT. *Introduction to Conflict Management: Improving Performance Using the TKI*. The Myers-Briggs Company; 2002.

by public health leaders in the Institute cohort they assessed were avoiding, accommodating, and compromising. Few scholars in the cohort preferred competing or collaborating.[15(p187)]

The low self-assessment result of the collaborating preference among the public health cohort is concerning because it suggests that despite organizational emphasis on partnership and collaboration with community members around public health priorities, public health leaders have work to do in managing and handling conflict through the collaboration mode in their workplaces, in the communities in which they work, or both. Barriers to collaboration include the time and commitment needed to create satisfactory resolution to difficult problems, but the payoff of a mutually satisfactory and perhaps better resolution that could be obtained otherwise certainly can make the investment of resources worthwhile. Continuing to strengthen the knowledge, skills, and abilities of public health professionals to collaborate and resolve conflicts through the collaborating conflict-handling mode should be a priority of public leaders if similar low preference scores are found within their teams after being similarly assessed on the TKI.

While it is important to identify the source of conflict, how conflict is handled in organizations is critical to organizational performance and success. The sources of conflict described by Gallo (relationship, task, process, and status) are helpful to understanding how conflicts arise and where to focus efforts to address and resolve them.[5] The conflict-handling modes developed by Thomas and Kilmann are well-described ways to manage interpersonal conflict.[1] EI provides a crucial set of skills that can be used to manage individual responses to the behavior of others, especially in conflict.[6,7] These insights all lead toward employing more effective approaches to handling conflict.

CONFLICT RESOLUTION

At the root of all conflict resolution is the need to make underlying interests and perspectives known so that individuals can better understand one another and adapt, evolve, innovate, or transform their positions with the interests of others. As with negotiation overall, the ability to understand the other parties' interests and motivations informs the negotiation process and can lead to a more satisfactory outcome for all involved. Without a clear understanding of the other's interests, negotiations may be based on misperceptions, misunderstandings, and assumptions about the needs and desires of others that may not be correct. Of course, this does assume that both parties are interested in a successful resolution. Resolving conflict with a rigid, unbending fighter not willing to consider alternatives is unlikely. Resolving conflict takes time and dialogue, and a commitment to achieving an outcome that is satisfactory to both parties. If the goal of a resolution is not shared but rather one or both sides want to merely push for their position, no opportunity to resolve the conflict exists. That is why avoiding conflict is so destructive: it provides no opportunity for resolution and positive relationship building. Many of us choose to avoid conflict, thinking it will be easier than getting involved in a difficult conversation. However, avoidance is likely to make the situation worse by allowing conflict to go unresolved. This lack of resolution can lead to further misunderstandings and resentments and make future resolution that much more difficult.

Empathy, or the ability to feel what another person may be feeling, is a critical skill to develop to effectively resolve conflict. Understanding others' feelings and then acting upon that information allows for fuller understanding of the issues at hand and how to respond to them. Empathy differs from sympathy: empathy is being able to take the position of the other and experience what they are experiencing from their point of view. Sympathy means understanding the other's position from the individual's own point of view but not putting oneself "in the other's shoes." Empathy allows one to consider alternatives to their own point of view by validating another's interests or perspectives, even if they disagree with them. From there, dialogue on potential approaches to resolving the conflict can begin through a conversation of interests and opportunities.

Conflict resolution involves negotiation, but true resolution is often not a negotiated "settlement" or compromise.[8(pxxxi)] Settling can fail to produce a satisfying outcome for either or both of the parties and is akin to the "compromising" conflict-handling mode described previously in the overview of the TKI.[1] Because either or both of the parties may feel that the conflict was not fully resolved in the settlement they reached, there may be lingering issues to address after the parties finish their negotiation and continue to work together in the future.

James Sebenius describes several characteristics of effective negotiators that are applicable to conflict resolution.[16] As previously discussed, effective negotiators are able to understand the interests and point of view of the other and consider them as part of the resolution to the issue at hand. Effective negotiators know the difference between the other parties' position and their actual interests, much like the iceberg figure illustrates (Figure 13.1.). Uncovering those below the surface items that might be contributing to the visible issue is a successful tactic in dialogue to resolve a conflict because it makes all the factors known. Sebenius also describes situations in which effective negotiators may have to walk away from the negotiation and the instances when no resolution, or no deal, is reached because the parties may be too far apart in their interests or searching too hard for common ground that is not obtainable.[16(p91)] There may be some conflicts so difficult to resolve that they might require multiple attempts at resolution, and the contributions of a skilled facilitator, arbitrator, or negotiator to help support the process.

Adapting Rune and Flanagan's work on conflict competent leadership to public health management, Fick-Cooper and Baker describe "7 Habits of Conflict Competent Managers" that summarize the skills needed for effective conflict management.[15] These seven responses help structure responses to conflict and promote constructive resolution; they are[15(p188)]:

1. Taking on a different perspective
2. Creating solutions
3. Expressing emotions
4. Reaching out
5. Thinking reflectively
6. Delaying a response
7. Adapting

These habits build on the insights of EI and conflict-handling described earlier in this chapter and provide concrete activities that can be used in approaching conflicts at the interpersonal and organizational level.

Taking on a different perspective (habit 1) refers to one's ability to empathize as well as practice the social awareness and relationship management competencies that are part of the practice of EI. Creating solutions (habit 2) relies upon the collaborating conflict-handling mode that is part of the TKI approach and speaks to the synergy and learning that results from sharing interests and assumptions and generating new ideas or options as a result. Expressing emotions (habit 3) is the ability to surface the factors that may be at play in the conflict such as feeling disappointed, disrespected, or angry, and describing why. This involves stating feelings openly and honestly, not irrationally confronting another using the fight response. By expressing positive emotions, such as a commitment to the relationship or to the community and one's sincere desire to resolve the conflict, individuals can potentially uncover resolution options and demonstrate the vulnerability needed to build trust that Lencioni suggests in his *Five Dysfunctions of a Team* model.[12]

Reaching out provides the opportunity to engage in dialogue and initiate the process of reaching a potential resolution (habit 4). Thinking reflectively (habit 5) refers to the inward self-assessment that is needed to effectively manage and resolve conflict. Like EI's self-awareness and self-management, reflective thinking is the practice of observing our thoughts and feelings as they are experienced and then reflecting upon them to help understand the reactions and emotions that result. Reflective thinking may also allow for the discovery of new approaches to conflict by allowing oneself time to assess their emotional reaction to conflict and manage the response to it. Delaying a response (habit 6), similar to the avoiding or accommodating conflict-handling mode, suggests the need to allow time to process a potential reaction and resolution to conflict. This response is helpful when a conflict is emotionally charged and time is needed to allow those emotions to settle, or when a rushed resolution is not optimal. Delaying acknowledges the situation is not going to produce an ideal resolution and that more time is needed to develop it, unlike avoiding in which a potential resolution is never reached because efforts to resolve it are never made. Adapting (habit 7) includes openness and flexibility needed to achieve a successful resolution, unlike the competing, or a "my way or the highway,"[15(p187)] conflict-handling mode.

CONFLICT ESSENTIALS FOR PUBLIC HEALTH AND HEALTHCARE PROFESSIONALS

As discussed, management and resolution of conflict requires several different skills and abilities. Managerial and leadership competency in conflict resolution is essential to a high-performing organization. This section of the chapter describes five skills that can be used to manage and resolve conflict at work. Building on the material previously discussed, these skills are described, and examples are provided of how to apply them in practice.

TAKE AN OPEN MINDSET

An "open mindset" approach to conflict management and resolution is an important place to start a dialogue. Open mindset refers to an individual's belief that they can grow and learn from interactions with others, and they are curious about why things are the way they are and what they could be. An open mindset allows for an opportunity to consider alternatives and solutions to a conflict versus hardening one's position. A closed mindset does not allow space for curiosity about another individual's point of view, or a desire to learn and grow from interactions with others. An open mindset combined with empathy for the other provides the foundation for a constructive conversation about the issue at hand, as well as the chance to uncover other factors that may be at play in the conflict situation. Helpful questions for taking an open mindset and empathetic approach include:

- *Am I open to the possibility that I might be wrong? Am I open to the possibility that I might have to change or do something differently to resolve this conflict?*
- *Why am I feeling this way in this situation? What prior experiences do I have with feeling this way, and what caused those? Is this related or unrelated to the conflict at hand?*
- *What might be going on with [the other person] that is driving this conflict?*
- *What do I value about my relationship with [the other person] and have I shared that with them?*
- *If I was looking at this interaction for the first time, what would I see?*
- *What is my role in this conflict, and what might I need to change to resolve it?*

UNDERSTAND THE SOURCE OF THE CONFLICT

Another crucial skill in managing and resolving conflict involves assessing the actual source of the conflict itself. As Cloke and Goldsmith describe, the conflict issue may not be the true source of conflict one is experiencing.[8] Uncovering the true source of the conflict means discovering and appreciating those factors below the surface in the iceberg pictured in

Figure 13.1. Once the true source of the conflict is revealed, resolution is possible because the issue at the source of the disagreement can be addressed. Questions that might clarify the sources of conflict include:

■ *Could this conflict be about something more than the issue at hand?*

■ *What else might be driving my disagreement or dispute with [this person]?*

■ *If someone else was observing in this conflict, what would they say it is about?*

■ *Have I addressed this issue before? How was that issue resolved?*

CLEARLY DEFINE THE SHARED OR COMMON GOAL

Achieving agreement on a shared goal is important to resolving a conflict. Unclear goals and direction may be contributing to conflict because individuals involved may have different understandings of what they are trying to achieve. The leader's challenge is to clearly artic- ulate a team's or organization's purpose, help set direction toward that purpose, and mo- tivate others to achieve it. If the purpose is unclear, objectives and implementation may be similarly unclear and require further discussion to reach clarity. It is important to distinguish between conflict around the goals themselves (what we are here to do) versus the process (how we are to reach them). Questions you can ask that can help clarify goals include:

■ *I understand our goal/purpose to be [your understanding of the goal/purpose]. What do you see as our goal/purpose?*

■ *I think we are all here to accomplish [goal/purpose], but we have different understandings about that. What do you think?*

■ *I appreciate that we are both here to do [purpose/goal]. However, I think it would be important to make sure. What do you see as the [purpose/goal] of our work?*

COMMUNICATE USING "I" MESSAGES AND ACTIVE LISTENING

The previous questions about defining shared goals are all "I" statements, a style of commu- nicating that enables the clear expression of the feelings, beliefs, or experiences of an individ- ual. "I" statements allow the individual to state what they see or observe, or believe or are feeling, in a way that does not blame the other, misattribute responsibility, or accuse another person of doing something (or of not doing something). After all, one can never know what another person is thinking without them revealing it directly. Think about the difference between these two statements:

Statement #1: You really screwed up that presentation to the boss. I know I could have done better than you with those slides and I would have caught all those mistakes beforehand. Now we really have a mess on our hands.

Statement #2: I am disappointed that the presentation to Joan did not go as I thought it would because the data were presented with what I think are errors. In the future, I would like the chance to review the slides beforehand and to practice the presentation with you.

The second statement is clear, provides a rationale for how the individual might be feeling, but it does not blame. It allows space for a discussion of perspectives, and for the other person to understand where the other is coming from without necessarily feeling defensive. A constructive dialogue can follow from the second statement, but probably not the first which might shut down constructive conversation and lead to hurt feelings and potentially further conflict.

Critical to any conflict resolution is the need to actively listen to the position and perspec- tive of the other even if they are feeling upset, stressed, or disagree. Active listening is not just letting the other talk, it is actively processing what they are saying and processing what is being heard to better understand the other's position and potential way forward. Discussion prompts that can help promote active listening include:

- *What I hear you saying is [this]. Is that accurate?*
- *So, to confirm what I am hearing you say, you are thinking [this]. Is that true?*
- *When you say [that], I think you mean [this]. Is that correct?*

Active listening is more than just hearing: it is listening to understand the other with empathy and with an aim of understanding. Unfortunately, in many conflicts, individuals often talk past each other because they are not actively listening to what each other is saying. Conflict resolution requires active listening to truly understand the other and to clearly communicate interests, needs, and potential solutions. (See Chapter 1, "Dialogue: A Foundational Skill for Effective Health Leadership," for more on active listening.)

ATTEMPT TO REACH A COLLABORATIVE RESOLUTION

A win–win solution is a collaborative solution, one that takes the collaborating conflict-handling mode described in the TKI.[1] What is important about a win–win solution is that both sides are fully satisfied in the resolution. This does not always mean that both parties get exactly what they wanted when they entered into the negotiation or resolution process. Instead, it means that both parties discuss what resolution looks like and develop solutions together that allow both sides to gain. In some cases, this means creating new solutions that are the product of discussion, exploring what is important and significant, and asking questions that lead to the creation of new outcomes and positions that the parties were not aware of individually beforehand (appreciative inquiry). What is important about a win–win solution is not just that an individual may feel better through collaborative resolution, but that the solution may be optimal to the original position because it was collaboratively developed and incorporates the thinking and sincere commitment of both parties to obtaining a positive outcome.

To reach a collaborative solution, consider the following:

- Do you understand the interests of the other individual, and are you sincerely committed to resolving the conflict to your mutual satisfaction?
- Do you have adequate time to develop the win–win solution together?
- Are you in an appropriate space to facilitate reaching an agreement (i.e., free of distractions, on "neutral" ground)?
- Are you prepared to use "I" messages and actively listen to the other?
- Do you have a process to raise both your thoughts on the issue at hand, but also those things that are under the surface (e.g., the iceberg of conflict) that may be impacting how you are thinking and feeling?
- Do you have a process to brainstorm or develop new ideas, not just restate what you already believe to be the case?
- Are both parties able to commit to a resolution and to evaluate the resolution post-hoc, and make adjustments as needed together?

If the answer to these statements is yes, one may be successfully set up for a discussion to reach a win–win, collaborative resolution. However, if the answer to any of these statements is "no," one may want to set up another time that might be more conducive for discussion (ideally soon after the conflict), or to use another conflict-handling mode such as compromising or accommodating. Importantly, at the end of the discussion and when a successful resolution is reached, both individuals must agree on the solution and commit to a future evaluation of the resolution and potentially discuss what might be helpful strategies to prevent potential similar conflicts in the future.

SUMMARY

Public health and healthcare managers and leaders need to be fluent in conflict management and resolution to ensure the effective functioning of their teams. Conflicts over ideas are important to developing new and valuable programs, policies, and services for communities. However, conflict between individuals or within teams can have a negative impact on organizational performance. This chapter provides an overview of ways to address conflict at work. While most team members seek to avoid conflict, it is important to address conflict and leverage the opportunity it presents to strengthen relationships on the team and the ideas that the team is generating. When conflict is genuinely and sincerely addressed, it builds trust within a team, which contributes to accountability and improved results. The information in this chapter can help leaders and managers better understand the importance of conflict and how to constructively manage it to achieve organizational goals and strengthen team relationships.

DISCUSSION QUESTIONS

1. What are the five conflict-handling styles and how do they differ? What do you think is your dominant or most common conflict-handling style? What does this mean for how you handle conflict?
2. Explain how diversity can improve organizational performance but may also create conflict in an organization. What is your experience working in diverse organizations? How do you think you would best manage conflict over systemic or organizational issues in your organization that might be identified by groups that are marginalized at work and are seeking organizational change?
3. Describe the four domains of EI. Why is EI so important? Which domain do you think is most important in managing conflict? Why?
4. Think about a recent conflict between you and a coworker. How did you resolve it? After reading this chapter, what might you do differently? What did you do that was helpful in resolving the conflict? What material in this chapter supports your response?

CASE STUDY: COMMUNICATING PERFORMANCE FEEDBACK CONSTRUCTIVELY

It is performance review time in your agency, and you have to share some feedback with a subordinate whom you supervise. You are concerned about the poor quality of several work products they submitted to you. Over the last 2 years, this person has responded poorly to performance feedback and has become very upset when any of their work is criticized by any member of the team. This person has attributed prior negative feedback as personal attacks and ignored suggestions for improvement.

CASE STUDY QUESTIONS

1. Given this situation, what are some ways that you can plan for a constructive conversation with this individual? What do you want to make clear in the conversation?
2. If the individual gets upset, what are some ways you can help make the conversation productive?
3. What material in the chapter can you use to prepare for this interaction and plan for a useful dialogue with this person?

CASE STUDY: MANAGING DISAGREEMENT ON PUBLIC HEALTH POLICIES

You are the health officer of Smith County, a medium-sized city in Anystate, USA. Given increases in COVID-19 infections in your county and a recent Centers for Disease Control and Prevention (CDC) recommendation that all individuals wear face coverings in all indoor public spaces even if they have been fully vaccinated, you believe it is critical that your county's schools mandate the use of masks indoors for all students, staff, and visitors to prevent transmission of the virus. Several parents in the community disagree with such a mandate and have stated that they do not want a mandate in schools because it violates their civil liberties. The president of the county's board of education is taking the position of the parents and not planning on issuing a mask mandate for the school year. You have requested a meeting with the president and are preparing for a discussion about the mandate. The president said she wanted to speak with you first before making a final decision and is open to dialogue about how to best resolve this conflict.

CASE STUDY QUESTIONS

1. Apply the five conflict-handling modes described by Kilmann and Thomas[1] to this scenario. What are some of the potential outcomes of the discussion with the board president using each mode?

2. Using Figure 13.1 (the "Iceberg of Conflict"), reflect on the position of the board president. What might be some of the "below the surface" factors that are influencing her decision?

3. Using the five conflict essentials described at the end of the chapter, how might you approach this conflict? What questions will you ask? What resolution will you propose? How will you evaluate a successful resolution?

LEADERSHIP AND MEASUREMENT TOOLS

1. The TKI Instrument

   ■ The TKI is a widely used approach to measuring and describing the different ways individuals behave when experiencing interpersonal conflict and preferred conflict management styles. The TKI is based on the work of Kenneth Thomas and Ralph Kilmann, who describe two main dimensions of conflict behavior: assertiveness and cooperativeness. The TKI can be found on the Kilmann Diagnostics website: https://kilmanndiagnostics.com/overview-thomas -kilmann-conflict-mode-instrument-tki/

2. *The Five Dysfunctions of a Team* Assessment

   ■ Fear of conflict and the other four dysfunctions of a team as described by Patrick Lencioni are easily assessed using the questionnaire included in his book *The Five Dysfunctions of a Team*. The book is widely available from online booksellers.

A robust set of instructor resources designed to supplement this text is located at http://connect.springerpub.com/content/book/978-0-8261-4924-4. Qualifying instructors may request access by emailing textbook@springerpub.com.

REFERENCES

1. Thomas K. *Introduction to Conflict Management: Improving Performance Using the TKI*. The Myers-Briggs Company; 2002.
2. Ollove M. The pandemic has devastated the mental health of public health workers. *Pew Stateline*. August 5, 2021. https://www.pewtrusts.org/en/research-and-analysis/blogs/stateline/2021/08/05/the-pandemic-has-devastated-the-mental-health-of-public-health-workers
3. Halverson P, Yeager V, Menachemi N, Fraser M, Freeman L. Public health officials and COVID-19: leadership, politics, and the pandemic. *J Public Health Manag Pract*. 2021;27(suppl 1):S11–S13. doi:10.1097/PHH.0000000000001281
4. Sanders B, Mobus F. *Creative Conflict: A Practical Guide for Business Negotiators*. Harvard Business Review Press; 2021.
5. Gallo A. *Dealing With Conflict: Assess the Situation, Manage Your Emotions, Move On*. Harvard Business Review Press; 2017.
6. Goleman D. *Emotional Intelligence*. 25th Anniversary ed. Bantam Books; 2020.
7. Bradberry T, Greaves J. *Emotional Intelligence 2.0*. TalentSmart; 2009.
8. Cloke K, Goldsmith J. *Resolving Conflicts at Work*. Revised ed. Jossey-Bass; 2005.
9. Markham A. The problem-solving process that prevents groupthink. *Harvard Business Review*. November 25, 2015. https://hbr.org/2015/11/the-problem-solving-process-that-prevents-groupthink
10. Emmerling T, Rooders D. 7 strategies for better group decision-making. *Harvard Business Review*. September 22, 2020. https://hbr.org/2020/09/7-strategies-for-better-group-decision-making
11. *The Emperor's New Clothes*. SDU H.C. Andersen Centret, The Hans Christian Andersen Centre. September 19, 2019. https://andersen.sdu.dk/vaerk/hersholt/TheEmperorsNewClothes_e.html
12. Lencioni P. *The Five Dysfunctions of a Team: A Leadership Fable*. Jossey-Bass; 2002.
13. Hewlett SA, Sherbin L, Gonsalves T. Innovation, diversity, and market growth. 2013. https://coqual.org/wp-content/uploads/2020/09/31_innovationdiversityandmarketgrowth_keyfindings-1.pdf
14. W. K. Kellogg Foundation. Truth, racial healing & transformation: implementation guidebook. December 1, 2016. https://wkkf.issuelab.org/resource/truth-racial-healing-transformation-implementation-guidebook.html
15. Fick-Cooper L, Baker E. Building conflict competency. *J Public Health Manag Pract*. 2011;17(2):187–198. doi:10.1097/01.PHH.0000394666.06764.5a
16. Sebenius JK. Six habits of merely effective negotiators. *Harv Bus Rev*. 2001;79(4):87–168. https://hbr.org/2001/04/six-habits-of-merely-effective-negotiators

Chapter 14

Crisis Leadership

J. Bennet Waters and Claude A. Jacob

INTRODUCTION

Crises are a reality for 21st century organizations, and the ability to lead effectively during a crisis is a fundamental leadership skill. It is one thing to manage the consequences of a crisis or significant event; it is quite another to leverage core leadership principles to antici-pate, prepare for, mitigate against, and recover quickly from all hazards. Doing so requires effective crisis leaders to understand the role of threat, vulnerability, and consequence in the context of risk management; be able to assess and quantify each component of the risk equation to prioritize efforts, resources, and personnel in a risk-based way; and know how to build resiliency within a complex organization. It is also imperative that leaders commu-nicate frequently, clearly, and transparently with both internal and external stakeholders to ensure unity of effort during a crisis. This requires interpersonal fortitude and organizational agility to respond swiftly and effectively during times of chaos. Leaders are expected to pro-vide strategic direction while paying close attention to the operational impact and making the necessary adjustments. This also requires recognizing the parallels between events (e.g., COVID-19 vs. climate change) as well as having a perspective of the systemic challenges of acute episodes that are anchored to chronic health and social conditions (e.g., legacy of institutional racism).

This chapter explains the concepts of risk and risk management; differentiates between leadership and management of crisis situations; provides strategies for effective commu-nication during crises; and includes a case study that demonstrates the concept of meta-leadership in the context of COVID-19.

OBJECTIVES

By the end of this chapter, the reader will be able to:

- Provide an overview of core principles of risk management, the components that make up risk, and how to identify and prioritize an organization's highest risk scenarios.
- Discuss how leaders might effectively anticipate, prevent, prepare for, mitigate against, respond to, and recover from complex organizational crises.
- Explain the concept of resiliency in the context of crisis leadership.
- Describe strategies for preplanning crisis communication materials and communicating with relevant internal and external stakeholders during and after a crisis.
- Introduce the concept of "meta-leadership" and provide a case study illustrating the concept in action through a local health department's experience during the 2019 coronavirus global pandemic.

CRISIS LEADERSHIP AND RISK MANAGEMENT

Crisis leadership is a complicated combination of skills, experiences, and techniques that enables an individual to "grasp a puzzle, shape a strategy, and courageously guide others on a path barely seen"[1(p8)] during times of incredible disruption and uncertainty. At its very core, crisis leadership requires one to understand the relationships—both temporally and causally—between potential risks and those which manifest themselves as crisis. It follows, then, that understanding how to lead in times of crisis first requires a foundation in risk management.

Effective risk management begins with a common syntax, framework, and conceptual understanding of risk itself. Not only is risk the possibility of loss or harm, it is also something or someone that presents a threat of loss or harm.[2]

To some, risk is an amorphous word that generates anxiety and trepidation. As with most acquired competencies, leaders can and should prepare themselves to manage risk proactively in order to maximize the efficiency of time spent dealing with actualized risks that take the form of crises.

From a public health perspective, risk is often expressed as "absolute" or "relative," with the distinction being on factors one can reasonably control (relative) to lower overall (absolute) risk. This chapter will focus first on how to determine absolute risk; it will also discuss the importance of interventions (preparedness, mitigation) that can help reduce this risk.

In practical terms, the seemingly complicated notion of risk can be simplified into a fundamental algebraic equation defined as the product of *threat*, *vulnerability*, and *consequence*. In other words:

$$R(isk) = T(hreat) \times V(ulnerability) \times C(onsequence)$$

In the context of this equation, each element is defined as follows:

- **Threat:** Threat refers to any entity or process that poses harm to another entity.
- **Vulnerability:** Vulnerability describes the relative level of preparation for, or mitigation against, a particular threat.
- **Consequence:** Consequence reflects the impact or outcome of a threat to a vulnerable entity.

All three inputs contribute equally to the product, and both the presence and magnitude of an element dramatically affects overall risk.

As with basic math, any number multiplied by zero results in a product of zero. The same is true in evaluating risk. If there is no threat, there is no risk. If there is threat but no vulnerability, there is no risk. It follows, then, that threat and vulnerability in the absence of consequence results in no risk. The magnitude of each element also drives risk proportionally, so the higher any individual component, the larger the overall risk. The following pages contain a case study illustrating risk in the context of COVID-19, and how threat, vulnerability, and consequence manifested themselves in the real-world of modern-day public health.

Armed with a fundamental understanding of the three dimensions to risk, one can take the mathematical concept a step further. By evaluating threat and vulnerability as independent yet linked variables, it is possible to re-express the combination of threat and vulnerability as probability—that is, the likelihood of a bad thing happening.

One is left, then, with two variables: probability and consequence (or similar taxonomy such as "likelihood" and "impact"). Using ordinal numbers on a Likert-type scale to reflect the magnitude of each variable, they can be plotted on X and Y axes from low (e.g., "0") to high (e.g., "5" or "10") as in Figure 14.1.

In broad terms, the graphing exercise produces four possible scenarios:

- **Low probability, low consequence:** An event that is unlikely to happen, and to be largely devoid of significant consequences if it does happen.
- **High probability, low consequence:** An event that is more likely to happen, but still likely to result in few if any consequences.

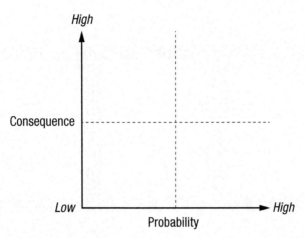

FIGURE 14.1: Probability–Consequence Graph.

- **Low probability, high consequence:** An unlikely event, but one that would have significant consequences should it occur.
- **High probability, high consequence:** Those things that are very likely to happen, and to have catastrophic consequences when they do.

Of course, both the X and Y axes require some subjective input regarding magnitude (i.e., what defines "low" versus "high" in each dimension), as well as a time reference. Pandemics, for example, are "low probability" if the time period is days, weeks, or a few years; on the other hand, they are exceptionally high probability if the time period is "centuries."

The overall concept of mapping threat, vulnerability, and consequence into mathematical equations and charts is significant because it allows the effective risk manager to prioritize time, effort, and resources accordingly, both in terms of preparation and mitigation. Low probability, low consequence risks can be largely ignored. On the other hand, high probability, high consequence risks should receive the most attention for obvious reasons: they are likely to happen, and the impact will be significant. Within this category, it is possible to assign the same framework to prioritize among the highest risk scenarios those that are most likely or most consequential.

In 2005, then-President George W. Bush issued Homeland Security Presidential Directive #10: Biodefense for the 21st Century. The directive divided biodefense activities into four pillars of activity, as shown in Figure 14.2.

In fact, and with minor modifications, the same four pillars are applicable across all categories of potential risks, not just those related to biodefense.

- **Risk awareness:** In addition to threat, and as previously discussed, the effective risk manager will also evaluate vulnerability and consequences to inform an overall picture of risk.
- **Prevention, preparation, and mitigation:** Risk managers obviously focus first on preventing crises from happening at all, but in some circumstances (e.g., hurricanes), it is not possible to prevent the crisis entirely. In those cases, the focus turns to preparing for those things that cannot be prevented, and to mitigating the consequences for those events that do occur.
- **Surveillance and detection:** Risk managers should develop, deploy, and continuously monitor any combination of people, sensors, systems, or other data collection techniques to accelerate the determination (or predictive analytics) of if and when a particular "bad thing" is likely to happen, is happening, or has just happened. Risk managers often speak of "getting left of boom," which refers to efforts to predict or anticipate events to guide their prevention, preparation, and mitigation activities.

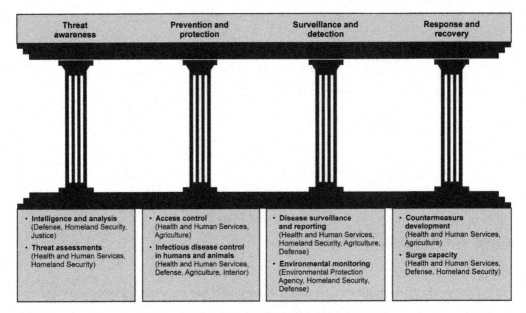

FIGURE 14.2: Homeland Security Presidential Directive #10.
Source: Currie C. The Nation Faces Multiple Challenges in Building and Maintaining Biodefense and Biosurveillance (GAO-16-547T). April 14, 2016. https://www.gao.gov/assets/680/676757.pdf

In public health parlance, this is referred to as "lead time" or the period between identifying a public health threat and having to face its consequences.

▪ **Response and recovery:** Once a crisis has occurred, risk managers shift focus to the overt steps taken during and immediately after the event begins, with the objective of recovering from and returning to normal operations as soon as possible.

Organizations that operate seamlessly across all four pillars are said to be resilient. Resiliency refers to the ability to adapt to or recover from change. Resiliency in the organizational crisis setting is chiefly about getting back to steady-state or normal operating parameters and doing so should be the ultimate objective of the effective risk manager following a crisis incident.

The final realization of the effective risk manager is an appreciation for the axiomatic nature of how success is defined. Risk management is just that: risk *management*, not risk *elimination*. The only way to eliminate risk entirely is to avoid all behaviors with potential negative consequences for an organization, which in most commercial settings is impractical. Instead, leaders should embrace the opportunity to manage risk proactively and build resiliency against all hazards. By systematically evaluating each component of the risk equation, plotting probability against consequence, leaders can prioritize resources and activities to manage crises and return to normal operations quickly, efficiently, and effectively.

LEADERSHIP VS. MANAGEMENT

Noted author and Harvard Business School professor emeritus John Kotter has written extensively about the difference between "leadership" and "management."[3] Kotter asserts that management is chiefly about systems, processes, and procedures that result in predictability. Leadership, on the other hand, is about vision that "creates organizations in the first place or adapts them to significantly changing circumstances. Leadership defines what the future should look like, aligns people with that vision, and inspires them to make it happen despite the obstacles."[3(p25)]

In *Leading Change*, Kotter summarizes the differences between leadership and management as shown in Table 14.1.

Kotter is not alone in drawing such distinctions. Nearly 45 years ago, Abraham Zaleznik published "Managers and Leaders: Are They Different?" Zaleznik's observations were later distilled into an executive summary in *Harvard Business Review on Leadership*:

> *Managers and leaders are two very different types of people. Managers' goals arise out of necessities rather than desires; they excel at diffusing conflicts between individuals or departments, placating all sides while ensuring that an organization's day to day business gets done. Leaders, on the other hand, adopt personal, active attitudes towards goals. They look for the potential opportunities and rewards that lie around the corner, inspiring subordinates and firing up the creative process with their own energy. Their relationships with employees and coworkers are intense, and their working environment is often, consequently, chaotic.[4(p61)]*

While seemingly academic, the distinctions between leadership and management are critical to any discussion about crisis leadership. This chapter is specifically *not* about crisis *management*—that is, the systems, processes, and procedures used to manage an actual crisis . . . it is about crisis *leadership* and the vision and prospective changes made to prevent, prepare for, and mitigate against the inevitable crises that cannot be avoided. It is precisely this proactivity and willingness to push organizations into an environment of continuous change that creates and enhances resiliency.

In *Crisis Leadership: Planning for the Unthinkable*, Ian Mitroff underscores this differentiation and asserts crisis leadership "attempts to identify crises and prepare an organization systematically, i.e., as a whole system, *before* a major crisis has happened."[5(p10)] Mitroff further argues that most managers employ "conventional" thinking that examines components of a system, whereas leaders become adept at "critical" thinking that appreciates the complexities and interrelationships of the whole:

> *In conventional thinking, the overall system will be taken care of if each of the parts is designed and functions well. In contrast, critical thinking insists that a system is always more than, or less than, the sum of the individual parts. The fact that each of the individual parts is designed well and performing well does not ensure that the overall system will work well.[5(p12–13)]*

Finally, the effective crisis leader must understand the potential value of experience. Mark Twain is widely credited with the notion that "good decisions come from experience, and that experience is acquired through bad decisions." Cognitive psychologist Gary Klein sought to explore this notion, and in 1985 began following first responders, emergency physicians, military aviators, and others in high pressure jobs that require split-second decisions to learn more about the role of experience in human cognition. In *Sources of Power*, Klein

TABLE 14.1: Management Versus Leadership

MANAGEMENT	LEADERSHIP
Planning and budgeting	*Establishing direction*
Organizing and staffing	*Aligning people*
Controlling and problem-solving	*Motivating and inspiring*
↓	↓
Produces a degree of predictability and order and has the potential to consistently produce the short-term results expected by various stakeholders (e.g., for customers, always being on time; for stockholders, being on budget)	Produces change, often to a dramatic degree, and has the potential to produce extremely useful change (e.g., new products that customers want, new approaches to labor relations that help make a firm more competitive)

Source: Adapted from Kotter J. *Leading Change*. Harvard Business Review Press; 2012.

describes the process by which experienced professionals call upon experience in times of crisis, and he highlighted the importance of intuition:

> *Intuition depends on the use of experience to recognize key patterns that indicate the dynamics of the situation. Because patterns can be subtle, people often cannot describe what they noticed, or how they judged a situation as typical or atypical. Therefore, intuition has a strange reputation. Skilled decision makers know that they can depend on their intuition, but at the same time they may feel uncomfortable trusting a source of power that seems so accidental.*[6(p31)]

Klein's work includes a vignette in which a fire commander orders his firefighters out of a house described as "a perfectly standard building with nothing out of the ordinary," but in which the lieutenant "starts to feel as if something is not right."[6(p32)] Though he could not pinpoint his reasoning, he later shared with Klein that several factors did not fit a pattern he would have expected in a small house fire. Moments after the firefighters exited to reassess the situation, the first floor of the house collapsed (the fire had been in the flooring system).

Klein and his team debriefed the firefighters extensively following the experience, and he summarized their findings in the context of intuition:

> *This incident helped us understand how commanders make decisions by recognizing when a typical situation is developing. In this case, the events were not typical, and his reaction was to pull back, regroup, and try to get a better sense of what was going on. By showing us what happens when the cues do not fit together, this case clarified how much firefighters rely on a recognition of familiarity and prototypicality. The commander's experience had provided him with a firm set of patterns. He was accustomed to sizing up a situation by having it match one of those patterns. This is one basis for what we call intuition: recognizing things without knowing how we do the recognizing.*[6(p32–33)]

Klein's work has significant implications for the effective crisis leader. The ability to "predict" future events is based, at least in part, on past experiences and the brain's ability to synthesize such experiences and draw upon them quickly to inform future decisions in similar—if not exact—circumstances. This promotes informed proactivity in situations calling for split-second decisions with high stakes consequences, and it is a key attribute for those building resilient organizations.

Of course, in a data-driven world, it is equally important to find quantitative information to inform decision-making. In his "Maxims on Leadership," the late Retired General Colin Powell suggested "Part I: Use the formula P=40 to 70, in which P stands for the probability of success and the numbers indicate the percentage of information acquired. Part II: Once the information is in the 40 to 70 range, go with your gut."[7(p260)] Restated, Powell points out that having less than 40% of the information is idiomatically "going off half-cocked." Conversely, waiting for more than 70% of the information creates the potential for "paralysis of analysis" in which leaders or their organizations fail to act out of fear of uncertainty.

Taken together, Powell and Klein offer powerful lessons for crisis leaders. First, it is both impractical and unwise to expect perfect information, and particularly when time is precious and circumstances call for immediate action. Second, there is a justifiable place for experience as an influential factor in one's decision-making, but not the *only* factor. The art of crisis leadership is in finding the balance between available quantitative information and the "gut instinct" of experience, which must then be coupled with a fervent attention to ongoing surveillance and additional data gathering. Having made a decision, leaders must remain open to new information and an iterative process of refining—even to the point of overturning—previous decisions as new data becomes available.

COMMUNICATING IN TIMES OF CRISIS

Communicating effectively during an incident is one of the most important responsibilities of the crisis leader. According to Coombs, "Crisis communications can be defined broadly as the collection, processing, and dissemination of information required to address a crisis situation."[8(p20)]

Different types of organizations have different measures of success for crisis communication efforts; as a result, there are numerous strategic approaches. Beginning in 1995, Coombs and colleagues pioneered what is now known as Situational Crisis Communication Theory (SCCT). "The premise was very simple: crises are negative events, stakeholders will make attributions about crisis responsibility, and those attributions will affect how stakeholders interact with the organization in crisis."[8(p38)] Whereas many crisis communication strategies are focused solely on reputation management as the critical objective, "SCCT has not limited itself just to reputation as a crisis communication outcome."[8(p40)] To be clear, protecting an organization's reputation is important during a crisis, but so is the responsibility to communicate effectively with internal stakeholders (who are typically less concerned about reputation) or those potentially in harm's way because of the crisis.

Much like the risk management approach described previously, the crisis communications continuum can be divided into three phases:

- **Phase 1: Before the crisis:** In the pre-crisis phase, communication efforts should be focused on anticipating the types of crisis communication materials that might be required for higher-probability or higher-consequence events. By preparing core messages, identifying distribution channels, and table-top exercising crisis communication strategies—just like any other preparedness activities—organizations can avoid having to "think on the fly" when time and initial information will be in short supply. In the same way sports teams practice repeatedly before games, crisis leaders should plan, test, evaluate, and iteratively improve their scenario-specific crisis communication materials before they are needed in real-world events.

- **Phase 2: In the crisis:** During the crisis, leaders should communicate early, often, and consistently with all involved stakeholders, both internally and beyond. While it will be tempting to focus first on avoiding or shifting blame (crisis communication theory lists denial, scapegoating, attacking the accuser, excuses, and justification as common approaches in this regard),[8(p36)] leaders should instead remain focused on communicating the facts of the event itself, how the organization is responding, and what stakeholders should expect to happen in the near-term.

- **Phase 3: After the crisis:** Once the crisis has resolved, future communication efforts should focus on the process by which the incident was thoroughly dissected (causes, effects, lessons observed); how observed lessons will be applied going forward; and what stakeholders can expect in terms of steps taken to avoid further instances of the same type.

In communicating effectively with stakeholders, credibility, trust, and reliability are among the crisis leader's most important intangible assets. Because they are intangible, each is a by-product of performance over some period, and they are measured subjectively from the perspective of different stakeholders. COVID-19 provided numerous examples of crisis communication and the role of intangibles like "trust" and "credibility" . . . some good, others less effective.

Without asserting fault or passing judgment on the rightness or wrongness of his actions, one can examine former New York Governor Andrew Cuomo's handling of certain aspects of COVID-19-related communications. Recent issues related to his resignation notwithstanding, Governor Cuomo's actions offer an example of the inherent complexities of both making decisions and communicating effectively once those decisions were enacted and additional information became available.

Cuomo received wide acclaim in the early days of the pandemic as he held daily press briefings and seemingly appeared to be the quintessential crisis communicator. Major television networks began carrying his news conferences and he was nationally praised for his honesty, clear message, and command of the situation in New York. In early 2021, however, reports emerged that perhaps things were not as they seemed, and in fact Cuomo may have deliberately withheld information.

On January 28, 2021, New York Attorney General Letitia James issued a report finding significant inconsistencies between what Cuomo reported to the public and what her investigation uncovered (New York Attorney General Press Room, 2021). Numerous media outlets have since chronicled the ongoing investigations, and STAT News reporter Rachel Cohrs succinctly summarized the turn of events:

> *Cuomo's fall from grace is a cautionary tale of the perils of policymaking during a public health crisis. Making the right decisions in the early days of battling a novel virus is incredibly difficult, and leaders shouldn't fear retribution for tough choices they made in good faith, five ethicists and public health experts told STAT. But that doesn't absolve leaders from taking responsibility for their missteps.*[9(para3)]

Cohrs' summary provides the basis to frame two very important points about leadership and crisis communications:

1) Leadership is an imperfect art, and while decisions will always be prone to retrospective analysis enhanced by the benefit of time and better information, leaders must be willing to act without all of the information (as Powell suggested in his "get P between 40 and 70" maxim); and

2) While it is imperative that leaders take action during times of crisis, they must also be open to new data and remain willing to amend, reverse, or otherwise reconsider prior decisions as that information comes to light.

Leaders *must* be capable of admitting when a prior decision did not work as planned and outline how they will apply lessons learned to inform future decisions. Just as it is important for leaders to display the courage required to make hard decisions with imperfect data, it is even more important that leaders recognize and embrace the fallibility of human decision-making such that they quickly and transparently acknowledge changing information, take remedial action based on that information, and communicate transparently in the process. General Powell aptly made this point, saying "Never let your ego get so close to your position that when your position goes, your ego goes with it."[7(p259)]

In sum, the effective crisis leader will develop, exercise, and continually hone communication skills to anticipate and respond to stakeholders' needs for information following a significant incident. Key areas of focus should include:

■ **Anticipation:** As with the difference between management and leadership, do not wait for a crisis to develop initial crisis communication templates. The process of executing a crisis communication plan is a management action defined by policies and procedures. Developing those policies and procedures should be the outcome of deliberate leadership efforts to prepare for potential crises. Effective crisis communications thus requires proactive thought and effort to anticipate events, and especially those determined to be higher-probability or higher-consequence scenarios.

■ **Stakeholder and perspectives identification:** It is critically important to identify and understand both internal and external stakeholders, and their unique perspectives. It is said that "perceptions become reality," and this is particularly true during times of crisis. Humans have an innate need for information, and just as nature abhors a vacuum and seeks stasis, so do people when they feel threatened or otherwise at risk. Crisis stakeholders will voraciously seek information, and it is incumbent on the leader to provide that information honestly, clearly, and frequently.

■ **Clarification:** In today's hyperconnected world, crisis leaders will often deal with information overload as opposed to information deficits; however, the *quantity* of information should never be confused with the *quality* of those data. The term "fog of war" is often used to describe the lack of clear, reliable, actionable information in the early moments of a conflict or crisis. This challenge has been magnified in a world of "fake news," deliberate disinformation, and the pervasive use of social media that results in torrents of unverified information in near-real time. Leaders must prospectively build processes and systems to help obtain, characterize, validate, synthesize, and distribute actionable information quickly and efficiently.

- **Simplification:** Effective crisis communication requires finding the right balance in simplifying without restricting information flow to stakeholders. This is a delicate balance to be sure. On one hand, leaders will always have more raw information than they can or should release to the public; on the other, there is an incumbent responsibility not to delay or withhold relevant information. Prospectively identifying stakeholders, understanding their perspectives, and developing scenario-specific crisis communication templates is key to striking this balance.

- **Repetition:** People receive and process information in myriad ways. Some stakeholders will "get" crisis-related information quickly; others will require multiple iterations to absorb the same information (and particularly if the news is not overly positive). It is thus imperative that crisis leaders communicate early, often, and via consistent methods with their stakeholders.

- **Authenticity:** Above all, effective crisis communicators must be honest and authentic. Leaders should not attempt to "shape" messages or facts, or to be interpreted as telling stakeholders what to think. Crisis communications is not crisis marketing, and part of authenticity is allowing stakeholders to form their own conclusions once provided with a set of facts about what has happened, is happening, and is anticipated to happen going forward.

While leaders face many choices during a crisis, the need to communicate is not a "choice" at all; it comes with the job. Mishandled communications will almost certainly erode stakeholder trust; create further financial, operational, or public relations issues; and result in long-term damage to the organization. On the other hand, effective communications in times of crisis offers enormous opportunities to build (or rebuild) trust with stakeholders, minimize disruption, and contribute directly to the resiliency of the organization in returning to normal operations as quickly as possible.

META-LEADERSHIP

Significant crises that extend beyond traditional organizational boundaries challenge even the most effective leaders. In their 2019 book *You're It*, Leonard Marcus et al. propose the concept of "meta-leadership," which they axiomatically describe as encouraging leaders to "learn to look at problems, opportunities, and solutions from a 'meta-' perspective," that is, in a way that incorporates the bigger picture of a crisis.[1(p3)] Marcus et al. go on to describe three critical dimensions of this holistic view of leadership: (1) the person, (2) the situation, and (3) connectivity among the stakeholders involved. With parallels to chaos theory, the authors underscore the nature of interrelatedness even in complex environments, and they assert the need for systems thinking in all aspects of one's approach to leadership in crises. They write:

> Through your meta-leadership, you are seeking a wider perception and a deeper understanding of people, their experiences, and what affects them. That understanding—through connectivity—allows you to find patterns of behavior, reaction, and response. The intersection between what occurs in your surroundings and its impact on people becomes clearer. You take and guide actions in this broad human panorama.[1(p255)]

While arguably applicable to leadership generally, the meta-leadership concept is particularly important in the context of extra-organizational crises. Just as Kotter espoused the differences in "leadership" versus "management," crises that extend beyond one's direct sphere of influence or control require additional skills and expertise that call upon the leader's abilities to look beyond the organization itself, and across the broader ecosystem in which that organization exists. By expanding one's focus to include the perspectives of both internal and external stakeholders, the specific attributes of the impending or evolving crisis, and the myriad interrelationships among those potentially responsible for, involved with, or affected by a crisis, meta-leaders can overcome complexity, align interests, and accelerate solutions at scale.

In March 2020, Claude Jacob, then health director for the City of Cambridge, Massachusetts, faced an unprecedented crisis that clearly transcended organizational, city, state, and national borders: the beginning of the COVID-19 pandemic. Without yet having the benefit of reading *You're It*, Jacob quickly realized that he and his team were, in fact, "it" when it came to managing the public health implications of the brewing crisis. The following case study describes his experience and how he called upon many of the core concepts of meta-leadership for a particular experience that occurred over the course of an 8-month period.

SUMMARY

This chapter offers a framework for crisis leadership. It summarizes core concepts of risk management; differentiates between crisis managers and crisis leaders; discusses the importance of risk communications during times of crisis; and includes a case study demonstrating the concept of meta-leadership in practice, and in the context of COVID-19.

In developing the content, examples, lessons, and additional resources, the authors present a range of tools and information for those charged with leading organizations during crisis situations. As with any new set of tools, however, it is incumbent upon the user to become facile with those tools, practice their application, and continuously refine their utilization.

Effective crisis leadership is rooted in a fundamental understanding of risk and the three component inputs (threat, vulnerability, and consequence) that determine an organization's exposure to disruptive events. By understanding the range of threats potentially facing an organization, one can develop scenarios for the most likely risks and identify the competencies, resources, and capabilities required to respond when actual events occur.

Second, and leveraging the previous understanding of risk, crisis leaders must think proactively about creating resilient organizations. Using an effects-based, capability-oriented planning system, leaders should identify potential crisis scenarios; take steps to prevent as many of those scenarios as possible; prepare for those that are not preventable; mitigate the impact of events that do occur; and have robust capabilities to respond quickly and return to steady state as soon as possible. This "cycle of preparedness" should underpin the anticipatory nature of crisis leadership.

Third, those entrusted with navigating organizations through crisis events must understand and be able to apply the different skills required to create and sustain a vision that shifts the paradigm to one of proactivity (versus managing the effects of an event). Fundamental skills in crisis management are indeed important, but they are insufficient in elevating an organization beyond simply dealing with the impact of a crisis. As previously noted, this chapter is specifically not about crisis *management*; it is about crisis *leadership* and the vision that enables an organization to leverage an environment of continuous change to build and sustain resiliency.

Fourth, the successful crisis leader must be an adept negotiator and communicator. Perhaps never before has the need for effective, bidirectional communication been so important. The lessons of COVID-19 have made clear the necessity of fidelity, transparency, and authenticity in crisis communications. Crises are not linear events: facts evolve, data improve over time, and as more information becomes available, it is imperative that crisis leaders have the trust capital of their stakeholders when communicating with them. Through understanding stakeholders' perspectives and anticipating, clarifying, and simplifying messages in a way that inspires confidence, crisis leaders can build and trade upon such trust capital.

Finally, and as Claude Jacob experienced in the example as the Cambridge, Massachusetts public health director during the beginning of COVID-19, crisis leaders must themselves be resilient. They must practice and be prepared to demonstrate the concept of "meta-leadership" and rise above the chaos, uncertainty, and fears created by organizational crises. They do so by developing and maintaining emotional intelligence, forging relationships with internal and external stakeholders, and rising above the fray to create sustainable change and a vision for the future that guides a return to steady state.

As noted at the beginning of this chapter, organizational crises are a fact of life in the 21st century. Whether or not a leader will encounter crisis is not the question; rather, the challenge—in fact, the opportunity—for such leaders is how they will respond.

DISCUSSION QUESTIONS

1. Provide an example of a tool or resource you have found to be effective in helping you respond to an organizational crisis. Why was it helpful?
2. Describe a situation where you had to apply the principles of risk management to address a delicate situation. What principles did you apply, and what did you learn from the situation? What does the concept of resiliency mean to you in the context of a global crisis? Please explain your answer.

CASE STUDY: CRISIS LEADERSHIP IN ACTION

INTRODUCTION

Imagine yourself as director of the Cambridge (Massachusetts) Public Health Department on March 19, 2020. A public health emergency has just been declared in the city of Cambridge as a result of three reported COVID-19 cases among residents and a cascade of leadership challenges present themselves. Among these challenges is providing compassionate care and protection for the city's homeless individuals. Some questions to ponder:

- *What might you imagine would be the nature of these challenges?*
- *How might you envision an approach that could protect homeless individuals from contracting COVID-19, developing severe illness, and then transmitting the disease into the broader community?*
- *What might the role of the health department leader be in addressing these challenges?*
- *How might the leader develop a shared vision among community leaders and community members to address this challenge?*
- *Once a shared vision is crafted, how might the health department move to create strategies to realize that vision and then manage a process of effective implementation?*

All of these questions presented themselves to Claude Jacob, the chief public health officer of the Cambridge Public Health Department (CPHD) at that time. To make matters even more challenging, he was faced with a need to make decisions rapidly in the face of considerable uncertainty on multiple fronts—uncertainty regarding the behavior of the virus as well as uncertainty about the behavior of the community and community leaders. During the following weeks, Mr. Jacob was guided by a deep set of values and beliefs as he provided leadership in Cambridge. As a career public health leader, he was committed to the central belief that public health is grounded in social justice and is actualized by concerted action, often in the face of uncertainty and conflicting values. Given that foundation, he led a process of creating a shared vision and strategies while managing operational realities on the ground.

SHARED VISION

In his role as "social architect," Mr. Jacob visualized a *safe facility* which could house homeless individuals with appropriate protective measures designed to reduce or eliminate COVID-19 infection. This vision was developed not just by one person but also by a series of conversations designed to create a shared vision such that "others could see it." Once this shared vision was then "socialized" in Cambridge, core strategies were developed to realize the vision with the support of key community partners and stakeholders.

ACTIONS AND RATIONALE

In March 2020, the city manager appointed an Emergency Task Force ("ETF") and charged the group with identifying a temporary location to shelter and protect homeless individuals from COVID-19. ETF members included representatives from public health, public safety, public works, public schools, human services, elected officials, marketing and communications, and the city manager's office. This allowed ETF members to "zoom in" to address the possible clinical scenarios and the environmental strategies to mitigate the spread of COVID-19. This approach also allowed the group to view different dimensions of this project and to integrate a shared knowledge in its decision-making algorithm. The ETF provided strategic oversight while deferring to designated departments to take on more managerial or logistical functions to ensure the success of this ad hoc project. Claude's role was to *map* the alignment of these systems by "connecting the dots" across different networks in the city.

Due to the intensity of the COVID experience and the seismic disruption for area residents, it became clear early on that the team needed to secure a readily available space while also factoring in the ability to return the site to normal post-use. The War Memorial Recreation Center ("War Memorial"), which is adjacent to the Cambridge Rindge and Latin School ("CRLS") campus, is a facility that serves as the designated site for emergency preparedness. The War Memorial is the only city facility that has been previously certified as an emergency shelter location by the American Red Cross and is designated by the Cambridge Health Alliance as part of its emergency preparedness plan. For these reasons, the War Memorial was selected as the ideal site to address this time-sensitive need. This site has been used on previous occasions to conduct mass flu clinics and emergency drills here in the city.

The War Memorial site required only minimal construction of temporary clinical structures in the facility's sublevel/garage area that were also easily removable. Deep cleaning of the entire facility had to be conducted quickly to comply with environmental cleaning and disinfecting standards as defined by the Centers for Disease Control and Prevention (CDC) as well as the Massachusetts Department of Public Health. These factors allowed the facility to be returned to normal operations when school and recreational programming were reinstated in October 2020.

In the end, the planning process included input from various city departments, clinicians, and area service providers to support these vulnerable residents on a temporary basis while being committed to returning the facility to its original use. As chief public health officer, Claude had the unique perspective to think through the engagement of key stakeholders and the arc of this ad hoc project. This allowed him the opportunity to demonstrate the influence that public health as a discipline may have in shaping a "system-level" intervention anchored to the city.

RESULTS

The activation of the temporary emergency homeless shelter included a "pre-screening" program to rule out COVID-19 positive individuals to have them referred to a designated isolation and recovery center prior to admission. Over 200 individuals were reached through a mobile testing and shelter-based screening program which focused on the city's areas of highest need based on the incidence and prevalence of reported cases. In the end, over 100 unique clients registered for admission to the War Memorial's field house space over the course of an 8-month period. At its peak, the field house space averaged 60 clients for overnight stays during this period. More than 40 COVID-19 positive individuals (including staff) were referred to the state's designated regional isolation hotels.

The success of this surveillance system depended on synchronizing provider networks by managing the client referrals effectively from the area homeless shelters. There were negligible levels of COVID-19 transmission within the temporary shelter site itself, which may be attributed to clinical support provided by the city's healthcare for the homeless program as well as the oversight provided by an anchor social services agency that established clear protocols and practices to monitor the health and well-being of the shelter residents.

As an agent of the health department, Claude had a unique *view from the balcony* to support the coordination of activities across different networks in the city which included ensuring the early identification of COVID-19-positive individuals within this cohort, coordinating the seamless transfer of these individuals to the state's designated isolation and recovery centers, and supporting the longer-term behavioral health needs of this clientele. A major challenge was having access to data in *real-time* to make critical decisions. The ETF relied heavily on the health department's nimble nursing staff and epidemiologists to access and analyze the data in a timely fashion by coordinating with area service providers, public safety partners, and state agencies.

LESSONS LEARNED

Key leadership lessons included:

1. *Prompt action* in the face of uncertainty was essential.
2. *Situational awareness* included not only case surveillance but also maintaining an awareness of the public's understanding and concerns over time by CPHD's leadership.
3. Amplified and *consistent communication* with elected officials and community members was invaluable.
4. *Adaption. Alignment. Affirmation.* Recognizing the challenges while remaining steadfast in adherence to effective procedures needed to protect all homeless individuals and the staff serving them was critical.

PERSONAL REFLECTIONS

Claude Jacob

This case study provided a framework and vocabulary for describing what occurred over the course of 400+ days as illustrated within the three dimensions of meta-leadership; it also served as a powerful exercise for reflecting on my experiences from February 2020 to June 2021. I took advantage of an opportunity to act promptly in the face of uncertainty during the Spring of 2020. I gained even more insight about the data that helped inform the situational awareness needed for surveillance. I also maintained an awareness of the public's understanding and concerns over time made by key decision-makers. I feel that my personal, academic, and professional experiences helped me to become a more adaptive leader by ensuring the alignment of existing systems both municipally and regionally.

In addition, this experience has affirmed my role as a "public health architect" through the application of the broader tenets of adaptive and situational leadership. This allowed me to take a step back to determine the best approach while zeroing in on the day-to-day adjustments to ensure the successful implementation of this ad hoc project. This entailed time to adjust personally and professionally to the demands of this exercise *(Becoming the Person of the Meta-Leader)*, the design of a time-sensitive intervention to address the immediate needs of homeless individuals within the community *(Grasping the Situation)*, as well as leveraging networks across the city to address its municipal and regional needs and logistical pressures *(Building Connectivity)*.

Finally, this experience helped me to be more cognizant of the inherent challenges that impact the quality of life of one our most vulnerable populations when calamity strikes. It was also one of the most acute and demanding experiences, which involved managing the expectations of superiors, colleagues, and stakeholders. The end result is a case study that illustrates the importance of having a systematic way of assessing risk, of applying the tenets of evidence-based leadership frameworks, and the perspective of a practitioner in the field.

CASE STUDY QUESTIONS

1. What did Mr. Jacob do well in this situation? Please use examples from the case study and tie them to material in the chapter.

2. Is there an aspect of the case study where you would have taken a different approach? What would you have done differently, and why?

ADDITIONAL RESOURCES

- Crisis Leadership Podcasts by FOCUS Training: https://podcasts.apple.com/us/podcast/the-crisis-leadership-podcast/id1505796670
- What Leaders Need to Know to Lead Through a Crisis: https://www8.gsb.columbia.edu/video/videos/what-leaders-need-know-lead-through-crisis
- Q&A: Jeff Katz on Leading and Managing Through a Crisis. https://www.phocuswire.com/Travel-leadership-coronavirus-crisis
- Prioritize People in Times of Crisis: An Interview With the CEO of BHP: https://www.mckinsey.com/featured-insights/asia-pacific/prioritize-people-in-times-of-crisis-an-interview-with-the-ceo-of-bhp

SUPPLEMENTAL CONTENT

Impact as a Leader (The Cambridge Story)

The following highlights reflect the acknowledgements from a national foundation as well as affirmations by the leadership and key stakeholders in the City of Cambridge, Massachusetts, which were in large part attributed to the lessons learned and the execution of this ad hoc project. This experience was made possible because of the vision and support of the Cambridge city manager and commissioner of public health, the unconditional commitment by colleagues and area service providers, and the tireless dedication of the fantastic staff at the CPHD.

- CDC Foundation Story—*A Bed for the Night: Helping the Most Vulnerable During a Pandemic*

  https://www.cdcfoundation.org/stories/bed-night-helping-most-vulnerable-during-pandemic

- 2020 Mitch Snyder Award

  https://cambridgema.iqm2.com/Citizens/Detail_LegiFile.aspx?Frame=&MeetingID=2689&MediaPosition=&ID=12757&CssClass=

- City of Cambridge City Manager / City Council Recognition

  https://www.wickedlocal.com/story/cambridge-chronicle-tab/2021/06/22/cambridge-honors-outgoing-public-health-officer-claude-jacob/5303151001

- State Association Spotlight. New Chapter Begins.

  https://mhoa.com/mhoa-spotlight-claude-jacob

 A robust set of instructor resources designed to supplement this text is located at http://connect.springerpub.com/content/book/978-0-8261-4924-4. Qualifying instructors may request access by emailing **textbook@springerpub.com.**

REFERENCES

1. Marcus LJ, McNulty EJ, Henderson JM, Dorn BC. *You're It: Crisis, Change, and How to Lead When It Matters Most.* Public Affairs; 2019.
2. Merriam-Webster. Risk. In: Merriam-Webster, ed. *Merriam-Webstercom Dictionary*; 2021.
3. Kotter J. *Leading Change.* Harvard Business Review Press; 2012.
4. Zaleznik A, ed. *Managers and Leaders: Are They Different.* Harvard Business Review; 1998. Review HB, ed. *HBR on Leadership.*
5. Mitroff I. *Crisis Leadership: Planning for the Unthinkable.* John Wiley & Sons; 2004.
6. Klein G. *Sources of Power: How People Make Decisions.* MIT Press; 1999.
7. Harari O. *The Leadership Secrets of Colin Powell.* McGraw-Hill Publishing; 2003.
8. Coombs, WT. Parameters for Crisis Communication. In SJ Holladay, & WT Coombs, editors, *The Handbook of Crisis Communications.* London: Blackwell Publishing Ltd.; 2010: pp17–53.
9. Cohrs R. Andrew Cuomo's COVID-19 nursing home fiasco shows the ethical perils of pandemic policymaking. STAT; 2021. https://www.statnews.com/2021/02/26/cuomos-nursing-home-fiasco-ethical-perils-pandemic-policymaking

Building and Leading Teams: Essential Approaches and Practical Tools for Improving the Health of Populations

Kathleen Colville and Trissa Torres

INTRODUCTION

Developing teams is a lifelong journey that draws on leaders' intellectual and interpersonal skills to accomplish two fundamental goals: get the work done well and take good care of the people doing it. Distilled from organizational and developmental literature, the authors describe five behaviors that cultivate cohesion: using a "person-in-environment perspective" to understand individuals in context and to take action to modify environments; an "asset-based approach" to ground organizational processes in respect for people and their range of strengths; the principle of "investment in relationships" to cultivate psychological safety to drive innovation and quality; "cultivating a shared vision and purpose" to provide guidance to everyday tasks and at times of crisis; and "pursuing equity and sharing power" to acknowledge and disrupt bias and structural oppression. The authors offer practical descriptions of tools useful for managing task performance, such as intentional meeting design, the project management approach, and systematic problem identification.

OBJECTIVES

By the end of this chapter, the reader should be able to:

- Promote reflective practices among team members and leaders.
- Identify the impact of environmental and structural issues on individual and team performance.
- Analyze tools used by leaders to foster team psychological safety.
- Present techniques and tools used to facilitate the foundational dimension of team effectiveness.
- Present techniques and tools useful in coordinating the everyday needs for effective communication, distribution of tasks, and shared decision-making.

TEAM LEADERSHIP IN PUBLIC HEALTH AND HEALTHCARE

People who work in public health and healthcare do not shy away from the toughest societal challenges but instead run headlong toward them. They lead the fights against global pandemics, tirelessly work to unlock interventions that improve well-being and increase life expectancy, eradicate disease through brilliant science and creative fieldwork, and compassionately heal the sick and the injured. These are not solitary pursuits. In addition to leveraging extensive subject-matter expertise, health leaders must also be effective members and leaders of strong, capable teams that coordinate their talents and tasks to accomplish ambitious goals with precision, courage, and care. Team leadership is a craft that is burnished and honed over the long arc of a career. Teams and their leaders struggle, shine, stumble, learn, and shine some more.

This discussion of building and developing effective teams is grounded in five cross-cutting concepts that represent mindsets, principles, and intentions that are useful in a wide variety of organizational settings—large and small teams, whether focused on policy or practice, or oriented toward clinical care or public health interventions (and on beyond these dichotomies!). The person-in-environment perspective and asset-based approach represent mindsets that shape a team leader's assessment of individual and team dynamics, and which lend themselves to a multitude of constructive avenues for change and improvement, rooted in respect for people. Two grounding principles—investment in relationships and cultivating a shared vision and purpose—focus on the interpersonal aspects of team success, and the investment of time and resources necessary to cultivate connections between team members and the team's goals. The fifth cross-cutting concept, pursuing equity and sharing power, regards the interpersonal, environmental, and material aspects of diversity, equity, and inclusion, with a call for leaders to pay attention to both inclusive team processes *and* equitable outcomes.

In designing this chapter, the authors thought deeply about their own development as team leaders and how they have improved their skills over decades of engaged practice. They agree with the claim by leadership scholars Jackson and Parry[1] that "the point has been well and truly established that the most effective leaders will achieve a balance between the twin challenges of getting the job done and looking after the welfare of the workers."[1(p27)] This chapter seeks to offer guidance on both aspects. Building effective teams is not a competency to be mastered, checked off, and considered "complete"; leading people is a life-long journey of learning and continuous improvement. Key ingredients and commitments include (a) learning about theoretical frameworks and research on team effectiveness, often by reading books and articles from a wide variety of disciplines; (b) investing significant time in reflection on team dynamics and the roots of team problems; (c) talking with peers and mentors about how they approach team leadership, and peppering the leaders with questions to tap their expertise through stories of their experiences; and (d) developing the ability to identify and use practical tools to improve self-awareness, interpersonal understanding, equitable practices, group facilitation, and task organization. These ingredients are included in this chapter.

Specifically for this book chapter, the authors interviewed 10 people and culled memories and stories from dozens more to distill the wisdom of practitioners whose work and approaches they viewed worth emulating. For the interviews, people were selected who represent a balance of early, mid, and late career experience. They are now or have previously served in local, state, and federal governmental health agencies, community and academic medical centers, public health training programs, nonprofit population health agencies, and health policy and advocacy organizations. In this process, the authors were conscious of race, ethnicity, and gender, and intentionally sought to oversample the perspectives of women and people of color. It is important to note that both authors identify as mid-career White women. They acknowledge that these aspects of their identities shape their views of what is important in team leadership and invite readers to interpret their offerings with that in mind. Interviewees were promised anonymity to allow them to speak openly about their experiences. Several composite stories were created with details modified to both maintain the integrity of their accounts and to respect their privacy. All names used in stories, vignettes, and examples are fictitious.

This chapter foregrounds the stories of health practitioners because stories are one of the most accessible and enduring ways that humans assimilate new information and use it to accomplish complex tasks. The *homo narrans* model of the human asserts that we think in stories, with characters, plots, morals, and settings forming the structure of our cognitive on-ramps.[2] In addition to being an effective pedagogic tool, stories are fun, interesting, memorable, and, importantly, they underscore the core belief that team leadership is a skill that ripens and deepens while facing new challenges over a lifetime.

FIVE CROSS-CUTTING CONCEPTS FOR EFFECTIVE TEAMS: MINDSETS, PRINCIPLES, AND INTENTIONS

PERSON-IN-ENVIRONMENT PERSPECTIVE

The visible and invisible values, rules, and norms of the environments in which people work (whether the office, the larger organization, or whole societies) both enable and constrain choices and opportunities. Drawn from professional social work practice, the person-in-environment perspective holds that a person's behavior is best understood—and influenced—by assessing an individual's strengths and challenges in light of how the particularities of any given environment shape those factors.[3] This perspective also appreciates the influence that individuals can have in shaping and changing their environments. When teams or individuals struggle, sometimes there are key improvements that individuals can make to their skill base, such as improving time management or public speaking. Sometimes, those skills already exist but a current practice, structure, or system is blocking their progress. The person-in-environment perspective helps us avoid a reflexive tendency to blame individual deficits for group problems and focus instead on systemic changes to increase success for all.

An extensive internal study of teamwork at Google debunked the idea that effective teams are achieved by assembling a group of hyper-talented individuals. Their research found that team effectiveness is shaped by how members interact and structure their work, and that the most successful teams share five key traits: psychological safety, dependability, structure and clarity, their belief in the meaning of their work, and their perception of the impact of their work.[4] Adopting the person-in-environment perspective can be instrumental in building these traits, especially in developing team psychological safety, the trait that Google researchers identified as most critical for team success. Team psychological safety is understood as the ability of team members to trust that their intelligence, skills, and perspectives are respected, and to use that base of trust to take interpersonal risks, such as admitting mistakes, asking for help, offering a different perspective, or trying out a new idea.[5] These behaviors are important to team success because they help to drive change, improvement, and innovation.

One community health leader whose work involved collaborating with stakeholders in a variety of settings reported feeling valued and respected in racially inclusive community-based organizations that tended to have diverse representation and respect for professionals who were able to build trust with community leaders. The same leader felt less esteemed in clinical settings within traditionally White institutions where medical degrees and educational attainment were highly prized. She interacted very differently with her peers in these two settings. She was seen as a "rock star" among her community health colleagues, known for her innovative insights, work ethic, and creativity, but was often observed as "very quiet" by clinical colleagues, who remained unaware of her ideas and leadership potential.

Leaders who adopt a person-in-environment perspective avoid the tendency to diagnose problems as attributable to individual behavior and place blame on one person. They also recognize that many organizations continue to propagate legacies of structural exclusion, but that those mechanisms of exclusion may be invisible, especially to those who belong to dominant groups. These leaders look for ways to intervene in the operating environment to promote team psychological safety, such as fostering appreciation for diverse skills sets and implementing meeting formats that provide more inclusive opportunities for participation. This is important and difficult work, and a section of this chapter is devoted to a more detailed description of structural bias and team effectiveness. Leaders seeking to disrupt and dismantle exclusionary structures will find additional tools in this chapter's section on pursuing equity and sharing power.

Reshaping the environment can also involve changes to the actual physical space in which a team works. Office design can reflect organizational values, such as assigning better and bigger offices to certain team members, intentionally creating inviting collaborative spaces, or providing work-from-home flexibility. The shift to work-from-home that began in early spring of 2020, an acute response to the global pandemic, required rapid adaptation, and demonstrated that people could find ways to move forward even in very different circumstances. Though many decried the shift to work-from-home necessitated by the pandemic as a threat to working relationships and cohesiveness, others experienced significant benefits, such as time saved commuting, closeness with family, and ability to practice self-care.

FA, a nonprofit community health practitioner, confided in her leader that she feels at her best working from home. Throughout her life, FA has experienced social anxiety and being physically present in the office required significant energy to be constantly "on." Working from the comfort of her own home allowed her more control over the timing and duration of her interpersonal interactions, increased her comfort level, and had a positive effect on her engagement, creativity, and productivity. This change was noticed and appreciated by her colleagues. FA's experience illustrates a long-standing tenet within public health practice: environments shape behaviors. While we may often work on environmental change in communities to promote physical activity or access to healthy foods, environmental changes for our work teams can also produce meaningful change.

Leaders may also reshape the operating environment by questioning assumptions and modifying the dominant narratives that prevail within a team's ethos. The swirl of values, biases, myths, and stories in which we operate constitutes an environment of sorts, as these narratives form powerful foundational belief systems. TF, a nonprofit leader, noted that the office assistant was undervalued in his role and was the object of negative office talk. Because he was physically separated from the rest of the employees and did not really "belong" to any one functional team, few people had taken time to understand his job or his capabilities, or to observe him in action. TF saw deeper potential in him and decided to intervene in the prevailing narrative that the assistant was inadequate and expendable. She began talking up the assistant's skills and intelligence to the rest of the office and suggesting that they engage him in some of their projects: "I flipped the script. I was sowing seeds of positive narrative because that's what I believe. He needed development, but he is quick-minded, and I knew he would take the initiative to learn." The assistant rose to the opportunities created for him when the organization's leader modeled respect for his skills and encouraged others to examine their assumptions about him. Understanding that our biases, gossip, and dominant narratives can themselves become an obstructive aspect of our organizational environments, the leader chose to make a change in how the group thought about this individual, and, as a result, improved behaviors and interactions followed that mindset shift.

Evaluating and modifying the environments, systems, and structures in which a team operates is an important responsibility for a team leader. Often a team will develop a process early on and continue to proceed in that way for no better reason than "because we've always done it this way." Sometimes we unquestioningly, begrudgingly, or despairingly accept things—such as our current office space design or our existing organizational hierarchies—that can appear to be set in stone but are in truth modifiable to produce a different or better outcome. Asking "Why do we do it this way?" and "Is there a better way to do this?" will often evoke important structural changes. In some cases, those same questions will also help clarify the advantages of existing processes. The person-in-environment perspective reminds us to explore changes in larger structures to drive team success.

ASSET-BASED APPROACH

Like the person-in-environment perspective, the asset-based approach spends little time blaming individuals for team problems. The asset-based approach is not about staying relentlessly (or nonsensically) positive or ignoring difficult issues; rather, leaders with this approach are focused on unearthing and developing the latent capabilities of team members and organizing them for group success. PM joined an existing team as a leader where the prior leader was beloved and revered. She had many ideas about changes and improvements that she wanted to make; however, if she focused solely on those, she risked alienating her team, ignoring the perspectives that they could bring, and ultimately impairing the ability to advance their goals together. PM was operating within a deficit-based mindset. She could see—vividly—all the problems that needed to be fixed, and these issues crowded out everything else. There was no room on her radar screen for her team's skills, characteristics, and positive values, despite the fact that these existed in abundance and would be the raw materials for creating change.

An asset-based approach focuses on strengths rather than needs, and systematically catalogues and connects those strengths to create positive change. John McKnight and John Kretzmann championed asset-based community development (ABCD), a population-level methodology that focuses on leveraging the strengths in a community, based on the premise that all communities have resources that can be identified, developed, and elevated to achieve sustainable outcomes.[6] They pointed out that practitioners who approached communities—often low-income communities of color—with a deficit mindset tended to bring a savior mentality, ignored or minimized the positive attributes in a community, and could do harm to and in those communities through short-term, externally driven fixes. The same can be true in teams. Leaders can do harm by ignoring the current skills and future potential of their existing team members, always wishing for "better people" and lacking capacity to effectively develop the skills of their current employees. In his 1989 classic *The 7 Habits of Highly Effective People*, Stephen Covey coined the term "abundance mentality" or "abundance mindset" which he defines as "a concept in which a person believes there are enough resources and successes to share with others."[7(p220)] This is in contrast to a scarcity mindset which tends to foster a win–lose and either-or approach. On the other hand, leaders can cultivate an asset-based approach by intentionally adopting mindsets and attitudes that shift their focus toward building on team strengths.

JJ had a similar experience to PM as a new leader but was able to shift to an asset-based approach. She recommends that leaders new to a team start from a position of curiosity, asking "What have you done before? What worked well? What didn't work? What improvement opportunities do you see?" JJ suggests that leaders listen thoughtfully to these answers, validate the experiences shared, adopt the language and phrases that team members use, and cultivate dialogue with team members rather than lecture to them. The goal, according to JJ, is for colleagues to experience new ideas as aligned to their own interests and goals, rather than as a critique of their past performance. In this way, leaders walk the delicate line between honoring the past and making needed improvements.

Many of the leaders whom we spoke to in the field emphasized the importance of leveraging all assets. KT described one of the successes that she celebrated in using an asset-based approach to help a team innovate. This team was delivering a community diabetes education program, and had reached a plateau in participation and engagement, with many participants dropping off before completion. In the past, one person was responsible for program evaluation, but KT took a different approach to better leverage the assets of the team. In order to drive improvement, she first started by approaching those closest to the problem, asking for ideas from the staff who delivered the program. They, in turn, listened to and engaged the voices of program participants to better understand the challenges and envision solutions. KT encouraged the program staff to take risks and try out their new ideas; these improvements ultimately led them to serve more people, become more sustainable, and be recognized as a national model of community diabetes programming. KT felt a key part of that success was that she had assured the team that failure was an acceptable outcome. She created a learning environment that did not allow itself to fixate solely on identifying and fixing problems, but rather saw abundance and opportunity. The asset-based approach cultivated team psychological safety and allowed employees to freely share their ideas and assets.

An asset-based approach can be helpful even when everything appears to be falling apart. EM and her small team were responsible for designing, hosting, and facilitating a meeting of high-level health leaders from across the country. From a logistics perspective, all that could go wrong did: in the cold of winter, the venue's heat was not functioning; the room was not set up; the supplies that were sent ahead never arrived; and the coffee urn caught on fire, triggering a fire alarm and evacuation. As the senior leader on the team, EM felt responsible for the success of the meeting, and for the problems and experiences of the event participants. It would have been easy for her to fall into the trap of trying to solve all the problems herself and get caught in a cycle of self-blame. Instead, she realized that the people around her could help, wanted to help, and would do a good job. She turned to her team and the meeting participants and asked for their support to resolve the many issues facing the group. One team member went in search of supplies. Another found blankets. Another helped shift the agenda to account for time lost. Participants joined in to help and even continued leading their discussion groups while standing outside waiting for the "all-clear" from the fire alarm. EM attributes the success of the day (and upon reflection she calls it a success) both to the collaboration of her team and participants and to her own willingness as a leader to share responsibility for the solutions and leverage all assets.

In another example, YL was coaching a community coalition striving to improve health outcomes by addressing food security. The plan was to establish a "food as medicine" program to increase Medicaid consumers' access to healthy food. The coalition had been together for several months but had experienced several starts and stops and frequently experienced tension among the members. YL recognized that the assets of the target population of this work were not being recognized, as no one from the Medicaid consumer group was included in the intervention design. YL started by asking, "Who is not at the table?" The coalition was made up of representatives of various organizations including healthcare providers, food service agencies, and social service agencies, none of whom had ever experienced food insecurity.

YL asked the members to identify potential candidates for the coalition that would be able to use their past or current experiences of food insecurity as an asset and a source of insights into how to create an effective program. It is important not to paint a rosy picture of the lived experience of food insecurity, but rather to assert that people who are directly impacted by a social or health challenge bring a unique skill set to intervention design and this expertise is an important asset. Once the food security coalition membership was more inclusive, YL realized that they needed to adopt practices that would cultivate team psychological safety and avoid privileging socially legitimized expertise such as medical degrees over the insights of lived experience. YL invited folks to adopt a mindset that starts from the belief that people are "naturally resourceful, creative, and whole from the start."[8(para2)] The richness of ideas and assets brought by those community members initially excluded became invaluable to the progress of the work.

INVESTMENT IN RELATIONSHIPS

In order for a team to move beyond the status of "work unit" and into higher levels of collaboration and performance, members of a team must get to know each other and get familiar with each other's habits, skills, frailties, and foibles. Knowing others and being known, warts and all, is a key to the development of "psychological safety," a state which opens up team members to take the interpersonal risks necessary for learning, innovation, and improvement.[9] This starts with investment of time and attention to relationships.

AB was an experienced leader who was appointed to direct a federal health agency. Upon arrival, he quickly observed that many employees had low morale and there was little synergy between the efforts of various departments and initiatives. AB realized that he would be able to accomplish very little unless he developed a personal connection that gave him information about how to help people re-gain their passion for the agency's important work. AB implemented daily rounds; each morning he would visit a different department and meet the employees, listen to them, learn what mattered to them, and get to know them by asking about their interests, or pointing out a photo on a desk and asking about it.

These are simple concepts, but AB found that they meant a lot, primarily because when he asked employees about their lives, he was genuinely interested in the answer. If he had been doing this to "check the box," his disingenuous motivations would have been quickly suspected and he would have lost trust. AB was and is tremendously curious, and employees experienced his attention as warmth and esteem. The impact was significant, and morale quickly improved. Work became more focused, intentional, and synergistic. Ultimately the team, which had previously struggled to collaborate effectively, worked together to create landmark legislation expanding healthcare coverage and new payment and delivery models across the country.

This team's shift from low-morale-to-landmark-legislation did not happen overnight, but it was the result of intentional cultivation of the types of relationships that create trust between team members. Team members who have attained psychological safety are willing to ask questions, admit mistakes, ask for help, take risks that may result in failure, and use these opportunities to grow. Some scholars differentiate the concept of psychological safety from trust, which is the willingness to be vulnerable to others' behaviors.[10] In feeling psychologically safe, one assumes that team members will give the benefit of the doubt, even when mistakes are made. When one extends trust, one offers fellow team members the benefit of the doubt, effectively investing in one another.

Scholars point to the concept of the "vulnerability loop" as a key component of trust-building.[11] One person might start this loop by providing a "cue," or statement of vulnerability, such as, "Gosh, I just can't figure out how to solve this. I keep messing up." If the response is supportive, trust grows—and it grows even more if the responder offers a vulnerability statement of their own, such as, "I find this project really tough, too." The confidence that nurtures this reciprocal vulnerability is the result of intentional team activities to cultivate self-awareness, interpersonal understanding, and caring for each other. Leaders who invest in relationships prioritize time for one-on-one meetings (that foster connection, not just provide task performance guidance), group learning activities, and celebrations, and pay attention to the details of team dynamics, such as how well the team is fostering inclusion, cultivating healthy debate, and demonstrating appreciation of each other's unique qualities.

Working practitioners who were interviewed repeatedly emphasized how critical it is, as a leader on a team, to attend to the human side of change, sharing touchstone phrases such as "We are people first" and "Relationship before task." JF's team took this advice to heart from the start of an ambitious multi-year project to improve 100 million lives (Box 15.1). Multiple teams needed to build trust and working relationships across differences, so from the onset project leaders established a set of principles around how they wanted to work together successfully. They referred to these principles as "touchstones" for their work.

The teams were able to use these touchstones in a variety of ways to strengthen their relationships and commitments to one another. They would often refer to them at the beginning of each meeting and reflect on which one was particularly resonant or challenging. When conflict arose, they would return to these touchstones to help them navigate to resolution. JF found the creation and use of touchstones was a very powerful way to hold a complex team together and advance their goals.

In another example, AP described a technique to strengthen authentic relationships that they had seen used successfully. It was having each person share the story of their name.[13] AP, too, had worked with community coalitions across the country. A few months in, after some struggles, they did this exercise. AP observed that this "softened our hearts, broke down title and power, and allowed us not to objectify one another." With those barriers out of the way, their work both accelerated and became more joyful.

Box 15.1: 100 Million Healthier Lives Touchstones for Collaboration[12]

- Be present as fully as possible. Speak your truth from your heart and mind.
- Listen generously to each other's truths. Trust that we all hold a piece of the puzzle, and we need each other's pieces to understand the whole picture.
- Embrace differences and be open to learning from each other.
- When the going gets rough, suspend judgment, and get curious. Be quick to forgive and ask open questions to understand.
- Honor each other's learning and resourcefulness. Trust we each will learn and contribute in our own way, that there is no need to "fix" each other.
- Make space to pause and reflect to deepen our thinking.
- Be willing to have meaningful conflict to create unprecedented goals and solutions. When needed, seek council for help with conflicts.
- Allow your ideas to be developed further by others.
- Seek common ground. When we can't fully agree, commit to a unified decision, and see what happens with a humble posture of learning. If we have made the wrong turn, we will discover it together and turn the right way together.
- Accept that we will sometimes fail, but we will learn together and move forward.
- Help each other to have the confidence to spread our wings, be creative, and take on new roles.
- Balance our yearning for change with patience for the process of change and growth.
- Make the way we work together an example of what is possible.

Source: Institute for Healthcare Improvement. 100 million healthier lives touchstones for collaboration. http://www.ihi.org/resources/Pages/Tools/100-Million-Healthier-Lives-Advancing-Equity-Tools.aspx

Subsequently, AP was serving on a new leadership team in the organization where they had worked for more than a decade. The majority of leaders on the team along with AP had also been at the organization for a similar period of time. Because these leaders had worked in the same organization for so long, they skipped the early phases of team formation. It wasn't long before the team was floundering, falling back to their comfort zones, and primarily working in silos. AP recognized that having known each other for so long, it was too easy to make assumptions about one another. AP invited their peers to go back to re-learn about one another as people. They used the "story of your name" exercise as a starting point to re-build authentic relationships. It is important to note that these techniques seek to build connection on a personal level as unique people, shifting the emphasis from professional contribution and skills to each person's intrinsic value and specific perspective. GH describes a practical approach that she uses with nearly all her teams, which she calls "a regular check-in as humans," such as starting a meeting with a question like "What is one thing that brought you joy in the past week?" She frequently reminds herself and her teams that they can be "serious about their work, and not take themselves too seriously." She finds that the leaders that she admires most and chooses to emulate are those who "inspire, not from a place of fear, but from a place of authentic relationship."

CULTIVATING A SHARED VISION AND PURPOSE

NW, who is a deeply talented collaborator, is asked to serve on many different multi-sector coalitions working to improve health in her local community. The contrast between two of the coalitions on which she currently serves is startling. Compare her descriptions of these groups:

People come back week after week after week. The commitment level is just amazing, honestly. Some of the success that we've seen in that group stems from that commitment. People know our purpose, they understand it, they are very clear about it and they are clear about why they

are at the table. They know why they are there, they know the work that we're doing and how they contribute to that. Since they have that sense of clarity, it's easy to know why we're coming back together week after week after week.

and

The statistical data on this health problem is very, very small and the numbers are going to remain small. So I always kept wondering, 'Why do we even need this group?' It just made it seem like one of those 'Let's check the box' kind of things; I think this group was put into one of those 10-year or 5-year plans for the city a long time ago. Now it's like 'We are going to make recommendations' but City Council has no obligation to accept these; there is no funding moving forward for this statistically small issue. There are a lot of folks who just don't understand why they are at the meeting, where this group is going. I think what makes it hard is the uncertainty. No one in the leadership of the team is making the connection of saying 'This is why this is important and this is the work that we have done in the community to know that it's important to the community.' That's why it feels to a lot of people in the community like, 'Hmm, what are we really doing at this table?'

NW uses the terms "clear" and "clarity" multiple times to describe the first group, which is aligned on a shared sense of purpose and a focused vision of its collective goals and how their own contributions are instrumental to achieving them. NW struggles to understand the purpose of the second group, which seems to have little legitimate justification for its existence—no funding, no special status with elected officials, no deep ties to community grassroots, and unconvincing data. It appears at this point to be meeting just to meet, while flailing and failing to articulate a meaningful purpose. This sounds like a familiar story—a group that struggles to explain its reason for being, but can't seem to let go, either.

Hopefully many practitioners are also familiar with and have experienced the satisfaction of serving on a clearly defined and focused team like the first group. NW reports that this group is so tightly attuned to their purpose (promoting health equity in access to medical care during the COVID-19 pandemic) that they don't even use an agenda or send out minutes; up to this point, they just haven't needed those tools to stay on track. CD, a health system leader, details another attribute of a strong focus on shared vision and purpose—the belief that when this is solid, many other things seem to fall into place:

When you constantly keep it at the forefront, people don't forget what your 'Why' is. What are we doing? Why are we doing it? Why is it important to be doing it? When we do have those rough patches, we can always recall and say, 'This is why we're doing what we're doing.' And that takes the emotions out of it.

In CD's experience, a clearly articulated sense of "the Why" behind the work serves the team in its everyday tasks and in the "rough patches." While the Tylenol-tampering deaths of 1982 were much more than a "rough patch," the lessons that CD shares about how her team leans on their shared sense of purpose during the tough times is highly relevant to that tragedy. Seven people in Chicago died after taking Tylenol that had been laced with cyanide; this was prior to the development of tamper-proof pill bottles, and the poison was introduced after the product was on shelves, making people across the country feel vulnerable. Johnson & Johnson, the manufacturer of Tylenol, called for an immediate nationwide recall of all products still on the shelves (at a cost of $100 million) and developed safer packaging within 6 weeks. Johnson & Johnson's response is considered among the most effective examples of crisis management and is recognized by Coyle in *The Culture Code: Secrets of Highly Successful Groups* as an exemplar of the value of attention to shared purpose.[14]

Johnson & Johnson's founder wrote a statement called "The Credo" in 1943 in which he stated, in four paragraphs, the company's purpose, values, and commitments; it begins with "We believe our first responsibility is to doctors, nurses and patients; to mothers and fathers and all others who use our products and services."[15] The Credo was displayed on company walls and subjected to regular "Credo challenges" at all levels of the company, where employees would be invited to challenge the document, and either change it or commit to its principles. Then-Johnson & Johnson President James Burke credits those discussions with creating clarity and steadiness in the midst of the tampering crisis:

> *"We had to make hundreds of decisions on the fly; hundreds of people made thousands of decisions," Burke said afterward. "If you look back, we didn't make any bad decisions. We really didn't. Those thousands of decisions all had a splendid consistency about them, and that was that the public was going to be served first, because that's who was at stake. So the reason people talk about Tylenol when the Credo discussions come up is the Credo ran that. Because the hearts and minds of the people who were J&J and who were making the decisions in a whole series of disparate companies . . . they all knew what to do."[14(p177)]*

CD stated that a clear sense of purpose reduced the emotional stress of the "rough patches" for her team. James Burke describes how the Credo guided the J&J team's complex decision-making during a charged and uncertain period. NW describes how her coalition's shared vision of health equity drives its members' high level of commitment. This is clearly a critical element of team success. So how does a team leader go about assuring that team members are aligned, focused, and in agreement on their purpose and vision?

There are multiple websites, consulting groups, and articles readily available to help guide leaders seeking to cultivate this common agenda within their teams. Many will suggest that teams invest time in developing statements related to the team's charter, mission, vision, values, or possibilities. These statements often have a future-focused orientation and typically include the population involved, the principal values under which the team will operate, and the desired results and aspirations. This is valuable work that reflects the aspirations and motivations of the individuals crafting these statements. Mark Friedman, in his book *Trying Hard Is Not Good Enough* lauds the passions of the many people who work on the most wicked problems; nevertheless, he contends that discipline must accompany passion in order to make progress on these tough issues.[16] The tenets of Friedman's results-based accountability (RBA) provide an organizing structure to help people working for population-level change within multi-sector coalitions develop a clear set of shared goals and complementary actions.

The RBA process begins with detailed group exploration and articulation of the conditions that communities want to experience. Rather than "We need a new medical clinic" (which is a possible strategy, not a result, in RBA-parlance), RBA-trained practitioners will gather to identify the population and the results (defined as "conditions of well-being stated in plain language"[16(p39)]) that the coalition wants for this population. Results are simple: jargon-free statements express conditions of populations, not programs or data, such as "Children in St. Louis are born healthy" or "The West End Neighborhood is safe and nurturing." RBA lays out a systematic process for community partners to develop a shared agenda, beginning with the Seven Population Accountability Questions (Box 15.2).

Box 15.2: Results-Based Accountability's (RBA) Seven Population Accountability Conditions

1. What are the quality-of-life conditions we want for the children, adults, and families who live in our communities?
2. What would these conditions look like if we could see them?
3. How can we measure these conditions?
4. How are we doing on the most important of these measures?
5. Who are the partners that have a role to play in doing better?
6. What works to do better, including no-cost and low-cost ideas?
7. What do we propose to do?

These questions typically take multiple sessions to answer fully, a process that builds consensus among coalition members about critical decisions in problem-solving, such as what needs to change, what can be done about it, and who is responsible. RBA teams continue to use clear, simple tracking systems like posters and score cards to monitor progress.

As these examples attest, from local public health practice to national manufacturing, teams thrive when they have thoughtfully considered their purpose. They will return to their shared core vision for guidance during everyday tasks and during stress and crises. These guiding principles provide steadiness and the basis for enduring commitment.

PURSUING EQUITY AND SHARING POWER

DD, a graduate student of color, was a student in a master of public health program at a predominantly White university when the coronavirus pandemic emerged and quickly shut down his campus for in-person learning. DD and his fellow students immediately became very isolated, attending class virtually, studying from their rooms, often far from their families and friends. When George Floyd was murdered and racial tensions across the nation magnified, student stress heightened, particularly for students of color. DD expected faculty and leadership in his MPH program to acknowledge these events and create space for students to process the impact. To his shock, disappointment, and anger, this did not happen. DD recognized the need for people to support one another, so along with a couple of classmates he convened a group of students virtually to share their experiences. Their goal was to create a space where everyone felt a sense of belonging, particularly students of marginalized identities, and to counteract the isolation and alienation of being one of the few people of color in the department.

This lack of response from the school's top leadership can be contrasted with the way that RG, a new nonprofit leader and the first Black woman to serve in her position, communicated with her team after she realized how much the murder of George Floyd was affecting her and her team. "It was a weight. I'm feeling emotionally heavy, obviously the team was, and I sent something to the staff that acknowledged my pain and gave everybody the okay to take a day. If my whole staff had said they needed a day, I would have closed down that day. I didn't do that to get brownie points; I did that because that's how I am as a person. They saw me as a person of character and integrity and that alone helped me to start crafting the team that I need to bring our agency to its success." RG made a breakthrough with her team not by buttoning up, silencing her emotions, and soldiering through the trauma of this event, but rather by disclosing her vulnerability and inviting her team to share their needs openly.

There is significant literature and thought leadership that address diversity, equity, inclusion, intersectionality, systems of oppression, power, and related topics. This chapter focuses on how those issues play out in the experiences of teams. Camara Jones, scholar, activist, and past president of the American Public Health Association, published a theoretical framework in 2000 on the levels of racism that she framed in the allegory of "A Gardener's Tale."[17] She describes three levels of racism: institutionalized, personally mediated, and internalized. The three levels reinforce one another, resulting in a system of advantage and disadvantage based on race. Whether attending to racism or other forms of oppression, understanding them as multilayered systems can help us think about levels of action necessary to dislodge the underlying attitudes, behaviors, and structures that perpetuate them. Teams are often thought of as made up exclusively of interpersonal interactions. These are indeed important aspects of teams. In addition, team members bring their own internal beliefs, values, and attitudes that shape interactions. Teams function in environments steeped in cultural norms and practices built on inequities. In this way, all three levels of racism play out in teams. To improve equitable experiences in teams and begin to dismantle these structures, it is critical to attend to all levels—the individual journey, how things play out interpersonally, and the policies and practices in place that perpetuate the status quo. There are many techniques and practices that leaders can use to address these many layers.

Make the Implicit Explicit

DD helped create a sense of belonging among his MPH classmates by speaking honestly about his own perspective and the dynamics at play in his environment. He started by acknowledging his own privilege as a male from middle class financial means. He went on to acknowledge who was in the room—welcoming colleagues of color, White colleagues, students of all genders, and so on. He acknowledged people who were missing or underrepresented. He acknowledged the diversity, lack of diversity, systems of oppression, and power in the room, what he refers to as "recognizing the room." As DD states, "There is always an elephant in the room. If we start by naming it, at least we can begin from seeing the same reality." Through this approach, the students were invited into the space, began to experience a shared sense of power and purpose, and leaned in to support one another. Unfortunately, they continued to experience a disconnect with formal institutional leadership.

In another example, MG, a mid-career White woman, was serving on an executive leadership team. She was experiencing déjà vu. How many times had she experienced this before? She would offer an idea and be dismissed. A few minutes later, a male colleague would offer the same idea, and both he and "his" idea were celebrated. While some would dismiss these as unimportant slights ("Who cares who gets the credit as long as the ideas get out there?"), this is a very concrete example of the layers of oppression that Jones explained. This is an example of an underlying system of oppression (in this case gender-based) influencing the interpersonal level of interaction; people of color, particularly women of color, frequently report similar experiences.

In order to change this pattern, MG knew she needed to make the implicit explicit. Her underlying assumption was that this was not intentional, but that it was important. Her colleagues generally respected her and acknowledged her value to the team. Even though they had similar positional power as peers, there was varying power in their various identities. They needed dialogue about it. But how MG brought this into the open mattered. If she challenged individuals, particularly in front of the group, they would most likely get defensive and either lash out or shut down. MG asked for a pause. MG shared that she was experiencing a negative interaction and wanted to discuss it as a team. The initial (predictable) response was denial. But they had established some ground rules for interaction, which helped them to acknowledge the pattern and commit to change.

Taking it one step further, the team came up with behaviors to support that change. One example was using a structured approach to brainstorming. Everyone takes 1 minute to think quietly, 1 minute to write down all their ideas, and then all share the ideas simultaneously via the chat function when connected online (whether in the room together or working remotely). This simple approach eliminates the problem of who talks most, loudest, first, or last, and assures people's names are connected with their ideas. By drawing their awareness to the challenge and creating structures around it, it helped set the team up for success in the future. In addition, they had shared ownership for solving the problem.

LP's experience illustrates the layers in Jones's model of racism: institutionalized, personally mediated, and internalized. When LP was hired as a manager at a local health department, she was the only person of color on the team. At first her colleagues and her supervisor seemed to welcome her, though always keeping a distance. The supervisor, who was White, began to praise LP's work in front of the team; while presumably well-intentioned, the supervisor did not acknowledge that, over time, this created resentment among LP's colleagues. She recalls a time when her supervisor made a decision that was unpopular with the team. As the team began to push back, LP was quiet. The supervisor pointed out that LP was the only one who was not complaining and causing problems, which further alienated LP from her colleagues. Later, as the team functioning deteriorated even more, the supervisor blamed LP for the underlying discord. Senior leaders in the organization who were aware of the problem did nothing to intervene.

Unfortunately, this is not an uncommon occurrence for women of color. The pattern is so prevalent that the Centre for Community Organizations (COCo) published an infographic on this phenomenon within nonprofit organizations that went viral.[18] In doing so, COCo chose to make the implicit explicit in hopes of helping others to recognize this pattern and break the cycle. COCo's diagram, entitled "The 'Problem' Woman of Colour in the Workplace," identifies a honeymoon period followed by the reality period (a time when the organization is experiencing challenges and the woman of color is experiencing microaggressions), followed by a response to challenges that blames the woman of color, and questions her qualifications, communication, and ultimately her "fit" at the organization. To promote learning, COCo advises that organizations ask themselves three questions: *What is the impact of this dynamic on the woman of color in the organization? What is the impact of this dynamic on the organization? What is the impact of this dynamic on the community sector at large?* Thoughtful leaders use questions like these to deepen their awareness of these patterns, heighten their awareness of these traps, and break these harmful cycles.

Take an Equity Pause

MG took a risk in asking the team to pause to attend to her experience. NT, a mid-career woman of color, describes a situation where, in a team she was leading, they institutionalized the expectation for an "equity pause." In each weekly meeting as a standing agenda item, a rotating member of the team came with a reflection question for all to examine and discuss. Some examples included:

■ In your personal equity journey, what is one thing that you have had to unlearn?

■ Reflect on a work situation in the past week that made you uncomfortable. What was the source of your discomfort? How did you address it?

■ When do you experience feeling most powerful? least powerful?

■ How are we doing on each of our touchstones/equity agreements? What can we do better?

Regularly inviting dialogue regarding issues of equity and power also helps to make the implicit explicit. Taking an equity pause addresses several challenges simultaneously. It encourages and normalizes dialogue on these critical issues, and it slows us down, an important counterbalance to the ever-present sense of urgency embedded in dominant culture.

That sense of urgency is magnified during crisis/critical situations when attending to equity and sharing power gets even more difficult, and likely more important. In the initial weeks of the COVID-19 pandemic, NZ was working on a project team. It became urgent to get services to partners and complete tasks on an accelerated timeline and under new and stressful conditions (e.g., people working remotely, stressful background situations, fear for the health of themselves and their families, unreliable technology). Recognizing that these conditions increased the pressure for speed and productivity on all team members, NZ chose specific behaviors to counter that.

They started by pausing to ask themselves, "What other things can I feel, instead of urgency, to get the work done?" They chose to link back to their shared sense of purpose; serving others during these challenging times became the motivator, rather than urgency, anxiety, fear, and obligation. In addition, NZ took the opportunity to make the implicit explicit; for example, naming "This is really hard" and explaining change honestly: "Though our norm is to make decisions in a collaborative manner, during this time there may be several decisions that I will make unilaterally. I will tell you when that is going to happen and why." This also serves as an example of acknowledging power as an impactful leadership behavior.

Do the Internal Work

RM, a mid-career White woman, believes that leaders must commit to their own internal equity journey. This is a critical part of the work, regardless of the stated purpose of the team. Addressing bias, power, and privilege are critical and ongoing leadership practices, whether the work is to run an organization, create a new program, solve a problem, improve a service, generate revenue, or advocate for policy change. This can be done authentically by reflecting on the sources of internal biases and assumptions that drive behaviors on a very personal level. Ruth states that "These are *not* the 'soft skills.' These are the hardest skills." She has found that during her most challenging times she often has to "let go of her own negative self-talk." She described a reel in her brain that was telling her all the ways she was failing. If she had listened, her own needs to have her ego soothed would likely have gotten in the way. Instead, she invested in critical internal work to quell that negative voice so she could bring her best self in support of her team.

Leaders can start by examining their own identities, how these influence their behaviors and choices, and the impact of these on the people around them. To prioritize this internal work by all team members, leaders create the time and spaces for all team members to think, talk, read, and explore issues of identity, power, and privilege, and *not* after hours. Failing to do so results in damaged relationships, impeded work, and the risk of causing more harm. These foundational opportunities for individual and group reflection are not "one-and-done" tasks; rather, an ongoing commitment to regular reflection will deepen interpersonal understanding, structural analysis, and capacity for effective change. Leaders and teams need resilience and humility for the long haul.

Nobody Does Not Count

KR, a late-career White male, was a leader in the field who joined an existing team as a consultant. The team leader demonstrated behaviors that excluded some of the voices in the room—primarily women, people of color, and people serving in roles deemed insignificant. KR decided to take a different tack. He intentionally asked the opinion of those who had not spoken, including the notetaker and the audiovisual technician (people who many others in the meeting had not considered to have relevant opinions). He would invite them to contribute by stating, "I'm interested in hearing what your experience is like" and then listening intently and affirming their comments. By validating their contributions, he effectively lent some of his power as a "subject matter expert," assuring that their comments were taken seriously and not dismissed.

The hospital safety movement has taught the importance of creating a "culture of safety" that encourages anyone on the team to alert others to a potential safety issue. For example, on a well-functioning surgical team, the scrub nurse or anesthesia tech needs to feel safe enough to point out the errors of more senior and powerful team members. The senior members, such as the surgeons, need to feel safe enough to admit their errors and thank the team member for the alert. This is implemented through a structured approach where each team member is authorized to call for a pause if they see a potential issue to be reviewed.

Both KR's impromptu intervention and the intentional cultivation of a safety culture are examples of strategies of inclusion and valuing all perspectives. Organizational policies and practices such as pay equity, promotions, assignments, and access to mentorship and growth are all critical elements that can either contribute to or detract from team members' experience of inclusion and value. If leaders do not have the power to change these directly, naming and acknowledging the inequities can be an important step toward a shared understanding of the problem and shared commitment to change. While many people work in hierarchical settings with levels of responsibility and power, it is important to recognize the challenges of these structures and intervene when they become oppressive and harmful. Within these structures, some have little power and others are expected to be all powerful; both are dehumanizing. Understanding that "nobody does not count" and committing to practices that share power are beneficial to all.

Move the Table

Efforts to work together to tackle health inequities often involve inviting a representative from an historically excluded group to serve on a team. Though well intended, this is most often insufficient and can be harmful. BT, a mid-career White woman, offers guidance that

"People with lived experience of inequity must be centered and leading this work—not tokenized (just one or two invited to the table). Instead, we need to move the table." BT describes her experience in serving on two teams, both with an aim to improve Black maternal outcomes. The first was a group of mostly White clinicians at a hospital, who initially were focused on very technical solutions, such as blood pressure screening. The second was a community-based organization founded and run by women of color. The latter focused on creating communities of support to better understand and meet the needs of those around them. Though the technical solutions proposed by the first team should not be dismissed, BT's experience (as a White woman) was that the second group championed by those experiencing the inequities had much more potential to leverage their power to drive meaningful, sustainable system change. As leaders of teams, it is critical to move toward a shared commitment to change based on an understanding that equitable process and outcomes benefit us all. In the words of Lilla Watson, an Aboriginal leader, "If you have come here to help me, you are wasting your time. If you have come because your liberation is bound up with mine, then let us work together."[19(para1)]

These five mindsets, principles, and intentions (the person-in-environment perspective, asset-based approach, investment in relationships, cultivating a shared vision and purpose, and pursuing equity and sharing power) are foundational practices that foster teams that can identify and resolve conflict, connect authentically, share power, and commit to a shared sense of purpose. These practices are also critical to accomplishing concrete tasks. While many teams are evaluated on their sense of cohesion, engagement, and morale, they are more frequently judged on whether they are getting the work done well. The previously described concepts could be understood as commitments that teams make to foster a healthy culture that leads to success. To accomplish their goals, these teams must also work with a well-stocked toolkit of skills and practical abilities. The remainder of this chapter focuses on specific tools for effective teamwork, techniques that enhance a team's ability to manage the organization and completion of tasks to fulfill its mission.

TOOLS FOR EFFECTIVE TEAMWORK

SYSTEMATIC PROBLEM DEFINITION AND PROBLEM-SOLVING PROCESS

All teams, whether they know it or not, have methods for defining problems and solving them. Conflict arises when each member does this differently, as very soon it feels like everyone is going off in different directions, often working toward different outcomes. To prevent this, teams invest time up front to develop consensus on the answer to the very-basic-yet-very-complex question of "What is the problem we are trying to solve?" This is a critical step in the process phase of "understanding the problem," which may also use techniques of root cause analysis such as the "Five Why's" and fishbone diagram to identify multiple contributing factors. After defining the problem, teams follow a methodical process of implementing countermeasures, such as Lean's A3 process or the Plan-Do-Check-Act cycle. Intentional processes keep all team members aligned on the sequencing, goals, strategies, and resources involved in working together successfully.

> **For Further Learning**
>
> ▪ The Institute for Healthcare Improvement's (IHI) take on how to implement the Five Why's and the Plan-Do-Study-Act cycle
> ▪ Colorado Department of Healthcare Financing and Policy's collection of resources for Lean management
> ▪ Wisconsin Division of Public Health's Overview of A3 Thinking

PROJECT MANAGEMENT APPROACH

There are many wonderful metaphors to describe one of the key aims of the project management approach: making sure we're all on the same page, singing off the same sheet of music, and getting on the same wavelength. Project management is a complex field with numerous tools dedicated to the technical aspects of organizing the tasks, timelines, and communication surrounding a set of work. It is less important which tools you choose and more important that the team identifies consistent ways to engage with one another relative to managing the phases of complex work. The project management approach helps with several key aspects of teamwork. Project management can reduce team conflict by clarifying steps and responsibilities, and it can help promote on-time task completion (and open discussion of barriers and delays) when team members can understand how their responsibilities are connected to other team members' tasks and needs. It also helps people see the "big picture" of how the parts come together (and why) and understand the importance of their own contributions. Practical and effective project management is particularly important in a virtual space where asynchronous contributions are expected. Creating shared timelines and work plans helps assure transparency, shared expectations, distribution of workload, leveraging all assets, and ultimately contributes to the success of a project team.

PERSONALITY, STRENGTHS, AND LEADERSHIP ASSESSMENTS

Assessments of individual strengths and tendencies can serve as a tool for self-awareness and growth, as well as illuminating possible sources of differences that drive both team strengths and conflicts. There are a multitude of assessments available, and they tend to focus on traits, leadership behaviors, or situational challenges (such as managing conflict); a few of the more well-known assessments are listed in the text that follows. Ideally, leaders will use assessments to assure that a diversity of strengths are represented on the team and that all members are respected. Each assessment tool varies in emphasis and is based on different theories of personality, but the process feels similar: participants respond to a series of statements or questions; responses are analyzed to identify an individual's best-fit personality typology or traits; and discussion illuminates the strengths of those tendencies and how they can come into conflict at times. These assessments can help engage a team's empathic understanding. For example, a team member might be initially frustrated by what is perceived as another team member's rigidity, but also draw on their understanding of these assessments to remember that the same person's conscientiousness and organization are valuable assets that make a meaningful contribution to the team's success. Teams can also use these tools to assemble strong project teams and to assign responsibilities to the members best suited to the tasks.

For Further Learning

- The DiSC Profile analyzes alignment with the four domains of dominance, influence, steadiness, and conscientiousness.
- The Big Five Personality Test scores people along a spectrum based on their propensity toward the traits of extraversion, agreeableness, conscientiousness, negative emotionality, and openness to experience.
- CliftonStrengths identifies an individual's strengths among 34 themes (such as connectedness, focus, ideation) that converge in four leadership domains of strategic thinking, relationship building, influencing, and executing.
- The Thomas-Kilmann Instrument (TKI) assesses leaders' use of five conflict-handling modes: collaborating, competing, compromising, accommodating, and avoiding).

MEASURING REAL-TIME EFFECTIVENESS

From a leader's perspective, it is important to understand the progress a team is making. This provides the opportunity to make real-time adjustments to increase the likelihood of success.

In healthcare, joy in work has been tied to patient satisfaction and safety, thus underscoring how critical it is to understand and improve the experiences of team members. Something as simple as using weekly huddles to invite team members to share a "feeling word" (or "How are you feeling about your work this week?") can provide actionable information to focus support where needed. This type of real-time feedback can be particularly critical in a predominantly virtual environment as was experienced during the global pandemic. Teams may choose to track metrics over time that relate both to progress toward their goals and also the strength of relationships on their team. For example, a team that is tasked to recruit participants for a new program may choose to create a dashboard of metrics that includes outreaches made (process metric), participants recruited (outcome metric), and team members' sense of connection to one another and to the work.

For Further Learning

- The success of a team might be measured on all three aspects of the results, process, and relationships triangle as described by the Interaction Institute for Social Change—results, process, relationships triangle.

- IHI describes three approaches to local level measures of Joy in Work: Daily Visual Measure, Three Daily Questions, and the Pulse Survey. Joy in Work Measures

INTENTIONAL MEETING DESIGN

Thoughtful attention to the purpose and design of meetings helps teams to use time effectively, builds connection and trust, and allows for dynamic sharing of ideas and feedback to improve quality. While many meetings may take place just because they are already on the calendar and use an agenda slapped together minutes beforehand, a well-planned meeting stands out when its convener has clearly put thought into assuring that the right participants have been invited, the purpose of the meeting is clear, and all aspects of the meeting serve that purpose. The activities on the agenda will accomplish the purpose when the facilitators lead participants through activities (such as reflection, brainstorm, timeline development, process mapping) that elicit deep engagement. Well-designed meetings also include a thoughtful process for following up on the commitments made at the meeting, documenting highlights of group discussion, and sharing key information and insights. Though people often think of meetings as in-person interactions, all these principles apply equally, if not more so, to virtual meetings.

For Further Learning

- Harvard Business Review provides tried-and-true basic tips for the components of an effective agenda.

- Liberating Structures offers a menu of activities designed for inclusive dialogue and reflection.

- Find tools for developing captivating questions for group discussion in the classic article "The Art of Powerful Questions."

LEADING VIRTUAL TEAMS

During the COVID-19 global pandemic, many organizations and teams made a very rapid shift from in-person work environments to working virtually, often from home. Some teams have worked completely virtually for many years; sometimes these are referred to as "distributed" teams or organizations. There are pros and cons to working virtually. Many describe drawbacks such as difficulties picking up on body language, fewer informal spontaneous interactions, challenges engaging emotionally, "screen fatigue," and disrupted work–life balance. Others extol the virtues of virtual work including lower travel costs and time commitments, improved work–life balance, overcoming geographic barriers, leveraging synchronous and asynchronous participation, and employee retention.

Leading a virtual or hybrid team creates a different context, yet the five cross-cutting concepts described in this chapter still apply, although they may require intentionality in their application. For example, it may be important to flexibly accommodate variables in the personal work environment of team members (e.g., parenting responsibilities, connectivity issues, shared workspaces) in order to help optimize their function and contributions. Being virtual may present an opportunity to engage new team members where travel would have been a barrier to participation, thus leveraging previously untapped assets. Investing in relationships remains critical and often can be accomplished with similar approaches to the in-person environment: hearing all voices, listening, engaging the head and the heart, making space for emotions. Helping all team members connect to purpose may become even more important, particularly if some feel their connection to people has loosened. Opportunities to address equity and share power abound in both in-person and virtual contexts and there may be some opportunities created by the virtual environment that invite us to make even bigger strides in creating safe and equitable spaces for our teams and team members to thrive.

While the performance of distributed teams is a growing area of investigation, consensus is emerging that there are several areas of attention important for consideration by leaders of hybrid and virtual teams; three are highlighted here: cultivating internal team culture, making the most of meetings (and using them sparingly when other methods of information sharing would suffice), and task transparency. Some hybrid or distributed teams may set aside specific time for virtual "coffee breaks" to promote team connection, or develop a Slack channel for social messaging, chat, and urgent messaging. Others schedule in-person days, whether weekly, monthly, quarterly, or annually, to attend to tasks that just work better when people are together. One fully distributed company, Automattic, with employees in 65 countries, commits to a full week of in-person meetings annually, known as the Grand Meetup. The words of their CEO, Matt Mullenweg, speak to the principle of investment in relationships:

> Despite being a fully distributed company, I believe it's still important to meet face-to-face— just not every day, in the same office. The Grand Meetup is our chance to get to know the people behind the Slack avatars and build relationships that can carry us through the other 51 weeks of the year. . . . It's so much easier to hear the nuance in someone's chat message or p2 posts if you've hung out with them at Harry Potter World, or learned about their family, pets, and hobbies during a flash talk.[20(para2)]

As Mullenweg's comments illustrate, appropriately combining in-person and remote work environments can maximize the benefits of both. Business scholars advise against categorical demands for or against a specific type of environment and suggest thoughtful analysis of a project or task's goals and the type of work environment that best achieves them. Ringel cautions against scheduling every interaction, and asking yourself, "Should this be a meeting? Are my meeting goals relationship-based or task-based? How complex are my objectives?" among other criteria to determine whether a meeting should take place in-person, virtually, or at all.[21]

Lastly, technology tools abound, and though not solutions in themselves, when leveraged appropriately, they can help leaders and their teams manage the challenges of working virtual environments. These tools can be especially helpful in managing a critical challenge of virtual environments: task transparency. This refers to the concept that team members who are not able to pop their heads into each other's offices for a quick check-in need other ways to understand what tasks are in progress, stuck, or moving full speed ahead. Not everyone needs to be an expert at all the tech tools, but leaders can invite those experts on their teams to contribute their assets to help all learn and grow.

For Further Learning

- An article in *Psychology Today* offers 17 tips for leading virtual teams derived from leadership research (https://www.psychologytoday.com/us/blog/cutting-edge -leadership/202107/17-tips-leading-virtual-teams).

- This article in *Forbes* discusses five key leadership characteristics necessary for leading virtual teams (https://www.forbes.com/sites/forbescoachescouncil/2021/ 02/22/top-five-leadership-40-skills-for-managing-virtual-teams/?sh= 3066c85b8502).

- Ideas for improving the joy and satisfaction of hybrid and remote teams can be found in this article (https://www.gartner.com/smarterwithgartner/making-hybrid-work -more-permanent-set-some-ground-rules).

- This blog discusses ways to build culture in a remote team (https://inside.6q.io/ building-culture-in-a-remote-team).

SUMMARY

Investing in teams can bring leaders joy, purpose, and success. Many find meaning in shared impact, shared purpose, shared commitment, and shared experiences, even when these occur under conditions of extreme stress. During the COVID-19 global pandemic, public health and healthcare teams have solved challenges previously unknown, dedicated long hours, risked exposure, witnessed significant losses, and endured numerous stressors. Though exhausted, many describe a source of energy generating from the sense that "We are all in this together."

Achieving that level of synergy and cooperation is a complex endeavor that demands creativity, patience, persistence, and flexibility from team leaders. Drawing from the rich experience of practitioners in the field, this chapter has shared tools, techniques, frameworks, and approaches for leaders to use in building and strengthening their teams. Leadership is a longitudinal learning journey. The authors, believing it is critical to model what they promote, chose to use the opportunity of drafting this manuscript to reflect on where their current practice as team leaders could be improved, and are using some of their own ideas to help their teams better understand each other, organize their work, and move forward. Team leadership is truly a lifelong process of reflection, experimentation, and learning. If the purpose of this chapter is realized, your practice, too, will benefit from the wisdom of practitioners and researchers that has been gathered here.

Leadership of teams is not a passive pursuit. It requires intention, passion, and discipline. Adept leaders use these traits to foster an environment of shared vulnerability, trust, and psychological safety. They lead meaningful reflection and change systems in order to dismantle historic systems of oppression that impair the function of teams. They seek to understand the environmental influences that facilitate or hinder, to harness the assets of all team members, to learn what matters most to one's colleagues, and to align that with shared purpose. And through these efforts, leaders can build strong successful teams that support one another and together move mountains.

DISCUSSION QUESTIONS

PERSON-IN-ENVIRONMENT

1. What are the structures, processes, and systems that appear unchanging and unchangeable in your work environment? Why do you do things that way? Can and should they be changed?
2. What aspects of your work encourage your own psychological safety and willingness to take risks? On the other hand, what have you seen leaders and other team members do that shut down the free and comfortable exchange of ideas?
3. What existing mindsets or narratives enable or inhibit the success of our team? How might we amplify or modify those mindsets for improved impact?

ASSET-BASED APPROACH

1. How are you engaging those closest to the work? Who is not at the table?
2. How are you uncovering hidden assets? How are you creating a safe learning environment for folks to share their assets and ideas?
3. What mindsets might you need to shift to better leverage the assets of others on the team?

INVESTMENT IN RELATIONSHIPS

1. How can you and your team members better learn about each other as people? How can you better understand what matters most to each and what brings them to this work?
2. What techniques can you use to demonstrate vulnerability and invite vulnerability in return?
3. Can you collaboratively create with your team touchstones for your work that will guide and ground you in authentic relationships over time?

CULTIVATING SHARED PURPOSE

1. What techniques have you used, as either a team member or leader, to help teams clarify their purpose and answer the question, "Why do we even need this group?"
2. Think of a time that you have been on a team that was rudderless, continuing to meet but lacking direction. Why do you think the team continued to meet? Looking back, what might you do with the team or ask of the team in order to either help it end or move forward productively?

PURSUING EQUITY AND SHARING POWER

1. What techniques can you use to help create a sense of belonging for all? To assure all voices are valued?
2. What opportunities can you identify to slow down, uncover broken systems, and begin to shift norms and practices?
3. Where might it be helpful for you to examine your own assumptions and beliefs and advance your own learning?

CASE STUDY: BUILDING THE FOUNDATION FOR A SUCCESSFUL TEAM

JK is a leader at an organization that works to support community-based public health projects. She is tasked with pulling together a team from individuals across the organization to serve on a new project. The team will support a newly formed local community-health system partnership in their community health improvement efforts. Historically, to form her team, she might have sought applicants for a project manager, a data manager, and a clinician leader role and received the following interested candidates:

ROLE	POSSIBLE CANDIDATES
Project Manager	AM DF
Clinician Leader	SZ JM
Data Manager	JF JC

JK was concerned that this approach, which prioritizes titles and positions, tends to elevate the same folks again and again and may not get her the best team for this work. Instead, she wanted to take a more asset-based approach. JK started by creating a matrix of skills and attributes that she felt were needed to support this project. She expected the new partnership between community and health system would require a fair amount of team building and she wanted to prioritize these skills. After interviewing each candidate, she mapped their talents like this:

CANDIDATES	FACILITATION SKILLS	BUILD TIMELINES AND WORK PLANS	CLINICAL INSIGHT	ANALYZE AND INTERPRET DATA	PRESENTATION SKILLS	STRENGTHEN CROSS CULTURAL RELATIONSHIPS
AM	x	x			x	
DF		x		X		x
SZ	x		X		x	x
JM			X	X		
JC				X		x
JF		x		X		

Using this approach helped her select SZ over JM, because though both brought clinical insight, SZ brought several assets beyond the technical. Because JK felt strengthening relationships was a high priority, she selected JC over JF to specifically augment this strength. Originally, she thought she just needed one person in a project manager role, but she discovered that DF's and AM's assets were quite complementary. She rethought the approach and was able to bring them both onto the team. Her focus on assets and strengths allowed her to build a stronger team.

During early team formation, JK invited them all to share with her and one another, "What brings you to this work? What do you want to learn? How do you want to grow?" This both served to uncover hidden assets and to strengthen commitment to one another and the work. In this process, JK discovered that JC wanted to build her facilitation skills, so she created opportunities for JC to partner with AM and SZ to practice these techniques. JK observed that commitment grew when she started to intentionally align each team member's contributions with their professional development goals and passions. JK still had much work to do to build and align her team, but she knew they had the foundation for success.

CASE STUDY QUESTIONS

1. How might the asset-based approach that JK uses in her team selection potentially help counter historical structural inequities?

2. What pushback might JK receive in her organization for using this different approach to team selection? How might she respond?

3. What approaches might JK use to help her newly formed team build their relationships and align to purpose? How might those same approaches be used with the community and health system partners?

ACKNOWLEDGMENTS

Inspiring leaders from a variety of backgrounds helped shape the content of this chapter. They have decades of experience in local, state, and federal health leadership, nonprofits, government, and philanthropy. Each generously shared their successes, missteps, and insights honestly and openly. Thank you to Christina Gunther Murphy, Yazmin Garcia Rico, Ninon Lewis, Jamilla Pinder, Mathew Pavlovic, Josie Williams, Don Berwick, Beverly Scurry, Shannon Welch, and Marianne McPherson. The authors are also grateful to Emily Hooks for her insights and research into leading virtual and hybrid teams.

 SPRINGER PUBLISHING CONNECT™ | A robust set of instructor resources designed to supplement this text is located at http://connect.springerpub.com/content/book/978-0-8261-4924-4. Qualifying instructors may request access by emailing textbook@springerpub.com.

REFERENCES

1. Jackson B, Parry K. *A Very Short Fairly Interesting and Reasonably Cheap Book About Studying Leadership*. 2nd ed. Sage; 2011.

2. Jones M, McBeth M, Shanahan, E. Introducing the narrative policy framework. In: Jones M, Shanahan E, McBeth M, eds. *The Science of Stories: Applications of the Narrative Policy Framework in Public Policy Analysis*. Palgrave Macmillan; 2014:1–25.

3. Kondrat M. Actor-centered social work: re-visioning "person-in-environment" through a critical theory lens. *Soc Work*. 2002;47:435–448. doi:10.1093/sw/47.4.435

4. Rozovsky J. The five keys to a successful Google team. [Google website]. November 17, 2015. https://rework.withgoogle.com/blog/five-keys-to-a-successful-google-team

5. Edmondson A. Psychological safety and learning behavior in work teams. *Adm Sci Q*. 1999;44:350–383. doi:10.2307/2666999

6. Kretzman J, McKnight J. *Building Communities From the Inside Out: A Path Toward Finding and Mobilizing a Community's Assets*. ACTA Publications; 1993.

7. Covey S. *The 7 Habits of Highly Effective People*. Simon & Schuster; 1989.

8. It's time for a new language of leadership. [Co-active Training Institute Website]. https://coactive.com/about/new-language-of-leadership

9. Frazier M, Fainshmidt S, Klinger R, Pezeshkan A, Vracheva V. Psychological safety: a meta-analytic review and extension. *Pers Psychol*. 2017;70:113–165. doi:10.1111/peps.12183

10. Edmondson AC. Psychological safety, trust, and learning in organizations: a group-level lens. In: Kramer RM, Cook KS, eds. *Trust and Distrust in Organizations: Dilemmas and Approaches*. Russell Sage Foundation; 2004:239–272.

11. Coyle D. The most important four words a leader can say. [Daniel Coyle Website]. http://danielcoyle.com/2017/10/03/the-most-important-four-words-a-leader-can-say

12. Institute for Healthcare Improvement. 100 million healthier lives touchstones for collaboration. http://www.ihi.org/resources/Pages/Tools/100-Million-Healthier-Lives-Advancing-Equity-Tools.aspx

13. PRACTICE: Preventing radicalism through critical thinking competencies. Activity 1: the story of my name. [PRACTICE Website]. https://practice-school.eu/activity1-story-of-my-name

14. Coyle D. *The Culture Code: Secrets of Highly Successful Groups*. 1st ed. Bantam; 2018.

15. Johnson & Johnson. Our Credo. [Johnson & Johnson Website]. https://www.jnj.com/credo/

16. Friedman M. *Trying Hard Is Not Good Enough*. 3rd ed. CreateSpace Independent Publishing Platform; 2015.

17. Jones CP. Levels of racism: a theoretic framework and a Gardener's tale. *Am J Public Health*. 2000;90(8):1212–1215. doi:10.2105/ajph.90.8.1212

18. The Centre for Community Organizations. The "problem" woman of colour in the workplace. [The Centre for Community Organizations Website]. https://coco-net.org/problem-woman-colour-nonprofit-organizations

19. Lilla: International Women's Network. About. [Lilla: International Women's Network Website]. https://lillanetwork.wordpress.com/about

20. Mullenweg M. The importance of meeting in-person. October 16, 2018. https://ma.tt/2018/10/the-importance-of-meeting-in-person

21. Ringel R. When do we actually need to meet in person? Harvard Business Review. July 26, 2021. https://hbr.org/2021/07/when-do-we-actually-need-to-meet-in-person

Chapter 16

Talent Management:
A Leadership Imperative

Lynn "Stevie" Sesslar McNeal

INTRODUCTION

This chapter leverages the leadership competencies and traits discussed in previous chapters by applying those insights in an integrated, thoughtful, and disciplined manner to leading and managing individual employees for optimal results. The importance and value of talent management—and the amount of leadership time and attention invested in it—grows exponentially as leaders progress through their careers due to increases in span of control, resource allocation, and scope of influence. Truly successful leaders embrace the concept of "flipping" the traditional organization paradigm from a pyramid with the leader at the top telling people what to do, to an upside-down pyramid in which the leader enables the people in the organization to radiate their talents.

To that end, a successful talent manager must recognize the criticality of people management, understand their organization's approach and strategy to people management, and then invest the time and effort to successfully engage and manage their employees in an authentic and robust manner.

OBJECTIVES

By the end of this chapter, the reader will be able to:

- Highlight the growing leadership imperative to effectively unleash the power of the workforce in an increasingly competitive public health (PH)/healthcare (HC) industry.
- Provide a brief overview of the organizational components of human resource (HR) strategies/people management and how they impact the leader's approach to talent management.
- Introduce a toolkit for enabling leaders to "unearth, polish, and deploy" their employees' skills, talents and aspirations in a manner that creates value for the organization, the customer/patient, and the employee.

THE TALENT MANAGEMENT IMPERATIVE IN PUBLIC HEALTH AND HEALTHCARE

Over recent decades the U.S. economy has shifted from traditional manufacturing to a service-based economy driven by the digital revolution which blurs the lines between products and services. As noted by Derek Thompson in *The Atlantic*: "No sector provides clearer evidence of today's ongoing economic transformation and the rise of services than the need for quality health care, which has risen to fill the economic void left by industries like manufacturing. 'In 2000, there were 7 million more workers in manufacturing than in health-care. At the beginning of the Great Recession, there were 2.4 million more workers in retail than health-care. In 2017, health-care surpassed both.'"[1(para9)]

One key result of this shift is that the source and durability of a healthcare organization's competitive advantage no longer rests primarily on product, brand or reputation, process, and location advantages. Rather, sustainable differentiation—and hence organizational success—requires an entity to be able to attract, develop, engage, and retain the talent to survive and thrive in an exponentially competitive job market.

And there is no sign that the demand for healthcare workers will abate. To the contrary, trends within the healthcare industry point to increasing staffing challenges and competition in the future. The U.S. healthcare sector accounted for 18% of GDP in 2020 (the highest among developed countries by 30% to 75%) and is forecasted by the Centers for Medicare and Medicaid Services (CMS) to continue to grow at over 5% per year through 2028.[2,3] While there are myriad factors driving this growth, the following are worth noting:

- aging and increased wellness and comorbidity challenges of the U.S. population
- emergence of global pandemics and lack of readiness to address large scale challenges quickly and adeptly
- systemic industry complexity in terms of decision-making, choice, access, cost, innovation, speed of change, fragmented processes, information flows, personal health information (PHI), and a unique lexicon
- traditional silo thinking across diverse set of players—providers, payors (public and private), technology, pharmaceuticals, research, and government—often with contradictory incentives and motivations

At the same time, the talent pool to address these unprecedented needs is insufficient. According to the U.S. Bureau of Labor Statistics, the healthcare sector is forecasted to need an additional 2.3 million workers between 2018 and 2025 across all sectors of the industry.[4] And while the overall numbers may be daunting, the impact on key delivery roles is even more acute. For example, by 2030, there will be a deficit of nearly 105,000 doctors in the United States, according to the Association of American Medical Colleges.[5] Additionally, two-thirds of executives at hospitals with more than 1,000 employees are currently facing a nursing shortage or expect one within 3 years, according to research from The Economist Intelligence Unit commissioned by Prudential Retirement.[6]

In addition, critical public health roles are experiencing shortages,[6] exacerbated by the heightened demand due to COVID-19. The Center for State and Local Government Excellence highlighted the workforce shortage, stating that many governments were facing vacancy rates of up to 20%. The fact sheet noted a particular need for public health nurses, epidemiologists, and environmental health professionals.[6]

Further exacerbating this challenge is the changing needs and expectations of public health and healthcare workers. Potential healthcare workers are finding it difficult to access the necessary education and preparation to have a successful healthcare career as pipeline programs are too expensive, too time-consuming, and too competitive.[7,8,9] Current public health and healthcare workers report strenuous work conditions and high levels of burnout–especially in areas of chronic understaffing.[10] Additionally, numerous roles report low compensation and benefits, especially in the public health/government sectors which often have limited compensation and recognition flexibility due to funding and policy constraints. And the older public health and healthcare workers are nearing retirement age. Most recently, these trends have been exacerbated by the impact of COVID-19 and increased turnover among healthcare workers as evidenced by a McKinsey survey of 100 large private sector hospitals who reported that nursing turnover increased 4% to 5% during 2020.[11] The net result is that many workers are dropping out of the public health and healthcare workforce and current pipelines appear unable to backfill current needs while preparing for the increased demand being forecasted.

In this hypercompetitive staffing landscape, the talent management mandate for the successful public health or healthcare leader is clear. The "call to action" is compelling. Fulfilling individual and organizational missions and aspirations will require emerging talent to become effective people leaders and managers. Building the requisite toolkit to attract, engage, and retain the right talent is essential to survive and thrive into the future.

THE ORGANIZATIONAL TALENT MANAGEMENT STRATEGY CONTEXT

By definition, no leader works in a vacuum. Identifying and understanding the human resources (HR) context in which a leader is operating is essential to be effective and efficient as a talent manager. While the approach of an organization's HR function will vary based on its needs, size, and maturity, a leader needs to understand both the explicit and implicit HR goals and strategies. While this HR context provides the foundation for successful talent management, it is not sufficient. At a minimum, HR should provide a roadmap and guideposts to ensure appropriate compliance, equity, and consistency across the organization. At its best, an organization's HR strategy will enable and support great talent managers.

To begin, it is important to understand the different roles HR functions play. At the simplest level, HR functions are responsible for identifying, hiring, paying, and supporting the human assets of an organization. These are the "necessary" functions for basic operations as well as ensuring consistency and regulatory compliance and reporting (e.g., Equal Employment Opportunity Commission [EEOC], Occupational Health and Safety Administration [OSHA]). All organizations need to ensure that the basic HR management functions are being achieved. Depending on the size/maturity of the organization, some of these functions can be outsourced to ensure appropriate expertise and minimize fixed expense. The bottom line is that these functions are "table stakes" for operating any public health or healthcare entity.

In addition to these basic roles, most organizations recognize the importance of developing a more formal people management strategy. Taking a strategic approach helps heighten the organizational visibility and importance of people management by engaging organizational leaders in thoughtful and integrated planning for future HR needs based on an assessment of the people needs, strengths, gaps, and opportunities. As a small or young/start-up organization, these strategic objectives might be discussed and owned by the board, the executive director, or entrepreneur; however, as an organization grows and matures, the articulation, documentation, and systemization of these components becomes more formal. In addition, many health departments, clinics, and satellite offices will have HR policies and practices dictated by the larger organization or government entity. Regardless of organizational maturity and size, the recognition, alignment, and competitive positioning of the key elements of "people management" are essential to organizational sustainability and success. In this section, we will briefly highlight the key strategic dimensions of a people management strategy as these components provide a "solution space" in which the public health or healthcare leader can maneuver and implement their own talent management approach. In doing so, keep in mind the "call to action" for talent management and consider how these different components could be designed and aligned to create an attractive and mutually beneficial employment offer.

ORGANIZATIONAL DESIGN

Organizational design speaks to how an entity organizes its work and people to achieve its goals and deliver the mission and vision of the organization. The overall "structure" of an organization will evolve over time, especially as an organization grows. A small entity can be more informal as key information, decisions, and actions can be quickly and informally communicated between the small number of employees; however, even in small operations, it is important to document and understand who is responsible for basic functions and overall decision-making roles and processes. As an organization grows, aligning the work and responsibilities into a more formal structure is essential for effective and efficient operations.

As a public health or healthcare leader, understanding not only the basic structure but what it implies for who does the work, how it gets done, and how resources are allocated is important as it enables a leader to more effectively design roles and manage and coach staff for success. While organizations can be structured in a number of different ways (e.g., functionally, geographically, by product or service, by customer type), discerning where the "true" locus of power lays is essential. This can be discerned by asking two questions:

- **How does the organization determine its strategy and goals for the foreseeable future?** To truly understand how this works, consider the who, what, when, and how. Who is involved and at what point in the process? This is particularly important as it often reveals what matters to key decision-makers and what is perceived as the most critical activity or source of competitive advantage. What is the time frame and level of goal iteration? When and why is it changed? Is the process more top-down, bottom-up, or a hybrid?

- **How are the major work tasks and people organized to deliver the mission, vision, values, and goals?** A quick review of an organization chart will provide a sense of the organizing paradigm (e.g., by function, by product) as well as the chain of command (who answers to whom); however, talking to the people in the organization will provide key insights as to how the company really works and where there may be heightened importance and visibility. For example, does the finance function drive key decisions through budget allocation or do research/development needs dictate priorities? Most organizations experience friction between organizational areas and understanding the nature of those tensions helps define the organizational context.

JOB DESIGN

Job design addresses how work is structured into specific jobs and roles and defines individual scope of responsibility. The scope and design of roles can enhance or hinder the degree to which employees find meaning and growth opportunities, which is becoming increasingly important to attract and retain the talent of the future.[12,13] In smaller organizations, job design often requires employees to wear multiple hats, which has some benefits as well as limitations. In larger organizations, the reverse can be true: jobs may be so narrowly focused that they lack meaning and challenge, resulting in retention issues. While job design and descriptions generally fall under the purview of HR, an effective people leader should provide input that ensures the role is accurate and attractive. Among the key considerations for job design are the following:

- What are the goals and objectives of the role (i.e., the scope of the role)?
- What level of education, training, and experience are required to perform that role (i.e., minimum requirements)?
- How dependent or integrated is the role with other areas or other roles within the organization? How many layers for decision-making? Who decides what (i.e., level of autonomy)?
- What is the target span of control (i.e., how many employees per leader)?
- What kind of flexibility does the role have in terms of when and how the role is accomplished? The recent rapid transition to remote working for many roles has created unprecedented pressure on organizations to rethink and accelerate their ongoing level of workplace flexibility.

RECRUITING AND ATTRACTING TALENT

Recruiting and attracting talent includes elements that are owned by both the HR function and the hiring manager. This section will focus more on the HR organizational responsibilities; the public health or healthcare leader's role will be addressed in more depth in the next section.

At the highest level, HR often partners with hiring managers at least annually to forecast recruiting and headcount needs. This is typically an outgrowth of the annual planning process and helps an organization think more strategically about how much recruitment activity will be needed in light of growth and projected turnover.

Next, one of the most visible and, at times, controversial elements of HR is the pricing (compensation levels) of jobs/roles. If not well thought out, documented, and understood, this component can lead to employee frustration and dissatisfaction. At a minimum, the corporate HR function will provide guidelines and parameters for how much the entity will pay for specific roles. Many organizations use "market pricing" in which they set compensation ranges based on comparable jobs in the industry and adjust those ranges periodically using new market data and trends. These ranges define the minimum and maximum an organization will pay for a role. The specific placement of an employee within that range is often a function of education, experience, and results. HR will usually define what components of total compensation the organization will use and to what extent. For example, how much of total compensation is fixed (i.e., salary) versus variable (i.e., incentives, commissions)? When are sign-on or retention bonuses merited and for how much? Do certain roles require premiums due to scarcity, location, or other factors?

In addition to compensation, HR is critical in defining other elements of the "total rewards" package an employer provides to their staff, which can be significant in attracting candidates. This includes a number of noncompensation benefits including vacation and sick leave (paid time off), health insurance and benefits, retirement programs and contributions, tuition reimbursement, relocation assistance, and employee assistance programs. Understanding what is offered and how it compares to competitors will be important for making attractive job offers.

When the need arises to fill an open position, HR is responsible for implementing a legally compliant process for posting the job and soliciting candidates. This begins with ensuring an up-to-date job description that clarifies minimum hiring requirements. Then HR will often partner with the hiring manager to implement an agreed-upon approach for solicitation that includes ideas on where and how to attract viable candidates as well as exploring traditional versus nontraditional hires (e.g., career switchers). This can include paying for postings, advertisements, job fairs, and maintaining relationships with schools and search firms to find difficult-to-fill or highly competitive/scarce skill sets.

Lastly, HR develops and maintains the interviewing process to ensure an equitable, timely, and compliant approach. This process includes mechanisms to efficiently screen and communicate with the applicant pool, train interviewers, schedule interviews, collect feedback, and consult with the hiring manager to create and extend offers. In addition, HR often consults with leaders on additional ways to identify and recruit a diverse set of candidates to address the growing diversity needs and challenges.

ENGAGING AND SUPPORTING TALENT

Engaging and supporting talent is primarily owned by the public health or healthcare leader. That said, the HR organization provides an infrastructure and approach that enables the leader to be successful through the following activities:

- **Orientation to the company:** Ensures a consistent onboarding of new employees and builds a common culture and set of expectations.
- **Standard training and development programs:** Includes both internal and external programs and events necessary to ensure the requisite skill sets.

■ **Performance management process and requirements:** The minimum expectations for when and how employees receive feedback on job performance.

■ **Rewards and recognition:** Linking performance management to the monetary and non-monetary outcomes (e.g., sets ranges for raises and awards, celebrates outstanding contributions).

■ **Employee relations and support:** The ongoing mechanisms for employee feedback and issue escalation necessary for a positive employer/employee relationship.

SUCCESSION PLANNING

Succession planning is the process of ensuring sufficient talent to fill critical leadership roles as current leaders move or exit the workforce. Succession planning is both an individual leader and organizational responsibility to ensure a viable pipeline of critical talent to accommodate turnover while providing realistic career expectations and trajectories for high potential employees.

EMPLOYER BRAND AND REPUTATION MANAGEMENT

Employer brand and reputation management focuses on actively building and cultivating an attractive employment brand that enables the organization to successfully attract, engage, and retain the right complement of employees. This often includes participating in external surveys and reviews, gathering and assessing employee or applicant feedback, analyzing key data points such as applicant-to-hire ratio, reviewing voluntary and involuntary turnover trends, pursuing publication, and monitoring social media mentions.

The most effective leaders invest in creating positive working relationships with their HR organizations across all these dimensions. At the same time, recognizing the opportunities and limitations created by the organization's model is essential for leaders to be able to effectively manage their talent pools.

THE LEADER'S TALENT MANAGEMENT TOOLKIT — THE GEM MODEL

For most established public health or healthcare organizations, there will be a clear distinction between the organization's overarching HR/people management responsibilities and how great talent managers specifically lead their people and departments within that broader organizational construct. Regardless of the broader organizational context, every leader has the opportunity to help form and shape the organizational approach while ensuring alignment with their own talent management philosophy.

This section introduces a toolkit for enabling leaders to "unearth, polish, and deploy" their employees' skills, talents, and aspirations in a manner that creates value for both the organization and the employee. In doing so, it is helpful to draw an analogy from the field of precious minerals—that is, GEMs. Gemology is the science of identifying, studying, shaping, evaluating, and positioning precious minerals to optimally realize their full value. Successful gemologists and jewel-smiths are quick to discern both the visible and invisible traits and properties of a raw mineral and decide how to customize their approach to unleash the full potential. Successful people leaders can do the same by creating and maintaining their own GEM toolkit for how best to manage their most valuable assets: their people. In addition, applying this thoughtful and disciplined approach will help address unintentional biases and foster a more diverse and inclusive approach to talent management

In the GEM model, it is helpful to think about three distinct aspects of talent management within the construct of a precious cut gem (Figure 16.1).

1. **Goals and expectations (G):** The top face of the gem really defines how the employee is seen and valued within the organizational setting.

2. **Engagement and execution (E):** The side facets of the gem showcase the employee through successful job performance.
3. **Management and motivation (M):** The corner "anchor" facets heighten and spur the employee on to higher levels of achievement over time.

Table 16.1 compares the different roles of the organizational HR entity and the leader's talent management role. It is important to note that the different roles should be integrated and mutually reinforcing.

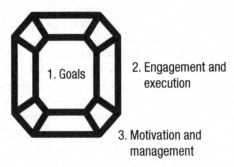

1. Goals

2. Engagement and execution

3. Motivation and management

FIGURE 16.1: The GEM Model of Talent Management.

TABLE 16.1: Comparison of Organization and Leader Roles in Talent Management

ORGANIZATIONAL HUMAN RESOURCES ROLE	PUBLIC HEALTH OR HEALTHCARE LEADER'S TALENT MANAGEMENT ROLE
● Compliance, processing, and reporting	Adhere to compliant processes and standards and provide input for reporting purposes
● Organizational design, job design ● Recruiting and attracting talent	**Goals** - Meaningful and clear role - Specific goals and expectations - Cultivation and selection of the "right" candidates
● Engaging and supporting talent	**Engagement and Execution** - Employee onboarding - Regular and meaningful dialogue - Goal planning, refinement/refresh - Coaching and development
	Motivation and Management - Assessing total performance - The performance management discussion— critical conversations - Tools for performance intervention - Rewards and recognition
● Succession planning ● Employer brand management	- Career planning - Leader-specific talent management brand

GOALS AND EXPECTATIONS FOR THE EMPLOYEE (G)

Setting and communicating a *meaningful, measurable, feasible* set of expectations for an employee is the foundation for talent management. This is the process in which the "raw stone" is identified, selected, and positioned for success. It begins before an employee is hired and is an ongoing focus of successful talent managers as goals and expectations will shift over time due to organizational, competitive, and personal realities.

Meaningful Role

While HR does play an important role in job design, a hiring manager should be equally involved in reviewing, updating, and revising job descriptions to make sure they meet the needs and objectives of both the organization and the target candidate pool. HR is responsible for maintaining a cadre of job descriptions and ensuring that they are consistent with organizational guidelines and policies. The hiring manager is responsible for articulating and tailoring the role description to highlight why the role is necessary and the overall objectives. Focus on conveying the attractiveness of the role in terms of the level of impact on the health and well-being of individuals, communities, and people, as that can be a uniquely attractive dimension for the emerging talent pool in the public health and healthcare sector. At a minimum, the leader should clearly articulate how the role contributes and links to the broader organizational and divisional aspirations to improve health and illustrate how the role fits within the broader organizational processes and any upstream or downstream impacts. Do not assume the value or impact of the role is clear, as many employees can feel like a "cog" in a larger process and not appreciate the criticality of their contributions, or conversely, the negative impact from failure to deliver. Lastly, be explicit about how the job impacts external constituencies (e.g., patients, communities/public, regulators, funders, board, suppliers, distributors).

Role-Specific Goals

With the broader role definition providing a sense of meaning and relevance for the employee, the next step is to translate that into the specific "what" in terms of goals and objectives for each area of responsibility within the job description. In other words, what are you asking the employee to accomplish in this role and what does success look like? It is also important to clarify how those objectives should be accomplished, which enables a leader to reflect not only the values and culture of the organization but of their respective department and team as well. A common and useful approach to goal-setting is to focus on goals that are specific, measurable, attainable, relevant, and time-based (SMART).[14]

Cultivation and Selection of the "Right" Candidate

One of the pivotal responsibilities in talent management is ensuring the identification and selection of the best candidate to fill your role. This can be particularly problematic as many leaders fall into predictable habits that can limit their team's longer-term success such as requiring unnecessary education/experience levels, limiting job postings, or "hiring in their own image."[15,16]

Hiring Requirements

Make sure you start with a clear and necessary set of hiring requirements. While certain qualifications and degrees are absolutely necessary in many healthcare roles, there is a tendency to ask for more education or experience than is needed in an attempt to attract a higher caliber candidate pool.[17,18] This can actually backfire in that you may miss a number of high-potential candidates that get screened out upon initial review. It may be true that someone who has done the same job for a number of years will hit the ground running and require less initial coaching; however, you may miss high-potential candidates who bring a fresh approach and energy that will eventually surpass the experienced hire. Similarly, as the customers/patients of many public health or healthcare organizations grow increasingly diverse, adding requirements to roles that reflect a need for understanding and ability to work with diverse populations is essential.

Recruiting

While job postings and searches are a necessary component of any hiring, great "talent managers" actively build and cultivate a network of potential employees through deliberate actions and behaviors. One of the most powerful tools is maintaining an ongoing relationship with previous employees and colleagues who can be powerful and authentic referral sources. Active membership in industry, functional, and diversity organizations is another effective means by providing broad access across companies, industries, locations, and populations. An individual's profile can be further heightened by taking on visible leadership roles and speaking opportunities at conferences and events. Additionally, there is value in staying in touch with related colleges and universities that place not only new graduates but assist alumni with career progressions as well. While the previous information will help to cultivate a candidate pool, beware the trap of limiting a search to "tried and true" sources. In our increasingly diverse healthcare space, the need to think more wholistically about how to identify and meet the needs of diverse populations challenges us to continually rethink how we identify and assess potential candidates.

The Interview Process

A thoughtfully planned and prepared interview approach helps ensure an objective and professional interaction that identifies the best candidate while creating a positive impression on all interviewees. It is also a powerful opportunity to drive diversity and inclusion into the selection process. The business case for diversity is compelling with recent research demonstrating that organizations that achieve gender, ethnic, and cultural diversity on their leadership teams better fulfill their organizational goals and objectives. That is, they simply outperform those organizations with lower diversity.[19]

To begin, make sure to consider *who* should be involved in interviewing and that they are properly prepared to engage and provide meaningful feedback. While the hiring manager is ultimately responsible for the hiring decision, creating and preparing a diverse slate of interviewers who reflect an array of insights/expectations for the role will provide robust insights for both interviewer and candidate. For example, consider including employees one or two levels down in the organization, other departments who are internal customers or suppliers, a mix of newer and tenured employees, as well as employees with different backgrounds, genders, and racial/cultural diversity. A diverse set of interviewers mitigates the tendency to hire to an established "profile" that emulates what has "worked" in the past. Once you have your slate, make sure each interviewer is appropriately knowledgeable about the role and is able to share unique perspectives with the candidate.

In conducting the interview, use a disciplined interviewing approach to ascertain skills and fit. All interviewers should follow a structured and relatively consistent approach to minimize potential bias and ensure equity in the process. New techniques such as "blind" resume reviews and interviews in which potential indicators of a candidate's gender, race, and culture are eliminated are proving helpful to eliminate implicit bias.[20] Selection criteria can be as simple as weighting the hiring criteria and assigning points or can draw upon more established methodologies such as STAR in which candidates are asked to describe a situation(S), their task(T), the action they took(A), and the result achieved(R).[21] Additionally, be sure to allocate sufficient time to understand the candidate's career goals, expectations, and work style and give them time to ask questions about the role, organization, risks, and concerns.

After completion of all the interviews, it is important to step back and collectively rate and rank the candidate pool in terms of technical and behavioral fit with the job. Each interviewer should provide independent written feedback on the candidate, then engage in a roundtable discussion so interviewers can share feedback and calibrate ratings, as well as provide an explicit opportunity to "check" any implicit biases that may be in play. Among those, be sure to explicitly consider the experience vs. potential trade-off and have a realistic expectation of the length of commitment. For certain roles, hiring someone who may only stay a couple years can make sense, especially if you have a unique, time-boxed need such as a critical project or building a new product, service, or team. For other roles, investing more time and effort to develop an employee upfront may slow down the initial realization of results, but can lead to higher levels of performance in the long run and enable attainment of more meaningful diversity. Lastly, recognize that candidates may not always be 100% forthcoming with their level of commitment given the interview dynamic, which is why asking broader questions about career goals, personal goals, likes and dislikes, and employment history will provide key insights.

Make sure to manage the communication process and expectations with all viable candidates in recognition that this is building a "talent management" brand. Being prompt and professional creates a positive impression, thereby cultivating a future talent pool. Timeliness is important throughout the process, including how quickly candidates are notified, interviews scheduled, offers made, and how much time a candidate is given to deliberate/accept.

ENGAGEMENT AND EXECUTION (E)

Once the appropriate talent has been identified and recruited, the leader is responsible for ensuring this new "gem" is appropriately positioned and equipped with the tools, information, and support to achieve or exceed the position's goals on an ongoing basis and provide an enriching job experience for the employee. These steps create the "solution space" for the employee's success and shape the raw stone for the gem it will hopefully become.

Onboarding

The old adage "you never get a second chance to make a first impression" is particularly true when onboarding new talent. As previously discussed, larger, established organizations with an HR function will have a standard "organizational orientation" process that covers company-wide matters, policies, and procedures. That said, every hiring manager has the primary responsibility to ensure the successful onboarding of their new employee and should build a plan with the following elements to ensure your new hire gets off on the right foot.

Announcements and Communications

Set a schedule for proactively communicating—both written and verbally—within the team and the broader organization. Identify and draft key messages that include the role and expectations as well as introducing the professional and personal background, experience, and interests of the new employee prior to arrival.

Week 1 Schedule

Share a high-level schedule for the first days to week on the job including any organizational onboarding activities as well as a team or department welcome plan. At a minimum, schedule key introduction meetings across the organization, lunch meetings with colleagues, and daily checkpoints to assess how things are going.

Goals and Expectations Framework

Reiterate and reinforce the goals and expectations for the role and specifically how the employee will be assessed, both in the short term (i.e., a 30-, 60-, 90-day plan) and over the longer term. Describe what success looks like in the role and discuss how to balance and/or trade-off potential conflicts and challenges that may arise. In doing so it is particularly useful to clarify the levels of authority and autonomy the employee has regarding specific tasks and recognizing that those levels often evolve over time as knowledge and skill increase.

The "4 Levels of Authority" model[22] provides a simple framework for these discussions:

- **Level 1:** Act upon instruction (i.e., do what you are told)
- **Level 2:** Act after approval (i.e., recommend an action but seek approval before acting)

- **Level 3:** Decide on an action, inform, and act (i.e., decide on right action but inform your manager first)
- **Level 4:** Decide and act (i.e., full autonomy and accountability to take action based on proven knowledge and competence)

A new employee tends to operate in the lower levels of authority with an expectation that they will increase over time; however, for some tasks, a role may always operate at a lower level. For example, a supervisor's level of authority for a task impacts the degrees of freedom available to the subordinates.

While the focus in the onboarding process is on short-term goals, it is equally important to set expectations for the ongoing goal-setting process including the mid-cycle and annual goals and how they link back to broader departmental and organizational plans.

Meaningful Team Integration

A lynchpin in successful onboarding is quickly establishing a sense of belonging and cohesion within your team and organization. While planning cycles may not always coincide, the sooner new talent can be engaged in a teambuilding activity and—even more powerfully— a strategy/planning exercise, the more quickly the leader will benefit from fresh insights while solidifying the new talent's bond and inclusion in the team.

Regular and Meaningful Dialogue

While effective dialogue is covered at length in Chapter 1, how to structure opportunities for robust dialogue from a talent management perspective will be the focus here; specifically, how to create a disciplined approach that will enable effective employee communications, which are the basis of a valued relationship that becomes the foundation for talent management.

Team/Department Meetings

While scheduling regular and frequent (e.g., weekly, semi-monthly) team meetings is a common practice in almost all organizations, ensuring they are a valuable use of time for employees requires discipline and application of three basic tools.

- **Meeting agendas:** These should be distributed at least 24 hours in advance and include the meeting objectives, specific agenda items that are time-boxed, and indications of the desired outcome (e.g., awareness, discussion, input, action, decision).
- **Ongoing team reflection and feedback:** One of the most valuable tools in creating authentic dialogue and trust among a team is providing a regular mechanism for individual team members to assess how effective the team meetings are and offering suggestions for ways to improve. An easy-to-use approach is a "Plus/Delta" round robin session at the end of the meeting in which each team member says what went well (+) and what could be done better (delta), with those comments captured on a flip chart/whiteboard. The leader can then acknowledge positives and engage team members in improvement opportunities. Over time, the frequency of the Plus/Deltas may decrease but should be done at least quarterly as a leadership best practice.
- **Action items and tracking:** These create a "closed loop" and visibility on assignments. Together, the agenda and associated minutes become a mechanism to keep team members fully informed and on the same page going forward.

Individual 1:1 Meetings

Done well, 1:1 discussions become the vehicle for ongoing talent management. Similar to team meetings, these discussions benefit greatly from a structured approach while allowing more flexibility for the organic and personal discussions that build a foundation of trust. To that end, schedule 1:1 sessions on a regular basis and treat them as a high priority using a "lite" agenda format and following these "tips":

- Prepare by soliciting and agreeing on agenda topics in advance. While most sessions might follow a standard format (e.g., goal and activity updates, challenges and obstacles, upcoming milestones), it is important to give advance warning if a new or surprising topic needs to be discussed so both parties can be prepared.

■ Create an expectation of "upward management." Consistent with turning the organizational paradigm upside down, empower talent to manage upward by sharing their concerns and asking for specific help or support needed from the manager.

■ Manage the discussion for meaningful dialogue:

● Start with a general check-in—"*How's it going?*"—before jumping into agenda topics.

● Err on the side of listening more, especially at the beginning of the discussion.

● Playback discussion to make sure the employee feels truly heard.

● To the extent it is relevant, provide facts, perspectives, and insights to issues and concerns, especially related to the rumor mill or other "rumblings."

● When appropriate, share personal stories of similar challenges, actions taken, and lessons learned. Sharing hard lessons learned and mistakes is one of the most powerful tools for building trust and openness.

● Periodically ask for feedback, and treat it like a gift. "*What do you need from me to be wildly successful?*" and just as importantly, "*What don't you need from me?*"

● Provide reasonable transparency while recognizing not everyone can know everything at all times, especially related to other personnel and confidential organizational matters.

● Document key take-aways, actions, and agreements and share those with the employee.

■ Beware common pitfalls:

● Focus employees on what they can control or change rather than what everyone else is doing. Create a "no victimization" mindset by reinforcing that the only thing anyone can truly control is how to act, respond, and comport themselves on any given day in any given situation. (Note: This is not meant to disregard significant issues of bias, discrimination, harassment, or hostile work conditions. Those need to be raised and addressed in a timely manner and in accordance with company reporting and escalation policies.)

● Prevent triangulation by not engaging in discussions about other people without those discussions having first taken place directly with that person. When issues need to be addressed with others, schedule meetings with all parties present.

● Recognize the candor limitations created by "position authority." A leader may not always get an "unvarnished" answer or honest feedback from someone reporting to them.

Goal Planning, Refinement, and Refresh

One of the keys to inspiring talent over time is to ensure the goals remain meaningful, challenging—and, to the extent possible, provide new opportunities and experiences. While the organizational planning process drives the overall direction and priorities, every leader needs to engage their teams in identifying how their roles will contribute and potential trade-offs and concerns. The most effective planning processes are an annual top-down/bottom-up approach in which high-level aspirations are established and then vetted and refined through bottom-up feedback from departments and teams. A key part of the upward feedback is clarifying what resources and new skills will be needed to achieve the goals. Ideally, every employee will have an opportunity to provide some input into the annual planning process through departmental work sessions in which top-down aspirations are clarified and questions and concerns are discussed.

Not only does bottom-up participation drive buy-in, it kick-starts the individual goal-setting process. Similar to setting broad goals for a role, it is important to revise goals annually and to ensure that those goals are SMART (i.e., they are specific, measurable, attainable, relevant, and time-based).[6] Additionally, this process now becomes a dialogue between the employee and their manager to ensure the revised individual goals and performance levels meet the departmental priorities and that any new skills, resources, and support for goal attainment are identified and planned.

Coaching and Development Opportunities

While both the ongoing employee–employer dialogue and the formal goal-setting process are the formal foundation for the coaching and development of an employee, providing additional feedback and interactions are tools to help further polish your employee into a sparkling "gem."

Training and Development Investments

As part of the annual goal-setting process, identify additional skills and experiences the employee will require to continue to grow and contribute. These can be formal training plans or classes, participation in industry or functional conferences and events, as well as new assignments and projects within the organization. Be sure to explicitly discuss and agree on what those plans are for the year and when and how they can be fulfilled.

Focused Work or Problem-Solving Sessions

Look for opportunities to "get into the dirt" on tough problems by rolling up your sleeves and working side-by-side with the employee to address challenges. Offer tools, frameworks, and processes for how to handle tough situations. Share past experiences and lessons learned.

Real-Time Feedback

Few things are as powerful as catching someone doing the "right" thing and calling it out. The concept of "filling others' buckets" originated in early childhood education and has become a powerful leadership competency in which a leader looks for daily opportunities to publicly highlight the good work and contributions of others.[23] The key is being authentic and clear in the accolades and to focus on extolling what others have done or accomplished (i.e., "other's buckets") rather than what the leader has done (i.e., "leader's own bucket").

It is equally important to give constructive feedback on a real-time basis—albeit generally done in private. Quick and specific feedback on unacceptable behaviors and actions is essential to create and maintain a positive working environment and to signal what is valued and what is unacceptable on a consistent basis.

MOTIVATION AND MANAGEMENT FOR SUCCESS (M)

This section solidifies the goals and engagement created through talent management by discussing how performance management and rewards or recognition can enhance employee motivation and results. These "final cuts" by the skilled gemologist nuance the gem's shape while enabling its innate brilliance to shine.

Effective Performance Assessments

At a minimum, every employee should have a formal performance appraisal annually with checkpoints every 3 to 6 months. Typically, the minimum standards are set by the organization to ensure consistency across employees and leaders—especially as related to merit raises and rewards. That said, an effective leader manages the employee to ensure that the formal process is a natural and expected outcome of the ongoing dialogue and discussions.

Assessing Performance

Having engaged in regular 1:1 meetings with the employee in which discussion items and actions have been collectively documented now provides an audit trail by which to assess performance over the course of the year. An effective formal performance discussion should contain "no surprises" for the employee in that it is a natural culmination of the ongoing dialogue. That said, the formal performance discussion will benefit from additional input and data points to ensure a more wholistic assessment. To that end, consider the following sources:

- Employee self-assessments are highly recommended and helpful to review after completing a preliminary assessment but prior to discussion with the employee. While input from the employee can provide additional details resulting in modifications or additions to the assessment, it is even more valuable in helping prepare for the face-to-face discussion, especially if there are differing viewpoints.

- Internal and external customers/patients are a rich source of new perspectives. Consider asking these audiences for written feedback that can be either directly shared or summarized back to the employee.

- 360-degree feedback tools provide an even more comprehensive feedback mechanism. This tool collects and compiles anonymous feedback from peers, subordinates, superiors, and others across the broader organization that interact on a fairly regular basis. When considering when and how to deploy, assess the timing (when in an employee's tenure in a role), how the data will be shared, who will see the data, and the cost and time commitment to implement.

Balancing the "What" and the "How" of Performance

In assessing the overall performance of the employee, explicitly evaluate both "what" level of performance they achieved and "how" they achieved it. A helpful framework for this assessment is a 3x3 grid for plotting the level of results attained (horizontal axis) against the behaviors exhibited (vertical axis; Figure 16.2).[24]

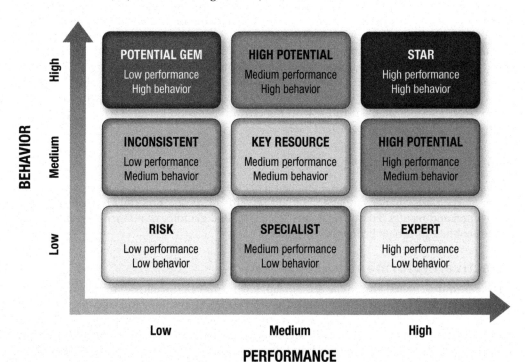

FIGURE 16.2: Employee Performance Evaluation Grid.

This approach helps the leader balance messages and reinforce the organization's culture and values. For example, achieving high results but with poor behaviors is shown in the lower right, indicating a performance risk to be actively addressed. At the same time, someone who achieves only moderate results while exhibiting high behavioral competency is an overall high performer. Additionally, even those with low results but high behavioral competency are not overall low performers. Rather, these employees merit additional support to address their results shortfall. For this tool to be effective, it is important to communicate the framework to employees upfront and then have specific data points to reinforce their placement on the grid.

Other Considerations

Lastly, in preparation for the performance management discussion, consider the following additional questions:

- Are any performance shortfalls due to a lack of the necessary skills that could be addressed in a development plan?
- Or, does the performance gap reflect a lack of will or commitment to do what needs to be done to be successful? Or, a combination of both skill and will?
- Are there any unique externalities that may be impacting performance (e.g., major industry or organizational changes; personal changes and challenges)?

Managing the Performance Discussion

Having completed the written assessment, the next step is to prepare and actively manage the performance discussion.

General Process and Agenda

It is highly preferable to separate performance discussions from any monetary discussions to enable a primary focus on how the employee is performing and what they can do to be even more successful. How that translates into merit increases and bonuses is largely governed by organizational practices with only a limited degree of talent manager flexibility. To enable a productive discussion and minimize angst, distribute the written performance assessment 1 to 2 days in advance of the meeting.

Create a meeting flow that best enables a productive and balanced discussion:

- Verify the employee has reviewed the document and ask for any overall reactions, in particular *"Were there any major surprises?"*
- Review and discuss the employee's strengths and give specifics. A great way to do this is by starting with *"What I value most about you."*
- Review and discuss performance shortfalls, both in terms of results and behaviors. Again, provide specific examples and concerns and not sweeping generalities.
- Discuss ways to improve performance and get to the next level. Be prepared to share specific ideas and react and respond to employee suggestions. Every employee should have a development plan that reflects not only the organization's needs but the employee's goals and preferences as well.
- Agree on specific action items and next steps.
- Wrap-up with the overall performance assessment/rating and follow-up quickly with the monetary (incentives, merit increases) discussion.

Tips for Having Tough Performance Management Discussions

The previous process provides a general roadmap for performance discussions. The following are some tips for when there is a performance issue and/or a difficult discussion.

- Ensure clear, written articulation of performance shortfall and gaps. Ideally, these should be measurable and provide specific examples. Illustrate the organizational and departmental implications of the shortfall (i.e., why it matters).

■ Clarify the potential employee consequences of not addressing the shortfall and the necessary time frame to demonstrate improvement. If the performance issue is severe enough to jeopardize employment, make sure that is clear and be definitive on the time frame for corrective action.

■ Probe on drivers of the performance shortfall, making sure to explore all aspects that may be coming into play (e.g., skill deficits, lack of understanding, exogenous factors or challenges, lack of motivation).

■ Allow "silent time" while being prepared for a wide gamut of emotions from anger, denial, sadness, hopelessness, frustration, and resignation.

■ Ask the employee to take several days to process and reflect, then schedule a follow-up discussion to agree on a plan for moving forward.

Interventions/Actions to Deal With Performance Issues

When there is a significant performance issue, both the employee and the manager collaborate to build a plan for success. This begins with mutually defining what success looks like and ascertaining whether the employee is interested and willing to do what is needed to perform at the level required. There are situations in which the employee may realize they are not in the right job and either a different role or separation from the company is the desired outcome. Be careful not to default to that conclusion too quickly by allowing "soak" time for both the leader and the employee. That said, there are situations in which the "fit" just isn't right and supporting a voluntary resignation can be the best outcome for the company and the employee.

Assuming there is a mutual desire to address the performance problem, the next step is to develop a "corrective action plan" (CAP). This is a formal written document that clearly articulates what the employee needs to achieve to address performance concerns and in what time frame. It is important to note that the CAP not only identifies a deadline for achievement but requires maintenance of performance at the target level going forward. While format varies, all CAPs should have:

■ clear statement of goal and result that needs to be achieved

■ specific actions employee needs to take

■ defined interim checkpoints

■ end date

An effective talent manager will work with the employee to identify and implement the specific actions that can help address the performance issues. While not exhaustive, the following tips provide a starting point.

■ Results shortfalls
  ● Review and document best practices for the role.
  ● Conduct a schedule or work process review to identify "black holes" that are consuming unnecessary time and effort (e.g., meeting mania, reporting overload).
  ● Shadow or interview employees in similar roles.
  ● Identify internal and external training programs to fill skill gaps.
  ● Develop job aids.

■ Behavioral shortfalls
  ● Conduct a "listening tour" in which the employee meets with a cross-section of colleagues to gather feedback.
  ● Implement a 360-degree survey.
  ■ Assign an internal mentor or external coach.

Together, the employee and manager should discuss which approaches make the most sense and when and how they can be implemented. Ideally, both parties agree on the specific actions; however, there may be times in which the manager will require the employee to take actions that the employee does not agree with. While it is important to listen and acknowledge the employee's concerns, the manager has the authority and responsibility to make that call while explaining the basis of that decision.

Throughout the CAP process, the manager and employee will be meeting to assess progress and make any necessary adjustments. Consequently, at the end of the agreed-upon time frame, there should be no surprise as to the outcome.

Rewards and Recognition

While performance assessments and ratings are the substance of talent management, nothing speaks louder than how those messages are translated into monetary and non-monetary rewards. As previously discussed, the organizational HR entity defines the broad parameters for how employees are rewarded. That said, the talent manager is responsible for implementing those programs in a way that ensures that the highest performers are rewarded significantly more than the average and lower performers. One of the most demotivating leadership mistakes is to use the "peanut butter" approach in which everyone gets basically the same percentage of merit increase and bonus.

Leaders must think wholistically about how to use the traditional reward levers—merit increases and bonuses—to send a coherent message about the employee's performance and value to the organization while being clear about future potential. At the same time, recognize that earning potential for most jobs has limits based on the market value for that job. Hence, if an employee wants to grow their earning potential, they need to be thinking about ways to expand their scope.

Additionally, leaders need to expand their reward and recognition toolkit to keep key talent engaged and motivated. As you continue to build employee relationships, invest the effort to create employee-specific motivation plans that are tailored to the needs, wants, and preferences of each person. There is an arsenal of non-monetary tools that can be as powerful as the monetary rewards when used appropriately and thoughtfully (e.g., public recognition, expanded roles, special projects or assignments, new title, enhanced work flexibility, new training opportunities, conference attendance, association membership). Make sure to use a variety of methods, especially in situations in which the traditional reward systems are limited (e.g., small or start-up organizations, government entities, unions).

Career Planning

While good talent managers are a great asset to an employee, employees own their career! It is their responsibility to define and reassess career goals and develop plans for how to achieve them. At the same time, a leader needs to be continually thinking about the talent they will need in their organization in the future and how best to ensure they have the requisite skills, whether through internal development or external recruiting.

There are times when the organization and the individual's career goals align such as supporting an employee to attain a promotion or a new job or helping them round out their skill set and experience through assignments; however, there are times when an employee's career aspirations and the needs of the team or organization conflict or diverge. At those times, career growth may require an employee to move to a new organization and a leader should be authentic and transparent about those conflicts or limitations.

The manager's role in an employee's career planning is to be a resource, sounding board, and—when it makes sense—enabler. That said, to be a useful career resource and coach, a manager must first understand what matters to the employee from a future career perspective, including:

- scope of responsibility
- earning potential
- type of work and challenge

■ continuous learning
■ flexibility
■ location

Armed with the knowledge of what the employee aspires to achieve, the leader can be an effective member of the employee's career development team by offering expertise, advice, and internal growth opportunities when available.

The Talent Management Brand

The GEM model is designed to leverage all the leadership traits, intangibles, and tools previously discussed in this book by providing a short and feasible set of priorities and checklists to build a talent management toolkit. How this toolkit is used will inevitably create a talent management "brand" or "persona" through everyday leadership actions and behaviors; that is, how a manager is perceived as a boss, a leader, a coach, and a teacher. The competition for public health and healthcare talent is increasing rapidly and those leaders who cultivate a positive talent management brand will be able to attract, engage, and retain talent in a way that delivers higher results for their organization and the community. To aid in this process, there are numerous additional books, papers, and frameworks for building a talent management brand[25] that can be incorporated into and augment the GEM framework provided in this chapter. Successful talent managers stay apprised of the latest thinking and insights and continually incorporate those learnings into an authentic, evergreen talent management brand.

SUMMARY

This chapter provides a "practitioners'" guide on how to lead and manage individual employees to achieve optimal results in the increasingly competitive and challenging public health and healthcare sectors. To that end, effective people leaders must understand both the organizational and individual components of talent management. The organizational context is created through the HR policies, programs, parameters, and expectations that provide the foundation upon which the talent manager will lead. The GEM Model of Talent Management provides an individual practitioner's toolkit that a leader can then tailor to their organizational needs and in a manner consistent with their own talent management philosophy. The GEM Model provides a short and feasible set of tools and tips focused on three distinct aspects of talent management: employee goals and expectations, employee engagement and execution, and employee management and motivation. The thoughtful and disciplined application of the GEM Model enables a leader to develop a positive talent management brand which is essential to attracting, developing, engaging, and retaining the right talent to deliver better results for their organization and community.

DISCUSSION QUESTIONS

THE TALENT MANAGEMENT IMPERATIVE

1. What are the critical skills your organization will need to achieve its mission, vision, and goals in the future? Be sure to consider both technical skills as well as non-technical skills such as communication, leadership, collaboration, and teamwork.
2. What specific recent trends or pressures do you see that will make attracting and retaining those skills more difficult?
3. What key factors or characteristics drive you and your peers and colleagues to seek employment at certain organizations? How has this changed over the last several years?

Exercise

1. Rank order job attributes in order of importance to you and ask three to five colleagues to do the same. While not exhaustive, some of the attributes to consider are:
   - job scope and title
   - compensation (salary and bonus potential)
   - traditional benefits (e.g., health insurance, paid time off, retirement plan and contributions, leave policy)
   - extra benefits (e.g., tuition assistance/reimbursement, employee assistance program, relocation assistance)
   - training and development programs
   - career path/opportunities
   - job flexibility (schedule, work location)
   - geographic location
   - company/entity reputation

2. Compare your results with your peers. Are there any surprises? What might cause the ranking of your attributes to change (e.g., life stage, experience, industry changes, education)?

3. Consider implications for how you could use these insights as a people leader. What might you do differently as a talent manager?

THE ORGANIZATIONAL TALENT MANAGEMENT "CONTEXT"

1. Which organizations or companies are the most successful in recruiting the skill sets you will need? Why?

2. When you think back on past jobs and roles, which companies or organizations have left the most positive lasting impression (focus here on the organization more than a specific individual or supervisor to the extent possible)? Why? How has that impression changed over time?

3. Which organizations have left the worst impression? What actionable advice would you give those organizations?

THE TALENT MANAGEMENT TOOLKIT

Every one of us has worked for leaders who we would gladly work for again and then others who we would avoid like the plague. Take a few moments to think about each of those experiences and answer the following:

1. Who were the "best" and "worst" bosses you have worked for? What did they do (or not do) that earned that rating?

2. What three adjectives would you use to describe the "best" and what three for the "worst?

3. What expectations or preconceptions did you bring to your role and how did that impact your boss–employee relationship? How did that change over time and why?

4. As a people leader, how would you want your employees to describe you to prospective recruits?

5. What do you anticipate would be the most difficult talent management situation for you to address in the future?

CASE STUDY: TALENT MANAGEMENT: FINDING LEVERS AND OPPORTUNITIES

The northwestern counties of North Carolina have long been known as the "lost provinces" due to their separation from the rest of the state by the Eastern Continental Divide with elevations of between 2,500 and 3,500 ft. and a lagging public road system which made access difficult, especially to more rural, mountainous locations. That isolation has abated in recent years as investments in roads, tourism, and the arts have made these counties increasingly attractive to visitors and new residents. The current demographic of this region is 85% rural and White, but Hispanic populations have increased to nearly 5%. The average age is mid-to-late 40s, and while over 85% of the population has a high school education, less than 20% of the population has a bachelor's degree.

It is in this bucolic setting that AS—a Boston-raised and -educated primary care physician—was recently appointed as the director of the Mountain Health Department (MHD). AS knew when she accepted the role that the clinic, as a government-funded entity, was struggling to attract and retain qualified clinicians to meet the need of an increasingly diverse yet transient population—and that challenge was greatly exacerbated by the recent COVID-19 epidemic. In addition, AS knew that the area had a low capacity of existing healthcare workers as evidenced by a physician-to-population ratio of 10.4/10k people, which is only a third of the national average.

In the first weeks of her new role, AS invested significant time gathering feedback from staff, volunteers, patients, and community leaders to develop a 90-day plan with priorities and specific actions. As AS reviewed her notes from her inaugural listening tour, she noted the following:

- The two major reasons for loss of clinical staff over recent years were low pay and poor job satisfaction.
  - MHD salaries tended to be 80% of comparable private roles but it was not clear how the roles fared with respect to the non-monetary aspects of the job.
  - Departing employees listed frustration with their inability to make a difference due to policy constraints and lack of sufficient training and preparation nearly as important as compensation in their decision to leave.
- The length of time a position remained open or unfilled has been trending upward over the last 5 years with recent postings remaining open for an unacceptable 9 to 12 months.
- The majority of the current staff has a significant personal and professional commitment and investment in fulfilling the department's broader social mission.
- Tension and conflict among staff have increased as departmental goals fall short and staff compete for scarce resources while working longer hours.
- Several long-tenured staff have been very outspoken and critical of MHD and have basically "checked-out"; in other words, doing the bare minimum to get their jobs done.
- Public funding for MHD has remained stagnant over the last 4 years with no pay raises or notable budget increases.
- Awareness and demand for MHD's services has grown slightly due to population growth and the success of public awareness and outreach campaigns.

As AS looked out her office window at the cascading mountain vistas of the region, she contemplated whether she could make the kind of positive impact she envisioned when she joined MHD. She had always considered herself a great people-leader and while she had some relevant experience in building a team, her challenge at MHD was daunting. Clearly, being able to attract, engage, and retain the right talent to rejuvenate MHD was priority one, but what levers and opportunities did she have to make a real difference?

CASE STUDY QUESTIONS

1. In addition to her listening tour, what other actions should AS take as soon as possible to make sure she understands the talent management landscape?

2. In a perfect world with a magic wand, what could AS do to address the talent shortfall?

3. Which of these "blue sky" opportunities are limited by AS's current environment and setting? How can these limitations be mitigated?

4. How can AS build trust and credibility with her new staff necessary to tackle these challenges?

5. How should AS handle the "squeaky wheel" staff?

6. What is a reasonable time frame for AS to develop and begin to implement some actions? What specific actions should AS take in the near term (90 to 180 days)? In the longer term (1 to 2 years)?

 A robust set of instructor resources designed to supplement this text is located at **http://connect.springerpub.com/content/book/978-0-8261-4924-4**. Qualifying instructors may request access by emailing **textbook@springerpub.com**.

REFERENCES

1. Citi. The American economy is experiencing a paradigm shift.*The Atlantic*. 2018. https://www.theatlantic.com/sponsored/citi-2018/the-american-economy-is-experiencing-a-paradigm-shift/2008

2. Statista. *Health Care Expenditures as Percent of GDP 1960–2020*. Jenny Yang; September 8, 2021.

3. Centers for Medicare and Medicaid Services. *NHE Fact Sheet*. United States Government; December 16, 2020.

4. Hobbib B. The state of healthcare recruitment: four major struggles facing healthcare staffing firms. *Recruiting Daily*. April 5, 2018. https://recruitingdaily.com/state-healthcare-recruitment-four-major-struggles-facing-healthcare-staffing-firms/

5. Heiser S. *New Findings Confirm Predictions on Physician Shortage*. AAMC; April 23, 2019.

6. Freeman M. Talent shortages present opportunities for U.S. hospitals, survey says. *Prudential Newsroom*. June 20, 2017. https://news.prudential.com/talent-shortages-opportunity-us-hospitals-survey.htm

7. Wong K. Top workforce challenges and trends impacting the healthcare industry in 2020. Achievers. December 4, 2019. Last updated January 21, 2020. https://www.achievers.com/wp-content/uploads/2020/10/Top-Workforce-Trends-Impacting-the-Healthcare-Industry-in-2020.pdf

8. McKinney C. High medical education costs extend past medical school. LLU Institute for Health Policy Leadership; June 1, 2020. https://ihpl.llu.edu/blog/high-medical-education-costs-extend-past-medical-students#:~:text=If%20you%20attend%20medical%20school,schools%20and%20%24242%2C660%20for%20private.

9. Kelly R. Why getting into medical school is harder than ever. *The Savvy Pre-Med*. April 22, 2019. https://www.savvypremed.com/blog/why-getting-into-medical-school-is-harder-than-ever

10. Keck School of Medicine. A closer look at the public health workforce shortage. University of Southern California, US; Public Health Online; February 26, 2020. https://mphdegree.usc.edu/blog/a-closer-look-at-the-public-health-workforce-crisis/

11. Berlin G, Lapointe M, Murphy M. Increased workforce turnover and pressures straining provider operations. McKinsey & Company. August 19, 2021. https://www.mckinsey.com/industries/health-care-systems-and-services/our-insights/increased-workforce-turnover-and-pressures-straining-pro-vider-operations

12. Abid AM, Sarwar A, Imran K, Jabbar A. Effect of job design on employee satisfaction. *Eur J Business Manag.* 2013;5(19):1–7. https://www.iiste.org/Journals/index.php/EJBM/article/view/7266

13. Truss K, Baron A, Crawford D, et al. *Job Design and Employee Engagement.* Engage for Success; 2014. https://engageforsuccess.org/wp-content/uploads/2021/01/Job-Design-and-Employee-Engage-ment-Katie-Truss-et-al-11.pdf

14. Doran G, Miller A, Cunningham J. There's a S.M.A.R.T. way to write management goals and objectives. *Manag Rev.* 1981;70(11):35–36.

15. Chamorro-Premuzic T. Should leaders stop hiring in their own image? *Forbes.* September 8, 2020. https://www.forbes.com/sites/tomaspremuzic/2020/09/08/should-leaders-stop-hiring-in-their-own-image/?sh=6966b516419c

16. Dhanda P. How to avoid hiring and promoting in your own image. *Technation.* June 3, 2019. https://technation.io/news/diversity-how-to-avoid-hiring-in-your-own-image/

17. Heinz K. How to write job requirements. *BuiltIn.* October 27, 2021. https://builtin.com/recruiting/job-requirements

18. Collamer N. Why so many job postings are so ridiculous. *Forbes.* September 22, 2014. https://www.forbes.com/sites/nextavenue/2014/09/22/why-so-many-job-postings-are-so-ridiculous/?sh=-222c16a35ad0

19. Dixon-Fyle S, Hunt V, Dolan K, Prince S. *Diversity Wins: How Inclusion Matters.* McKinsey & Company; May 19, 2020. https://www.mckinsey.com/~/media/mckinsey/featured%20insights/diversity%20and%20inclusion/diversity%20wins%20how%20inclusion%20matters/diversity-wins-how-inclu-sion-matters-vf.pdf

20. Knight R. 7 practical ways to reduce bias in your hiring process. *Harvard Business Review.* June 12, 2017. https://hbr.org/2017/06/7-practical-ways-to-reduce-bias-in-your-hiring-process

21. DDI; STAR method. DDI World; 1970s. https://www.ddiworld.com/solutions/behavioral-interviewing/star-method

22. MacLaren-Jackson RJ. Understanding the four levels of delegation when managing people in business. The Project Management Hut (PMHUT); October 1, 2012. https://pmhut.com/understand-ing-the-four-levels-of-delegation-when-managing-people-in-business

23. Clifton D, Rath T. *How Full Is Your Bucket? Positive Strategies for Work and Life.* Gallup Press; 2004.

24. Satija K. Performance evaluation: the best practices and the 3x3 matrix to measure employee perfor-mance. Seven Bosses Blog. June 25, 2020. https://sevenbosses.com/wp-content/uploads/2020/06/Employee-performance-evaluation-3x3-matrix-or-9-box-grid.pptx

25. Hanna T. The top 15 best talent management books. *Talent Management Solutions Review.* December 5, 2019. https://solutionsreview.com/talent-management/2019/12/05/the-top-best-talent-manage-ment-books/

Chapter 17

Creating Effective Public Health Messengers

Barbara Alvarez Martin and Gene W. Matthews

INTRODUCTION

Twenty years from now, today's public health workforce will be viewed with awe because they knew the world before the 2020–2021 pandemic and were part of the struggle to overcome it. It has become abundantly clear that effective communication of public health challenges and interventions is essential to an effective public health practice, and to leading change in a polarized political environment.

Historical and policy conditions have left public health at a disadvantage in recognizing and responding to the political pressures it faces. To serve as effective messengers, public health practitioners need deeper insight into the intuitive frameworks that shape how the public health workforce engages with its intended audiences, given diverse social, political, and cultural contexts.

This chapter addresses ways public health leaders at all levels can more effectively communicate to meet urgent community needs. It also offers practical strategies for public health to become more trusted and effective messengers to shape change during challenging times ahead.

In this chapter the use of the general term "public health" is intended to include both public health leadership and frontline workforce, as well as the larger circle of allied public health collaborators who serve as healthcare and community health leaders and professionals.

OBJECTIVES

By the end of this chapter, the reader will be able to:

- Recognize the historical and political conditions that currently challenge public health's ability to change law and policy in order to meet urgent community needs.
- Address ways in which public health and healthcare leaders can communicate more deeply and meaningfully with communities of all backgrounds, given the politically polarized culture.
- Apply practical communication strategies that public health can use internally to improve its political skill sets, as well as externally to nurture the voices of other non-public health allies to support common efforts.

HISTORICAL CONTEXT OF COMMUNICATION IN PUBLIC HEALTH

For generations, the United States has experienced wide swings in the cultural and political responses to significant public health events (Figure 17.1).[1] In 1954 the first Salk polio vaccine was welcomed into a United States cultural and political landscape that had long awaited a tool to prevent a dangerous, contagious disease that had haunted the world for centuries. Although the Eisenhower Administration was generally opposed to "socialized medicine," it responded to widespread demand of the United States public for immediate polio vaccine access. All levels of government then quickly mobilized to implement a federally financed national polio vaccine immunization program, and the subsequent public participation in it was for the most part cohesive and remarkable.

By contrast, a generation after the discovery of the polio vaccine, the first cases of what was to be known as AIDS were identified in June 1981, accompanied by no vaccine or even any effective treatment. All of public health had to deal collectively with a slow-moving and polarized political response that included blaming the victims and/or stigmatizing those infected. Almost a decade passed, and many died before a cohesive prevention response was funded, implemented, and accepted.

Two decades after the arrival of AIDS, the terrorist attacks of September 11, 2001, and the appearance of anthrax spread in the U.S. Postal System immediately triggered a relatively cohesive national emergency response at all levels of the U.S. government. In response to these sudden and unanticipated developments, significant resources were provided for several years thereafter to rebuild the capacity of public health systems in order to respond to the threats of both intentional bioterrorism and newly emerging infectious diseases. Most of these resources were supplied through bipartisan support for large federal public health emergency preparedness grants that met this dual threat of bioterrorism and emerging infections. Unfortunately, public and political attention decreased over the next 5 years, and those same new funding streams that supported public health capacity gradually faded away.

Fast forward to 2020, and another generation was again suddenly faced with the most challenging pandemic in a century, COVID-19. Yet at that moment the U.S. public health

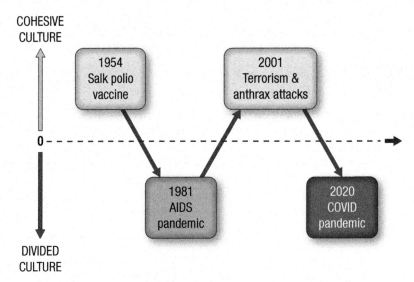

FIGURE 17.1: Swings in the Cultural Responses to Historic Public Health Events.
Source: Adapted from Matthews G, Martin B, Hunter D. Becoming better messengers to communicate public health: skill-building for public health advocacy. Presented at the Network for Public Health Law 2021 Conference; September 20, 2021; online.

systems found themselves under-resourced and unprepared to deal with key aspects of this event. Despite the most rapid, global effort to develop a highly successful vaccine in history, a sizable portion of the United States was skeptical. Many individuals chose to believe conspiracy theories spread by polarizing politicians and social media rather than being guided by the research and factual data reported by health experts.

These dramatic pendulum swings in the cycles of cultural and political history beg the question: *How can those working in public health become more effective and consistent communicators to community members and decision-makers?* Clearly, public health needs to do more than improve the words used in its messaging. Public health also needs to better understand and connect with the target audiences, and to build the necessary skill sets to become more trusted messengers to those being served.

INCREASING COMPLEXITY OF PUBLIC HEALTH ISSUES

Public health faces persistent and vexing population-level problems (e.g., the obesity epidemic, alcohol and substance abuse, and the opioid crisis). These problems have many contributing factors that span the community, institutional, and public policy levels. Underlying health inequities often lie at the root of these problems. Solutions to these more systemic issues are often socially or politically controversial. Stakeholders have differing opinions on how to address these problems, including whether —and to what extent—government has a role to play in solving them. Yet it often takes stakeholders across many sectors, working together, to address complex public health issues. Public health leaders need to engage diverse stakeholders to identify and carry out promising, synergistic, and sustainable actions to alleviate public health's greatest challenges.

Consider, for example, the obesity epidemic in the United States. Rates of obesity remain stubbornly high, and the economic and health impacts are immense. Experts continue to advocate for a broad array of evidence-based strategies that are community-based, and not just individually focused, to increase healthy nutrition and physical activity. Community-based solutions to reduce obesity are wide-ranging, from policies to improve school nutrition standards; zoning regulations to add bike lanes; and economic development in poor communities to combat "food deserts." Addressing these issues requires engaging many different stakeholders, including legislators, educators, the food industry, civic groups, government regulators, health leaders, and, most importantly, the impacted communities themselves. Yet these stakeholders may view the causes and effects of obesity very differently and disagree on solutions. For example, while some support regulating what can be served in public school lunches, others oppose this as government overreach.

COMPLEXITY OF COMMUNICATING ABOUT PUBLIC HEALTH

Not only are the public health and healthcare issues that leaders face more complex, communicating about them has also become increasingly daunting. The technology landscape for how public health distributes and receives information has changed immensely over the past few decades. People live in a time where 24-hour cable news, the internet, and social media channels offer endless information. If this were not challenging enough, unprecedented political polarization and the demonization of mainstream journalism as "fake news" have made it hard to know who—or what—to believe.

Public health and healthcare leaders must find ways to cut through the noise and effectively, persuasively communicate to stakeholders, no matter their political ideology. However, if public health leaders are to become more effective and consistent communicators with community members and decision-makers, they need to first wrestle with this question: *How does public health effectively communicate and garner buy-in with stakeholders who have different values, opinions, and agendas?* It is not as simple as agreeing that eating more vegetables is good for us.

THE PUBLIC HEALTH LEADERS' COMMUNICATION CRISIS

The 2020–2021 global pandemic was a perfect storm that engulfed public health and health-care. It exposed critical weaknesses in public health's ability to lead the country during the most daunting public health crisis of our time. It also became clear that local and state public health leaders had scarce resources and insufficient clout. Public health communication officials frequently must shape messages in a dynamic situation, without waiting for 100% data certainty, about issues that are evolving, complex, nuanced, and subject to unexpected change. In times of crisis, when new data and potentially conflicting information are emerging daily, public health leaders must be trusted messengers. Yet during the COVID pandemic, data-driven, evidence-based solutions like wearing masks and getting vaccinated were questioned, discounted, and even politically weaponized in the United States. Public health as a profession proved to be relatively unskilled at negotiating this complex political terrain and communicating effectively.

How did it come to this?

HOW WE GOT HERE: THE BACKSTORY

In the early 20th century, public health practice was more closely integrated into the U.S. political systems.[2] Local public health officials needed to have an effective political skill set to be able to implement community-wide infectious disease control measures such as ordering quarantines or closing public events. The first local boards of health were established by politicians both to gain the advantage of new expertise becoming available in health disciplines, and to provide themselves with some independent political cover when difficult policy choices became necessary. At the national level, U.S. Surgeon General Thomas Parran, in 1937, published a short book entitled *Shadow on the Land* to build broad U.S. support from industry, voluntary organizations, and the civic-minded to control syphilis.[3]

THE LONG DECLINE IN PUBLIC HEALTH'S POLITICAL SKILL SETS

Beginning in the middle of the 20th century, changes began to take place in the political orientation of public health, as illustrated in Figure 17.2. With the arrival in the 1950s of the availability of modern antibiotic treatments and the advent of the polio vaccines, the fear of dangerous contagious diseases diminished in the United States, and life expectancy increased.[4] Local health officers were less frequently called upon to use their political skill sets to implement quarantines and facility closures. Furthermore, in the 1960s large federally directed public health categorical grant programs began to emerge that were fueled by discretionary funding streams authorized by Congress. As these federal funding programs increased, public health departments became less dependent upon state and local political support for tax revenues appropriated by state and local elected officials.

Over time, the predominant mindset inside the public health profession during the 1970s and 1980s drifted in the direction of concern that too much engagement in politics might tarnish the independence, credibility, and scientific integrity of the research that formed the basis of public health actions. This internal perspective of "narrow public health" gained acceptance as a guiding principle, resulting in the public health workforce minimizing its engagement with political systems, legislatures, courts, and the business community. Public health became more insular and complacent with its comfortable niche in the governmental structures. (For more on this topic, see the 2012 article by Daniel Goldberg.)[5]

AWAKENING TO PUBLIC HEALTH'S COMMUNICATIONS GAP

As a result of this short-sighted philosophy, the political skill sets of public health leaders had atrophied by the time that taxpayer revolts (beginning with California's Proposition 13 in 1978) gained momentum to put limits on the amount of discretionary spending by

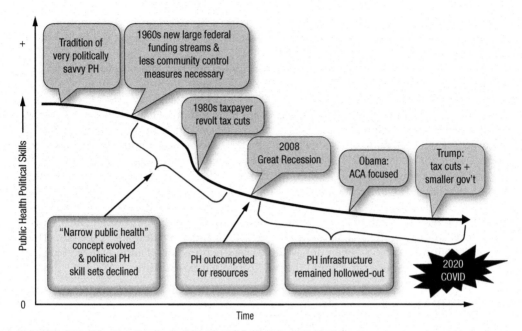

FIGURE 17.2: The Decline in Public Health's Political Skill Sets.
Source: Adapted from Matthews G, Martin B, Hunter D. Becoming better messengers to communicate public health: skill-building for public health advocacy. Presented at the Network for Public Health Law 2021 Conference; September 20, 2021; online.

governments. Eventually these popular taxpayer protections spread nationally, and public health then found itself unskilled to adapt and compete in this new landscape for their share of shrinking federal, state, and local budgets.

Meanwhile, the other sectors of government, like agriculture, education, and transportation, had always maintained their political skill sets and external allies to support them. Governmental agriculture agencies constantly nurtured close connections and political alliances to external organizations like the Future Farmers of America, 4-H Clubs, state fairs expositions, local and state farmer organizations, food processors, manufacturers, and bipartisan elected officials who could advocate for appropriation resources. Educational agencies had similarly maintained close alliances with teachers' unions, PTA organizations, schools and colleges, and the broader base of parents actively participating in the political process to improve the quality of education for their children. Transportation departments at the federal, state, and local levels retained and expanded their alliances with external advocates dating back to the days of the New Deal, such as construction industries, businesses seeking to improve supply chains, and communities seeking the jobs provided by large local public works projects. With the enactment of Medicare and Medicaid in the 1960s, healthcare providers, the pharmaceutical industry, medical device manufacturers, and even insurance companies developed increasingly robust advocacy components to make sure that government funding was available to support governmental healthcare reimbursement programs.[2,5]

In the face of the general reductions in discretionary spending in the 1980s, these other sectors of government could advocate more effectively than public health for appropriations at all levels despite tightening budget caps. A widening public health communications gap had emerged with both elected officials, as well as their constituents, about the fundamental role and importance of population health to their communities.

Other factors have further limited public health messaging and advocacy efforts. State preemption laws, limitations on agency appropriations, and internal rules of conduct for government employees have often been used by forces that seek to limit the authority and voice of public health leaders. The net effect has been a weakening of local public health authority, a chilling of public education and debate, a deceleration in the adoption of innovative public health policies, and even the sowing of divisions within the public health community itself.[6,7]

It is worth noting that there were some unanticipated and temporary infusions of funding into the public health sector in the form of the public health preparedness funding streams, which were in response to the September 11, 2001, terrorist attacks. By the time of the Great Recession of 2008, however, most of these preparedness resources had dwindled away. Public health still found itself without the political skill sets to anticipate and compete with other governmental sectors, like transportation, for the "shovel ready" spending projects that were expediently enacted and implemented to boost the U.S. economy in 2008 to 2010. The net result is that public health agency budgets at the federal, state, local, and tribal levels all remained hollowed-out after the 2008 recession.

Unfortunately for public health, in the subsequent years through 2016, the Obama Administration had to use all of its available political capital simply to protect against successive efforts to dismantle its signature policy achievement, the Affordable Care Act. There was little political flexibility for a public health-friendly presidential administration to effectively add federal resources to rebuild the public health infrastructure.

PUBLIC HEALTH AMID THE PERFECT STORM

In 2016 the Trump Administration was elected on a platform in part to cut government spending and dismantle "Obamacare," the previous administration's healthcare achievement. As a result, the problems for public health only increased with respect to the lack of traction for rebuilding public health resources and for communicating effective public health messaging.

Similarly, public health has struggled with the decreasing level of civil discourse in the recent U.S. cultural and political environment. The heart of public health is community coalition building. This is essential to identifying local needs and empowering communities to establish priorities for making change. Yet building coalitions and engaging in civil conversations becomes more difficult at the local level amid echo chambers reverberating across social media that encourage divisiveness and political polarization. In 2020, public health found itself being weaponized by both major U.S. political parties as the coronavirus pandemic became a driving issue in the run-up to the November presidential election. A current challenge continues to be that, in this era of 24/7 social media, the public's 21st century brains seem to prefer a simple lie over the complex truth. It is unfortunate that public health constantly deals with complexities in a dynamic environment, where simple and final answers are rarely available.

The net result is that by the time the coronavirus pandemic struck in early 2020, the U.S. public health systems found themselves seriously under-resourced, without internal political skill sets in persuasive communication, and without external allies to understand and advocate for public health in a polarized political environment.

AN OPENING FOR PUBLIC HEALTH LEADERS

If this history underscores anything for public health and healthcare leaders, it is this: your voice is vital. Public health cannot shy away from engaging with local political decision-makers; on the contrary, it is time to lean in. To do this, public health must improve its communications skill sets, build allies outside of public health, reach out to its splintered communities, and become more trusted messengers.

The good news is that public health and local elected leaders share a common goal: to take care of their communities. Local policy makers are more connected to their communities than those at the state or federal level. This presents an opening for public health. Just as former U.S. Speaker of the House Tip O'Neill famously said, "All politics are local," public health must get back to its roots and strengthen its relationships with local decision-making stakeholders. This will help overcome the sharp polarization that has politicized many health issues, like the opioid crisis and coronavirus pandemic. To strengthen those ties, public health and healthcare leaders need to develop stronger communication skills.

UNDERSTANDING COMMUNICATION

WHAT GOES INTO COMMUNICATION?

There are many challenges inherent in effectively communicating and securing buy-in among different audiences. McGuire's Persuasion Matrix[8] provides a useful framework for considering these challenges—and for identifying solutions.

According to McGuire's Persuasion Matrix, there are five inputs to communication: the *sender*, the *receiver*, the *message*, the *channel*, and the *context* (refer to the left side of Figure 17.3). Public health and healthcare leaders need to optimize each of these elements for their communications to be effective. First, as communication *senders*, leaders need to consider and assess their own interpersonal and communication skills, as well as their values and beliefs about both the public health issue and the stakeholders with whom they are communicating. Communication is often influenced by the sender's personal and professional credibility, their power and authority, and by their social capital (i.e., the networks and social connections they need to tap to effectively produce the changes they seek). Second, these influencing factors also exist for the intended *receiver*. Whether the receiver is a local politician, business leader, or other type of stakeholder, their receptivity to what is being communicated will be influenced by their own values, knowledge, and beliefs about the public health issue (the message), as well as their perception of the sender. Third, when public health issues are complex, *messages* can be complicated to construct. Effective framing is key. This is discussed in detail in the next section. Fourth, there are a variety of *channels* by which to deliver messages. Channels might involve traditional or social media, direct action advocacy, one-on-one communication, going through an intermediary, and so on. Finally, leaders need to consider the larger *context* in which their communication is occurring. Many complex issues compete for stakeholder attention. In addition, historical and cultural contexts around the public health issue, the current political climate, and other external factors can heighten or dampen the effectiveness of communication efforts.

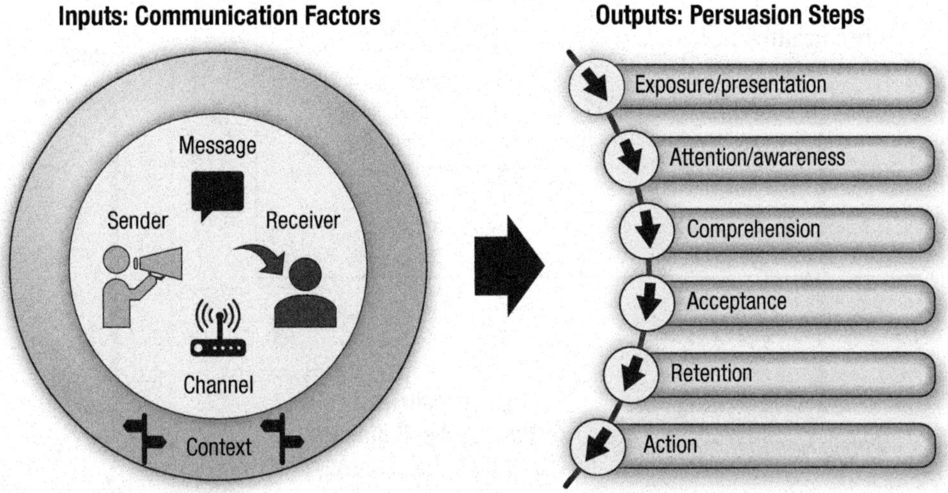

FIGURE 17.3: McGuire's Persuasion Matrix.

Source: Reproduced with permission from Martin BA. *Improving Public Health Communication in a Politically Polarized Environment: Exploring the Use of Moral Values in Message Framing*. Dissertation. 2021. University of North Carolina at Chapel Hill. https://cdr.lib.unc.edu/concern/dissertations/dj52wf88m

The right side of McGuire's Persuasion Matrix describes the outputs that represent the steps in the persuasion process: *exposure/presentation, attention/awareness, comprehension, acceptance, retention,* and *action.* The sequential and somewhat cyclical nature of the outputs reflect that communication is ever evolving and adjusting. Lessons are learned about what works and what does not. Often, the context changes. Messages need to be adapted.

THERE ARE DIFFERENT WAYS FOR PUBLIC HEALTH TO COMMUNICATE

There are multiple mechanisms by which public health and healthcare leaders communicate to the public to influence their social norms and behaviors (see Figure 17.4). As illustrated by the top arrow, public health can communicate directly to the public. This is often done through public awareness campaigns. Public health leaders can also influence norms and behavior by framing messages for the public and by using earned (i.e., free) media to make a topic more salient and "in the news." Looking one level down, public health can use additional routes to influence public norms and behaviors by communicating to—and through—stakeholders. Stakeholders can be a diverse collection of individuals, organizations, or agencies that have a relevant and significant interest in the causes, consequences, or impacts of an issue. Some stakeholders (e.g., advocacy organizations, the media, community coalitions) address public health issues by directly communicating with the public. Other stakeholders, like elected officials, hospital and business leaders, and judges, have the authority to adopt laws, institutional policies, regulations, or rulings. Public health leaders can leverage these laws and policies (e.g., smoke-free ordinances, city funding for greenways) as platforms to communicate to—and influence—the public about the norms and behaviors

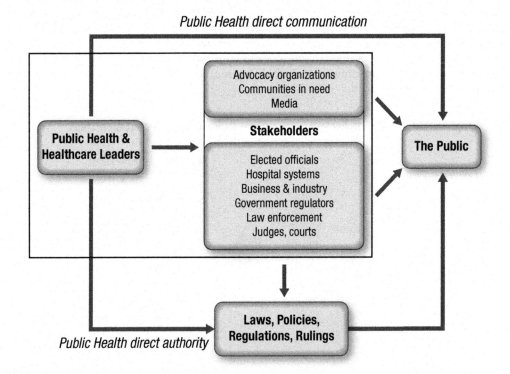

FIGURE 17.4: Ways for Public Health and Healthcare Leaders to Communicate.

Source: Reproduced with permission from Martin BA. *Improving Public Health Communication in a Politically Polarized Environment: Exploring the Use of Moral Values in Message Framing* [dissertation]. 2021. University of North Carolina at Chapel Hill. https://cdr.lib.unc.edu/concern/dissertations/dj52wf88m

that matter most. As shown on the very bottom arrow, there are also certain channels whereby public health has direct legal authority to communicate and influence public behavior through policy (e.g., COVID-related quarantines and mask mandates).

CHANNELS FOR EFFECTIVE COMMUNICATION

There are a variety of channels through which public health and healthcare leaders can reach policy-level stakeholders. Some general examples include holding a press conference, conducting media briefings, publishing op-ed pieces and letters to the editor in mainstream and online media, and meeting with newspaper editorial boards. Similarly, leaders can use educational and marketing tools like expert panels, polls, and online discussion boards to gather information. This material then can be targeted to stakeholders through public forums, dedicated websites, social media platforms, and other communication channels that are relevant and valued by the intended audience.

WHEN IT COMES TO COMMUNICATION, CONTEXT MATTERS

General wisdom holds that the larger political and cultural context plays an important role in the degree to which civic and government leaders support or oppose complicated community issues. Context can include historic, economic, or political circumstances affecting or experienced by a community, as well as the timing of the problem and its proposed solution. For example, in the 1980s political leaders began looking at the AIDS crisis differently after media attention about Ryan White, a young boy with hemophilia who contracted HIV from an HIV-contaminated blood transfusion. Shortly after his death, a major piece of AIDS legislation, the Ryan White CARE Act, was passed by the U.S. Congress to provide services for people living with HIV/AIDS. Context can also reflect deep-seated, implicit racial biases. For example, even though Blacks and Whites have long used illicit drugs in similar proportions, media coverage and policy and law enforcement responses have differed greatly.[9] When the focus of the opioid addiction of the 1980s and 1990s was on urban Blacks and Latinos, the War on Drugs response was to criminalize heroin injectors. By contrast, media coverage was much more sympathetic in the 2000s, when the face of the epidemic was suburban, White, prescription opioid users. Instead of pushing for the incarceration of users, policy responses focused on treatment, education, and cracking down on trafficking. Context matters.

CREDIBILITY WITH THE MESSAGE'S INTENDED AUDIENCE

Who delivers the message can be as impactful as the message itself. Key considerations are the sender's credibility with the intended audience and their skills as a communicator. Be aware of unintended effects. For example, physicians are viewed as authorities on health-related issues, so they are often sought out to be spokespeople and advocates. The public, however, often does not understand the difference between healthcare and public health, or the distinction between personal health and systemic factors. For a message that is intended to increase awareness and support for prevention or population-level changes, a public health champion may be a more effective sender than a medical provider. Another point: sometimes it is the *unexpected* stakeholder who can make a bigger impact as the message sender. Think of a chamber of commerce president speaking out in favor of a smoke-free ordinance, or a police chief advocating for increased funding for drug treatment and needle exchange programs. Such unexpected validators should be identified early and given a platform to advocate for public health.

Senders need to be skilled in how to be effective communicators. As mentioned earlier, the public health workforce has lost ground in its historical ability to effectively work with local political officials. As explained later in this chapter, recent research suggests that the public health workforce may have blind spots in their understanding of the intuitive values driving the judgments and reasoning among certain audiences.[10] Before introducing the concept of intuitive values, however, it is necessary to address certain aspects of framing.

MESSAGE FRAMING IS CRITICAL TO EFFECTIVE COMMUNICATION

Framing is defined as "selecting some aspects of a perceived reality and make them more salient in a communicating text, in such a way as to promote a particular problem definition, causal interpretation, moral evaluation, and/or treatment recommendation for the item described."[11(p52)]

There are different types of framing that can be strategically used for effective communication; for example, *diagnostic framing* focuses on what the problem is and how to define it, *prognostic framing* focuses on how to solve the problem, and *motivational framing* offers the call to action.[12]

> *[Message] framing is about the choices we make in what we say, how we say it, what we emphasize, what we leave unsaid, and how these choices shape how people think, feel, and act. Framing plays a major role in social change. . . . The way the media, political leaders, and advocates frame issues shapes how the public sees the world.*[13(paras1-3)]

It is important for public health leaders to recognize how to frame messages to maximize receptivity. Sometimes framing public health issues as a societal problem rather than only a public health issue can support political agenda setting. This is particularly important for policy stakeholders who are not already familiar or engaged with public health, so they can still find resonance with the issue. In other situations, health-focused talking points are not necessarily the most compelling frames by which to engage others. For example, obesity is too often considered a problem primarily for the healthcare sector to solve. Yet there are evidence-based policy solutions that illuminate the need for broader changes across society. Research suggests that when communicating about obesity, it may be more effective to frame it in terms of both individual responsibility for health *and* as a systemic issue with social and environmental causes. Such "co-framing" can help underscore the symbiotic relationship between individual choices and the influences that physical and social environments have on a person's behavioral choices.[14] Public health leaders need to be more open to and strategic about "co-framing" complex health problems—for example, as health *and* non-health-focused, or as impacting individuals *and* systems—in an effort to build more stakeholder buy-in. One important way to do this is by using a policy entrepreneur. These are highly motivated individuals who are often the driving force for change. They form coalitions to encourage dialogue and foster policy learning. They strategically serve as a bridge builder across sectors and to help find common interests with stakeholders. They are skilled at reframing issues to emphasize certain benefits to specific stakeholder audiences.

In effective communication, leaders can also frame problems and messages in ways that accelerate action on public health priorities. When a stakeholder says no to a public health policy solution, it is important to understand why. Public health leaders need to consider the underlying perceptions, motivations, and choices of that stakeholder. By clearly understanding these, one can then frame a problem in a way that gets the person to say "yes."

THE IMPORTANCE OF FRAMING FOR PUBLIC HEALTH

People with different political perspectives often view complex health issues differently. A study commissioned by The Robert Wood Johnson Foundation (RWJF) found there were differences in how Democrats and Republicans viewed the social determinants of health.[15] These variations were based on distinctions in the deep metaphor frames that people in these groups held. These types of frames influence how individuals view the world and largely function at an unconscious level.

Research by the FrameWorks Institute has found that the very concept of "health" is defined quite differently by public health professionals versus stakeholders in other sectors. Public health experts consider health to be a "positive state of integrated well-being." By contrast, leaders from other sectors like education, housing, business, and health systems thought of health as "the absence of illness." These other sector leaders also thought that public health professionals lacked the necessary skills and perspectives to meaningfully contribute to the work of their sectors.[16]

To help the public health profession more effectively communicate the value of public health, a resource called PHRASES—*Public Health Reaching Across Sectors*—was developed by communications experts (www.phrases.org). Drawing on robust polling and findings from focus groups, PHRASES provides evidence-based framing tools and resources to help public health professionals communicate and collaborate more effectively. Their goal is to foster a better understanding of public health and a greater willingness of other sectors to engage in cross-sector partnerships with public health professionals. PHRASES was designed with the strategic understanding that many sectors, including education, business, housing, and health systems, have roles to play in improving health outcomes and building healthier communities. Yet many leaders in these other sectors do not understand the value of partnering with public health. By providing public health professionals more training and skills in how to effectively communicate their value to other sectors, PHRASES can help motivate other sectors to support public health efforts.

PHRASES was developed by the de Beaumont Foundation in partnership with the Aspen Institute. The de Beaumont Foundation focuses on improving health at the community level by investing in tools, partnerships, policies, and the public health workforce.

As one resource example, the PHRASES tool kit offers a useful method for communication called The Narrative Structure.[17] Messages should include four elements to optimize their power to motivate: people, goal, problem, and solution. Each element needs to be framed in a way to tell the most compelling "story."

CRAFTING MESSAGES WITH THE INTENDED AUDIENCE IN MIND

To be effective communicators, public health and healthcare leaders must craft messages in ways that are most appealing to their intended audience. While this seems intuitive, many in public health and healthcare do not do this in practice.

Effective practices include creating messages that combine facts and data with emotional appeals, because frames that use emotional appeals are more compelling. Messages need to be culturally relevant, transparent, respectful, and flexible to change. Headlines (and subject lines) should be concise and easy to remember. Messages should be communicated in clear, simple language.

The practical problem is that many public health issues are just not that simple. There is often a vast web of factors that contribute to the problem, and there is rarely a single silver bullet solution. To be more effective in their communication, public health and healthcare leaders need to know how to acknowledge the complexity of issues while at the same time providing clear, tailored, and compelling messaging.

In the next sections, the chapter explores three areas that are vital for effective public health communication: the role of empathy, the importance of centering equity, and the use of intuitive moral values in framing messages.

THE ROLE OF EMPATHY IN BECOMING A BETTER MESSENGER[a]

Empathy is important in public health communications because it serves to build relationships, to reframe and connect with the audience, and to establish public health communicators as trusted messengers. Two key components of empathetic communication are active listening and storytelling.

Active listening requires the communicator to practice humility about one's own opinions and moral frameworks and to maintain a genuine curiosity about those of other people. (Refer to Chapter 1, "Dialogue: A Foundational Skill for Effective Health Leadership," for more on active listening.) In one-on-one conversation, the first step is to pause and not jump in with one's own opinions about the topic. Ask open questions like: *What is your perspective on this issue? Can you tell me more about that? Can you give me an example?* When you are called upon to speak, it is equally important to be candid about where you and your public health colleagues stand on an issue. State your view concisely and give the data or interpretations that may have informed your view. To keep the dialogue going, you might ask, *What am I missing?* or, *Do you see where I'm coming from?* It is also helpful to ask *yourself* questions to challenge your own biases and prompt empathetic framing before you engage; for example, *Why would a person who values care and fairness as much as I do believe what this person believes?*

As mentioned elsewhere in this chapter, *stories* are also very valuable because they can touch individuals and make them care. Dr. Neal Baer provides valuable insight to apply to public health: "Most people are not data-driven. They are driven by emotional stories. Only then, can we provide the data, give them context, give them evidence. But they need to be moved by the story first."[18(para3)] In framing stories, keep in mind themes, not just episodes or events. Avoid relying too much on the individual, especially heroic individuals overcoming all odds. Begin by providing context, trends, and/or an illustrative community problem needing change using your own words.

Whether in conversation or speaking to a wider audience, using empathy to develop effective messages requires one to:

- **Beware shaming and name calling:** Such adversarial approaches only drive the other person away and shut down the foundation for meaningful communication. Remember to avoid this on social media as well as in conversation with community members.

- **Offer individuals a sense of control:** Give the other person the opportunity to explain why or how they have arrived at their current viewpoint. If there's a specific action you want them to take, offer multiple pathways, emphasizing the validity of each.

- **Enlist trusted partners who may be unexpected validators:** One of the most valuable assets in communication and advocacy is discovering a person from a different political or social point of view who agrees with you on your particular issue. Let that person have the opportunity to be the unexpected validator to advocate for the issue. For example, use law enforcement officials to speak in favor of a sterile needle exchange program because such programs increase the safety for their police officers.

- **Emphasize benefits over threats:** Focus more on the positive aspects of your recommendation rather than the negative consequences of it not being followed, which may make the other person defensive and shut down.

- **Connect to what's meaningful to the audience, not to you:** Focus your message on the values and interest of the intended audience, not your own personal values.

[a]Acknowledgment: This section comes from a series of *Becoming Better Messenger* workshops and webinars developed and presented by Elizabeth Sureau Thomas of UNC in 2021.

■ **Remember that public health is a long game:** Even the best listening skills and messaging won't win over every audience member. By demonstrating that you care and that you're curious and empathetic, you will become a more trusted partner. This will pay dividends over time in your community.

CENTERING EQUITY IN PUBLIC HEALTH COMMUNICATION[b]

Centering equity is another valuable messaging tool that can contribute to the identification and elimination of structural racism in public health and healthcare. It requires focusing on both the *content* of the message and the *outcome* of the message. The reason for centering equity is to share solutions that ensure everyone has what they need, in the way they need it, in order to have the best health possible. Centering equity also helps reach people where they are and normalizes conversations about what leads to differences in health outcomes.

There are several components for creating a foundation for equitable messaging.

1. **Know your audience:** You may find your audience along a collaboration continuum that ranges between resistant, curious, aware, advocate, or champion. In addition, you may find your audience to be somewhere along another stakeholder management spectrum that ranges across unaware, resistant, neutral, supportive, or leading. Once you have a feel for your audience within these ranges, you may then have a better feel for the arguments or messages that will fit where they are located on these two spectrums.

For example, in discussing the need for a higher minimum wage, there are a range of choices to apply depending upon your knowledge of your audience that might best resonate with that particular topic:

■ **Reduced reliance on public benefits:** This approach may resonate better with fiscal conservative audiences.

■ **Protection for American workers:** This framing may appeal to working class audiences and the economically underserved.

■ **Increased consumer spending:** This choice may resonate better with free market and business communities.

■ **Better health outcomes:** This approach has the potential to appeal across the political and social spectrum.

■ **Economic stability for struggling families:** This choice resonates strongly with people in need.

■ **Fewer people in poverty:** Interestingly, this framing may resonate both to those in need and to fiscal conservatives.

■ **Black, Hispanic, Latino, and Indigenous employees will see reductions in pay disparity:** This approach has appeal to people of color as well as to all groups promoting social justice.

2. **Focus on systems, places, or conditions:** Identifying the systems, places, or conditions that affect health outcomes focuses the narrative on structural factors as points of intervention instead of a personal responsibility narrative. This is important because it recognizes that there are several factors that influence health outcomes aside from individual behaviors, and that changing individual behavior will not lead to systemic change. For example, instead of using a person-directed statement like, "African American people in this community have more cases of COVID-19," consider using a message focusing more on conditions: "COVID-19 is more common in communities that have a higher risk of asthma and chronic obstructive pulmonary disease (COPD) due to environmental hazards."

[b]Acknowledgment: This material is developed from presentations by Dawn Hunter, Regional Director, Southeastern Region, Network for Public Health Law during webinars with the authors at an ASTHO leaders workshop on July 14, 2021 and at the 2021 Public Health Law Conference on September 20, 2021.

3. **Use storytelling:** As previously discussed in the section on empathy, the use of an effective story can unlock the conversation and then connect people and their experiences to your data. Storytelling can be used to influence behavior by connecting information or data to personal impact, such as when people share stories of why they chose to get vaccinated or stopped smoking. Storytelling also provides an opportunity to highlight the strengths and assets of your community through the eyes and voices of the people who are impacted by policies, programs, and services. For example, a city might share information about free exercise zones in city parks, but a community member might share how access to those free exercise zones enabled them to stay active and engage their whole family during the pandemic. In addition, your own credibility is improved by stories that can expand the understanding of and buy-in to your organization by demonstrating your organization's value and impact. For public health, this means telling the story of how programs and services keep people and communities healthy.

4. **Be authentic:** In this same context use language that is meaningful to your audience and to you by recognizing relevant characteristics of your audience like age, affiliation (for example, a church community or professional association), languages used, education level, and other factors. Meaningful communications also connect content to values and personal experience; they are relatable to the audience. Frequently it is more effective to engage trusted community partners to deliver the message. Always be mindful to use translators and interpreters for the languages commonly spoken in your community. Above all, strive to center the voices of the impacted community members.

5. **Understand the opposition:** In all advocacy communications, it is essential to know who is likely to oppose you and anticipate what messages they may be using. Analyze various arguments and perspectives with a particular focus on understanding and seeking more information on positions that differ from your own. Keep in mind how your own communication responds to the context of the opponent's position, as well as how they might coordinate their own advocacy tactics. These steps can be informal or undertaken as part of a structured stakeholder analysis process that identifies stakeholders (audience members) and their interests and maps them according to factors like power, interest, and urgency. Whether you use an informal or structured process, taking steps to understand the opposition can allow you to anticipate responses, prevent misunderstandings, and identify ways to leverage relationships as part of developing and disseminating messages.

6. **Always be aware of your own limitations:** To prepare yourself for sensitive conversations relating to health equity and systemic racism, it can be helpful to do a self-assessment of your own cognitive biases that are part of your history. Questions you can ask yourself may include thinking about the following biases that challenge us all:

   ■ **Confirmation bias:** *What are your own preconceived notions about racial equity? About people of different races and abilities? How do these beliefs influence your message?*

   ■ **In-group favoritism:** *What groups do you belong to? How diverse are they? Does your audience look like any of the groups you belong to?*

   ■ **Framing effect:** *What kind of spin are you putting on the data? Why?*

   ■ **Authority bias:** *Who do people in your target group trust? Do people trust your organization? If not, what are you doing to build trust?*

In conclusion, in conversations on health equity, look to emphasize the common good. The improvement in the health of one group does not mean that another group's health will decrease. Health equity is not a zero-sum game. Everyone benefits from improving the health of the entire population.

USING MORAL FOUNDATIONS THEORY TO INFORM COMMUNICATION

INTUITIVE MORAL VALUES UNDERPIN COMMUNICATION

One important component for persuading stakeholders involves deeper insight into the way that messages speak to their moral intuitions. Research shows that social and political judgments depend heavily on quick (and largely unconscious) intuitive appraisals.[19] Public health leaders can benefit from a deeper understanding of the intuitive moral values of their stakeholders to ensure that public health messages reach and influence their intended audiences.

In particular, public health and healthcare leaders can be more effective communicators with external stakeholders if they maintain an awareness of what underpins effective communication—and then frame messaging to fit the moral foundations (and political world-view) of the audience.

There is promising, preliminary evidence that persuasive messages framed using moral foundations that align with the recipient's political views can be effective in increasing behavioral intentions and behaviors like recycling, charitable donation, or policy support.[20–22] One implication is that guiding people to consider certain moral foundations may be an effective way to promote self-control goals, such as sticking to a diet or exercise routine.[23]

WHAT ARE MORAL FOUNDATIONS?

In his 2012 book *The Righteous Mind*, Jonathan Haidt describes Moral Foundations Theory.[19] Based in evolutionary moral psychology, its premise is that one's thinking is primarily and first guided by one's intuitions; strategic reasoning comes second. This is particularly true for one's social and political judgments. Think of judgments like a rider and an elephant: 90% is guided by the intuitive elephant, and just 10% by the rational brain riding on top (Figure 17.5).

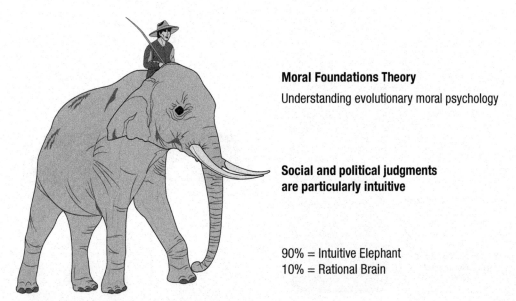

Intuitions come first, strategic reasoning second

Moral Foundations Theory
Understanding evolutionary moral psychology

Social and political judgments are particularly intuitive

90% = Intuitive Elephant
10% = Rational Brain

FIGURE 17.5: Moral Foundations Theory.
Source: Reproduced with permission from Matthews G, Martin B, Hunter D. Becoming better messengers to communicate public health: skill-building for public health advocacy. Presented at the Network for Public Health Law 2021 Conference; September 20, 2021; online.

Moral Foundations Theory posits that people's intuitions and reasoning are guided by six moral foundations: *care, fairness, loyalty, authority, sanctity,* and *liberty* (see Figure 17.6). *Care* refers to concern for the vulnerable and intolerance of harm or suffering. *Fairness* means an appreciation for impartial or just treatment, and a social intolerance for cheaters or "free riders." *Loyalty* refers to cherishing the group and despising those who betray it. *Authority* refers to a belief that legitimate authority should be obeyed and that it is wrong to subvert rightful leaders. *Sanctity* refers to feeling that some things are sacred and pure, and disgust for things that contaminate the mind, body, or spirit. *Liberty* refers to a preference for free choices and actions, and a disdain for bullies and dictators. People are more likely to engage in efforts that align with their moral values.

Research finds there is a relationship between people's moral values and where they fall along the political spectrum. Specifically, there are consistent differences in which moral foundations resonate for people, and these differences relate to whether the respondents are politically liberal (focused on helping those in need) or conservative (focused on preserving norms and traditional institutions).[24] Those who are politically liberal tend to resonate most with the individualizing moral foundations (care and fairness) and least with the binding foundations (loyalty, authority, and sanctity). Political conservatives tend to resonate with all six moral foundations and, in particular, with the binding foundations.

Care and fairness are categorized as individualizing foundations—meaning they use the individual as the starting point of moral value, and the focus is on protecting individuals from harm by other individuals or by societal systems. Loyalty, authority, and sanctity make up the binding foundations, which view the family as the starting point for society. The focus is on values that bind people into moral obligations and mutual accountability.

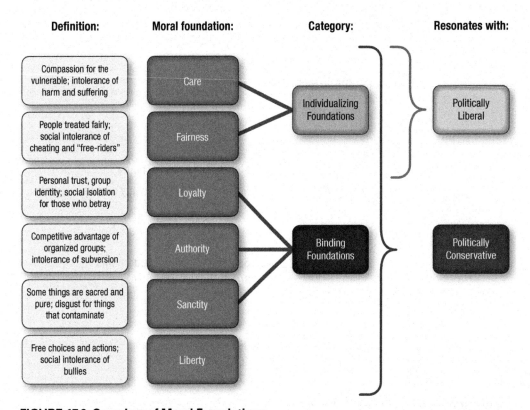

FIGURE 17.6: Overview of Moral Foundations.

Source: Reproduced with permission from Martin BA. *Improving Public Health Communication in a Politically Polarized Environment: Exploring the Use of Moral Values in Message Framing.* Dissertation. 2021. University of North Carolina at Chapel Hill. https://cdr.lib.unc.edu/concern/dissertations/dj52wf88m

THE PUBLIC HEALTH ADVANTAGE

In *The Righteous Mind*, Jonathan Haidt suggests that political conservatives have an inherent advantage because they resonate to some degree with all six intuitive moral foundations. Political liberals, on the other hand, strongly resonate with just two—care and fairness—and score significantly lower on the binding foundations (loyalty, authority, and sanctity).

Scott Burris and other thought leaders contend that public health can also authentically resonate with—and thus message on—all six moral foundations (see Figure 17.7).[25] This presents an advantage for public health leaders. Here is why: it is the authors' experience that in external messaging, public health almost reflexively resonates with the values of care and fairness, as well as liberty. Recent data, however, find that public health resonates quite well with the other three "binding" moral foundations.[10] This finding makes sense. The heart of public health is community coalition-building, which taps into loyalty. Public health has utilized its police power when necessary for quarantines, food inspection, and facility closures, which corresponds with authority. Public health altruistically embraces moving into disease situations to aid others even where there is personal risk, which draws on sanctity.

MORAL FOUNDATIONS PROFILE OF THE PUBLIC HEALTH WORKFORCE

A study in 2021 assessed the moral foundations of over 500 public health practitioners and local elected officials in one southeastern state in the United States.[10] There were several interesting takeaways:

1. The public health workforce seems to resonate with all six moral foundations. While it was expected that public health would connect strongly with care and fairness, it is useful to learn that the public health workforce connected with the other intuitive moral values as well (Figure 17.8).

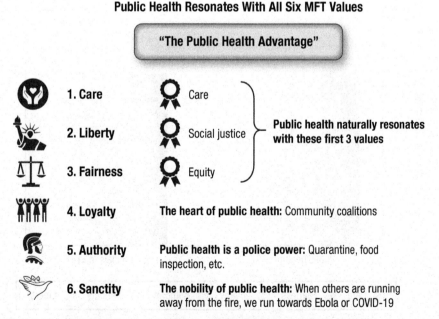

Public Health Resonates With All Six MFT Values

"The Public Health Advantage"

1. Care — Care
2. Liberty — Social justice
3. Fairness — Equity

Public health naturally resonates with these first 3 values

4. Loyalty — **The heart of public health:** Community coalitions

5. Authority — **Public health is a police power:** Quarantine, food inspection, etc.

6. Sanctity — **The nobility of public health:** When others are running away from the fire, we run towards Ebola or COVID-19

FIGURE 17.7: The Public Health Advantage. MFT, Moral Foundations Theory.

Source: Reproduced with permission from Matthews G, Martin B, Hunter D. Becoming better messengers to communicate public health: skill-building for public health advocacy. Presented at the Network for Public Health Law 2021 Conference; September 20, 2021; online.

2. Although public health and local officials had significantly different scores within each moral foundation, the overall *pattern* (higher in care and fairness, somewhat lower on the binding foundations of loyalty, authority, and sanctity) was quite similar (Figure 17.8). This suggests that when it comes to foundational moral values, public health has more in common with this important stakeholder than it might realize. When public health professionals do communicate with local officials, this research suggests they can and should message first around care and fairness. What comes naturally to public health also intuitively appears to resonate with local officials, at least on these two issues. Leaders cannot limit their communications to framing with those individualizing moral foundations. Leaders need to be mindful to speak to the intuitive moral values of their audiences, not just of themselves.

3. There were clear differences in moral foundations by political views (Figure 17.9). As expected, liberals were highest on care and fairness (the individualizing foundations). Conservatives were highest on loyalty, authority, and sanctity (the binding foundations), as well as liberty. Political moderates (shown in purple) were in between. This suggests that when communicating with stakeholders, consider framing using moral foundations that align with their political views.

4. Those with the lowest education level had higher scores for loyalty, authority, sanctity, and liberty—a moral foundations profile that looked similar to the pattern for political conservatives (Figure 17.10).

5. Older respondents scored higher across all moral foundations compared to the other age cohorts (Figure 17.11). The implication is that public health practitioners may have more opportunities to connect with older officials across a broader range of foundational moral values.

6. The youngest members of the public health workforce scored the lowest on loyalty, authority, and sanctity (Figure 17.11). Yet those are moral values that resonate for local elected officials (see Figure 17.8). They may have a blind spot when it comes to talking with political conservatives. This can be addressed through training and skills building.

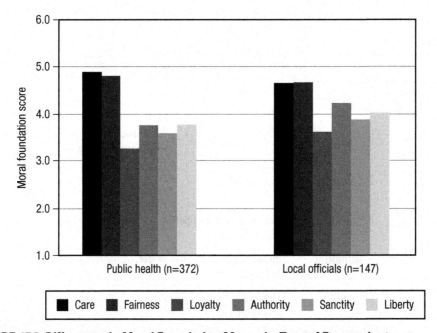

FIGURE 17.8: Differences in Moral Foundation Means by Type of Respondent.

Source: Reproduced with permission from Martin BA. *Improving Public Health Communication in a Politically Polarized Environment: Exploring the Use of Moral Values in Message Framing.* Dissertation. 2021. University of North Carolina at Chapel Hill. https://cdr.lib.unc.edu/concern/dissertations/dj52wf88m

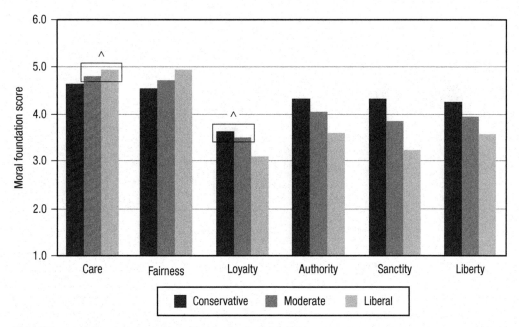

FIGURE 17.9: Moral Foundation Means by Political Views.

^Means for the pairs in the boxes were *not* significantly different from each other. All other pairwise comparisons were significantly different.

Source: Reproduced with permission from Martin BA. *Improving Public Health Communication in a Politically Polarized Environment: Exploring the Use of Moral Values in Message Framing*. Dissertation. 2021. University of North Carolina at Chapel Hill. https://cdr.lib.unc.edu/concern/dissertations/dj52wf88m

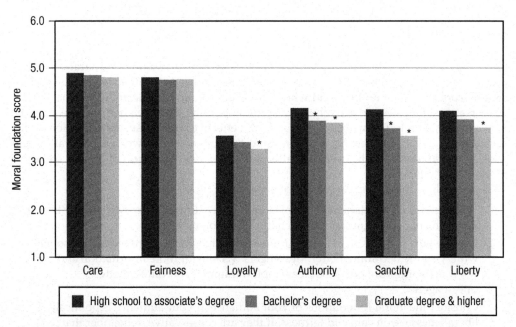

FIGURE 17.10: Moral Foundation Means by Education Level.

*Means were significantly different from those with high school (HS) to associate's degrees.

Source: Reproduced with permission from Martin BA. *Improving Public Health Communication in a Politically Polarized Environment: Exploring the Use of Moral Values in Message Framing*. Dissertation. 2021. University of North Carolina at Chapel Hill. https://cdr.lib.unc.edu/concern/dissertations/dj52wf88m

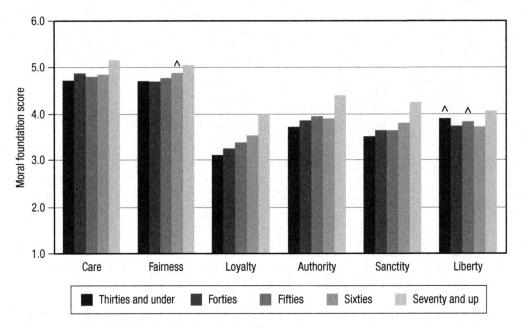

FIGURE 17.11: Moral Foundation Means by Age.

^Means were *not* significantly different from seventy and up. All other pairwise comparisons with seventy and up were significantly different.

Source: Reproduced with permission from Martin BA. *Improving Public Health Communication in a Politically Polarized Environment: Exploring the Use of Moral Values in Message Framing*. Dissertation. 2021. University of North Carolina at Chapel Hill. https://cdr.lib.unc.edu/concern/dissertations/dj52wf88m

PUTTING IT TOGETHER TO BECOME A BETTER MESSENGER

Changing laws and policies require interdisciplinary collaborations and strategic advocacy. When building those collaborations, public health needs to proactively engage decision-makers and communities. And when public health and healthcare leaders have these conversations, they need to actively listen for how intuitive moral values are revealed. The reasoning is that intuitive moral values underpin effective communication; intuitions come first, strategic reasoning second. Keep in mind the connection between moral values and political worldviews. Finally, public health must be aware of its individual and collective moral value "blind spots."

Here are three things you can do to become a better messenger

1. Take the Moral Foundations Assessment at https://tinyurl.com/MFTsurvey-book to learn which moral foundations you naturally resonate with.

2. Practice how to speak to the moral foundations that you *don't* necessarily resonate with. Visit the Becoming Better Messengers website for more information and tools: www.networkforphl.org/resources/topics/trainings/becoming-better -messengers

3. Consider the moral foundations of your audience. If your audience is politically liberal, message on care and fairness. If they are conservative, remember that conservatives resonate with all six intuitive moral foundations. This means they have multiple ways they think about the world. You may need to frame the message around care as well as authority or sanctity, for example. It is noteworthy that loyalty

appeared to be less resonant as a foundational value in the Martin research.[10] This finding is particularly interesting, given it was conducted in 2020–2021, during a time when rhetoric was used to inflame loyalty to tribalism, fear, and contempt for the "other." For this reason, public health may want to refrain from framing messages that rely heavily on the loyalty moral foundation.

SUMMARY

Public health issues are complicated and complex. Leaders need to engage diverse stakeholders to help solve these big problems. Yet these stakeholders may view problems and solutions quite differently. Communication has also become more complex, due to unprecedented political polarization and the proliferation of news and other information from mainstream and social media. Public health needs to cut through the noise. Yet underlying historical reasons make this task exceptionally challenging.

Public health and healthcare leaders need to develop their communication skills. To start, they need to consider the major elements in communication: the message, sender, receiver, channel, and larger political and social contexts. Careful attention to empathy and centering equity in your public health messaging can help to identify and reduce structural racism. The public health workforce also needs a deeper understanding of what underpins effective communication. When public health leaders tap into the intuitive moral foundations in themselves and their audiences, their public health messages are more likely to reach and influence the intended recipients.

The bottom line is there *is* no alternative; public health leaders must learn to message better. Who could have imagined that amid a global pandemic as the world faced in 2020, U.S. public health leaders would have encountered a political environment where public health itself became weaponized? Leaders have no choice going forward but to move deeper into how to message more effectively and to build allies in stakeholders who can assist in public health advocacy.

DISCUSSION QUESTIONS

1. Take the Moral Foundations Assessment at https://tinyurl.com/MFTsurvey-book to get your scores on the six foundational values. This will show the extent to which you resonate with each value.
   a. Does anything surprise you about the results of your own moral foundations profile?
   b. How do you think your profile differs from those of your friends, family, coworkers, and/or classmates?
   c. Where might you have gaps in your ability to resonate with the foundational values of audiences you want to reach?
   d. Do you think that your foundational values will change over time or in different contexts?
2. Identify a situation in which using empathy (or centering equity) could make your communication more effective.
   a. Can you think of a trusted partner or unexpected validator that could serve as an effective messenger in this situation?
   b. How might your approach to using empathy (or centering equity) be modified based on the setting (e.g., one-on-one vs. a group)?
   c. How might you use storytelling to relate with your audience and to connect their experiences to your data?

3. Revisit the section on centering equity and consider your own limitations:

   a. What are your own preconceived notions about racial equity? About people of different races and abilities? How do these beliefs influence your messages?

   b. What groups do you belong to? How diverse are they? Does your audience look like any of the groups you belong to?

   c. What kind of spin are you putting on the data? Why?

   d. Who do people in your target group trust? Do people trust your organization? If not, what are you doing to build trust?

CASE STUDY: FRAMING MESSAGES WITH MORAL FOUNDATIONS IN MIND

Imagine you are a leader of a public health organization in your community. Consider a complex public health issue that you or your community is wrestling with. For example, you could be addressing the opioid crisis, gun violence, substance abuse, or Medicaid expansion. Or perhaps you are advocating for increased resources for your chronically underfunded health department or community hospital. You are going before your Republican-majority board of county commissioners to advocate for a policy change or funding increase to address this issue.

CASE STUDY QUESTIONS

1. Map out your communication using the five inputs in McGuire's Persuasion Matrix (*sender, receiver, message, channel, context*). How can you optimize the effectiveness of your communication based on these inputs?

2. Describe the opposition. Who is likely to oppose you? What arguments might they make? How can you preempt, refute, or rebut these arguments? Can you identify ways to leverage relationships as part of developing and disseminating messages?

3. Develop framing points using each of the six moral foundations (*care, fairness, loyalty, authority, sanctity, and liberty*) to create messages in support of your policy change or funding increase.

4. Draft a message that focuses on *systems, places,* or *conditions*.

5. Describe how you might use empathy in your communications to build relationships and/or to reframe and connect with the county commissioners.

ADDITIONAL RESOURCES

LEADERSHIP MEASUREMENT TOOLS/EXERCISES

■ Moral Foundations Online Assessment Tool: https://tinyurl.com/MFTsurvey-book

■ Becoming Better Messengers message development worksheet, which can be found on page 27 on the PDF accessible here: https://www.networkforphl.org/wp-content/uploads/2020/01/Becoming-Better-Messengers-Series.pdf

REFERENCES

1. Matthews G, Martin B, Hunter D. Becoming better messengers to communicate public health: skill-building for public health advocacy. Presented at the Network for Public Health Law 2021 Conference; September 20, 2021; online.

2. Yong E. How public health took part in its own downfall. *The Atlantic.* 2021, October. https://amp -theatlantic-com.cdn.ampproject.org/c/s/amp.theatlantic.com/amp/article/620457

3. Parran T. *Shadow on the Land: Syphilis.* American Social Hygiene Association; 1937.

4. Cohen ML. Changing patterns of infectious disease. *Nature.* 2000;406(6797):762–767. doi:10.1038/35021206

5. Goldberg DS. Against the very idea of the politicization of public health policy. *Am J Public Health.* 2012;102(1):44–49. doi:10.2105/AJPH.2011.300325

6. Pomeranz JL, Pertschuk M. State preemption: a significant and quiet threat to public health in the United States. *Am J Public Health.* 2017;107(6):900–902. doi:10.2105/AJPH.2017.303756

7. Crosbie E, Schmidt LA. Preemption in tobacco control: a framework for other areas of public health. *Am J Public Health.* 2020;110(3):345–350. doi:10.2105/AJPH.2019.305473

8. McGuire WJ. McGuire's classic input–output framework for constructing persuasive messages. In: Rice RE, Atkin CK, eds. *Public Communication Campaigns.* SAGE Publications; 2013:133–145. doi:10.4135/9781544308449.n9

9. Netherland J, Hansen HB. The war on drugs that wasn't: wasted whiteness, "dirty doctors," and race in media coverage of prescription opioid misuse. *Cult Med Psychiatry.* 2016;40(4):664–686. doi:10.1007/s11013-016-9496-5

10. Martin BA. *Improving Public Health Communication in a Politically Polarized Environment: Exploring the Use of Moral Values in Message Framing.* Dissertation. 2021. University of North Carolina at Chapel Hill. https://cdr.lib.unc.edu/concern/dissertations/dj52wf88m

11. Entman RM. Framing: toward clarification of a fractured paradigm. *J Commun.* 1993;43(4):51–58. doi:10.1111/j.1460-2466.1993.tb01304.x

12. Benford RD, Snow DA. Framing processes and social movements: an overview and assessment. *Annu Rev Sociol.* 2000;26(1):611–639. doi:10.1146/annurev.soc.26.1.611

13. FrameWorks Institute. Five questions about framing. FrameWorks Institute. June 8, 2020. https://www.frameworksinstitute.org/article/five-questions-about-framing

14. Khayatzadeh-Mahani A, Ruckert A, Labonté R. Obesity prevention: co-framing for intersectoral 'buy-in.' *Crit Public Health.* 2018;28(1):4–11. doi:10.1080/09581596.2017.1282604

15. The Robert Wood Johnson Foundation, Lowe JI, Westen D. *A New Way to Talk About The Social Determinants of Health.* The Robert Wood Johnson Foundation; 2010. https://www.rwjf.org/content/dam/farm/reports/reports/2010/rwjf63023

16. L'Hôte E, Volmert A, Davis C, Down L. Public health reaching across sectors: mapping the gaps between how public health experts and leaders in other sectors view public health and cross-sector collaboration. FrameWorks Institute; 2019. https://www.phrases.org/wp-content/uploads/2020/07/Aspen-PHRASES-MTG-Report-2019.pdf

17. de Beaumont Foundation, Aspen Institute. *Motivating the Public to Support Public Health: A Toolkit for Communicating With Non-Experts.* de Beaumont Foundation; 2020. https://www.phrases.org/wp -content/uploads/2020/07/Public-Health-Communications-Toolkit-Final_.pdf

18. Baer N. Storytelling and public health: the power of emotion in science. Presented at the Yale School of Public Health; April 15, 2019; New Haven, CT. https://ysph.yale.edu/news-article/storytelling-and -public-health-the-power-of-emotion-in-science

19. Haidt J. *The Righteous Mind: Why Good People Are Divided by Politics and Religion.* Vintage; 2012.

20. Kidwell B, Farmer A, Hardesty DM. Getting liberals and conservatives to go green: political ideology and congruent appeals. *J Consum Res.* 2013;40(2):350–367. doi:10.1086/670610

21. Wolsko C. Expanding the range of environmental values: political orientation, moral foundations, and the common ingroup. *J Environ Psychol.* 2017;51:284–294. doi:10.1016/j.jenvp.2017.04.005

22. Feinberg M, Willer R. The moral roots of environmental attitudes. *Psychol Sci.* 2013;24(1):56–62. doi:10.1177/0956797612449177

23. Mooijman M, Meindl P, Oyserman D, et al. Resisting temptation for the good of the group: binding moral values and the moralization of self-control. *J Pers Soc Psychol.* 2018;115(3):585–599. doi:10.1037/pspp0000149

24. Graham J, Haidt J, Nosek BA. Liberals and conservatives rely on different sets of moral foundations. *J Pers Soc Psychol.* 2009;96(5):1029–1046. doi:10.1037/a0015141

25. Burris S, Matthews G, Gunderson G, Baker EL. Becoming better messengers: the public health advantage. *J Public Health Manag Pract.* 2019;25(4):402–404. doi:10.1097/PHH.0000000000001032

Chapter 18

The Evolution and Development of a Leader

Susan C. Helm-Murtagh

INTRODUCTION

Leaders evolve through a series of stages, and their development needs vary by stage. Understanding one's development needs at each stage, as well as the tools and techniques to address those needs, can help leaders maximize their full potential. This text covers a broad range of leadership approaches, skills, models, and contexts, which will provide students with both the concepts and the ability to apply those concepts in practice. This chapter presents development strategies for each of the four stages in the evolution of a leader, organized into six leadership development domains. Those development strategies specifically incorporate and reference the other material contained in this textbook.

OBJECTIVES

By the end of this chapter, the reader will be able to:

- Discuss the various stages of leadership.
- Identify the hallmarks of each leadership stage.
- Determine the development needs at each leadership stage.
- Develop and apply stage-specific development strategies.

LEADER STAGES AND DEVELOPMENT NEEDS

E. L. Baker identifies four stages in the evolution of a leader: the emerging leader, the early leader, the established leader, and the emeritus leader.[1] He also outlines the key development needs for leaders in each stage. The definitions of each leader stage and those key needs form the organizing basis for this chapter, and each are discussed in more detail.

To complement and enrich these development strategies, this chapter applies the "Warwick 6 Leadership Framework" to those leader stages.[2] This conceptual model, which Hartley and Benington developed initially to categorize healthcare-related leadership development literature, is also helpful in categorizing leadership development needs (Figure 18.1).[3]

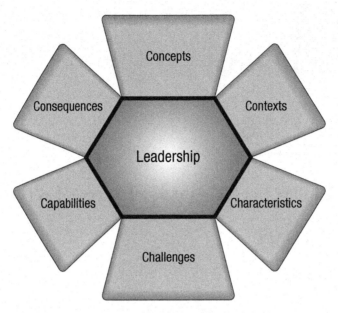

FIGURE 18.1: The Warwick 6 Leadership Analytical Framework.
Source: Reproduced with permission from Hartley J, Benington J. *Leadership in Health Care*. Policy Press; 2010.

As Hartley, Martin, and Benington point out, there is no one best way to develop leaders; effective leader development is context sensitive.[4] In other words, leaders must have the skills, attributes and characteristics that enable them to succeed within their organizational and environmental contexts (e.g., political, social, economic, and cultural). This adapted model incorporates context as a key consideration in recommending development needs. In addition, Hartley and Benington's model incorporates other relevant leadership development dimensions, including concepts, characteristics, challenges, capabilities, and consequences.

CONCEPTS

Leadership is a set of dynamic, interactive processes and it involves mobilizing action by many people toward common goals. Particularly in public health and healthcare settings, leadership takes place within and across groups, organizations, and networks of organizations. It usually involves diverse sets of stakeholders.

CONTEXTS

Organizational and environmental contexts shape leadership thinking and action; in turn, leaders interpret and influence their contexts through sense-making and the framing of issues and ideas. Contexts for public health and healthcare leaders include not only their organizations (internal contexts), which may be complex enough, but also include political, structural, technological, social, and economic contexts (external contexts).

CHARACTERISTICS

In the Warwick Model, the construct of characteristics of leadership refers to the variety of roles that leaders play and the resources to which they have access. Both vary by situation and can include the type of power the leader has (e.g., formal or informal, direct or indirect); the type of leadership role they play (e.g., clinical, managerial, political, community); and the context(s) in which they are operating.

CHALLENGES

Effective leadership requires the framing and analyzing of the challenges the leader faces, and adapting leader actions, decision-making, and stakeholder engagement accordingly.

CAPABILITIES

Leaders must develop the leadership capabilities required to use a range of different skills within different contexts and in pursuit of specific challenges.

CONSEQUENCES

In the Warwick Model, the consequences construct refers to the assessment of the impacts, outcomes, and consequences of leadership. From a leadership development standpoint, this involves understanding how effective one is as a leader; how one's actions, decisions, and behavior affect others and the organization; and one's strengths and areas for development.

A NEW MODEL FOR LEADERSHIP DEVELOPMENT

Hartley and Benington introduced an important additional construct, connectivity, to highlight the interdependence of each of the six leadership dimensions in the original Warwick Model.[4] For this chapter, the author has devised a model which incorporates Warwick's 6C Model, Baker's leader stages, and the added connectivity construct, as shown in Figure 18.2. At each of the four leader stages, the leader's development strategies incorporate each facet of the Warwick Model as a dimension for growth. In addition, the model adds two dynamic elements: career progression, which is represented by the gray chevrons, and mentoring, which is represented by the black chevrons.

Each of the six dimensions will be presented as a leadership development category, with implications and recommended development strategies for each leadership stage.

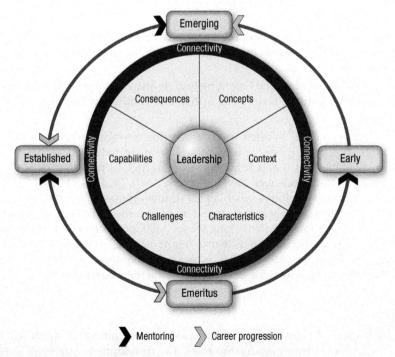

FIGURE 18.2: 7C Leadership Evolution and Development Model.

THE EMERGING LEADER

Definition

What is an emerging leader? Emerging leaders are not necessarily defined by age, but instead by where they are in their career progression. They can be new to leadership, new to a role, or new to an organization. Deb Calvert, an executive coach and trainer, offers the following hallmarks of emerging leaders.

1. **They are high performers in their organization:** This is generally the most common way to get recognized and promoted, but as Calvert points out, as emerging leaders progress, the ability to lead others becomes more important than their individual performance.

2. **They show high potential in their current role:** High potential refers to the emerging leader's ability to take on additional responsibilities and assignments.

3. **They informally influence others:** Even without formal authority, emerging leaders inspire others to follow them.

4. **They supervise others:** Supervisory or management responsibilities provide valuable opportunities for emerging leaders to apply, demonstrate, and hone their leadership skills.

5. **They are open to learning, failing, and growing:** Emerging leaders experiment, take risks, fail forward, and try again. They seek opportunities to be challenged and to challenge others.

6. **They have strong people-building skills:** Emerging leaders invest in developing others; they recognize the value of sharing knowledge, responsibilities, and development opportunities with others.

7. **They are centered by their core values:** Emerging leaders know who they are and what they stand for. They make decisions based on their core values and are clear and consistent in aligning their actions (principles) with those values.

8. **They see the possibilities for a better future state:** Emerging leaders remain focused on what can and should be done to improve both their organizations and the people and communities they serve.

9. **They unite others and help them see new possibilities:** Emerging leaders bring others together; they inspire and encourage those around them to envision and pursue a better future state.

10. **They want to become leaders:** Emerging leaders are committed to learning about leadership, developing the behaviors of a leader, and continually developing their leadership skills.[5]

The term "high potential" is often used to describe emerging leaders. What does that mean and, more importantly, how is it identified or measured? Harvard Business School professor Clayton Christensen and colleague Morgan McCall note that most methods for evaluating leader performance rely on "end states," or a leader's ability to demonstrate *acquired* traits, skills, and attributes, such as "is results-oriented" and "gives accurate and timely feedback."[6] Potential, they argue, should be a forward-oriented measure; it should be based on the demonstration of an emerging leader's *ability to acquire* the attributes needed for future leadership situations. Such measures might include, for example, "seeks opportunities to learn," "seeks and uses feedback," "is aware of what they don't know," "learns from mistakes." Potential, then, is learning-oriented versus achievement-oriented.[6]

Discussion

For emerging leaders, the development emphasis is on learning and acquiring the necessary attributes for larger, future leadership roles. The development strategies in each leadership dimension, then, focus on building the skills, experience, and knowledge acquisition required to advance to the early leader stage and beyond.

TABLE 18.1: Leadership Development Needs, Goals, and Strategies for Emerging Leaders

LEADERSHIP DIMENSION	DEVELOPMENT NEEDS/GOALS	DEVELOPMENT STRATEGIES
Concepts	Become attuned to leadership as a process; develop an appreciation for the role of stakeholders in accomplishing goals	Take on developmental assignments Acquire stakeholder analysis skills
Contexts	Build technical skills; develop an understanding of the contexts in which you, your team, and your organization operate	Invest in education/specialized training Build a network Create a personal learning cloud (PLC) Find a mentor/enroll in an organizational mentoring program
Characteristics	Be attuned to the types of roles and resources available to you and others in roles to which you aspire	Find a mentor/enroll in an organizational mentoring program
Challenges	Learn to frame and analyze challenges and create strategies to address them	Acquire systems thinking skills
Capabilities	Begin to build your leadership toolbox; gain an understanding of the behaviors and concepts related to the practice of leadership	Develop a leadership framework Create a development plan Acquire time management skills Create a personal learning cloud (PLC)
Consequences	Gain an understanding of your impact as a leader; your talents, abilities, and areas for growth	Mine feedback sources for insights: performance evaluations; self-assessments; mentor feedback and guidance

As Baker notes, a key development need for emerging leaders is that they must be identified as such. This highlights the importance of talent identification and management, both at the supervisor level and the organizational level (see Chapter 16, "Talent Management: A Leadership Imperative"). Further, emerging leaders must have a sense of their potential as a leader, as well as an awareness of what specific leadership talents and abilities they possess. Finally, emerging leaders must understand what effective leadership looks like.[1] In addition, Culvert, Christensen, and McCall all highlight the importance of learning in emerging leaders' development strategies. Those key development principles, combined with the adapted Warwick Model, suggest the development needs/goals and strategies for the emerging leader shown in Table 18.1.

Concepts

Emerging leaders, by definition, may not have had the experience of working in a leadership role, be it direct or indirect; they therefore may not be attuned to the concept of leadership as a dynamic, interactive process. What is the best way for emerging leaders to learn how to lead? There is a great deal of evidence that carefully structured and managed developmental assignments are effective methods to do just that.[7,8] Research indicates that the value of developmental assignments depends on the quality of the assignment. Such factors include the size of the assignment challenge, the degree of task variety, and the level of support provided.

Not surprisingly, providing emerging leaders with high-quality and timely feedback is also essential to the leadership development effectiveness of the assignment.[2] It is also important to include opportunities to influence peers, work across organizational boundaries, and develop an understanding of other parts of the organization.[9] Such opportunities also allow for emerging leaders to get comfortable taking risks and to learn from mistakes.

Leadership is not performed in a vacuum; it requires the support (or at least the effective management) of interested parties, or stakeholders. Stakeholders are the people and organizations that have a vested interest or concern in the process and/or the outcomes. Stakeholder analysis is the process of identifying key actors and assessing their knowledge, interests, positions, alliances, and importance related to the objective(s) at hand.[10] While stakeholder analysis and management is a critical leadership capability at every leadership stage, it is particularly important for emerging leaders to begin to develop competencies in this area.

Contexts

As previously noted, leadership contexts are bi-directional in nature. Organizational and environmental contexts shape leadership thinking and action, while leaders interpret and influence their contexts through sense-making and the framing of issues and ideas. Public health and healthcare leaders face enormously complex contexts; the healthcare and public health systems are highly fragmented and subject to profound political, social, economic, and structural forces. For emerging leaders, developing an understanding of those contexts is critical to their ability to successfully operate in and influence them.

Development strategies to support this include formal education (for example, pursuing a graduate degree in Health Administration or Public Health) and finding specialized training (through their organization or professional associations, such as the American Public Health Association or the American College of Health Executives). In addition, emerging leaders are encouraged to begin building a broad and diverse professional network, through alumni gatherings, volunteer work, social media, and online communities. This "network intelligence" can be an invaluable knowledge and career-building resource.

In addition, the "personal learning cloud (PLC)" refers to the growing variety of online courses, learning tools, and social and interactive platforms.[11] This content is often free (or inexpensive), can be accessed when and where it is most convenient for the learner, and can be personalized and self-paced. PLCs can be accessed through corporate training and development platforms, like LinkedIn Learning and Skillsoft, or through more individual-oriented platforms such as Coursera, edX, 2U, and MOOCs (massive open online courses). These platforms can be powerful resources to help emerging leaders build their knowledge and skill bases.

Characteristics

Mentoring is discussed in detail in Chapter 19, "Mentoring and Trusted Advisors." Traditional mentoring is defined as the personal relationship in which a more experienced (sometimes older) organization member acts as "a guide, teacher, role model, or sponsor of a less experienced (usually younger) member," and it has a long history of improving individual learning and career development.[12,13] Mentors can be invaluable in helping emerging leaders understand both the organizational and environmental contexts in which they are working. They can also provide introductions to key internal and external stakeholders and serve as advocates for emerging leaders.

Challenges

In the increasingly complex public health and healthcare contexts, successful leaders need to be effective systems thinkers. Systems thinking, which is addressed in Chapter 3, "Systems Thinking in Public Health," refers to the ability to see overall system structures, patterns of system "behavior," and system cycles (as opposed to seeing only specific events in the system).

Systems thinking enables the accurate diagnosis and solution identification of complex problems and is a critical skill for emerging public health and healthcare leaders to acquire.

Capabilities

The concept of a leadership framework and the process for developing one are addressed in Chapter 21, "Creating Your Leadership Framework." The objective of the framework is to provide leaders with a more reflective, practice-based, and integrative opportunity to elicit their understanding of leadership concepts and then to directly apply best practices and guiding principles to their own practice of leadership. This exercise will provide emerging leaders with the opportunity to create a solid, practical foundation from which to operate, including the opportunity to develop their core values. Although its complexion will change over time and will likely vary in content by stage of leadership, the leadership framework is a building block for each stage of leadership and thus remains a component in each stage's set of development strategies.

While leaders at all stages should have a development plan, it is especially critical for emerging leaders. Development plans are living, working documents that are created by the employee (the emerging leader, in this case) and their manager. They include both personal and career development goals, work development needs, and an action plan to achieve the goals and meet the development needs outlined. Plans should be discussed between the manager and employee on a regular basis (e.g., monthly or quarterly) and updated or modified accordingly. Development plans enable employees to actively enlist their manager in their career development.

Finally, time management is defined as "the decision-making process that structures, protects and adjusts a person's time to changing environmental conditions,"[14] and is an essential foundational skill for emerging leaders to develop. Establishing effective habits and methods to design and organize goals, plans, schedules, and tasks to effectively use time will enable greater productivity, more effective and deliberate prioritization, enhanced focus, and decreased stress levels.

Consequences

While feedback is critical for all leaders, establishing the mechanisms to solicit feedback and gaining the experience to filter, prioritize, and act on that feedback is essential for emerging leaders. Potential rich sources of feedback include performance evaluations, self-assessments (many of which are included or referenced in this text), 360-degree feedback, and mentor feedback and guidance.

THE EARLY LEADER

Definition

An early leader is charged with leading a team, with or without formal authority, and on a permanent or temporary basis. Early leaders can be supervisors, team leaders, project managers, front line managers, task force leaders, and so on. Throughout this career stage, leaders will face roles with increasing scope and complexity.

Discussion

At this stage in a leader's development, the focus begins to shift from technical proficiency and individual skills and competencies toward skills in team leadership, influencing, adaptive leadership, systems thinking, and strategic thinking.

Finally, early leaders should also begin focusing on developing their emotional quotient (EQ) and building out their set of trusted advisors, or their personal board of directors (see Chapter 19, "Mentoring and Trusted Advisors"). As their scope of influence broadens, the

TABLE 18.2: Leadership Development Needs, Goals, and Strategies for Early Leaders

LEADERSHIP DIMENSION	DEVELOPMENT NEEDS/GOALS	DEVELOPMENT STRATEGIES
Concepts	Begin to practice leadership as a process; develop an understanding of the role of stakeholders in accomplishing goals	Apply stakeholder analysis skills Acquire influencing skills Become proficient in effective dialogue
Contexts	Continue to build technical skills, while acquiring adaptive leadership skills; enhance and refine your understanding of the contexts in which you, your team, and your organization operate	Continue to invest in education and/or specialized training Tap into network intelligence Acquire adaptive leadership skills Develop moral courage
Characteristics	Be attuned to the types of roles and resources available to you and others in roles to which you aspire	Begin to build personal board of directors
Challenges	Learn to frame and analyze challenges and create strategies to address them	Acquire strategic thinking skills Acquire systems thinking Acquire change leadership skills
Capabilities	Begin to build your leadership toolbox	Refine leadership framework Refine development plan Acquire skills for building and leading teams Focus on building EQ
Consequences	Continue to assess your impact as a leader; your talents, abilities, and areas for growth	Mine feedback sources for insights: performance evaluations; self-assessments; 360-degree feedback; mentor; and personal board of directors

quality and diversity of sources of feedback becomes more critical for the early leader to develop an enhanced awareness of how others perceive them, as well as a clearer sense of their strengths and development needs. Key development needs/goals and strategies for the early leader are shown in Table 18.2.

Concepts

As the leader's scope of responsibilities and span of control increase, so does their reliance on getting things done through others. The stakeholder analysis skills acquired in the emergent leader stage can now be leveraged by engaging others through effective dialogue (see Chapter 1, "Dialogue: A Foundational Skill for Effective Health Leadership") and through influencing skills. According to the Center for Creative Leadership, there are four keys to influencing others:

1. Organizational intelligence, or an understanding of the organization's formal and informal structures. Organizationally intelligent leaders are "politically savvy"
2. Promotion of team and self, to draw attention to the work being done and the impact of that work

3. Building and maintaining trust, in order to gain the full buy-in and capabilities of the individuals and groups whose support the leader needs to accomplish organizational goals

4. Leveraging networks, or engaging the informal organizational structure (see "organizational intelligence") to span organizational boundaries and to create alignment, commitment, and support[15]

Contexts

As Baker notes, "Many early public health and health care leaders rely on technical skills they developed in training, such as epidemiology or clinical skills, when confronted with a challenge or framing a problem. These technical skills, while helpful and even sometimes necessary in understanding the nature of the problem, are often insufficient in the larger context, such as changes in practice and policy, needed to successfully address the underlying causes of a health problem."[1(p475)]

To do this requires the application of adaptive leadership skills (see Chapter 10, "Adaptive Leadership") to complement a leader's technical skills. Adaptive leadership skills enable leaders to "anticipate, react to, and navigate change; mobilize people to tackle evolving challenges; and help teams and organizations thrive in new realities." (Magaña-Valladares, Galea, and Casazza)

Early leaders face increasingly complex contexts and wider ranges of stakeholders and stakeholder interests, which can create competing objectives. As decision-making becomes more difficult, involving more issues, considerations, and options, early leaders will need to rely on a foundation of ethics and the deliberate application of those ethics, or moral courage (see Chapter 2, "Moral Courage in Public Health Leadership").

Characteristics

During the early leader stage, formation of a trusted set of advisors, or a personal board of directors, is vital to a leader's ongoing development (see Chapter 19, "Mentoring and Trusted Advisors"). These individuals can offer a diverse set of perspectives and insights, provide a safe "sounding board" for problems and challenges the leader is facing (particularly if these trusted advisors come from outside the leaders' organization and/or chain of command), and deliver candid feedback, which is especially important as the length and depth of the relationship progresses.

Challenges

Strategic thinking is a fundamental skill for early leaders to add to their toolkit; it enables leaders to identify, understand, and navigate continuous change (see Chapter 4, "Strategic Thinking: Rationale, Process, and Behaviors") and to create effective responses to challenges and opportunities, both internal and external. Leaders in this stage will be driving and leading change in both their internal and external contexts. Acquiring change leadership skills is another crucial addition to the emerging leader's toolbox (see Chapter 11, "Leading Change").

Capabilities

EQ, which is covered in Chapter 5, "Emotional Intelligence," has been positively associated with overall leadership effectiveness, even more so than IQ or personality. High levels of EQ better equip leaders to cope with uncertainty, lead with empathy, make better decisions under pressure, lead change, build trust, and maintain motivation levels—all critical capabilities for public health and healthcare leaders. Emerging leaders should invest in assessing and developing their EQ.

Emerging leaders will be called upon to lead larger, more diverse teams with increasing scope and visibility, and should thus develop skills for building and leading teams (see Chapter 15, "Building and Leading Teams: Essential Approaches and Practical Tools for Improving the Health of Populations").

Finally, participation in a formal, structured leadership development program may be helpful at this stage, whether it is part of an organizational training and development curriculum or is sponsored or supported by the organization. Such an approach can provide valuable opportunities for early leaders to assess and develop their leadership skills and gain new perspectives on leadership.[1]

Consequences

Early leaders will have had the opportunity to lead teams, influence others, and work within increasingly complex contexts. Seeking 360-degree feedback at this stage of their career can help early leaders develop a well-rounded sense of others' perceptions of them, their leadership strengths, and areas for development.

THE ESTABLISHED LEADER

Definition

The established leader has advanced in their career through hierarchical moves, movements between organizations, or, as is becoming increasingly common as organizational structures flatten, through movement across the organization. Career advancement involves taking on larger or new responsibilities, working in new organizational and environmental contexts, or both.

Discussion

Leadership success at this stage, while still somewhat dependent on technical skills (or the procurement of them in cases where the leader has moved into new roles and contexts), becomes increasingly associated with adaptive leadership skills. As Baker notes, "Established leaders must deal with ambiguity, conflicting demands, and a range of challenges that grow more complex over time . . . established public health [and healthcare] leaders are faced with major economic and political challenges along with a need to redefine the role of public health [and healthcare] in a rapidly changing health system."[1(p476)]

The term "established" by no means infers that a leader has arrived at their career destination. As Baker observes, "The most successful established leaders are those whose commitment to their own life-long learning is unabated during this most demanding stage of their career. Those who commit to their own development benefit not only themselves but others by setting an example and by improving their skills over time. As a result, established leaders continue to grow and to demonstrate the benefits of a life-long commitment to leadership development."[1(p476)]

The key elements of an established leader's development plan center on leveraging and refining their existing influencing, stakeholder management, and adaptive leadership skills; investing in and developing others through talent management and mentoring; and seeking new opportunities for leadership development and personal and professional renewal. These development strategies are outlined in Table 18.3.

Concepts

The established leader accomplishes goals and outcomes by inspiring and influencing others to carry out their vision. As they move into roles with increasing scope, responsibility, and complexity, effective leadership requires ever more facility with stakeholder management and influencing skills. Development plans at this stage should incorporate a recommitment to acquiring or honing those skills.

TABLE 18.3: Leadership Development Needs, Goals, and Strategies for Established Leaders

LEADERSHIP DIMENSION	DEVELOPMENT NEEDS/GOALS	DEVELOPMENT STRATEGIES
Concepts	Continue to leverage knowledge of leadership as a process and the role of stakeholders in accomplishing goals	Leverage stakeholder management and influencing skills
Contexts	Continue to hone and refine understanding of the contexts in which you, your team, and your organization operate	Continue to build and tap into network intelligence
Characteristics	Be attuned to the types of roles and resources available to you and others in roles that you have had, currently hold, and to which you aspire	Become a mentor Develop and manage organizational talent
Challenges	Learn to frame and analyze challenges and create strategies to address them	Continue to refine adaptive leadership skills Enhance strategic thinking skills Continue to refine change leadership skills
Capabilities	Commit to renewal	Refine leadership framework Reframe development plan Engage in reverse mentoring (see the text that follows) Pursue opportunities to engage in community service and enhance skills and knowledge
Consequences	Gain an understanding of your impact as a leader; your talents, abilities, and areas for growth	Mine feedback sources for insights: performance evaluations; self-assessments; 360-degree feedback; mentor, mentees, and personal board of directors

Contexts

In this stage, leaders will face larger, more diverse, and more complex internal and external contexts. Enriching and expanding their professional network can help established leaders connect with others who have valuable experiences and insights to offer.

Characteristics

Established leaders have a responsibility to invest in and develop others. They have experience, knowledge, and wisdom to offer, and should seek to actively engage in talent development and management, as well as mentoring others. Chapter 19, "Mentoring and Trusted Advisors," addresses both finding and being a mentor.

In addition, talent management—the identification, development, and nurturing of talent in others—is an imperative for established leaders. Chapter 16, "Talent Management: A Leadership Imperative," is devoted to talent management.

Challenges

Established leaders will continue to face new challenges, as their internal and external contexts change. Throughout this stage, leaders can expect to take on new or expanded responsibilities, experience job changes within or between organizations, lead different teams, report to different leaders, and be called upon to lead change in response to or in anticipation of shifts in their internal and external contexts. Accordingly, established leaders should continue to refine their adaptive leadership and change leadership skills and enhance their strategic thinking skills.

Capabilities

An established leader's toolbox should contain, above all else, the commitment to lifelong learning. The practice of leadership, like the practice of any other discipline, is one of continued improvement, curiosity, openness to new ideas and perspectives, and humility. This is particularly critical in the complex, dynamic and ever-changing contexts of public health and healthcare leadership.

As noted earlier in this chapter, leaders can accomplish this goal of continual renewal through regular refinement and updating of their leadership framework, as well as by reframing their development plan. These activities can be triggered by a periodic commitment (e.g., on a periodic basis to align with performance appraisals, operational planning, strategic planning exercises) or by career events (e.g., a promotion, assignment to a new role, career or organizational change).

One important source of input for established leaders is reverse mentoring. Reverse mentoring pairs younger employees with established leaders, and it can be a valuable way for senior leaders to refresh and reframe the ways in which they think about leadership, organizational culture, and even strategic issues. Jordan and Sorell found the following four main benefits of reverse mentoring for organizations and mentors:

1. **Increased retention of Millennials:** Millennials, defined as those born between 1980 and 2000, are forecast to comprise 75% of the global workforce by 2025.[16] Providing reverse mentoring opportunities for Millennials can provide them with the transparency and recognition from senior management they seek, which helps build their trust, engagement, and loyalty.[17]
2. **Sharing of digital skills:** As Jordan and Sorell point out, while this aspect of reverse mentoring should not be the sole focus of the relationship, it is often part of the dialogue and skills exchange.
3. **Driving culture change:** Millennials can help senior executives better understand current social and cultural issues, and the importance of social media and technology; they can also be invaluable in shaping effective Millennial recruiting strategies.[17]
4. **Promoting diversity:** Millennials are more likely to have been brought up in a more diverse, global world than established leaders. Reverse mentoring programs can help leaders better understand the needs of Black, Indigenous, and People of Color (BIPOC); Lesbian, Gay, Bisexual, Transgender and Queer (LGBTQ); and other marginalized groups of employees.

Finally, established leaders can continue their personal and professional growth, and "give back" to their communities through board service and volunteer opportunities. Established leaders can also expand the scope of their impact on current and future leaders by serving as guest speakers at conferences, writing books or articles, or serving as adjunct faculty at schools of public health or healthcare administration.

Consequences

To maintain their commitment to lifelong learning, established leaders must continue to carefully mine all of their valuable sources of feedback, such as performance evaluations, self-assessments, and 360-degree feedback. At this point in their career, the input from mentor(s), mentee(s), and the leader's personal board of directors becomes even more crucial. As a leader becomes more powerful and even more established, it may be more difficult to get candid feedback at this stage. Relying on relationships that have been developed over time, in which there is deeply embedded mutual trust, may be one of the few ways in which established leaders can get a true, unvarnished picture of their strengths and areas for growth.

THE EMERITUS LEADER

Definition

The emeritus leader may be officially retired from their formal leadership role, but they still lead in meaningful ways, mainly through influence and by providing guidance to emerging, early, and established leaders in the form of a sounding board, a coach, a mentor, or a member of a personal board of directors.[1]

As Baker notes, emeritus leaders "have their own needs. They need opportunities to share their wisdom and thereby continue to exert a positive influence on the unfolding of events. They also benefit from having their own peer networks as a way to remain in touch with current and future challenges."[1(p476)] Psychologist Erik Erikson, in his eight-stage theory of psychosocial development, describes this stage of an individual's life as one in which they face a choice between generativity and stagnation. Generativity "refers to 'making your mark' on the world through creating or nurturing things that will outlast an individual."[18(p73)] It also involves continuous learning. Stagnation, conversely, happens when the desire to contribute goes unfulfilled.[18] Emeritus leaders can meet their generativity needs by sharing their experience and wisdom through board service, teaching, writing, speaking, coaching, and mentoring.

Board service enables emeritus leaders to not only contribute their knowledge and experience in highly influential roles, but it also provides them with the opportunity to stay current on issues facing organizations, and to apply their skills and experience to causes or missions in which the emeritus leader has a personal or professional interest. This latter benefit is particularly true for those who choose to serve on nonprofit boards. Teaching, while it can require a significant investment of time, is both intellectually stimulating and rewarding; it provides exposure to the next generation(s) of leaders, emerging issues facing leaders and organizations, and new ways of thinking about those issues and challenges. Writing is also an excellent way to influence others on a broad scale, and to both share and gain knowledge, be it through books, articles, blogs, or regular posts on professional social media. Speaking engagements can provide emeritus leaders with the opportunity to expand their professional and social networks, revisit and reframe their experience through a more contemporary lens, and exert positive influence. Emeritus leaders may also consider becoming coaches for other leaders, either through informal relationships or by establishing a coaching practice. Finally, serving as a mentor and/or as a member of a personal board of directors enables the emeritus leader to play an important and vital role in the development and nurturing of the next generation of leaders.

SUMMARY

Development is essential at all stages of a leader's career, from the emerging leadership stage through to the emeritus stage. Specific development needs and strategies will change over time as the leader progresses and their contexts change, presenting new challenges. Understanding leadership development as an interconnected constellation of six dimensions (contexts, concepts, characteristics, challenges, capabilities, and consequences) can help leaders at each stage examine their strengths and development needs, identify their development strategies, and create a corresponding development plan. Throughout a leader's evolution, a commitment to continuous learning, development, and renewal are key to their continued success. Creating and maintaining stage-specific leadership development strategies can provide leaders with an intentional roadmap for growth.

DISCUSSION QUESTIONS

1. Based on the descriptions of the four stages of a leader, in what stage would you place yourself? Why?
2. Using the development strategies for your stage, identify your top three developmental needs. Explain them in terms of your own assessment of your level of development, your career goals, and your current role.
3. For each of the three development needs you identified, outline one key action that you can take over the next 6 months to address that need. Share your actions with a classmate and your instructor.

CASE STUDY: AN EMERGING LEADER

Cassidy sighed and looked at her watch again; it was almost 10 p.m., and she was still at the office. She did not think she would ever get this project done; honestly, she was feeling like she had bitten off more than she could chew. She wondered how she had gotten here, and how she could get the situation resolved.

Cassidy thought back to a little over a year ago. She had just gotten her undergraduate degree in public health and was eager to put her hard-earned degree to work. Although she had gotten offers from a health insurance company and a large national nonprofit, she had decided to take a job at a community-based organization in Philadelphia. She felt that the size of the organization would enable her to make more of an impact, and its mission (addressing health disparities in inner-city adolescents and youth) fit better with her interests and passions. She believed that public health often overlooked this age group, and she was eager to do something about it.

A lifelong athlete, Cassidy became passionate about health, well-being, and nutrition from an early age. When she got to college, she took a public health course on a whim and realized that health was much more than just the individual choices people make; so many factors contribute to a person's health, including the air they breathe, the food they eat, their access to health insurance and healthcare, the neighborhood they live in, and the policies in their city/state/country. She became interested in working in health disparities when she learned about how many people in America lack access to basic needs that affect their health.

Soon after she arrived at the organization, she immediately identified several programming improvements that she thought would help them reach more youth and cost less. She proposed the ideas to her boss, who immediately and enthusiastically told her to "go for it," and to let her know what Cassidy needed. "You're a rising star, Cassidy. From the minute you walked in the door, the creativity and energy levels have gone up. When you speak in staff meetings, everyone listens. You have a bright future here and anywhere you decide you want to go. I am sure that you will knock this project out of the park, just like you have everything else you've undertaken here."

That was 6 months ago. Her original timeline had her completing the project last month, but she had not anticipated the resistance she was getting from the facilities that they used and the parents. She also thought that the local grocery stores would be all in on her idea to sell their excess produce and other items at a smaller margin, but that was proving not to be the case. She was beginning to realize that she had oversimplified the problem and the solution. On top of all of that, she had no idea where the time went each day; it seemed as if just minutes after she sat down, everyone else was packing up to go home.

CASE STUDY QUESTIONS

1. Of the 10 traits of an emerging leader described in the chapter, which ones does Cassidy display?
2. Which of the development strategies for emerging leaders would you recommend for Cassidy?
3. How would you prioritize them, and why?
4. What advice would you have for Cassidy to help her resolve her current situation?

CASE STUDY: AN EARLY LEADER

Jaaziel was nervous. He was about to have his first annual performance discussion with his boss, Nina. He had only been in his role as nurse manager for a little over 11 months, and it was his first supervisory job. He had no idea what to expect from the meeting. As he waited for Nina's door to open, he reflected back over the past several years.

After getting his BSN (graduating near the top of his class) and his nurses' license, he had spent 5 years providing direct patient care at Dalebrook, a long-term care facility with several locations in the Chicago area. He found the clinical part of his job easy; when confronted with a patient care issue, it was almost as if he had a photographic memory of his coursework and could call up an instant replay of every similar situation he'd seen in practice—what to do came quickly and easily for him. The running joke with the rest of the nursing staff was, "Just do whatever you've seen Jaaziel do, and you will know it's right!"

No one was really surprised when he got promoted; he had gotten rave reviews from his patients, his colleagues could always count on him to step in when they needed help, and he was always upbeat, no matter how many hours he was into his shift or how many times Mrs. Jackson asked him if it was time yet for her medication. A few months into the nurse manager role, though, he noticed that people were reacting differently when he stepped in to help with patient care; what previously would have been met with a smile and relief was now met with a mumbled thanks and a glance at the floor or over Jaaziel's shoulder. In staff meetings, when the team was trying to solve scheduling issues or was having problems with another nursing unit, his upbeat manner and tendency to make light of problems was not going over well.

Then there was the issue with Regina. Everyone knew that she wasn't always on time for her shift, and her patient notes (if she left any) were impossible to decipher and usually so vague as to not be helpful. But she had been there forever and was a fount of knowledge about why things were done the way they were. She also knew who to talk to among the "higher-ups" to get new requisitions approved. A couple of Jaaziel's direct reports had come to him with complaints about her timeliness and shoddy patient record-keeping, but he just laughed and said, "That's just Regina for you!"

It was as if his staff expected something else from him, but he couldn't really put his finger on it.

Nina's door finally opened, and she waved Jaaziel into her office.

CASE STUDY QUESTIONS

1. What performance feedback do you think Nina will provide to Jaaziel? What are his strengths? His areas for development?
2. What development goals would you suggest for Jaaziel? How would you prioritize your suggestions, and why? What development strategies should he consider?

CASE STUDY: AN ESTABLISHED LEADER

Dr. Rochelle Walensky was appointed director of the Centers for Disease Control and Prevention (CDC) by President Biden on December 7, 2020. She inherited a monumental challenge: to restore the once internationally revered agency to its former status as a world leader in public health.[19] Battered by the COVID-19 pandemic, crippled by self-inflicted wounds, sidelined by the Trump Administration, and consistently undercut by the White House, the agency that is credited with eradicating smallpox globally and wiping out polio in the United States has "with breathtaking speed, become a target of anger, scorn and even pity."[20(p13)]

Dr. Walensky has a sterling reputation and credentials as both a physician and a researcher. She earned her MD from Johns Hopkins; has an MPH from Harvard; has been on faculty at the Harvard Medical School for 20 years; has served on numerous international, federal, and state-level advisory councils and panels; and been a division chief at Massachusetts General Hospital. Her appointment, in which she replaced outgoing CDC Director Dr. Robert Redfield, was initially praised by doctors and public health experts.

Nine months into her tenure, Dr. Walensky's initial goals remain unmet, and both she and the agency have continued to make notable and damaging errors in judgment. At one point, Walensky stated unequivocally that "vaccinated people cannot transmit the virus"; in May, the agency quickly reversed its initial guidance that vaccinated people could remove their masks indoors. Both of these incidents, along with Walenksy's failure to follow through on her sweeping promises to resuscitate the agency, have once again thrust the CDC into an unwanted, and unwelcoming, spotlight.

Meanwhile, as of early November 2021, 18 months after COVID-19 was declared a pandemic, the virus has claimed 760,000 American lives. The CDC's own Twitter feed starkly warns that "The #COVID19 level of transmission in the United States remains high."[21]

CASE STUDY QUESTIONS

1. Find at least three articles from credible sources that discuss the challenges that Dr. Walensky inherited and/or created. Choose the top three challenges and explain which leadership dimension they fall into. Explain your reasoning.
2. Based on your answer to the first question, what would you advise Dr. Walensky to do to address the leadership challenges she faces? Explain your reasoning.

ADDITIONAL RESOURCES

BOOKS

■ *Developmental Assignments: Creating Learning Experiences Without Changing Jobs,* by Cynthia McCauley

TRAINING

■ The National Academy of Medicine Emerging Leaders in Health and Medicine program (https://nam.edu/programs/emerging-leaders-forum)
■ Public Health Institute Center for Health Leadership and Practice (www.phi.org/our-work/programs/center-for-health-leadership-and -practice)

WEBSITES

■ World Health Organization, *Stakeholder Analysis Guidelines,* by Kammi Schmeer (www.paho.org/hq/dmdocuments/2010/47-Policy_Toolkit_Strengthening_HSR .pdf)
■ Using IDPs to Leverage Strengths, by Don Jacobson (https://govleaders.org/idp .htm)

REFERENCES

1. Baker EL. The evolution of a leader. *J Public Health Manag Pract.* 2011;17(5):475–477. doi:10.1097/PHH.0b013e318229ae3c
2. West M, Armit K, Loewenthal L, et al. *Leadership and Leadership Development in Health Care: The Evidence Base.* Faculty of Medical Leadership and Management; 2015. https://www.kingsfund.org.uk/sites/default/files/field/field_publication_file/leadership-leadership-development-health-care-feb-2015.pdf
3. Hartley J, Benington J. *Leadership in Health Care.* Policy Press; 2010.
4. Hartley J, Martin J, Benington J. Leadership in healthcare: a review of the literature for health care professionals, managers and researchers. *SDO.* 2008. https://njl-admin.nihr.ac.uk/document/download/2027538
5. Calvert D. 10 signs you are (or could be) an emerging leader. March 24, 2015. https://www.linkedin.com/pulse/10-signs-you-could-emerging-leader-deb-calvert
6. Christensen CM, McCall Jr. M. Identifying and developing capable leaders. Harvard Business School Background Note. September 2020 (revised December 2020).
7. McCall M, Lombardo M, Morrison A. *The Lessons of Experience: How Executives Develop on the Job.* Lexington Books; 1988.
8. McCauley C, McCall M. *Using Experience to Develop Leadership Talent: How Organizations Leverage On-the-Job Development.* Jossey-Bass; 2014.
9. Jacobson D. Making the most of developmental assignments: Q&A with author Cynthia McCauley. https://govleaders.org/development.htm
10. Schmeer K. Stakeholder analysis guidelines. In: Latin America and Caribbean Regional Health Sector Reform, ed. Policy Toolkit for Strengthening Health Sector Reform. Policy Toolkit for Strengthening Health Sector Reform; 2020:2-1–2-43. https://www.paho.org/hq/dmdocuments/2010/47-Policy_Toolkit_Strengthening_HSR.pdf
11. Moldoveanu M, Narayandas D. The future of leadership development. *Harv Bus Rev* 2019;97(4):40–48. https://hbr.org/2019/03/the-future-of-leadership-development
12. Leavitt C. *Developing Leaders Through Mentoring.* Capella University; 2011.

13. Harvey M, McIntyre N, Thompson Heames J, Moeller M. Mentoring global female managers in the global marketplace: traditional, reverse, and reciprocal mentoring. *Int J Hum Resour Manag*. 2009;20(6):1344–1361. doi:10.1080/09585190902909863

14. Dierdorff EC. Time management is about more than life hacks. *Harvard Business Review*. January 29, 2020. https://hbr.org/2020/01/time-management-is-about-more-than-life-hacks

15. Center for Creative Leadership. 4 ways to strengthen your ability to influence others. November 24, 2020. https://www.ccl.org/articles/leading-effectively-articles/4-keys-strengthen-ability-influence-others

16. Economy P. The (Millennial) workplace of the future is here—these 3 things are about to change big time. *Inc.* January 5, 2019. https://www.inc.com/peter-economy/the-millennial-workplace-of-future-is-almost-here-these-3-things-are-about-to-change-big-time.html

17. Jordan J, Sorell M. Why reverse mentoring works and how to do it right. *Harvard Business Review*. October 3, 2019. https://hbr.org/2019/10/why-reverse-mentoring-works-and-how-to-do-it-right

18. Erikson E, Erikson J, Kivnick H. *Vital Involvement in Old Age*. Norton; 1986.

19. Facher L. Rochelle Walensky said she'd 'fix' the CDC, but nine months in, she's faltering. November 8, 2021. https://www.statnews.com/2021/11/08/rochelle-walensky-cdc-faltering

20. Bandler J, Callahan P, Rotella S, Berg K. Inside the fall of the CDC: how the world's greatest public health organization was brought to its knees by a virus, the president and the capitulation of its own leaders, causing damage that could last much longer than the coronavirus. October 15, 2020. https://www.propublica.org/article/inside-the-fall-of-the-cdc

21. @CDCgov. The #COVID19 level of transmission in the US remains high. The 7-day average of new cases is 74,585, a 5.1% increase from the previous week. Get vaccinated. Twitter. November 10, 2021. https://twitter.com/cdcgov/status/1458547542778597377

Chapter 19

Mentoring and Trusted Advisors

Cynthia D. Lamberth, F. Douglas Scutchfield*, and C. William Keck

INTRODUCTION

Looking to others in one's profession for assistance in career and life decisions and guidance on how to show up as a leader is a time-honored leadership accelerator. One can derive valuable lessons by consulting with those who have walked the same or similar paths, which allows one to learn the successes and failures of others. Finding a mentor, establishing and maintaining successful mentoring relationships, and serving as a mentor to others are all powerful development skills. Additional self-reflective experiences include creating and maintaining a group of unofficial advisors—sometimes referred to as a personal board of directors (PBOD) or kitchen cabinet—and participating in seeking accountability partners, which are also vital resources for personal growth. These activities allow one to see their potential and capabilities through the eyes of others. This chapter guides leaders in building trusting relationships with mentors, advisors, and accountability partners as well as serving others in these roles.

OBJECTIVES

By the end of this chapter, the reader will be able to:

- Briefly describe the history and evolution of individual and group mentoring.
- Describe why mentoring is essential in today's dynamic public health and healthcare environments.
- Discuss how mentoring provides an organization with the opportunity to meet the needs of underrepresented staff.
- Describe the types of mentoring relationships.
- Explain how to find mentors, PBOD, and mastermind groups that match individual values and development needs.

THE HISTORICAL BASIS FOR MENTORING

The term "mentor" harkens back to the Homeric legend of the Trojan War.[1] When Ulysses (Odysseus), King of Ithaca, left to make war on the Trojans, he left his infant son, Telemachus, and his wife, Penelope, in the hands of Mentor, his friend and retainer. To a major degree Mentor was responsible not only for the boy's education, but for the shaping of his character, the wisdom of his decisions, and the clarity and steadfastness of his purpose. Ulysses was gone for some 20 years, so this relationship is frequently viewed as an example of essential elements of mentoring and guiding characteristics of a long and comprehensive mentoring relationship.

There is considerable literature on mentoring, much of it in the management and medicine professions.[2] There is powerful support for mentoring, and it is considered a critical component of many professional education programs to improve success. The evidence focuses on developing strong healthcare leadership[3] and suggests relationships with more

---

* Dr. Scutchfield passed away May 23, 2022, prior to publication of this text.

than one mentor[4] to bolster success. There is also a strong link between mentoring programs in helping underrepresented populations[5,6] bring their knowledge and cultural acumen to issues and solutions.[7] Attention is also given to the archetypical roles, including serving as a traditional or reciprocal mentor, coach, sponsor, and connector.[8]

The health, medicine, and management literature provides evidence on effectiveness and explores several models including the assigned, self-selected, group, reverse, and peer approaches, which are explored in this chapter.[9]

MENTORING MODELS AND THEORIES

The theoretical underpinnings of mentoring arise from three primary theoretical frameworks: developmental, learning, and social theories.[10]

DEVELOPMENTAL THEORY

Developmental theories on mentoring reflect an inherent hierarchic relationship between mentee and mentor within an individual's progressive development throughout many seasons of life.[11] The mentor provides practical support during a mentee's developmental transitions with effective mentoring relying on matching of career strategies to the mentee's core values, purpose, and desired outcomes. The focus is on the mentee's personal growth. Examples of the application of developmental theory include peer mentoring, reverse mentoring, and junior-senior faculty mentoring relationships.[12–14]

LEARNING THEORY

The concept of mentoring as a learning partnership is the basis of mentoring and is built upon transformative, action, and social learning theories. The mentor is a facilitator for the mentee's personal progress just as Mentor guided Telemachus.[15] Adult learning theory also emphasizes the facilitator role of the mentor, where both the mentor and mentee engage in a mutual learning process through self-reflection and critical discussion of past experiences and social roles.[16] This use of action learning approach using reflection is critical to mentor–mentee conversations. Similarly, transformative learning theory advocates for active discussion and critical thinking between mentor and mentee to explore career, work, and identity.[17] Learning theories of mentorship emphasize the role of the mentee as an active co-creator of their own development.

SOCIAL THEORY

The process of mutual development is also seen in social theory, which focuses on the process of learning through imitation.[10] Social theories of mentorship include socialization, human/social capital, social exchange, and social network theories, as well as communities of practice.[10] The various models of mentoring all identify the mentee as an active contributor to the relationship and this exchange of information and knowledge leads to success. Social exchange theory suggests that when there is a clear cost-benefit to both parties, based on values and individual purpose, a successful mentoring relationship evolves.[10] Communities of practice, including masterminds and accountability groups, create knowledge networks where mentoring is a partnership.[10]

THE MODELS AND TYPES OF MENTORING RELATIONSHIPS

Numerous studies provide evidence that those who have successful mentoring relationships perform better and are given more responsibility and promoted more rapidly.[18,19] The mentoring models of assigned, self-selected, group, reverse, and peer are most commonly explored in the literature.

- **Assigned mentoring:** Includes programs where the mentor is assigned to a mentee for a specific purpose. An example of this type of relationship is that of a medical or nursing intern and their assigned mentor for the year. The mentor is assigned to help the student learn the culture, protocols, structure, and resources of the organization as well as the ethics and values of their chosen profession.

- **Self-selected mentoring**: The mentee seeks out a mentor based on their career and personal goals using identified attributes to find a person who can guide their career decisions and bring out their best.

- **Group mentoring**: Includes masterminds, circles, and affinity groups all focused on personal development within a group setting. Group mentoring may be peer focused; however, many masterminds include individuals with both short- and long-term career experience.

- **Peer mentoring**: Refers to masterminds, circles, and groups that include a group of individuals who are peers in a profession or experience. For example, a group of candidates for a degree, or a group of new associates or employees, could be a peer mentoring experience.

- **Reverse mentoring**: A new associate, student, employee, or volunteer is engaged by a more senior colleague to reverse the knowledge transfer, allowing the more established worker to learn from the more junior person. This is particularly helpful in the technology profession, where cultural knowledge may be needed, and to understand the needs of newer and underrepresented staff. Reverse mentoring is a contemporary concept that relies on the reversal of the traditional roles of mentor and mentee and reverses the notion of the mentorship model as an apprenticeship or hierarchy. In reverse mentoring, a younger professional takes on the role of mentor and a more seasoned professional, the role of mentee. Reverse mentoring is founded in learning and social theories of mentorship and has been widely applied in information technology, business, and education fields; however, there is a role for reverse mentoring in medical education and the health sciences, particularly with the inclusion of innovative technologies in a changing health landscape, and the emphasis on interdisciplinary teamwork and improved workplace culture. Reverse mentoring is also helpful in bridging cultural gaps in health equity endeavors.

TYPES OF MENTORING RELATIONSHIPS

The formality of the mentoring relationship and length of intervention are often used to describe the types of mentoring relationships.[20] *Informal, short-term mentoring* is a series of meetings or calls for spontaneous advice or counsel without structure. *Informal, long-term mentoring* consists of being available as needed to discuss problems, to listen, and to share knowledge. *Highly structured, short-term* is a formally established relationship, sometimes assigned to meet specific objectives such as navigating a fellowship or residency. *Highly structured, long-term mentoring* is used for succession planning, grooming someone to take over a leadership position or public office, or to master a profession such as medicine, public health, or research. There are many instances where a mentoring relationship can morph into one of the other three quadrants based on the needs of the mentee and the desire of the mentor. Figure 19.1 shows this relationship.

- **Informal, short-term mentoring:** Occurs when a mentee seeks advice on a specific project or decision in their career. This might mean presenting the option to the mentor and then discussing the value, attributes, and drawbacks of each path. Once the decision is made, the mentoring would be considered complete.

- **Informal, long-term mentoring:** Occurs where a student may seek the advice of a senior faculty member as they are selecting studies, experiences, and courses in preparation for application to advanced learning or a terminal degree such as medicine, law, or PhD.

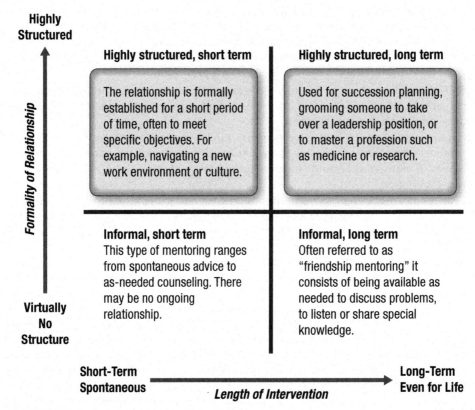

FIGURE 19.1: Types of Mentoring Relationships.
Source: Adapted from Shea GF. How to develop successful mentor behaviors. Crisp Publications, Inc. 2002.

■ **Highly structured short-term, self-selected mentoring relationship:** Occurs with public health and preventive medicine students where a faculty member serves as mentor for the capstone product. It differs from other mentoring activity as it is embedded in the rules of the university about research guidance to be provided by a professor. Nevertheless, in the long history of the relationship between student and teacher, this mentoring around a required research activity comprises at least one illustration of a university sanctioned and encouraged research mentorship between the student and a professor. Both freely enter this more formalized manifestation of tutoring in the quest for new knowledge of the process and practice of obtaining new scientific information. In this example, the mentor is consulted by the student mentee who must complete a "thesis" or "capstone" as a culminating exercise for the acquisition of a degree or completion of a program requirement for advancement in an educational program, such as an integrating experience, that the student will be able to call on and demonstrate the skills to organize and present a coherent and thoughtful product of their intellectual activity.

■ **Highly structured, long-term mentoring:** May span many decades and includes a deep personal relationship between both mentor and mentee for mutual benefit. The case study provided by Dr. Keck within this chapter is a perfect example of a highly structured, long-term mentoring relationship.

THE DIFFERENCE BETWEEN MENTORING AND COACHING

The terms "coaching" and "mentoring" are frequently used interchangeably and share some of the same goals; however, there are some differences worth noting. Coaching and mentoring both seek to help an individual grow, develop, and reach their potential. Coaching typically seeks to guide the individual by asking many questions and using tools that guide self-reflection so that the answers are discovered by the one being coached. Coaching is also used to focus on performance improvement, much like a sports coach analyzes skill and directs practice drills to increase skill. A mentor is typically someone who shares their knowledge, skills, and experience to assist in personal development; they communicate far more by telling than by asking questions. The mentor also serves to make connections, share personal experiences, review writings, and encourage bold decisions. The hybrid model of coaching with mentoring is frequently used, which allows the relationship to begin by asking many questions to fully understand the goals of the relationship and uncover areas of indecision or uncertainty that need to be addressed.

WHY MENTORING IS ESSENTIAL

Looking to others in one's profession for assistance with career and life decisions and guidance on how to show up as a leader is a time-honored leadership accelerator. One of the hallmarks of being a mentee is responding to the questions a mentor asks that encourage self-reflection, allowing a deep assessment of personal values, goals, and options.

Connecting with a mentor also helps those new to a profession connect with the history and legacy of their chosen path through a personal relationship with someone who has walked the path. The relationship is also reciprocal, meaning the mentor will also learn from the mentee and understand more about those new to the organization or profession.

Mentoring can also bridge the disconnect that may exist between senior leadership and more junior contributors; this happens in both traditional mentoring relationships and reverse mentoring created to accomplish this specific knowledge transfer. It is also an excellent support tool for underrepresented individuals in a profession or setting that may link women and Black, Indigenous, and People of Color (BIPOC) to resources and knowledge that address existing structural effects created by historical practices in education, hiring, and communities. In the past, mentors often sought to help women, people of color, and other individuals address cultural differences they may have had with the organization or profession they were entering in efforts to *assimilate* into the existing norms and practices. Today, however, mentors seek to learn from the mentee and discover how the brilliance of those cultural differences can add to the organization and help meet the needs of the clients and communities they serve. This is also an example of how reverse mentoring can benefit diverse cultures. For example, one of the author's student mentees had relocated from her home country and wanted to reach out to members of her new community who had relocated from the same home country in order to assist with knowledge of childcare and pediatric care, as well as provide training on how to protect children from environmental exposures. Others had made similar attempts, including pediatricians at the local clinic, but all failed to attract these immigrant families to events and classes. The mentee knew that in her culture a shamanic healer could influence whether mothers and families would welcome the knowledge offered; ultimately, she was successful in creating a bridge between her culture and the pediatric providers at the local clinic through a reverse mentoring relationship with one of the pediatricians. This bridge helped to secure the endorsement of the shamanic healer and members of the community began to accept the services offered by the local clinic. Mentoring is a reciprocal experience and gives the mentor an opportunity to learn from those whose lived experiences are different and include knowledge that may be critical to the success of the organization and both mentor and mentee careers.

HOW TO FIND, CREATE, AND SUSTAIN A PRODUCTIVE MENTORING RELATIONSHIP

To paraphrase William Arthur Ward, "The mediocre mentor tells. The good mentor explains. The superior mentor demonstrates. The greatest mentors inspire."[21] Looking for and finding someone who will inspire a person to greatness is seldom an easy task.

A productive mentoring relationship is built on mutual respect, strong listening skills, commitment to the journey, and accountability. In looking for a mentor it is important to consider if that person can serve in one or more roles described in the next section under creating a PBOD and the five types of members of your board (Table 19.1).

The first step is to identify individuals who may be a connector, maven, influencer, sponsor, or traditional mentor/coach. Selecting someone who is a role model, by observing their career, their accomplishments, and their communication style, is a start; however, the deeper skills of a mentor may not be obvious until the potential mentor and mentee have met numerous times.[22]

TABLE 19.1: The Five Types of Members of Your Board

The Connector	A connector is a "people person," one who knows and has great relationships with many people. These people love to open doors, make introductions, and help grow their network and the network of others. The strength of connectors is that they know and keep in touch with many people. "Connectors are people who link us up with the world. People with a special gift for bringing the world together."[22 (p38)] Is there someone who can't resist introducing you to the right people? Consider them for the role of connector. When asked a question, a connector will provide links to two or three others who know the answer.
The Maven	Mavens want to educate; they take delight in having knowledge about many things or knowing where to find it. This person typically has a finger on the pulse of what is going on in their profession or field and organization. This is the person to seek out when information about both history and new trends, ideas, projects, and opportunities is the goal. A maven is frequently the knowledgeable colleague everyone looks to for advice, or the colleague who is acting as a bridge between cross-functional teams or community partners due to their breadth of knowledge and established trust. The maven or informational powerhouse will also have great ideas of experiences to explore or books to read to enhance career trajectory and personal goals.
The Influencer	This person makes things happen. This person has a way of eliciting agreement and collaboration from teams, and can provide the heavy-hitting support that will influence project or program success. An influencer has earned the respect of the organization for their knowledge, professionalism, and work ethic. To identify an influencer, look for someone who is amplifying the voices of others, advocating for their suggestions and supporting them.
The Sponsor	A sponsor is an influential individual who can accelerate one's career by placing them in consideration for career opportunities including presentations, high-visibility assignments, committees, conferences, and positions. Unlike mentorship, sponsors usually see potential in someone and choose to assist. A sponsor typically chooses whom to sponsor; however, there are actions one can take to make it more likely that a sponsor will want to advocate. Showing an eagerness to learn and take advice, demonstrating outstanding job performance, making achievements known to leaders who have a track record of developing talent, and sharing individual goals with potential sponsors so that they know which opportunities might be a good match are all good practices.
The Mentor/Coach	This person supports the mentee's growth and development by providing advice, feedback, and guidance. A mentor also acts as a sounding board for career-related decisions and can help navigate challenging situations at work. This entire chapter is about good mentoring and mentee behavior so it is not necessary to repeat those here.

A common question is whether or not one should invite someone to be their mentor. In a non-assigned mentoring relationship, it is best to ease into the relationship by first asking for one meeting; if the conversation meets one's personal goals, then ask if the individual would be available to meet on a regular basis, either short or long term. Realize that many senior and/or seasoned professionals may need to limit the number of individuals they guide and advise, so they may not be able to commit to a formal mentoring relationship. Opening the dialogue for mentoring must include a clear list of goals, values, and expectations of the relationship. Tools to uncover personal values, goals, and expectations are all included as appendices to this chapter.

Knowing the expectations of the relationship and whether one is ready for mentoring are crucial to a productive relationship. The self-assessment mentoring audit is a good tool to use when considering a mentor or meeting with an assigned mentor (Appendix 19.1). A mentor may ask a mentee to complete a values inventory (Appendix 19.2) and vision planning (Appendix 19.3) to be clear on their desired outcomes.

Establishing the terms of the mentoring relationship means defining what success looks like. This is important for both mentor and mentee. The mentor will want to review an updated resume or curriculum vitae (CV), LinkedIn profile or academic publishing sites, and recent publications. Have these easily available for the potential mentor. Discussion of mentee values, goals, relationship needs, and expectations should be documented for both to review. Define what success looks like for the mentor and mentee. This includes sharing assumptions, expectations, and limitations with candor and confidentiality. Discuss options for learning, including a commitment to reading and discussing books and experiences. Like any good plan, it is not "cast in stone" but should be reviewed and modified along the way. Some formal mentoring experiences include a checklist or form to document this; however, a straightforward document agreed to by both mentor and mentee may be sufficient.

A review of what makes a good mentor (Box 19.1) and what makes a good mentee (Box 19.2) will provide a good checklist for finding a mentor and establishing a productive relationship.

Box 19.1: What Makes a Good Mentor?

Mentoring Best Practices

- Think of yourself as a "learning facilitator" rather than the person with all the answers. Help your mentee find people and other resources that go beyond your experience and wisdom on a topic.
- Emphasize questions over advice giving. Use probes that help your mentee think more broadly and deeply. If they talk only about facts, ask about feelings. If they focus on feelings, ask them to review the facts. If they seem stuck in an immediate crisis, help them see the big picture.
- When requested, share your own experiences, lessons learned, and advice. Emphasize how your experiences could be different from their experiences and are merely examples. Limit your urge to solve the problem for them.
- Resist the temptation to control the relationship and steer its outcomes; your mentee is responsible for their own growth.
- Help your mentee see alternative interpretations and approaches.
- Build your mentee's confidence through supportive feedback.
- Encourage, inspire, and challenge your mentee to achieve their goals.
- Help your mentee reflect on successful strategies they have used in the past that could apply to new challenges.
- Be spontaneous now and then. Beyond your planned conversations, call or email "out of the blue" just to leave an encouraging word or piece of added information.
- Reflect on your mentoring practice. Request feedback.
- Enjoy the privilege of mentoring. Know that your efforts will have a significant impact on your mentee's development as well as your own.

Source: Center for Health Leadership & Practice Public Health Institute. *Mentoring Guide: A Guide for Proteges.* Center for Health Leadership & Practice; 2003; Center for Health Leadership & Practice Public Health Institute. *Mentoring Guide: A Guide for Mentors.* Center for Health Leadership & Practice; 2003.

Box 19.2: What Makes a Good Mentee?

Mentee Best Practices
- Think of your mentor as a "learning facilitator" rather than the person with all the answers.
- Embrace using a variety of resources and discussing findings with your mentor.
- Seek discussion and input rather than advice. Look to your mentor to help you think more broadly and deeply.
- Apply the knowledge shared with you and discuss its application.
- Be open to your mentor's efforts to help you see alternative interpretations as well as approaches to decisions and actions.
- Remember that you are responsible for your own growth. If your mentor's style leans toward managing the relationship and directing your development, speak up diplomatically and maintain control.
- Be receptive to receiving constructive feedback.
- Ask your mentor to share with you successful strategies and resources they have used in the past that could apply to the challenges you face.
- Enjoy the mentoring experience. Know that the energy you invest will have a significant impact on your development. Your mentor will also grow from the relationship.

SUNSETTING MENTORING RELATIONSHIPS

There typically comes a time when the mentee and/or the mentor is ready to move on. Visiting the example of learning to play an instrument is helpful; at some point there may not be significant content the teacher can offer to the student. That does not mean the teacher or mentor does not want to stay in contact and celebrate career and life successes with the mentee, but both should acknowledge the formal advising meetings are no longer necessary and perhaps set up touchpoints to stay in contact. The use of social media is helpful here. There may also be instances where the fit between mentor and mentee may not be working based on changes in each of their responsibilities and careers. In some relationships, the mentee may feel like the mentor is overstepping by making decisions for them rather than helping the mentee create their own path. At any time in the relationship when either mentor or mentee feel there is no longer benefit, an exit strategy should be discussed and implemented. The most common of these is a plan to stay in touch and a heartfelt thanks from the mentee for the guidance and assistance provided.

SELF-DIRECTED LEADERSHIP

CREATING YOUR OWN PERSONAL BOARD OF DIRECTORS

Another highly effective approach to personal development is to create a "PBOD." This recent approach is one that responds to the need for more than one mentor. A PBOD, or as some call it "kitchen cabinet," is a group of trusted advisors that each serve a unique purpose. In a *Harvard Business Review* article, Priscilla Claman defines this unique set as "a group of people you consult regularly to get advice and feedback." Claman adds, "This is the wave of the future and may replace traditional mentoring relationships."[23]

With a personal board, no joint meetings are held, and it is not necessary to inform each person of their status as a board member. It is important to select the right advisors with unique contributions that add to thinking and decisions. A recent coaching client shared, "I would not have seen the rapid trajectory in my career if not for my personal board of directors and their support." In curating a PBOD, it is beneficial to include those individuals who fulfill a specific role as well as those who bring an extensive network of professional contacts. The importance of the board of trusted advisors is critical in situations when seeking advice from the formal organizational hierarchy is not appropriate. Another attribute of a PBOD is that it may include representatives from all aspects of your life: personal, professional, spiritual or religious, community, health, and financial.

The personal board may also include guidance from books and authors. This might include reading and re-reading a particular book that provides insight and may include guidance from leadership and self-development books, podcasts, blogs, and Twitter feeds as well. Several famous and successful businesspeople read *Think and Grow Rich*, the book written by Napoleon Hill after interviewing and spending time with the most successful people of that era.[24] Based on the suggestion of a valued mentor, this author regularly reads the work of Thomas Merton, which feeds spiritual goals.[25]

SELECTING PERSONAL BOARD OF DIRECTORS MEMBERS

Enlisting a personal board is a smaller ask than finding a single mentor, as the associated time commitment is less significant for each member. It is important to identify the specific input about a specific area of expertise each board member will fulfill. It is critical to not ask all board members for guidance on everything. This may lead to conflicting ideas and delays in decisions and actions.

Board members can serve as role models; however, when building a PBOD, these guidelines will assist in not only identifying the knowledge base and experience of individuals but the five types of people to consider (see Table 19.1).

MASTERMIND GROUPS

Mastermind groups, an approach introduced by Napoleon Hill in his time-tested book, *Think and Grow Rich*, is another self-leadership mentoring opportunity.[24] A mastermind group is designed to help one navigate through challenges using the collective intelligence of others.

Typically, a group of goal-oriented people meet weekly or monthly to tackle challenges and problems together. They lean on each other, give advice, share connections, and offer support to each other in congruent journeys such as starting a new practice, business, or working on community issues. It is very much peer-to-peer mentoring and those who participate in masterminds typically see a marked change in their life as the opportunity to add a group of knowledgeable eyes and ears on any situation can lead to better informed decisions and actions. Masterminds work best when the participants represent varied careers and aspirations to broaden the thinking. A formalized mastermind group may require an invitation from the members and can include an application process. There is also the opportunity to start your own mastermind group.

The positive aspects of participating in a mastermind include:

- Being part of a supportive and reciprocal community that sees you as far more capable than you might see yourself. Plus, the other members need you just as much as you need them.
- Experiencing advisement: No person is an island. Other members of the mastermind can become advisors on many life and career situations.
- Collaborating and co-creating with members can emerge as symbiotic relationships develop in the group.
- Extending your overall network as the mastermind members share their connections and solutions.
- Enjoying bigger thinking: Being in a mastermind group seeks to give you a master mind in that you cannot help but think bigger and stretch beyond your boundaries when surrounded by amazing people doing amazing things.

ACCOUNTABILITY

Accountability is about commitments and interdependence. Accountability starts with personal accountability to one's values and vision in all decisions. A newer version of peer mentoring is the use of accountability circles, introduced by author Sam Silverstein.[26]

This trusted group of accountability partners for your life, career, and vocation is a group committed to helping each other be clear on their individual standards that define one as a person and therefore define the standards of relationships with everyone. This reciprocal group supports each other in identifying and acting on individual purpose, mission, and values. The goal of the circle is to help one be a leader in their own life.

Silverstein goes on to identify 10 interrelated commitments that can help one notice and respond effectively to decisions and choices.[27] The 10 commitments are:

1. Commit to discover and realize your potential . . . and to help others reach theirs.
2. Commit to the truth.
3. Commit to the values.
4. Commit to "It's all of us."
5. Commit to embrace faults and failures as well as opportunities and successes.
6. Commit to sound financial principles (stewardship).
7. Commit to a safe place.
8. Commit to "my word is my bond."
9. Commit to stand strong when all hell breaks loose.
10. Commit to a good reputation.

The circle will support each member in keeping these commitments, personal values, and vision in focus for all choice work and decisions. The peer-guided support alleviates the "lone ranger" syndrome where we think we have to create our own solutions and hesitate to ask for help. Silverstein shares, "This vision of a self-reliant accountability is wrong. In fact, everything we have been taught about accountability is wrong. Accountability is not about having to prove ourselves, create some original idea, or live an independent life, and it is certainly not about "holding others accountable. Quite the contrary—accountability is all about commitments and interdependence. We need other people to help us to be our very best, and we need to help other people to be their very best. It is in helping others fulfill their potential that we identify and achieve our own true potential!"[26(p3)]

SUMMARY

Life is seeking growth: personal growth, career growth, spiritual growth, intellectual growth. A time-tested approach and leadership accelerator is the use of mentors and trusted advisors in all aspects of the path one walks in life. Looking to others for support and advice through mentoring, coaching, and peer structures in both informal and formal relationships fulfills a basic human need for connection and growth. Attending to the relationships with mentors, a PBOD, accountability groups, and mastermind groups enriches the professional journey for the mentor, mentee, and peers in groups. This chapter provides tools to find mentors and board members as well as peer structures of support. The outcomes of a good mentoring relationship are based on the strong participation of the mentee and a clear vision by the mentee that includes values, purpose, overall career vision, and accountability. Thinking that one can accomplish anything in life alone is a career and personal limitation; therefore, setting a personal vision and goals, and identifying individuals to serve as mentors and trusted advisors is key to success. We need other people to help us to be our best in life and career, and we need to help other people to be their very best. It is in helping others fulfill their potential that we solidify, identify, and achieve our own true potential. The noble act of serving as a mentor and advisor for others as one's career and life progresses is a valuable contribution to our world and our professions.

DISCUSSION QUESTIONS

1. If you are putting together a "PBOD" who are the five people you would select and what criteria would you use?
2. If asked to join a multidisciplinary mastermind group devoting 2 hours a week to this group, would you say yes or no and what would drive that decision?
3. Do you have a list of the five most influential books in your life and career? Would you suggest these to others in your field? If you do not have a list, create one now.

CASE STUDY: 1:1 MENTORING – LONG TERM

C. William Keck

AF made an appointment to see me in my office at the Akron Health Department in the spring of 1994. I was director of health for the city and chair of what is now the Department of Family and Community Medicine at the Northeast Ohio Medical University. I had first met AF when she was a medical student at the university. After graduation she had finished her residency in OB/GYN and gone into private practice in 1992. A year later she was reevaluating her goals.

AF explained to me that she wanted to do more than just see patients one-on-one, as the talk about healthcare reform at the time piqued her interest in enhancing health on a community basis. Since she really enjoyed educating patients on healthy living, she was interested in possibly setting up wellness programs for corporations. She had decided to leave her practice and spend some time and effort learning more about public health and about the business world to explore this option. To that end she had already enrolled in the master of business administration degree program taught in the evenings at the University of Akron and the master of public health degree program taught on weekends at The Ohio State University in Columbus. She came to see me because she was looking for a way to explore public health and support herself while she pursued those two degrees.

I was certainly intrigued. At the medical school I was often the "go to" source for medical students who wished to study medicine but were questioning whether their future should be in clinical service. I was used to helping students understand how flexible a medical degree is and the many nonclinical career options that are available, including public health.

I explained to AF that I had no physician positions open at the moment, but that I could offer her a part-time position as a health educator where she could focus on working with prenatal patients and also teach about breast and cervical health issues. Her acceptance signaled the beginning of a mentoring relationship that has lasted until the current day.

We discussed her goals and expectations and agreed that we should use the ensuing 2 years to give her as broad an experience in understanding local public health issues and services as time and circumstance would allow. Our expectation was that the combination of her degree courses and practical health department experiences would help her to more intelligently sort through her career options. I promised to involve her in public health policy discussions when possible.

Year One

The Health Department staff were delighted to have a personable OB/GYN physician involved with their female patients and AF was pleased with her experiences. During this year I became involved in leading an effort to develop a Federally Qualified Health Center (FQHC) in Akron that was a collaborative effort between three hospitals and the health department. It was an organizationally, politically, and financially complex project and I thought it a wonderful opportunity to show AF how this particular kind of "sausage" can be made (or not!). She gladly learned about the process, helped me proofread documents I had to produce, and attended planning meetings when she could. Her participation was real and helpful.

Year Two

As the first year came to a close, AF came to me with a new proposition. She was leaning more and more toward a career in prevention and public health and wanted to pursue a residency in preventive medicine. The Ohio State University had such a residency program and AF needed only a year of public health training to qualify for residency completion. Ohio State was willing to count AF's first part-time year with the health department as one-half of the public health year and would accept her second year with us for the remainder of the public health year if she could arrange a more targeted experience with a preceptor boarded in preventive medicine. I fit those qualifications and agreed to precept her using the FQHC development as her project. The result was a stronger presence for AF in both formal and informal sessions dealing with all aspects of the project, and a specific role in developing quality assurance policies.

During our discussions of progress toward meeting her goals and next steps for her, AF made it clear that what she loved most was teaching. I, meanwhile, was a bit in awe of AF's intellect and capacity for hard work. After all, in June of 1996 she had earned two degrees (MBA and MPH) and finished a preventive medicine residency in just 2 years. I was thinking about how to keep AF in the community.

I had been working several years at the college of medicine to develop an MPH program focused on providing a degree opportunity for working public health professionals and thought taking charge of it might interest AF. She accepted my offer in 1996 to become an assistant professor and the project director for this new program that would be a consortium effort between the college of medicine and three universities. She moved from working for me in the health department to working for me in the college of medicine, and immediately stepped into helping develop the organizational and functional details of a complicated partnership. As department chair, I remained the principal figure as negotiations proceeded, and AF began to learn about the personalities and egos involved, how to listen carefully to concerns, to craft compromises, and to resolve issues of administration, organization, and finance.

The Next Phase

During the next 12 years until my retirement from the college of medicine we focused on two major areas: developing and managing the MPH program and developing AF's standing in her profession. For the first area, our discussions centered on communication with the consortium partners, the medical school hierarchy, and the program's faculty and students. We successfully prepared for program accreditation, her promotion to program director, and her promotion to associate professor in 2005. We talked about when to go it alone and when to involve the "boss(es)," and as problems arose, there were clear discussions of what AF does well (teaching, service, program management) and what she is less fond of doing (research, personnel management). These discussions were important in assessing how to proceed and who to involve when issues related to program and career occurred. For example, working with professionals representing five universities was a challenge, both from a political and personal standpoint. I was able to demonstrate to AF that by consulting with allies, one can make progress toward goals. "Asking for forgiveness rather than permission" became a mantra when working through some unprecedented complex and sticky situations.

In the area of professional development, we reviewed the importance of cementing her professional credentials by passing the preventive medicine boards and becoming a fellow of the American College of Preventive Medicine, which she accomplished in 2003. Next was service to the community, institution, and profession, including the best way for AF to approach that area from the perspectives of her own professional growth and the importance of involvement in ways that would meet her goals for eventual promotion to the rank of professor, which she achieved in 2013. She looked within the university and at local, state, and national groups. She has been active with a wide range of university committees, local groups (FQHC, Akron Health Department, Coalition for Asian Health, etc.), state associations (Ohio Public Health Association, Health Policy Institute of Ohio, Ohio Research Association for Public Health Improvement), and many national professional associations (American Public Health Association, Association for Prevention Teaching and Research, Council on Education for Public Health, American College of Medical Quality, Council on Linkages Between Academia and Public Health Practice, Council of Graduate Programs in Public Health, and the Association of Schools and Programs of Public Health). My role, particularly early in her career, was to help her sort out where to best spend her energy and to help introduce her to these organizations, many of which I was active in. She quickly rose to leadership positions in a number of these groups and gradually had a diminishing need for my advice.

My role as a mentor did not stop with professional development. I often found opportunities for AF in my other roles. She went to Cuba three times to study their medical system and culture through my ties with Medical Education Cooperation with Cuba. She developed her bicycle riding skills so that she could accompany our riding group to go to see the Ohio Light Opera in Wooster. She recorded several videos in my Media Mentoring project. She was also the subject of one of the chapters in my book about collaboration. Throughout all these experiences, she felt comfortable enough to let me know about her personal life, which included topics of family, relationships, and health.

Role Evolution

My relationship with AF began as teacher/student and evolved through health director/employee to department chair/faculty member and eventually to colleague and friend. It has always been a mentoring relationship that has benefitted us both. I was able to help AF find a career that suited her well and provide some guidance as her career evolved. In return, I was rewarded through pride in her achievements and growth of my College of Medicine Department fed by her excellent stewardship of its MPH program. After my retirement, the roles reversed somewhat as AF did her best to keep me up-to-date with happenings in public health and continued to involve me in MPH teaching. She has mastered her profession well and is now the teacher and mentor to medical and public health students and young professionals.

CASE STUDY QUESTIONS

1. In reviewing the case study from Dr. Keck with his protegee AF, how would you describe the changes in their relationship over time?
2. What could you do in your mentoring relationships as the protegee to realize this positive outcome?
3. What examples from the case show Dr. Keck's ability to help AF see the best use of her time and energy based on her goals?

CASE STUDY: 1:1 MENTORING—SHORT TERM

F. Douglas Scutchfield

An interesting and rewarding experience in mentoring occurs as students in public health and preventive medicine come to the end of didactic experience and begin to think about their research required for a degree, either a capstone paper or a more formal research experience with the preparation of a thesis or its equivalent.

As the result of this experience, I have had a series of opportunities to mentor students developing the thesis or capstone experience in their academic area. I benefit in my own scholarship, as we are likely to be jointly exploring an area of interest for me, as the student has come to me with an anticipation that I am knowledgeable or interested in their understanding of the research. I may not be knowledgeable, and the student's work is likely to expand my own depth of knowledge in the appropriate area. Moreover, in many cases, this relationship has developed into a longer term, more involved mentorship and relationship with the student.

PC was a student in an honors college class I taught on Thomas Merton. She had done well and seemed to come out of a shell as the course progressed and she became more engaged. She went from a wallflower to an active contributor, which is always gratifying to a professor to see in a student. I was surprised by the email from her asking if she could visit with me the next year. I am happy to meet and visit with students about whatever they wish to discuss. I suggested a lunch at the faculty club. It was at that lunch that she indicated she would like to do research on Appalachian health, specifically focused on Kentucky. We talked at length about what she would like to investigate. She was working in her hometown, Hazard, as a pharmacy tech on weekends when she returned home from college to earn extra money for college. She talked about the patients she had met with, dispensing medicines that had been filled by the pharmacist, and the difficulty in explaining to patients the directions and character of the medicine, and she was never sure whether they took the medication and used it appropriately or not. I suggested that her interest sounded like an area of interest known as "health literacy." I suggested that I would put her in touch with a medical health science librarian to help her read some literature that might enhance her knowledge, but also suggest that there may be research opportunities in this area if she were interested or inclined to pursue it further. She was interested, so following the lunch I emailed an introduction of PC to the health sciences librarian who had been helpful to me in the past on literature searches. The two began a collaboration in developing a set of journal articles that PC reviewed and further developed with the librarian into a solid literature of the topic in Appalachia. The student learned to use EndNote as a part of this search and had the literature well laid out when she followed up our introductory meeting with the suggestion for another lunch. At this lunch she outlined what specifically she was interested in, health literacy in Appalachia Kentucky. She pointed out that they, she, and the librarian had failed to find a reference on the prevalence of health illiteracy in Appalachia Kentucky and that she would like to study that question.

This prompted the development of a new proposal, which would become the capstone required for all honors college graduates at the University of Kentucky. We had discussed a few steps, including the clarification of her specific aims for the study, a mechanism that I use to get students to narrow to a manageable topic and question. We worked through this exercise to develop an understanding of how we might approach the question and we agreed that she would prepare a proposal for the topic at our next meeting. I suggested that the proposal include a literature review that she had completed with the librarian and include a methodology for the next steps on her process, putting in place a first draft of the eventual introduction and methodology for a paper to come from her work on the topic.

Our next meeting allowed me to raise with her some questions about PC's research protocol. Her specific aim was to develop a measure of the level of health literacy and its characteristics in patients in Appalachia Kentucky. We discussed what instrument she would use to determine the level of health literacy, what was most commonly used, and if it had gone through the appropriate validity and reliability evaluations to assure it was a good tool. I suggested that she might even draw up "dummy tables" to help her understand how she would display her data at the completion of the study. When I asked her about how she would further analyze the data, she had not given it much thought. I suggested that she consider talking with and opening a discussion with a statistician who I knew would take the time and effort to work with PC to refine and develop the tables and data collection procedures to complete her study. I had a long-standing relationship from my own work with a very good biostatistician that I was able to put in contact with PC about her research and data management. This resulted, as expected, with better ideas about data collection and how it was to be used to portray her work.

She was anxious to get started with her data collection, but I asked her if she wanted to publish the results of her work, as we had found no data in the literature on the level of health literacy in Appalachia Kentucky. She was anxious to get it published, if we could do a good job on the manuscript. As a premedical student she was anxious to publish the work as it might improve her opportunity to successfully compete for a medical school slot by showing her research interest and acumen. This allowed me to point out that if she wanted to publish her work, as well as assure its acceptance, she needed to get the UK Institutional Review Board's (IRB) approval for the work and suggested that she meet with another colleague in our Office of Research Integrity to discuss IRB approval of the project or at least an exemption from that office for formal approval. I also asked about where she planned to collect data for the project. She was not sure, but when I suggested FQHCs in Appalachia, she quickly agreed that would be ideal. Again, I had a good friend who I had worked with who was the CEO of the Kentucky Primary Care Association, which represented all the FQHCs in Kentucky. An electronic introduction worked, and we received the help of several Appalachia Kentucky FQHCs as the CEO of KPCA asked them for their help, facilitating a relationship for the project and its outcome which would be shared with all the Kentucky FQHCs. With that she began her data collection to achieve the number of participants that she and her biostatistical consultant had agreed would be sufficient to meet the calculated power level for significance. This study has completed data collection and the statistician is helping the student frame what they can or cannot say about health literacy and its impact on patients. With that and some work with the results and discussion section of an MS degree, the student will have done a thorough and effective piece of research in health literacy in Appalachia Kentucky.

CASE STUDY QUESTIONS

1. What did PC do well as the junior researcher/student to assure a successful outcome?
2. Is the mentoring experience of PC a good example of matching the mentor's passions to the goals of the mentee? What did the two have in common and how did they capitalize on this?
3. How did Dr. Scutchfield fill the roles of connector, maven, influencer, sponsor, and traditional mentor/coach for PC?

A robust set of instructor resources designed to supplement this text is located at http://connect.springerpub.com/content/book/978-0-8261-4924-4. Qualifying instructors may request access by emailing textbook@springerpub.com.

REFERENCES

1. Homer. *The Odyssey*. Simon and Schuster; 1969.
2. Willbur J. Does mentoring breed success? *Train Dev J*. 1987;41(11):38–41.
3. Hawkins J, Fontenot HB. Mentorship: the heart and soul of health care leadership. *J Healthc Leadersh*. 2010;2:31–34. doi:10.2147/JHL.S7863
4. Chopra V, Edelson DP, Saint S. Mentorship malpractice. *JAMA*. 2016;315(14):1453–1454. doi:10.1001/jama.2015.18884
5. Atkins K, Dougan BM, Dromgold-Sermen MS, Potter H, Sathy V, Panter AT. "Looking at myself in the future": how mentoring shapes scientific identity for STEM students from underrepresented groups. *Int J STEM Educ*. 2020;7(1):1–15. doi:10.1186/s40594-020-00242-3
6. Predoi-Cross A. Inclusive mentoring and leadership, and the many roads to success. *Can J Phys*. 2020;98(6):ix–xvii. doi:10.1139/cjp-2019-0291
7. Beech BM, Calles-Escandon J, Hairston KG, Langdon MSE, Latham-Sadler BA, Bell R. Mentoring programs for underrepresented minority faculty in academic medical centers: a systematic review of the literature. *Acad Med*. 2013;88(4):541–549. doi:10.1097/ACM.0b013e31828589e3

8. Chopra V, Arora VM, Saint S. Will you be my mentor?—four archetypes to help mentees succeed in academic medicine. *JAMA Intern Med.* 2018;178(2):175–176. doi:10.1001/jamainternmed.2017.6537

9. Crisp G, Baker VL, Griffin KA, Lunsford LG, Pifer MJ. *Mentoring Undergraduate Students.* ASHE Higher Education Report. ASHE; 2017.

10. Dominguez N, Hager M. Mentoring frameworks: synthesis and critique. *Int J Mentor Coach Educ.* 2013;2(3):171–188. doi:10.1108/IJMCE-03-2013-0014

11. Levinson D. *The Seasons of a Man's Life.* Random House; 1978.

12. Darwin A, Palmer E. Mentoring circles in higher education. *High Educ Res Dev.* 2009;28(2):125–136. doi:10.1080/07294360902725017

13. Clarke A, Burgess A, van Diggele C, Mellis C. The role of reverse mentoring in medical education: current insights. *Adv Med Educ Pract.* 2019;10:693. doi:10.2147/AMEP.S179303

14. Voytko ML, Barrett N, Courtney-Smith D, et al. Positive value of a women's junior faculty mentoring program: a mentor-mentee analysis. *J Women's Health.* 2018;27(8):1045–1053. doi:10.1089/jwh.2017.6661

15. Zachary L, Fischler L. *The Mentee's Guide: Making Mentoring Work for You.* Jossey-Bass; 2009.

16. Marquardt M, Waddill D. The power of learning in action learning: a conceptual analysis of how the five schools for adult learning theories are incorporated within the practice of action learning. *Action Learn Res Pract.* 2004;1(2):185–202. doi:10.1080/1476733042000264146

17. Clutterbuck D. Mentor competences: a field perspective In: Clutterbuck D, Lane G, eds. *The Situational Mentor.* Gower; 2004:42–56.

18. Lunding FS, Clements CE, Perkins DC. Everyone who makes it has a mentor. *Harv Bus Rev.* 1978;56(July/August):89–101.

19. Scandura TA. Mentoring and career mobility: an empirical investigation. *J Organ Behav.* 1992;13(2):169–174. doi:10.1002/job.4030130206

20. Shea GF. *Mentoring.* Crisp Publications; 1992.

21. Ward WA. William Arthur Ward quotes. 2020. https://libquotes.com/william-arthur-ward/quote/lbx8c9t

22. Gladwell M. *The Tipping Point: How Little Things Can Make a Big Difference.* Little, Brown; 2006.

23. Claman P. Forget mentors: employ a personal board of directors. *Harvard Business Review.* October 20, 2010. https://hbr.org/2010/10/forget-mentors-employ-a-person

24. Hill N. *Think and Grow Rich.* Jeremy P. Tarcher; 2007.

25. Merton T. *Thomas Merton: Essential Writings.* Orbis Books; 2001.

26. Silverstein S. *The Accountability Circle: Discovering Your True Purpose, Potential, and Impact ... With Accountability Partnerships.* Sound Wisdom; 2020.

27. Silverstein S. *I Am Accountable: Ten Choices That Create Deeper Meaning in Your Life, Your Organization, and Your World.* Sound Wisdom LLC; 2019.

28. Lamberth, C. Values clarification exercise. January 2020. https://www.exudeu.com

29. Sinek S. *Start With Why: How Great Leaders Inspire Everyone to Take Action.* Portfolio Penguin; 2011.

30. Sinek S, Mead D, Docker P. *Find Your Why: A Practical Guide for Discovering Purpose for You and Your Team.* Portfolio Penguin; 2017.

APPENDIX 19.1: SELF-ADMINISTERED MENTORING AUDIT

A self-audit completed by the mentee is a great tool to help set the plan for the mentoring relationship. The purpose is to self-reflect on readiness to be mentored. Using the following Likert scale table, check your readiness:

	1 (NEVER)	2 (SOMETIMES)	3 (DEPENDS)	4 (FREQUENTLY)	5 (ALWAYS)
I am goal oriented					
I seek challenges					
I take initiative					
I am eager to learn					
I am a good listener					
I accept personal responsibility for my growth					
I am overly self-promoting					
I am frequently too busy to meet with someone to just talk					
I am not focused on the mentor's area of expertise					
I expect my mentor to solve all my problems					

Scoring Interpretation: A total score of 40 to 50 implies complete readiness. A score of 30 to 40 implies the mentee is well positioned to benefit from a mentoring relationship. Anything below 30 indicates that the mentee would benefit from additional self-reflection and development before entering into a mentoring relationship.

APPENDIX 19.2: VALUES CLARIFICATION[29]

VALUES

Take time to think about what you value and why you value this. There may be a story behind many of your values. For example, if one has experienced lack of resources in their life, they may be more cautious about spending, and thus value security. There is no set number of values. It is up to you to create what captures your heart and who you want to show up as every day.

Examine five sets of values—foundational values as well as values in each of the four life areas. Use the attached list to circle or highlight values that speak to you and then place some in the categories we use to create our vision. Developing a healthy mentor–mentee relationship requires the mentee to be clear about their values.

Foundational Values

- What is the one thing or things that you will never compromise on?
- What character traits do you value in yourself and others—those fundamental and distinctive values that are unchangeable?

- What values are non-negotiable—a positive standard that respects others, our world, our communities?
- Are there ONE or TWO values that guide your overall approach to life? This may be your credo or your spiritual foundation that will come into play in each of the four life areas that follow.

Health and Well-Being

- What are your values around healthy choices and self-care?

Love and Relationships

- What do you value about your family and friends' relationships?
- What values do you think your family and friends see in you?
- What values do you want in your closest partner, mentor(s), or PBOD?

Vocation/Creative Expression

- What values do you need in your workplace or creative pursuits?
- What values can you embody to be the best in your career/job/position?

Time and Money Freedom

- What do you value in your community and how can you make your community better?
- How, and on what, do you like to spend your free time?
- What would you do with more time and money freedom?

Source: Lamberth C. *Values clarification exercise*. 2020. https://www.exudeu.com/

APPENDIX 19.3: PERSONAL VISION PLANNER

A personal vision statement is a mission statement of what you want to accomplish in your life, both personally and professionally. As a mentee, it is important for the mentor to know your "Why" as this, along with your values, will be the basis of many decisions the two of you will discuss. Being crystal clear on what matters most to you in life will help your mentor provide guidance in the right direction. The personal vision statement can be used as a guide when determining the career to pursue, making important life decisions, planning how you'll accomplish goals, and realizing your life dreams. Simon Sinek calls this vision statement *Your Why*[29] and offers this formula to write one:

"To _____ (contribution) so that _____ (impact)."

Garnering your purpose into one short sentence is a challenge. The process of discovering your purpose[30] is best accomplished with a partner and includes the following steps.

1. Make a list of memories that you return to over and over that may have influenced who you are today.
2. Find a partner who is willing to listen to your memories and help you dig deeper into why these experiences are important, looking for themes and threads that pull the stories together.

3. Schedule listening sessions with your partner to explore the stories.

   a. What lessons were learned from this memory/experience?

   b. Why is this story important to you?

   c. Did someone say something or speak about something that stayed with you?

   d. What is it about this story that you absolutely love?

   e. How did this make you feel?

4. Look at the themes and feelings from each story to determine your personal vision statement.

Some vision statements that may help you uncover your own:

■ *To support what respects and enhances freedom* (Nelson Mandela)
Nelson Mandela was an anti-apartheid revolutionary who spent 27 years in prison to fight human rights abuses, and was the president of South Africa. He is a worldwide symbol of resistance to apartheid.

■ *Allow humanity to propagate into the future by using better sources of energy* (Elon Musk)
Elon Musk is an entrepreneur, engineer, inventor, and CEO of Tesla and SpaceX.

■ *Unite people and promote equality* (Martin Luther King, Jr.)
Martin Luther King, Jr. was an American Baptist minister, activist, humanitarian, and leader in the African American Civil Rights Movement. He is best known for his role in the advancement of civil rights using nonviolent civil disobedience based on his Christian beliefs.

■ *Equip and IN-power LEADERS to be the best version of themselves, living a life they love, so they may serve their community, family, tribe, country, world* (Cynthia D. Lamberth)

Chapter 20

Leadership Intangibles

Paul C. Erwin

INTRODUCTION

Leadership intangibles are essential traits and practices that equip public health and health-care leaders to lead change through complexity and turbulence; they include attributes such as mindfulness, self-restoration, courage, compassion, humility, kindness, generosity, and finding balance. These are elements that leaders draw on across the spectrum of their role, from managing the day-to-day tedium of routinized work, to those times when they are overwhelmed by professional and personal crises. Intangibles are, in many respects, responses to the proverbial question, "What makes a good leader?" But they also serve to answer the question, "What is your go-to trait or attribute when you feel at risk of going off the rail?"

OBJECTIVES

By the end of this chapter, the reader will be able to:

- Explain the concept of leadership intangibles and why they are essential leadership attributes.
- Identify several leadership intangibles.
- Compare different perspectives on leadership intangibles.
- Describe methods for building, acquiring, and maintaining leadership intangibles.
- Analyze leadership intangibles through personal reflection.

APPLICATION OF INTANGIBLE LEADERSHIP QUALITIES

Richard Davis, author of *The Intangibles of Leadership: The 10 Qualities of Superior Executive Performance*,[1] describes leadership intangibles as qualities or subtle behaviors that "often fall between the lines of traditional leadership models, so they can be hard to identify and even harder to develop."[2(para1)] The following is his list of 10 leadership intangibles:

- wisdom
- will
- executive maturity
- integrity
- social judgment
- presence
- self-insight
- self-efficacy
- fortitude
- fallibility

Considering that all the chapter authors in this book are leaders, and therefore possess and exhibit a range of leadership qualities, the approach to identifying and describing leadership intangibles was to invite all the chapter authors to choose from a list of leadership intangibles—or add their own—and participate in an interview about their selected intangible. The interviews were conducted via videoconference in the summer of 2021, with the following questions sent ahead of time:

1. From a list of leadership intangibles, you selected [fill in]–why?
2. Describe a situation where you drew on this intangible. What led you to apply [the intangible], and what was the outcome?
3. How have you seen other leaders model this intangible?
4. What lessons have you learned from practicing [intangible]? (These could be both positive and/or "constructive" lessons.)
5. For those seeking to acquire or hone this intangible, what guidance can you provide?

What follows is a brief summary of these interviews, covering 19 different intangibles.

MINDFULNESS: CYNTHIA LAMBERTH

Mindfulness is something that Cynthia Lamberth practices every day: "I begin and end each day in a state of mindfulness." Cynthia describes two definitions of mindfulness: a trait—mindfulness is the quality of being conscious or aware of something, and a mental state—being achieved by focusing on the present, while being aware of your thoughts, feelings, and environment; being present in the moment, not ruminating about what happened yesterday or worrying about what might happen tomorrow. For her, mindfulness as a leadership intangible encompasses both the trait and state. In practicing mindfulness, "I begin *in gratitude* before my feet hit the floor . . . in silent meditation, prayer, and journaling. I write both my to-do list for the day, as well as my *to-be* list: How will I show up and who will I become as a result of my thoughts and actions?" And at the end of the day, Cynthia checks in with herself on her to-be list, being grateful for what she experienced during the day.

Cynthia calls on mindfulness when in stressful situations, as when someone is challenging her or what she is doing. It reminds her of her purpose, her *why*, and, as such, becomes her anchor. One of her colleagues at the University of Kentucky was a surgeon who described how he brought mindfulness into the operating room. He used the analogy of an airplane pilot, in the pilot's check-through pre-flight, during flight, and post-flight, and that everyone wants to have *that* mindful pilot flying their airplane. And the pilot, on the other hand, if they are on the operating table, wants to make sure that everyone in the operating room has gone through *their* mindfulness "check-list." Prior to, during, and after each surgery, the surgeon led his team in a practice of mindfulness, which elevated his team's effectiveness and improved surgical outcomes.

"The biggest lesson I have learned is that mindfulness is absolutely critical in achieving my *why*, my *purpose*." And what is Cynthia's purpose? "My purpose is to serve people, specifically to equip and empower leaders to be the best version of themselves, living a life they love, so that they may serve their community, their family, their friends, their tribe, their country, their world." Her advice to the aspiring leader who wants to begin a practice of mindfulness: try it, read about it, create a morning routine that speaks to you. Commit to it for 30 days, starting off with gratitude, and see how different you feel at the end of 30 days. Then add the bookend at the end of the day. Mindfulness, in the end, is about consciously living in the moment, because *this* moment is the only one you can control—you cannot control the past or future.

SELF-RESTORATION: BILL KECK

For Bill Keck, *self-restoration* is important for attaining and maintaining balance in mind and body: "it keeps you focused, and some don't do it enough!" He pursues this through a variety of hobbies and outside interests, including working with his hands (leather-carving, building a radio receiver, building a car in Hazard, Kentucky), traveling, long-distance bicycling, music, and theater. Traveling with his wife of 60 years, Ardith, took hold when they acquired an old Land Rover to make the drive from Bolivia back to the United States, following Bill's almost 3 years there in the Peace Corps (1966–1969). Travel introduces you to people you might not otherwise meet or come to know, and thus enriches your life and the experience. "You just rent a car and go! That has proved interesting!"

Self-restoration also comes through cycling long distances—Bill has lost count of the number of times he has crisscrossed the United States—but it is those long days in the "saddle," the pavement beneath his tires as the road undulates to the horizon, where his mind and body find that balance. Close friends model this for him; he is joined on many of these rides by a public health physician friend from his time in the Peace Corps, Ron St. John. "Sometimes riding on a bike, I solve problems, because the work never really leaves you."

The lessons learned include contemplating the risks—the risks of biking, of traveling—while anticipating that the advantages far outweigh those risks, and that through this pursuit of self-restoration, "life is much more fun!" For the younger person aspiring toward leadership, Bill advises that self-restoration must be intentional; setting aside the time will not happen on its own. "It's just important to take breaks from the routine and do something that is gratifying and fun and different. Be willing to explore and exploit your talents—use them but have fun with it!"

COURAGE AND FALLIBILITY: BENNET WATERS

Courage and fallibility, for Bennet Waters, are two different but interrelated "intangibles" that are both a part of the work of crisis leadership. Courage is trying things with uncertain outcomes, while fallibility is accepting failure while still rewarding those for trying (but not for the same failures, repetitively!). Courage without the recognition of fallibility, though, "is a dangerous thing." Learning courage and fallibility comes from experience, and one experience that Bennet described was in the aftermath of Hurricane Katrina. Working at the U.S. Department of Homeland Security at that time, Bennet observed courage and fallibility firsthand in how newly appointed Secretary Michael Chertoff responded: he did not re-assign blame, he focused internally—"We will learn from this and get better"—and two summers later, with multiple hurricanes on the Gulf Coast and raging wildfires in the western United States, the lessons learned paid off through much more effective and efficient responses.

Bennet's most important learning has been understanding "calculated courage and risk-taking," in other words, "not blindly running into an unknown environment with absolutely no sense of the potential outcomes . . . .but making decisions with eyes wide-open, and then constantly surveilling and monitoring to observe cause and effect . . . and to hone our decisions over time." Bennet takes the example of General Colin Powell's calculated decision-making: doing so with 40% to 70% of information needed, because to wait for more than 70% of the needed information results in a "paralysis of analysis," while making a decision with less than 40% of the required information available has one "going off half-cocked."

The young leader wanting to hone courage and fallibility must be willing to "practice, practice, practice . . . and have a willingness to embrace fallibility." Such practice, in Bennet's discipline, comes through tabletop exercises, the most valuable of which are actually engineered to fail, "so you can learn, repeat, then fail again in another way." Over time, through continually refining and learning, we never fail for the same reason, but we find "a newer and more elegant reason to fail, and over time we squeeze the relative error rate down to something that becomes more acceptable." For Bennet, "the human condition is imperfect, and recognizing our imperfections and continuing to learn is just the beginning of the journey."

COMPASSION: SANDRO GALEA

"I have increasingly come to feel that *compassion* is a higher order attribute than empathy," so states Sandro Galea, with empathy conveying what it is like being in someone else's shoes, while compassion does not require you to be in someone else's shoes in order to want good things for them. Compassion, for Sandro, is one of the three cardinal character traits of leadership (with the other two being hard work and sincerity–integrity). Leaders have to make decisions that impact many people, and for most of these people, the leader does not really know what is going on in their lives, and compassion is required to make decisions in such a way that respects where people are. "The act of compassion—to aspire to the betterment of lives around one, even those one does not understand—strikes me as perhaps the highest calling of leadership."

Sandro has drawn on compassion in his relationships with faculty, as the expectations for higher level scholarship are not necessarily the expectations under which some were hired. Being compassionate with such faculty allows for them to retain a sense of dignity, of meaning, of purpose in making a living. One model for Sandro is Martin Luther King, Jr., who said, "Compassion is not flinging a coin to the beggar, it is asking him why he is a beggar in the first place." He sees other examples in political leaders who recognize that there is a fundamental problem with gun regulations in this country vs. those who engage in "performative shows" of prayers and condolences to victims of gun violence. "The former is compassion; the latter is moral grandstanding."

Practicing compassion, where everyone is afforded dignity and the opportunity to flourish, can be deeply rewarding; however, in efforts to combat some of the structural forces that stand in the way of bettering the human condition, some people will respond to compassion antagonistically. The leader must rise above that. Honing compassion requires a deliberate action. It is a deliberate "habit of mind," an act of will that requires careful thought.

HUMILITY: SUZANNE M. BABICH

Sue Babich conceptualizes *humility* as *cultural humility* as she reflects on her work on the global stage. She notes that for many health leaders, globalization presents new challenges and opportunities for growth: "Exercising cultural humility is one of the ways I continue to learn. When you demonstrate cultural humility, you acknowledge that you don't have all the answers. Others, in fact, may know of better ways to address a problem than you may have thought of." One of the benefits of cultural humility is that it opens us up for novel approaches to solving common problems.

Having an attitude that is at odds with humility, on the other hand, can shut down the conversation before you can fully share, because it conveys that "I have nothing to learn from you." This is the loss of the opportunity to learn and grow as a leader. Bringing an attitude of, and a capacity for, openness—open ears and heart—gets to the core and the power of diversity: humility allows us to engage diverse voices, and diversity equals excellence, which is the path to improving our global collective health and well-being. A mentor for Sue, William Roper, modeled humility in seeking to understand the nature of an organizational problem that Sue felt she had allowed to spiral out of control. "Help me understand what happened" she recalls him saying. This was an open invitation to a conversation without blame.

Practicing humility creates opportunities to learn and be inspired; for Sue, this is the reward of humility. "Staying truly open, you may end up with an idea you never would have thought on your own." How do leaders bring along others who do not practice humility? Model it. Practice humility with *them*. "This builds trust and camaraderie." Humility as a skill can be honed through listening more and talking less, committing to never stopping to learn, relaxing and letting go, accepting that in any given situation, we may not have all the answers and there may be a better way.

KINDNESS: DONNA PETERSEN

Leading the COVID-19 response for the University of South Florida, Donna Petersen experienced first-hand the multiple differences in attitudes, knowledge, and capabilities across faculty, staff, students, parents, and the community, and the ability to lead in this arena "all stemmed from *kindness*." If you are kind, you seek to listen and understand. Responding with kindness to a parent's opposition to requiring COVID vaccination for students, rather than responding only with facts, allowed a conversation and meeting to happen: "Are you going to require students to be vaccinated?" asked a parent. "We look forward to welcoming your daughter to campus" was Donna's immediate response, which, in an attitude of kindness, made a difference for this concerned parent. "It's not what you say, it's how you make them feel."

As a leader who is the last stop for the person—employee or student—whose behavior is negatively impacting the institution, "it is not your job to *understand* the behavior, but to *manage* it, and to do so with kindness." And in situations where the truth may hurt, "I don't lie; I tell them the truth, but kindly. It is a *kindness* to tell the person the truth. It's not about being nice," which is a different behavior. In Donna's experience, unfortunately, many of us never work with a leader to learn kindness, but we can learn it from others in observing and paying attention to how they make you feel. "When all is said and done, we need to treat each other with kindness," this is what matters, what people remember. They remember how you made them feel, not what you said.

GENEROSITY: EDUARDO SANCHEZ

Part of being a leader, for Eduardo Sanchez, is playing the role you expect others to display when it comes to *generosity*: being generous not only with your time, but having a generosity of spirit, as well as being kind, understanding, and unselfish. Eduardo experienced the power of generosity during his time as commissioner of the Texas Department of Health in working with public health partners in Mexico. Although there had been long-standing relationships between Mexico and the four border states (California, Arizona, New Mexico, and Texas), the interactions were mostly transactional. In pursuing Sister City Public Health Preparedness, Eduardo recognized his counterparts' English proficiency was limited. By translating documents from English to Spanish and meeting 1-on-1 with his Mexican counterparts (and conducting those meetings in Spanish) before the meeting with the larger group of border state participants, the manner of interactions became transformational. This was the generosity of language: a cultural generosity. The new ways of building relationships allowed Eduardo and his Mexican colleagues to exchange information and address needs related to cross-border issues such as multi-drug resistant tuberculosis, HIV/AIDS, and mosquito-borne diseases.

Eduardo experienced generosity in how former U.S. Surgeon General Rich Carmona worked with him in the immediate aftermath of hurricanes Katrina and Rita, assigning the senior health officer from the Centers for Disease Control and Prevention (CDC) to work directly as part of the Texas Department of Health leadership team. This was Dr. Carmona's generosity; Eduardo's reciprocation was to assign the health officer to a position within Texas that gave him direct access to both state and federal assets. This unusual working arrangement between state and federal public health officials facilitated the efficient acquisition, deployment, and management of federal assets. He has also seen generosity in other leaders he admires, including Dr. Julio Frenk—currently president of the University of Miami and former dean of the Harvard T.H. Chan School of Public Health—who was the minister of health of Mexico during Eduardo's time as commissioner of the Texas Department of Health. This was a generosity of thought and thoughtfulness in how to streamline going through customs to move important materials such as medicines.

Generosity is about leading by example and is one of the ways to exude confidence. This is in contrast to leading through control, which, for Eduardo, is the antithesis of generosity. For those aspiring to positions of leadership, "meet people where they are, understand context, and have empathy." Listen more than you talk, and doing so will bring insight, allowing for real and meaningful change. Fundamentally, generosity as a leader is now, for Eduardo, about generosity of time, and "generosity begets generosity."

INTEGRITY: KATHERINE L. TURNER

Integrity is the number one leadership attribute for Katherine Turner, a prized value that is "cherished as most dear in my life—I am constantly striving to *live in* integrity, ensure that my work is *in* integrity, and that I am practicing integrity in everything I do." For Katherine, integrity is a person's most important attribute, and it should guide and inform all of their lives, their decisions, and their behaviors. Integrity is so core and central to who she is as a person, and is her standard, that it is ever present in whatever work she is doing. In her work as a consultant on diversity, equity, and inclusion, she will ask herself, "As a White person, how can I conduct this work with integrity? Am I the best person to conduct this work, or is there someone else better positioned to do this particular work, who I can recommend?"

It is important to surround oneself with fellow truth-seekers and challenge each other to be our most authentic self: "being *in* integrity is being true to ourselves." Alignment—at the individual level as well as the organizational level—is integral to integrity: alignment of values, of vision, of mission. Accountability, for self, for others, for our organizations is also integral to integrity, and that means admitting to mistakes when we make them. "What we do when we make mistakes, how we respond, how we learn from that and grow from that and vow to do better, is really what defines us as people as well."

A model of integrity for Katherine was her grandfather, who came from humble roots but ascended to a position of authority and power at a senior leadership position in a large corporation. He remained connected to all types of workers at a very human level, never seeing himself above or better than anyone, but equal. "That really informed a lot of my thinking around integrity." Her father also provided lessons in integrity. Katherine once asked him to bring home pens and stationary supplies from his workplace so she could have what she saw her friends having, and he asked, "You're asking me to steal, from my workplace?" That lesson at a young age taught her about the *obligation* to be *in* integrity. Another model for Katherine is President Barack Obama: "we can disagree about certain policies or decisions he made, and certainly I do, and yet there's never been any question in my mind but that he's an honest, decent person with great integrity."

For the person at an earlier stage of leadership development, Katherine emphasizes *practice*. Develop a set of habits and skills that you practice every day. Read, listen, watch, educate yourself, stay open to new ideas, and develop meaningful relationships with diverse people. Ask hard questions of yourself and practice accountability. Be a part of leadership communities and networks that can help you hone integrity through practice and self-reflection.

PRESENCE: JOHN WIESMAN

For John Wiesman, there are three components to *presence*: showing up, being attentive and engaged, and managing your behavior and inviting the best of others. "People notice when you aren't paying attention." Being on the leading edge of the COVID-19 pandemic—as the secretary of health for Washington State, John was the person at the other end of the phone line when the CDC called to confirm the first positive case in the United States in a person in his state—John *had* to be *fully present*.

As an example of intentionally being present, John described a 2-day health summit held every other year by Tribal Leaders of the 29 Tribes in Washington State. As the secretary of health, John had a single, specific presentation, and it would have been typical of those in his position to come in, deliver his presentation, then leave. But instead, John stayed for the whole 2 days. The message that this conveyed was "this summit is important to you, therefore it is important to me, as I value your health." It was an act of respect that earned John respect, acknowledged with the gift and honor of a ceremonial blanket at the end of the 2 days. This made a great difference in how the Tribal Leaders engaged him over the span of 7 years that he served as secretary of health. It bought him goodwill, and it allowed the Tribal Leaders to be more forgiving when John made mistakes, as we all do.

As a model for presence, John describes how Washington State Governor Ensley interacted during conference calls, Zoom meetings, and in-person meetings. He modeled presence in the way he valued others' time and the work they were doing: rather than multitasking, if another urgent call came in during a meeting, he *asked permission: May I take this call?* The lessons learned in practicing presence are chiefly about building relationships: you learn if you are present, if you stop and listen. This also builds capital for the times you will need to ask for forgiveness. To hone this skill, the leader must begin with building time in their schedule that allows for full presence. Put down the phone, close the laptop, truly listen, actively learn. Asking questions will invite people into the space. This is the essence and reward of presence—"if you have it, you can be much more successful in your work; if you blow it, it can de-rail your career."

SELF-ACTUALIZATION: KATHY COLVILLE

One of the attractions to *self-actualization* for Kathy Colville is that it is "so elusive and inspiring as a concept" and it speaks to her of the importance of a career to her personal values, sense of self-worth and identity, and a source of meaning. Although self-actualization may rarely be attainable, it is always a goal, and there are moments along the way when she understands that she is "doing the right thing" with the skills and the gifts that come to her and that she is growing in being able to make a meaningful contribution in her work.

It can be profoundly moving to *see* self-actualization in others when they are doing *exactly* the right work they were meant to do. Her work as a leader is to help others become aware "of the particular gifts and capabilities they have and to optimize those rather than trying to fit them into some other idea of what a leader should be." She sees something magical when people begin asking, "Who am I? What are the things that come easily? What are the things that come with more difficulty? And how do I become the best version of myself?" Being able to identify one's own tendencies is a prerequisite for thinking about others: self-knowledge can lead to self-actualization, which in turn can allow the leader to "optimize" others' capabilities. This is a part of what Kathy sees as one of her fundamental purposes as a leader: to make other people feel known.

Kathy saw self-actualization modeled in a previous role she had with an international consulting firm whose work mantra was that there are many paths to leadership, "and our expectation of you as a leader is that you make your path, you know it, you seek to understand self." She carries what a former boss told her, that most successful leaders spend 20% of their time working on themselves. "I love that . . . and especially as you get higher and higher you might spend *more* time working on yourself." She has learned that one of the most valuable things she can do as a leader is to allow both her peers and direct reports to *see* her process of learning—"warts and all"—not to cover up her mistakes, but to show others *how* she learns from them—"the value of showing self-doubt." This is not foreign to, but a part of the process of self-development, awareness, and actualization.

For the leader aspiring to self-actualization, focus on self-awareness, work ethic, and attitude, and if you can sharpen those, "all of the subject matter piece tends to fall in by itself." In Kathy's experience, those who exhibit excellence in these characteristics get more opportunities. And in the end, self-actualized people have a sense of humor about their own and others' flaws, an anti-perfectionist view that it is not our job to make everything perfect but to become more aware of what is in the job for self and others.

FORTITUDE: CLAUDE-ALIX JACOB

For Claude Jacob, *fortitude* signals *staying power, stamina, resiliency.* As a French speaker, Claude knows the word "fort" means strength, with its root in the Latin *fortis.* It is no coincidence that Claude quotes the motto of the Olympic Games—*Citius, Altius, Fortius*; Faster, Higher, Stronger—as his mantra for getting through the COVID-19 pandemic (while also making a major career move). As a local health department leader, Claude has witnessed fortitude in his elected officials' behaviors and most notably in his public health nurses: "literally watching them slog it out; no claim, no ego, but in their humility serving others."

One of the keys to building fortitude is pacing. Becoming resilient does not happen overnight and one needs to develop a sense of patience to make it through the rough times. A tag line in Claude's household is "This too shall pass." The opposite of fortitude for Claude is not weakness, but *hubris*, letting ego get in the way. One actually gains fortitude through humility: There is a lot that we do not know about COVID-19, and being respectful, mindful, and humble allows us to build fortitude. "It is ok to say we don't know what we don't know, because it acknowledges the blind spots. It is not ok to say I don't know, and I don't care because it discounts the blind spots." Paying attention to our blind spots through being humble is what an aspiring leader can do to build fortitude. Claude circles back to the importance of pacing in maintaining fortitude, reminding us of Aesop's fable of the tortoise and the hare: slow and steady wins the race. "You know that hare suffered from a lot of hubris."

LISTENING: DOUG SCUTCHFIELD*

People come to you—the leader—with a problem, issue, or concern, not that they want or really expect a solution; rather, it is a reflection that they need something from you, and what they need most from you is simply for you to **listen**. And for "Scutch," if you are thinking or worried about what *you* are going to say next, you cannot listen, you are not listening. "I have to listen before I can understand. I have to understand before I can respond." The art of listening for Scutch begins with listening to yourself. Do not fire off that flagrant email or memo; let it rest on your desk for a week. This is what he has learned through emulating someone important to him. A mentor early in his career, Bill Willard, took Scutch with him when he left Kentucky for the University of Alabama. "He would sit in a room full of people, thumbs in his belt, seemingly asleep, but he was *busy listening,* and when everyone had their say, Dr. Willard would begin with 'Well it seems to me that" And then everyone else in the room says, "Well of course, that's it!"

It is a hard lesson to learn but Scutch emphasizes the critical skill of listening as a means to *understanding,* not just *knowing.* In addition to not thinking about your own next words, listen with your eyes, look at the nonverbal messages, and, when possible, prepare ahead of time through quiet reflection in order to better listen. For Scutch, the classic listener was Socrates: allowing the person to know what they already knew anyway through listening.

PACING: KAYE BENDER

Kaye Bender equates *pacing* with *pausing,* and "it's probably the most difficult intangible for me but one of the most important." Pacing is important for preventing burnout, and it will keep you from adding to the stress of a team. Kaye mentioned a quote that she kept on a "sticky note" on her computer during her entire tenure as the executive director of the Public Health Accreditation Board (PHAB), from Charles Fred who observed that "Pause is not a delay, but a discipline." (Charles Fred follows, "It's not a waste of time; rather, it affords us the time to *deliberate before we act.*"[3(para4)]) Practicing pacing at PHAB, more often than not, before they made big decisions about accreditation systems change that would have national impact, Kaye would say to her staff, "I'm going to go home and do two things: pray, and have a glass of wine." This was her way of pacing, of pausing, taking a breath, taking time to reflect. It is a pause, *not* a stop. She has seen, too many times, people who are trying so hard to *exercise* their leadership—even promote themselves—that they get far ahead of their team, community, legislators, stakeholders, and partners, and they become more of a barrier than facilitator. Pacing is simple to talk about, but in practice, it requires a great amount of self-discipline and self-awareness.

---

* Dr. Scutchfield passed away May 23, 2022, prior to publication of this text.

Kaye related a recent experience with COVID vaccination as another example where pausing became important. The state's National Guard was assisting with the vaccine clinics with good community participation, but they noticed that very few Hispanics were coming to the clinics. The clinic managers came to understand that Hispanics were not interested in driving into a clinic where the people registering them were in military uniforms. So, they had to take a pause, re-think the clinic logistics, and develop another approach. This took longer than anticipated, but the pacing was critical for not getting out ahead of the communities of concern.

A mentor who modeled pacing for Kaye was former Mississippi State Health Officer Ed Thompson. Dr. Thompson loved to sail, and when he was on his sailboat for 2 weeks at a stretch, he was not reachable (this of course was in the era before cellphones). "Well, that drove me crazy, because as his deputy it meant the buck stopped with me. As I matured, I saw that people who took time to pause, to pace, came back with bigger, better, stronger, and more positive ideas." One of the case studies that Kaye uses in Chapter 3, "Systems Thinking in Public Health," is on Healthy San Diego, an example of a sustained systems change that has been going on for 25 years. When Kaye interviewed the leadership of Healthy San Diego to explore their longevity, one of the first things they mentioned was pacing. Finally, as another example of the importance of pacing, Kaye mentions her organization's renewed work on equity, with a particular focus on institutional racism. "What I have learned in the year and a half we have been working on equity is how pacing matters for building a high level of trust. We work together for a while and the emotions can get raw, on all sides, and so we pause, we take a breath, and we reflect some more and come back." Pacing allows time for trustworthiness to build.

For the up-and-coming leader, Kaye advises that the person have a strong sense of awareness, that you don't have to be connected 24/7 in order to be an effective leader. She thinks that the younger generation of leaders already has a stronger sense of work–life balance than our baby-boomer generation did when we were all younger. "Whatever your pause is—riding a bike for 125 miles or 'vegging' on the couch—build that into your whole leadership professional development." Look around for mentors who have perfected pacing and emulate them. And keep returning to the notion that pacing is a deliberate act, a discipline.

RESPECT: GENE MATTHEWS

The sad reality for Gene Matthews is the obverse of *respect*: "we are living now in an age of disrespect." The heart of public health for Gene is *community*, and community coalition building requires community dialogue. And the heart of this is respect: without the capacity for civil conversation, we have no community dialogue, and thus we have no community. Public health practitioners are obligated to serve *all* communities, and those who aspire to leadership must recognize that respect is the currency through which they can engage with communities irrespective of politics. As a public health lawyer, Gene ponders how we can change laws in order to more effectively address the COVID-19 pandemic and be able to respond to the next one, when what we are experiencing is an atmosphere that makes "reaching across the aisle" seemingly impossible. Public health has become "weaponized" by *both* sides, and *respect* and the capacity for civil conversation has been lost. "Our 21st century brains prefer a simple lie rather than the complex truth; 'wear a mask, don't wear a mask' becomes a political message rather than a reflection of the evolving science of COVID."

Mentors for Gene who have modeled respect include former CDC Director William Foege, who taught that public health decisions are by nature political decisions, and in order to accomplish the mission of public health, respect must be at the heart of this decision-making. Gaining and sustaining respect requires listening: Gene describes the work of a county health department director in North Carolina—a very divided state on politics—who was leading an effort to establish a needle exchange program. "You just have to shut your yap and listen. To the person who really believes the sky is orange and not blue, ask 'Why do you see it this way? Tell me more.' Shutting your yap and listening is the first step in gaining respect." Honing the political skill sets that allow for respect to emerge takes practice—"don't be afraid to fail!" Find a mentor, find someone to mentor, and practice respect.

RESILIENCY: LAURA MAGAÑA

Resiliency is one of the most important leadership intangibles for Laura Magaña, because it allows you to maintain the level of energy you need to be your best self in leading your organization daily and supporting others to thrive. Building and maintaining resiliency begins with that attention to self: just as the airline steward reminds us that in the event of a loss of cabin pressure, place your own mask first before assisting others, practicing self-care allows resiliency to take root and expand.

Leaders need to take proactive, self-protective steps to strengthen and build resilience and reserves. Recharging is an important strategy for resiliency; it is, in fact, what allows us to *prepare* to be resilient. "If we recharge our cell phones and computers every day because they lose energy—why don't we recharge ourselves daily, if we also lose energy?" The everyday practice of resilience prepares us to be resilient in the face of adversity. And for the leader, it is not about if, but when adversity will come, because it *will* come. One week before the 2020 annual meeting of the Association of Schools and Programs of Public Health (ASPPH), the COVID-19 pandemic declared itself, and the 3-day meeting had to be moved entirely to a virtual platform. "To be able to focus, adapt, and move forward, I had to be resilient, and this helped others become resilient as well." And when faced with setbacks or extreme hardships, such as natural disasters, a financial crisis, or the COVID-19 pandemic, it is your resiliency that will allow you to move forward and inspire others to do the same. "You don't wait for others, assuming others will act."

Laura reminds us of the basic truths on the path to being resilient leaders: "Slow down, practice gratitude and generosity, and be present! Restore and raise your well-being by proactively and intentionally creating the opportunities to improve your physical, social, emotional, and spiritual life and see how you improve your resiliency!"

GRATITUDE: BARB MARTIN

Barb Martin chose *gratitude* because "the leaders who practice gratitude are the ones I respect the most, and I want to emulate those who are the best, the most capable, and most successful leaders." Gratitude is an action, and one that allows the leader to stay grounded, as well as to be humble and appreciative. In that sense, gratitude is related to humility and generosity, but it is more: it is "paying it forward." Barb has experienced this in her work, where in team meetings during the COVID pandemic, attention to what one is grateful for completely changes the narrative and helps turn the conversation from a negative one to one of hope. Keeping a daily gratitude journal is another way Barb practices gratitude, writing down at least three things she is grateful for. Practicing gratitude has proven benefits for a range of conditions, from better sleep, to a greater sense of well-being, and an ability to manage problems better. Gratitude plays a large role in how a leader can build a greater sense of purpose for an organization, group, or team.

As a model for gratitude, Barb describes the acts of her cancer center director, who often acknowledges the "small things" from others; for example, the administrative assistant who has pulled meeting minutes together. "What he is often times doing is making the invisible, seen." Practicing gratitude can also allow you to wrestle away a bit of control from what might be an uncontrollable situation. Barb mentions the word "practice" many times, as previously reflected, and for the up-and-coming leader to sharpen their sense of gratitude, it begins and ends with practice. It is "a habit to be nurtured."

TOUCH: PETE GINTER

Pete Ginter first suggested adding *control* to the list of leadership intangibles but realized that what he was actually wanting to convey was better expressed as *touch*. The right touch is what a leader must have to create a culture that allows for innovation, creativity, individuality, and growth: "if touch is too heavy and control is too far-reaching it fosters bureaucracy and smothers effectiveness, and if it is too weak there are unnecessary inefficiencies, a lack of direction, and difficulty in achieving goals." Having the right touch is often a "tug of war" between effectiveness and efficiency. A leader with the right touch, or the right amount of control, puts the organization somewhere "between complete stability and complete chaos."

In leading people within an organization, it is useful to put boundaries around thinking, which is what a vision, a mission, and values provide, "but we don't want to get the boundaries so tight that we take away thinking, particularly concerning *how* to accomplish these things." "It's a little bit like cooking . . . some sauce: some spice adds to the flavor, but too much is overpowering and ultimately ruins the dish." One of the most challenging aspects of leadership is that the right touch will vary across programs, across situations, and across individuals, so the leader must constantly adjust and fine-tune control. Where Pete has seen a sense of too much control, too heavy a touch, is the "100% solution for a 1% problem;" for example, a late-to-work policy that effects 100% of the people when it is only one individual who is habitually late. "If you have enough 1% problems and you solve all of them with 100% solutions, pretty soon you have a whole lot of rules, regulations, and policies that restrict the behaviors of everyone," behaviors that might otherwise be freed to focus on creativity and change. In advising the person aspiring to positions of leadership, Pete states, "Think before you act . . . too many leaders react with a new rule or policy," rather than assessing how much touch is required in any particular situation. "Too many routines, rules, and policies drive out innovation and flexibility. When it comes to touch, less is usually best."

HUMOR: JACK DUNCAN

"If *humor* is so pervasive in work groups and social groups, what function does it serve?" This question that Jack Duncan posed to his MBA students led to a series of investigations and published papers on humor. Quoting Gary Traylor, Jack observed that "Humor and person-focused joking defines and re-defines social groupings, reinforces social rankings, clarifies status relationships among group members, and provides a number of other functional leadership characteristics to a group."[4] And because of this, the leader who dismisses humor—"Work is serious business and allows no room for joking"—makes a big mistake in Jack's view.

As an interim dean, faced with the chaos of an organizational structure that had gone off the rail, in a very tense meeting with staff and department chairs, a single perfectly timed, but spontaneous quip about someone's sunburn—"Did you put on suntan oil or barbeque sauce?"—immediately removed the tension and frustration, and allowed the group to address the serious issues at hand. For humor to work, it must be spontaneous and not planned—"If you have a sense of humor, use it; if it isn't in your nature, it's best not to call on this leadership intangible very frequently." Underlying humor is trust: things can be funny if people trust you.

Jack's research on humor—yes, peer-reviewed, published research—indicates that humor can increase group cohesiveness, and in settings where high performance is the norm, increasing cohesiveness can result in greater productivity. Humor can increase a sense of belongingness, which can improve organizational culture; however, there is a danger to using humor—the proverbial double-edged sword—and knowing the distinction between making a joke *of something* vs. making *someone* the butt of a joke is critical.

To return to an earlier theme, Jack emphasizes that before humor can be something of value in the leader's toolbox, the leader must first be trusted. Developing a sense *for* humor, the leader must be sensitive to individual differences. And there are absolute limits and boundaries to using humor: never to have an ethnic, gender, or race target. Humor should never be used aggressively, as in put-downs. Patterns of such insensitive jokes can cross over into workplace harassment or become a violation of Title VII of the Civil Rights Act. "It is better to be cautious than needing to be sorry." Self-focused humor, on the other hand, can reduce workplace tension and frustrations. Most important for Jack, simply, is that "humor makes work fun, and I think work *should be* fun!"

WISDOM: STEPHANIE BAILEY

For Stephanie Bailey, *wisdom* is the culmination, the pinnacle of all the characteristics and facets of leadership, and is transportable across person, place, and time. In leading the Office of Public Health Practice at CDC, Stephanie endeavored to discern who in the organization had wisdom, to differentiate them from who (especially in the popular media) was considered an "expert." She came to understand that anyone with wisdom can speak to any topic without necessarily being the expert: "evaluate, speak coherently, and move the conversation forward." Her mentors modeled wisdom primarily in *how* they made decisions. A decision *pattern* that is consistent, reliable, thoughtful, and not dependent on which way the wind is blowing. "It takes courage to decide through wisdom, and it takes faithfulness." Wisdom is humbling, not arrogant or boastful, and requires patience and reflection; it is the melding of knowledge and understanding. The lessons of wisdom are lessons in "knowing thyself": self-awareness of your desires, attitudes, behaviors, boundaries, and limits. Growing wisdom can also be done through being observant: "watch the room, the people, the interactions." At the heart of wisdom, for Stephanie, is integrity: to become wise, one must first own not knowing.

HONING THE INTANGIBLES

LEADERSHIP COACHING

While some leadership intangibles may be innate, all of them can be practiced, refined, and sharpened. One approach to honing these leadership intangibles is through leadership coaching, which in this context is synonymous with executive coaching (EC). Leadership coaching can be defined as "A collaborative solution-focused, results-oriented and systematic process in which the coach facilitates the enhancement of work performance, life experience, self-directed learning and personal growth of the coachee."[5(para1)] Grant describes coaching as "essentially about helping individuals regulate and direct their interpersonal and intrapersonal resources in order to create purposeful and positive change in their personal or business lives."[6(p149)] Leadership/EC has been a professional pursuit for at least 40 years, with the Association of Coaching (based in London) having thousands of members in over 85 countries. In the United States alone there are numerous coaching associations, including the Association of Corporate Executive Coaches, the International Association of Coaching, and the International Coaching Federation. These and other organizations provide Accredited Coach Training Programs, which is a coaching certification process.

The literature—both scholarly and popular—is rich regarding both the processes and outcomes of leadership coaching. While this chapter is not meant to provide an exhaustive review of the literature, drawing the reader's attention to a few reviews may serve as a springboard for more detailed exploration. In a contribution to the *SAGE Handbook of Coaching*, Grant describes a Multiple Perspective Model of coaching research, which includes the experiences and outcomes from the perspectives of the coachee, the coach, and the organizational sponsor, as well as other stakeholders.[7] Capturing these multiple perspectives is critical to a comprehensive and inclusive research agenda on leadership coaching.

In a 2018 systematic review of EC, including 110 articles published in 37 peer-reviewed journals, Athanasopoulou and Dopson focus on both the processes and outcomes related to EC from multiple perspectives (as suggested by Grant), and reframe it "as a social rather than an individual intervention—one where the organization, the coach, and the coachee co-create new meanings embedded and shaped by the social context within which the intervention is applied."[8(p48)] They note the change in the focus of EC, from the mid-2000s when coaches were hired primarily to address toxic behaviors of leaders, to a decade later when the emphasis was on developing high-potential performers. Athanasopoulou and Dopson found three types of positive outcomes for the coachee: personal development, behavioral changes toward others, and work performance. EC also impacts organizational performance in non-ROI terms (e.g., increased employee satisfaction, productivity, leadership effectiveness. and coaching culture).

Based on their findings, Athanasopoulou and Dopson provide the following recommendations[8]:

- The coach should develop a curiosity about the coachee's social context.
- The coach can reframe the demands of the job for the coachee as choices, and then determine the choices that the coachee is making and whether these are actually serving the coachee and the organization.
- It is important to determine if there is alignment on views of leadership across the coachee, the coach, and the sponsoring organization.
- Rather than focusing on weaknesses, a coach's use of psychometrics—such as 360-degree feedback—can help empower the coachee for positive change.
- Coaches should explore how coachees seek knowledge and how their perceived social desirability and social utility of coaching goals may affect the EC outcomes.
- Organizations and coaches should determine how coaching can be better integrated within other leadership development initiatives of the sponsoring organization.

Finally, in a 2021 article that assessed coaching specific to a public health agency, Spears-Jones et al. examined the effects of leadership coaching among team leads and branch chiefs within the CDC.[9] In the federal government, *leading change* is one of five executive core qualifications used in developing leaders, comprising six competencies: creativity and innovation, external awareness, flexibility, resilience, strategic thinking, and vision; the focus of the Spears-Jones article included the first four of these competencies.[9] For this specific leadership development initiative in the CDC, leaders were provided two 360-degree multirater leadership assessments (before and after the coaching intervention); six leadership coaching sessions; a leadership coach survey; and two post-coaching program evaluations, one 3 to 6 months after leadership coaching (Phase 1), and another 18 months or more after the Phase 1 evaluation (Phase 2).[9] In-person and telephone interviews were conducted among first- and mid-level leaders who completed the leadership development program. In total, 94 of the 96 participants completed one or more interviews, and 74 (79%) reported improvements in their ability to lead change in three of the four *leading change* competencies: creativity and innovation, flexibility, and resilience. These self-reported improvements in leadership as a result of coaching are consistent with other reports in the literature, indicating that "coaching can contribute to an increase in the effectiveness of self-awareness, self-efficacy, resilience, hope, and goal attainment among leaders."[9(p8)]

360-DEGREE EVALUATION

Another approach to honing leadership intangibles is through peer and self-assessments, with the most popular being the 360-degree evaluation. This is a management tool used to assess leadership from the (confidential) perspectives of the leader's direct reports, their peers, their supervisor, and their own self-perspectives—hence the 360-degree label—using a quantitatively-based multi-item questionnaire (Figure 20.1).[10] Bracken et al. define 360-degree feedback (now copyrighted as 360° Feedback) as a "process for collecting, quantifying, and reporting coworker observations about an individual (i.e., a ratee) that facilitates/enables three specific data-driven/based outcomes: (a) the collection of rater perceptions of the degree to which specific behaviors are exhibited; (b) the analysis of meaningful comparisons of rater perceptions across multiple ratees, between specific groups of raters for an individ-

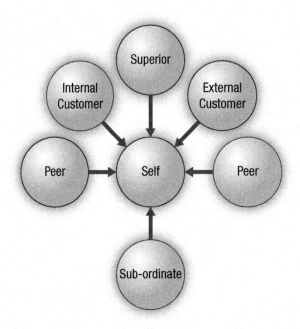

FIGURE 20.1: The 360-Degree Assessment.
Source: U.S. Office of Personnel Mangement. 360-degree assessment: an overview. 2021. https://www.opm.gov/policy-data-oversight/performance-management/performance-management-cycle/rating/360assessment.pdf

ual ratee, and for ratee changes over time; and (c) the creation of sustainable individual, group, and/or organizational changes in behaviors valued by the organization."[11(p764)] Typically, a leadership coach will ask the leader to identify individuals at these various levels and the coach will provide them with a questionnaire and then collate responses. While Bracken et al. describe multiple uses of a 360-degree assessment,[11] the predominant uses are either for the purposes of leadership development or performance management/appraisal, or both.[10] The coach provides the leader with results, and the leader can use these different perspectives to improve identified leadership shortcomings, build on identified strengths, and change leadership behaviors as appropriate. While such a *multi-rater feedback* approach may have value in providing the leader with different perspectives, there are inherent risks in using this assessment. While the questionnaire responses are meant to be confidential, clearly, the leader has only one supervisor. Direct reports may fear disclosure of their identity because of what they include in their responses; thus, they may temper their answers to certain questions. And there may be a bias regarding the leader's selection of peers to be included in the 360-degree assessment, choosing only those peers who may provide more favorable opinions of the leader.

TRAINING PROGRAMS

Engaging in various training opportunities is a third way to hone leadership intangibles. In the public health arena, the most popular leadership training programs are the legacies of the original CDC-funded National Public Health Leadership Institute (PHLI). Established in 1991, the PHLI was a year-long leadership training targeting national and state-level public health leaders, with 50 to 60 participants in each cohort.[12] Highly sought after in its first several years, not only because of the quality of the program, but also because it was essentially the only type of this training available to leaders in the public health workforce,

PHLI spawned similar regional and state-level public health leadership institutes, culminating in the establishment of the National Network of Public Health Leadership Institutes.[13] The special value of participating in the PHLI, in this author's view as an alum of the 1995–1996 cohort, is the network it helped to establish: two other chapter authors (Bender and Sanchez) were in that same cohort and two chapter authors (Baker and Scutchfield) were involved in establishing PHLI. While the PHLI as originally formulated is no longer in existence, the CDC and the Public Health Institute of California manage the National Leadership Academy for the Public's Health (NLAPH), which provides a year-long training to four-person multi-sector teams that advances leadership skills with a special focus on health equity.[14] Both the Association of State and Territorial Health Officials (ASTHO)[15] and the National Association of County and City Health Officials (NACCHO)[16] offer leadership training to public health leaders. The Regional Public Health Training Centers under the Health Resources Services Administration (HRSA) is yet another resource for leadership training for the public health workforce.[17] The ASPPH provides the Academic Public Health Leadership Institute for deans, associate deans, directors, and other leaders in academic public health.[18]

In the healthcare arena, the leadership training opportunities are almost too numerous to list. The American Hospital Association (AHA), the Association of American Medical Colleges (AAMC), AcademyHealth, and the American College of Healthcare Executives (ACHE)—to name but a few—all provide an array of leadership training programs and activities focused on healthcare.[19–22] The Council on Education for Public Health (CEPH)—the accrediting organization for schools and academic programs in public health—lists 12 doctoral programs with "leadership" in the title and one accredited Master of Public Health (MPH) program in Leadership in Practice.[23] And we would be remiss not to mention that one of these academic programs—the Executive Doctoral Program in Health Leadership at the University of North Carolina in Chapel Hill—is the "home" for this textbook and the alma mater of the two editors.[24]

SUMMARY

Leadership intangibles are essential traits and practices that equip public health and healthcare leaders to lead change through complexity and turbulence. From a list of more than 15 leadership intangibles, chapter authors from this book each selected one intangible, and each was interviewed to explore how they have seen the intangible modeled, lessons they have learned in practicing and applying the intangible, and guidance for those who aspire to positions of leadership. Leadership coaching and 360-degree feedback or evaluations are two approaches to honing these leadership intangibles. There are numerous leadership training programs in public health and healthcare that provide opportunities to develop and optimize leadership intangibles. There are also several public health academic programs that provide master's and doctoral degrees in leadership, providing the skills and knowledge for the next generation of leadership scholars to further establish the evidence-base for value of leadership intangibles.

EXERCISES

1. Develop your own list of "Top 10" leadership intangibles. Which of your top 10 are not included in the 19 that are the focus of the interviews with chapter authors? For your intangibles not among these 19, identify leaders who you believe exhibit the leadership intangible, and interview them, using the interview questions at the end of the Introduction section earlier in this chapter.

2. In Richard Davis' book, *The Intangibles of Leadership*, for each of his 10 described intangibles, he includes sections titled, "How Do You Know It [the Intangible] When You See It?", "How Do You Get It?", and "Why It Matters." Among your top 10 leadership intangibles, especially for those also included in this chapter, select three and write a brief paragraph for each of Davis' three sections.

3. What is the one leadership intangible on which you wish someone would interview you? Identify a supervisor, a peer, and someone you supervise, and ask each to interview you, using the earlier referenced interview questions. If possible, record the interviews, then compare and contrast your responses to the questions across the three interviewers. They are bound to be different. Why?

4. Develop a self-assessment tool for measuring one or more of the leadership intangibles described in this chapter. Share this with the editors of this textbook, and you may be invited to contribute to this chapter in the second edition!

ADDITIONAL RESOURCES

▪ The recorded interviews with John Wiesman (presence) and Barb Martin (gratitude) are available online at http://connect.springerpub.com.

 A robust set of instructor resources designed to supplement this text is located at **http://connect.springerpub.com/content/book/978-0-8261-4924-4.** Qualifying instructors may request access by emailing **textbook@springerpub.com.**

REFERENCES

1. Davis RA. *The Intangibles of Leadership: The 10 Qualities of Superior Executive Performance.* John Wiley & Sons; 2010.

2. Davis R. The intangibles of leadership. American Management Association. January 24, 2019. https://www.amanet.org/articles/the-intangibles-of-leadership

3. Fred C. The 24-Hour Rule: Leading in a Frenetic World. Magnusson-Skor Publishing; 2019. As quoted in Lead on Purpose, https://leadonpurposeblog.com/2019/12/30/the-power-of-pause-in-leadership/

4. Traylor G. Joking in a bush camp. *Human Relations.* 1973;26(4):479–486. doi:10.1177/001872677302600405

5. Association of Coaches. Coaching defined. https://www.associationforcoaching.com/page/Coaching Defined

6. Grant AM. An integrated model of goal-focused coaching: an evidence-based framework for teaching and practice. In: Passmore J, Tee D, eds. *Coaching Researched: A Coaching Psychology Reader.* 2021:115–139.

7. Grant AM. Coaching as evidence-based practice: the view through a multiple-perspective model of coaching research. In: Bachkirova T, Spence F, Drake D, eds. *The SAGE Handbook of Coaching.* Sage Publications; 2017:62–84.

8. Athanasopoulou A, Dopson S. A systematic review of executive coaching outcomes: is it the journey or the destination that matters the most? *Leadersh Q.* 2018;29(1):70–88. doi:10.1016/j.leaqua.2017.11.004

9. Spears-Jones C, Myles R, Porch T, Parris S, Ivy-Knudsen M, Dean HD. Leading organizational change: improved leadership behaviors among public health leaders after receiving multirater feedback and coaching. *Workplace Health Saf.* 2021;69(9):400–409. doi:10.1177/21650799211001728

10. Toegel G, Conger JA. 360-degree assessment: time for reinvention. *Acad Manag Learn Educ.* 2003;2(3):297–311. doi:10.5465/AMLE.2003.10932156

11. Bracken DW, Rose DS, Church AH. The evolution and devolution of 360 feedback. *Ind Organ Psychol.* 2016;9(4):761–794. doi:10.1017/iop.2016.93

12. Umble K, Steffen D, Porter J, et al. The National Public Health Leadership Institute: evaluation of a team-based approach to developing collaborative public health leaders. *Am J Public Health.* 2005;95(4):641–644. doi:10.2105/AJPH.2004.047993

13. National Network of Public Health Leadership Institutes. https://nnphi.org

14. Center for Health Leadership and Practice. The Leadership Academy for the Public's Health. ASTHO Leadership Institute. https://www.astho.org/members/ali/

15. Association of State and Territorial Health Officials. ASTHO Leadership Institute. https://www.astho.org/Member-Services/ASTHO-Leadership-Institute

16. National Association of County and City Health Officials. Change management and adaptive leadership. https://www.naccho.org/programs/public-health-infrastructure/performance-improvement/change-management

17. Health Resources and Services Administration. Regional public health training centers. https://bhw.hrsa.gov/funding/regional-public-health-training-centers

18. Association of Schools and Programs of Public Health. Academic Public Health Leadership Institute. https://www.aspph.org/aphli

19. American Hospital Association. The leadership summit. https://leadershipsummit.aha.org

20. Association of American Medical Colleges. Leadership development. https://www.aamc.org/professional-development/leadership-development

21. AcademyHealth. National change leadership programs. https://academyhealth.org/about/programs/national-change-leadership-programs

22. American College of Healthcare Executives. Leadership. https://www.ache.org/about-ache/our-story/our-commitments/social-responsibility/leadership

23. Council on Education for Public Health. Accredited schools and programs. https://ceph.org/about/org-info/who-we-accredit/accredited/

24. University of North Carolina. Executive doctoral program in health leadership. https://sph.unc.edu/hpm/hpm-drph

Chapter 21

Creating Your Leadership Framework

Susan C. Helm-Murtagh

INTRODUCTION

This chapter guides students through a structured, self-reflective process to develop their unique, sustainable leadership foundation (their leadership "framework") and apply it to their leadership practice. It draws on the topics and approaches presented in the preceding chapters of this text, as well as almost a decade of instructor and student–leader experience teaching, developing, applying, refining, and reflecting on the concept. The chapter presents an overview of the framework concept, describes the six key constructs of the framework, and offers strategies for development of each construct. Finally, students who have developed and applied their frameworks offer insights and guidance from their experience.

OBJECTIVES

By the end of this chapter, the reader will be able to:

- Explain the purpose and objectives of a leadership framework as a tool for leadership development and reflection.
- Describe the component elements of the leadership framework.
- Demonstrate the processes of constructing, applying, and maintaining the framework.
- Evaluate lessons learned and experiences from other leaders who have developed and used their own frameworks.

THE LEADERSHIP FRAMEWORK DEFINED

OVERVIEW

The concept of a leadership framework is not a new one; an internet search on the term in November 2021 yielded more than 600 million results, while a PubMed search yielded 5,072 articles. Organizations of all types, from the National Health System (NHS) in the United Kingdom, to the National Education Association (NEA) in the United States, to major consulting firms worldwide, have leadership frameworks. They are often a component of development programs or used to illustrate how an organization models leadership. In general, these frameworks provide a conceptual model for understanding and, in some cases, operationalizing the relationships between such constructs as theories, values, behaviors, competencies, and outcomes.

The word "framework" means an essential supporting structure, and that is the overarching goal of the leadership framework concept described in this chapter, which was first developed in 2013 by the author for a graduate-level public health leadership course. The concept and underlying constructs have been continuously refined and adapted since, based on student feedback and instructor experience. The objective of this leadership framework is to provide students with a more reflective, practice-based, and integrative opportunity to elicit their understanding of leadership concepts and then to directly apply best practices and guiding principles to their own practice of leadership; in other words, to develop their own unique essential supporting structure for their leadership practice. The key difference between this leadership framework and those described previously is that students are asked to be the architects of their own structure rather than to adapt or use an existing structure; to extend the analogy, students choose their own building materials and their own style, they make decisions about how large and complex the structure is, and how and with whom they will build it and maintain it. Along the way, students are asked to envision leading from this structure that they have built.

As such, each student develops their own framework. Given the highly individualized nature of the framework, the overall structure and length is discretionary; however, students are asked to include six basic constructs:

1. Their core values upon which they will build their framework (core values)
2. Self-insights gained through the course and throughout their leadership journey (self-reflection)
3. The leadership models or approaches that will serve as the building blocks for their framework (theoretical bases)
4. What stakeholders they will involve in the development and maintenance of the framework (stakeholder identification and involvement)
5. Their plan to keep their framework current (maintenance)
6. How they will continually self-assess progress against and alignment with their framework (self-assessment)

Students are encouraged to address the constructs in the same order as dispalyed in the previous list, as each step builds on the insights gained from the previous one. Each of these concepts will be explored in more detail in the section that follows. See Figure 21.1 for a conceptual model of the framework.

Before finalizing the framework, students present their work in progress to their peers and instructors. These presentations are not assigned a grade; rather, their purpose is to help students articulate and evolve their thinking, to gain input and garner support from their peers and instructors, and to serve as sources of inspiration and framework guidance for their peers.

Approximately 2 years after completing their coursework, students are asked to reflect upon how their leadership framework has changed over the course of the graduate program, addressing at least three of the six constructs included in their original framework. Themes and direct quotes from those reflections (used with permission) are included throughout the chapter to help illustrate how students have built, used, and learned from their frameworks.

To inform this chapter, the author conducted a survey of program graduates regarding their post-graduate experiences with the framework. The survey asked about the utility of the framework; the frequency with which respondents read, reviewed, and updated the framework; any impediments respondents had encountered in doing so; and any guidance they might have for students embarking on their own framework development. The results are summarized later in this chapter, and more detail is provided in Appendix 21.1.

As a final introductory note, each semester, when the assignment is initially discussed, students ask for examples of other students' frameworks. To make this exercise as self-reflective, unique, and meaningful as possible to the students, and to avoid being overly prescriptive for something as personal as this framework, those examples have not been provided in the course or in this chapter. The pages that follow do contain references to

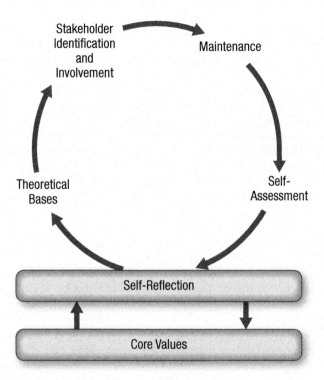

FIGURE 21.1: The Leadership Framework Conceptual Model.

more commonly used approaches; more importantly, the students' experiences, told in their own voices from their frameworks, post-coursework reflections, and the survey, have been provided to help illuminate both the concepts themselves and their utility.

CORE VALUES

DEFINITION AND BACKGROUNDS

Core values are the foundation of the leadership framework. They are the immutable bedrock upon which a leader operates; they guide a leader's behavior, clarify who a leader is (to self and others), articulate what a leader stands for, and serve as guideposts for decision-making. A strong set of core values provides a leader with a clear purpose and solid grounding from which to navigate change, uncertainty, and complexity. Drawn from the principles of authentic leadership and heavily reliant upon emotional intelligence, they require deep self-awareness and self-reflection.

The concept of core values, albeit in an organizational context, gained popularity in 1994 with the publication of *Built to Last* by Jim Collins and Jerry Porras. In their quest to determine what makes a company great, the authors embarked on a 6-year research project, in which they identified 18 companies that they deemed "visionary" and compared them with a control group of "successful-but-second-rank" companies.[1] "Visionary" companies had to be at least 50 years old, have an outstanding global brand image, and feature a long-term track record of outperforming the stock market. According to Collins and Porras, the key differentiator between these two groups is that "visionary" companies are able to successfully manage both continuity and change, and that ability is closely related to the ability to articulate a vision. Vision is based on two key constructs, core ideology and an envisioned future, which they represent in *yin* and *yang* fashion. The core ideology, which consists of core values and core purpose, is unchanging (*yin*). (Core values and visioning are also addressed in Chapter 20, "Leadership Intangibles.") The envisioned future, which consists of a 10- to 30-year BHAG (or Big, Hairy, Audacious Goal) and a vivid description of the future, is *yang* (Figure 21.2).[1]

In Collins and Porras' model, the core ideology is both defining and enduring. In their view, a core ideology is transcendent across time and is based, at least in part, on core values, which they define as "a small set of timeless guiding principles, [that] require no external justification; they have *intrinsic* value and importance to those inside the organization."[1]

While Collins and Porras' model is aimed at organizations, their core ideology construct is valuable in illustrating the role that core values play for leaders. Leaders are called upon to play a variety of roles (leader, follower, coach, mentor, teammate, teacher, and student), lead in different organizations and contexts over time, develop new skills and perspectives through experience, continuously navigate both positive and challenging change, and develop and manage relationships through the course of their leadership journey. Just as a "visionary" organization centers itself on its core values, leveraging the *terra firma* of continuity to manage change, so too does an effective leader.

In 2015 Bill George, the former MedTronic executive whose work on authentic leadership is covered in Chapter 8, "Authentic Leadership," published a book entitled *True North*. To understand how people can become and remain authentic leaders, George and his team interviewed 125 leaders, ranging in age from 23 to 93, from emerging leaders to senior executives. Interviewees were selected based on their reputations as effective and authentic leaders; these men and women represented different generations, nationalities, races/ethnicities, and socioeconomic backgrounds. They also hailed from a diverse array of organization sizes and types.[2]

To their surprise, the researchers found no consistent set of personality traits, leadership styles, behaviors, skills, or attributes that define effective leaders. Instead, there were several common denominators these leaders demonstrated; among them were that they learned from their life story, they had deep self-awareness, and they practiced their core values and principles.[2] This is the recipe for developing and maintaining a durable and consistent set of core values—through exploration and analysis of one's formative experiences, constant and meaningful self-reflection, and honing those core values through continuous application and testing.

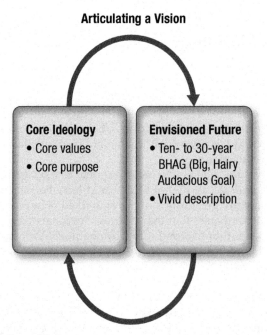

Articulating a Vision

Core Ideology	Envisioned Future
• Core values	• Ten- to 30-year BHAG (Big, Hairy Audacious Goal)
• Core purpose	• Vivid description

FIGURE 21.2: Articulating a Vision.

IDENTIFYING AND DEFINING CORE VALUES

How does one go about identifying and defining their core values? Consistent with George's findings, students report that a deep examination of their formative experiences, extending from childhood through the present day, provide useful insights into how culture, religion or faith, family, society, and life experiences have shaped their values. These factors often include their relationships with immediate and extended family, the students' role in their family, the occupations held by parents or other influential family members, the extent to which culture and faith or religion played a role in their lives, professional experiences, and lessons learned from role models and/or mentors. Impactful formative experiences can also include trauma; students who have experienced trauma and are comfortable examining its role in shaping their worldview report that such reflection leads to deeply enhanced self-understanding and, in many instances, an appreciation for the ways in which that experience compelled them to grow or develop.

Extending one's core values into principles is a powerful way to activate, test, and refine those values. Principles, according to Bill George, are values translated into action.[3] For example, a core value of "integrity" can be translated into a leadership principle such as "I am honest, open, and truthful in my words and my actions." Similarly, the core value "life-long growth" can be translated into "I regularly reflect on my experiences, the lessons I have learned from them, and how I will change as a result of those lessons."

Identifying and defining core values also provides a helpful lens through which to examine one's own decisions and actions, as well as those of others, be they individuals or organizations. These observations provide continual opportunities to reflect on and refine those core values, as one student describes:

> The values I outlined in my framework were People and Relationships, Adaptability, and Humility. These values will continue to serve as my core values, and I will add Empowerment and Credibility. The COVID-19 pandemic has propelled public health into the spotlight, both positively and negatively, and the values in my framework have never been more relevant. When the pandemic hit, the entire world began to continuously adapt to an evolving 'new normal.' Public health, business, government, and school leaders, along with the general public, were constantly adapting to new science, guidelines, restrictions, and mitigations strategies. To keep the public abreast and aligned with the current guidance, the government and public health authorities needed to focus on people and relationships. They needed to interact and communicate with the public, develop trusting relationships, listen, and engage. We did not do this well. The public also needed to be empowered to make informed decisions about their own health and their families. Information needed to come from credible sources, sources who followed the science and who could admit their wrongdoings. This rarely happened; humility would have gone a long way. The COVID-19 pandemic highlighted health inequities and disparities, social determinants of health, mental health issues, distrust in science, and an ill-equipped medical system. These issues were present long before COVID-19, but now they're front and center and action is required. As I address these issues in my own work, I will continue to be guided by the values laid out in my framework.

As another student notes, being intentional about one's core values helps reinforce and clarify them, for self and others:

> The process of actually thinking about my values and documenting them in my leadership framework only further reinforced them for me. Prior to documenting my values, I was still leading from them, but now when I make a decision or feel a certain way about a topic, I can better articulate why I think the way I do.

Another student beautifully illustrates the integration of culture, life experience, and family influences in forming their values:

> I grew up in a household with a strong social justice mission and values. As a first-generation islander who valued academic achievement and diligence, I found myself surrounded by family members who were clinicians, educators, and clergy, so—not surprisingly—it was expected

that my siblings and I "give back" to community as a part of the family ethos. In addition, I attended a Jesuit high school which pushed the philosophy of servant leadership. As a result, I developed an identity as the eldest son, high school "team captain" in two sports, and helper/ translator to my aging grandparents. This role extended to my volunteer activities.

Students are encouraged to develop a graphic or visual representation of their analysis and insights gained. Creating a "mind map" is an effective aid in understanding the relationships between life experiences, influential figures, lessons learned, and core values. This mapping also helps to deeply ground students' core values in their experiences, and to meaningfully activate those values into their principles.

IDENTIFYING YOUR CORE VALUES

- Begin by telling a story about yourself. Use pictures of family and events, along with anecdotes from key points in your life and career to help illustrate and bring your story to life. Identify which people and experiences have had the deepest impact on you. Include your childhood, youth, young adulthood, and early career experiences.
- Examine what you learned from those experiences, and how they shaped your values.
- Identify what you are most passionate about.
- Explain your core values, examine how they have changed over time, and note how those values have impacted your life and career choices.
- Translate your core values into leadership principles (behaviors).

SELF-REFLECTION

This component of the leadership framework focuses on careful deliberation and analysis of what students have learned about themselves over the course of their leadership journey. These can include insights gained from self-assessments, several examples of which are contained in this text, or third-party administered assessments (such as Myers-Briggs Type Indicator or MBTI, EQ-I, StrengthsFinder, Hermann Brain Dominance or HBDI, and DiSC Profile), leadership development training or coaching, other leadership coursework or self-study, performance evaluations, and the student's leadership experience. Constructing the framework may be the first time that students have had the opportunity to consolidate, reconcile, harmonize, and reflect on the various inputs that they have available to them. This step is particularly valuable when performed after the core values exercise, as that experience provides a helpful lens through which to self-reflect. For example, the realization that one's family or culture of origin was conflict-avoidant may help explain the results of a conflict management assessment and stimulate self-reflection on whether approaching and managing conflict differently may fill a key skills gap.

Students approach this component of the framework using different constellations of the inputs described previously. Developing a conceptual model can be helpful in distilling the various inputs and generating meaningful conclusions. Some students will use a SWOT (strengths, weaknesses, opportunities, threats) form of analysis to organize their thinking. This is also helpful in selecting the leadership styles, approaches, or models that will be incorporated into the framework, and for identifying elements to include in their self-assessment. As this student observes, developing self-awareness and framing that self-awareness with various leadership approaches helped inform their choices about their leadership practice.

Throughout . . . the various reflections and exercises, in learning about the different frameworks and approaches to leadership, I began to better understand my own leadership approach. In knowing and framing something, you can better understand and therefore mold something.

By knowing and framing my leadership at the beginning of this course—primarily a Servant Leadership approach—it helped me better understand my leadership choices. In understanding them, I was able to deliberately make choices to change them.

SELF-REFLECTION

- What have I learned about myself from:
  - Past performance appraisals?
  - Formal or informal feedback from peers, family members, or friends?
  - Past leadership development coaching or training?
  - Assessments I have taken?
  - My self-reflection practices, such as journaling?
  - This course?
  - The process of identifying and articulating my core values and leadership principles?
- What do I consider to be my strengths?
- What do I consider to be areas for further development?
- What opportunities do I see for myself, and how can I best take advantage of them?
- What are potential threats to my overall career satisfaction, well-being, and growth, and how can I best overcome them?

THEORETICAL BASES

Throughout this text and in the course of their leadership practice, students become exposed to a variety of leadership theories, models, and styles. Many bring additional perspectives from other leadership training, reading, or self-study. It is important to note that students may not always see themselves reflected in the leadership approaches presented; it is unfortunate but true that leadership studies have traditionally been focused on White males in Western cultures and that insights about the leadership experiences of women and people of color remain marginal in the field.[4] In addition, given that this is a highly individualized exercise, students are encouraged to "try on" various models and approaches from both the text and their own experiences, training, and study, and to select those elements that resonate with them and to reject those that do not.

As one student put it, after reflecting on their leadership framework:

I continue to feel that my approach to the theory of leadership is the one that is intuitive, organic, and best for me. The basis of this leadership framework continues to be the Authentic Leadership model we studied . . . although I've gotten away from referring to it as that in an explicit way, because I feel free not to tie myself to a particular academic theory for something (leadership) that is so hard to reduce to a theory.

Another observed:

There is no perfect form of leadership but having the ability to know your own style and how to adapt under others is critical.

And finally:

Each of the theories we studied made sense, but none seemed to be complete or relevant in my current leadership role. Some had elements that spoke to me, others seemed to omit important behaviors. I used authentic leadership as the primary approach but grafted pieces from other theories or approaches to arrive at what I think will result in maximum effectiveness at this stage in my leadership journey.

IDENTIFYING AND SELECTING YOUR BASES

As you identify leadership models and approaches from the preceding chapters or from other sources on which to build your own framework, you may find that you are drawn to more than one model. If so, attempt to distill the wisdom in whatever you select to create a synthesis of models from the texts to create your own model which captures your own set of leadership guiding principles. In addition to the theoretical models and approaches that you have studied, how have role models inspired you and influenced your career trajectory?

MAINTENANCE

This component of the framework challenges students to answer the question, "How will you keep your framework current?" This is analogous to the second half of Collins and Porras' formula for success: managing change. For the framework to remain meaningful, relevant, and useful as students grow and develop their leadership practice across different and changing contexts, it must grow and develop accordingly.

This, along with the self-assessment portion of the framework, is one of the most challenging aspects of framework development for students. Students are strongly encouraged to invest the time afforded them by the course and to leverage the resources made available to them over the course of the semester (e.g., course materials, peer and instructor support and guidance) to create a concrete, but realistic, plan for updating it. Students who have been most successful at keeping the framework current report that having identified "triggers" for updates, such as during their annual reviews or regular self-reflection periods, when changing jobs or roles, or experiencing other life changes, is the most effective and useful reminder method. Some students enlist stakeholder support to help keep them accountable for updates. Some lay out a specific maintenance "roadmap":

> As a means of keeping this framework fresh and relevant, I intend to utilize five strategies: 1) update the framework annually, 2) consume "leadership", 3) invest and involve myself in professional groups, 4) teach "leadership", and 5) develop "leadership" in my direct reports. Each year, during a spring one-week sabbatical that I take, I will go through the exercise of re-writing the framework. I will write as if it is a new document each time, letting the exercises and resources, which inform the framework, to arise from current experiences.

Other students adopt a more organic, continuous refinement approach.

> I have expanded my leadership library, soaking up books and podcasts in spare moments in between assignments and dissertation work. I have expanded my definition of what I consider a "leadership" book, because looking back, many of the books I have read for personal growth and inspiration have influenced my philosophy of leadership more than the books that are marketed for leadership. For example, I have read memoirs of women's journeys. . . . I see and hear myself in these stories, which helps me to amplify the power within me.

While a wide variety of maintenance approaches can be and have been adopted, students are encouraged to find the method that is most likely to work with their style, their needs, and their contexts, and (most importantly) one that will keep them accountable to their framework.

MAINTAINING YOUR FRAMEWORK

Consider ways in which you will renew yourself and your commitment to your lifelong development as a leader:

■ What will you do to reconnect with your core values and maintain the framework over time?

- How can your stakeholders support you in this?
- Are there identifiable "touchpoints," such as during your annual performance review, to which you can tie your maintenance plan?

STAKEHOLDER IDENTIFICATION AND INVOLVEMENT

This element of the framework asks students to identify their key personal stakeholders, those whom they will involve in the construction and maintenance of their framework. Students are encouraged to include a wide variety of stakeholders with diverse points of view, such as family; trusted friends; members of their faith or spiritual community; members of their cohort; past and current professional colleagues, supervisors, and direct reports; mentors; and mentees. Importantly, students should make sure they include a few stakeholders who can provide candid and honest feedback, and who can help hold them accountable to their goals. Students who have already formed a mentoring relationship or "personal board of directors" (PBOD; see Chapter 19, "Mentoring and Trusted Advisors"), will often include them. During this stage in their framework development, many students recognize gaps in their stakeholder group; for example, they may not have a mentor, a PBOD, or may not have considered stakeholders outside of their professional setting.

To the extent that they are comfortable doing so, students are encouraged to actively involve their key stakeholders in their framework development. Class presentations afford them the opportunity to involve their instructors and members of their cohort, and to practice how they will involve and articulate their framework to others.

The stakeholders included in my leadership framework were my life partner, graduate school and professional colleagues, and my . . . cohort peers. [These are] the people who support me, push me, and hold me accountable. In the framework I discussed why I chose these stakeholders (e.g., similar professional/educational experiences, personal history, and shared goals), but not how they contribute to my development as a leader. The most important way they do this is through conversation and reflection.

IDENTIFYING AND INVOLVING YOUR STAKEHOLDERS

As you think about your framework, consider the following:

- Who are the people whose needs and expectations you should consider?
- Who can provide support?
- Who can hold you accountable to your framework?
- Who can give you honest and caring feedback? Consider people in both your personal and professional contexts, such as friends, family, colleagues, and mentors.

SELF-ASSESSMENT

To ensure alignment with their leadership goals and to enable continued leadership development and growth, students are asked to address the following prompt: "How often and through what means will you get feedback on your performance as a leader?" Students who have translated their core values into principles (and thus actions) find this to be an easier task.

For example, one student mapped their chosen leadership models (Transformational, Adaptive, and Team Leadership) into values (Trust, Openness, and Respect) and self-identified leadership needs (Manage Up, Communicate, Teamwork). They then translated their values and leadership needs into behaviors (principles). Principles for Openness became "I listen to the group's ideas or concerns with an open mind," and "I reexamine critical assumptions to ensure that they are appropriate and relevant." Principles for Teamwork included, "I build in time to create a vision, plan, and organize," "I outline goals clearly," "I recognize the team in concrete ways," and "I share relevant environmental information with the team." These behaviors are then assessed through regular journaling, self-assessment, and 360-degree reviews.

Another student described their approach to self-assessment this way:

> *Again, it is important to me to make sure my intention and impact align. In order to actualize this goal, I use a pretty structured process to keep myself accountable. Specifically, I start and end each day with a self-check. I have added the four core values to my worksheet, asking how I intend to live into each value in the morning, and how I lived into each value and/or need to right the ship at night. I have also added the values, sub-values, and behaviors to my Friday-afternoon self-reflection. (Yes, I literally create worksheets for myself, second-grade style.) I will continue doing the annual solo retreat each year (usually the week after my birthday), and plan to add the leadership framework to the professional domain for review and updates. I will also continue to learn from my annual client survey, mentor meetings, and receptivity to feedback from my dear ones.*

ASSESSING YOURSELF

After you have established your own foundational set of guiding principles, identify those "best practices" that concretely translate theoretical models into the day-to-day practice of leadership. These practices can form the basis of your ongoing self-assessment and the involvement of stakeholders, mentors, coaches, and sponsors in the process of supporting your growth as a leader. In this way you can apply what you are learning in a more intentional way in the future. The key question is, "Are you practicing the best practices you have identified?"

GETTING STARTED: DEVELOPING YOUR LEADERSHIP FRAMEWORK

In responding to the author's survey, graduates offered several points of guidance to others embarking on the development of their own leadership framework. Those key points are summarized and illustrated by their direct quotes in the text that follows.

BE HONEST

This was the most frequently mentioned theme. Graduates advised students to address both strengths and weaknesses in their framework, as doing so will provide a solid, balanced foundation from which to grow. In addition, they strongly suggested that students root their frameworks in honest self-reflection: Who they are, what they stand for, and what type of leader they want to be.

- *Be honest! The framework is a great place to let your positive attributes shine, but you need to be just as honest about areas for improvement too. Putting that into writing can be freeing in a way.*
- *Be intentional about the leadership framework. There must be clarity about where the individual is around their leadership practice and where the individual wants to be. This will allow the individual to identify gaps in leadership practice and what needs to be done to improve.*
- *Be real to yourself about your weaknesses and find small wins that will enable you to improve on them.*

- *Be brutally honest about what's in the framework . . . it's YOUR [framework]. I was honest and included personal components and that is what made it still relevant for me even years later.*
- *Be real. Propose things that will advance your career and make you a better leader.*
- *Stay true to yourself and to what your gut tells you.*
- *Make sure it is informed by and infused with one's own ethics.*
- *This is really an opportunity to internalize and view yourself (and who you want to be) through the lens of management theories.*
- *Be open to the various leadership approaches and try to truly decide what your style is—even if it surprises you.*
- *Self-reflection is key. The various exercises leading up to thinking through the leadership framework were helpful (e.g., implicit bias, personality tests).*

INVEST (IN) YOURSELF

Graduates noted that the framework is both a personal and professional investment. They advised students to see it as a long-term, evergreen guide that can help inform and grow their leadership practice over time.

- *View this as a living document, and as a touchstone for future self-reflection: What elements fade into the background? Which elements are reinforced time after time?*
- *Prepare for the long game—this assignment is extremely practical if you really intend to become a leader in public health.*
- *It is worth the time and effort to develop the framework. I have shared it with many new leaders.*
- *Do it! It is a terrific self-reflection exercise and will help you evolve into a stronger leader as a result.*
- *The framework should not be seen as just part of the academic work but a personal evaluation and plan for improvement . . . it should not be rushed but adequate time [should be] allocated for the development to ensure it is well developed.*

PUT IT IN PERSPECTIVE

Graduates also advised students to approach the framework with a clear set of expectations about their purpose for the framework and to consider its application in their larger personal and professional contexts.

- *Consider what the goal of its development is in the first instance—[don't] over or under promise on its value. [It's] okay if it means different things to different people.*
- *Think about leadership not only from the perspective of who you are but the impact you want to make. For me, that means that I consider both the culture (work environment) and performance as well as my own leadership abilities. Organization wide, how can your leadership skills improve the performance and work environment?*

KEEP IT SIMPLE

Finally, as graduates evolved and applied their frameworks, they often found that distilling it to a set of key principles or a life philosophy helped them keep their frameworks both current and accessible.

- *Develop a life philosophy and everything can flow from that.*
- *Find a way to narrow it down to a few words.*

USING YOUR LEADERSHIP FRAMEWORK

Graduates were also asked how they had found the framework to be most useful. They identified the following key areas:

- Building self-awareness and self-confidence
- Building relationships
- Establishing and communicating clarity of purpose
- Evaluating their current and future career paths
- Supporting their growth
- Making difficult decisions

Those points are illustrated by their direct quotes in the text that follows.

BUILDING SELF-AWARENESS AND SELF-CONFIDENCE

- *The framework has also been useful in terms of thinking about how I will continue to grow as a leader, how I will know when I am doing a good job or need improvement, who those stakeholders are, etc. It has made me more purposeful in seeking feedback and looking for ways to improve.*

- *My leadership framework and style have continued to develop over the course of this program. During the time since I drafted the first iteration of my leadership framework, I do not think my overall preference for certain leadership styles has changed, though with practice, I think I have developed a better sense for which style to employ and when to try a different approach.*

- *To a large extent, it represented a self-actualization exercise for me. It provided an opportunity for reflection on some of the various theories that exist and how I see myself in them (at the time and as an aspiration).*

- *I have found it critical to have an intentional approach to my leadership style. It allows me to communicate more openly with my peers and team members, and also allows me to reconsider, evolve, and improve the way I engage as a leader.*

BUILDING RELATIONSHIPS

- *Taking inspiration from the framework, this program, and my leadership coach, I recently created a short one-pager describing how I am currently—and intend to continue to be—utilizing my specific strengths for the team. And I presented it to my team last month. For example, thanks to a battery of assessments I've done in the past few years (DiSC, Strengthsfinder, Myers Briggs, Berkman Method), I understand under what conditions I do my best work and I wanted to share those with the team and encourage them to do a similar sharing if they feel comfortable doing so. One outcome from this sharing is two team members felt "safe" enough to share that they prefer to work with their doors closed and for the extroverts on my team to not take offense by that. The team has grown closer through this sharing and the one-pager I wrote has helped me in refreshing my framework going into its 2-year anniversary. I have added this one-page synopsis of my preferred work style/strengths to my leadership toolkit. It's something I hadn't considered in my earlier framework.*

- *This year during a time when we had a few different transitions in management staff, I began sending an email to all new managers welcoming them to my leadership team. In this email I tell them what my leadership values are and what my expectations are for them as a member of the team, highlighting open and honest communication and encouraging them to bring forward new ideas that may be different from my own (that last part is in response to my 360 assessment). So far, I have received positive feedback from this email.*

■ *The framework provided some fundamental principles that have informed my approach to leadership and interaction with other stakeholders in my ecosystem.*

ESTABLISHING AND COMMUNICATING CLARITY OF PURPOSE

■ *I found the framework useful to me in terms of describing who I am as a leader, taking in all of the various aspects of personality, style, values, etc. In particular, the process of defining my values as a leader and having clarity around that has influenced my leadership positively.*

■ *I have found it critical to have an intentional approach to my leadership style. It allows me to communicate more openly with my peers and team members, and also allows me to reconsider, evolve and improve the way I engage as a leader.*

■ *It has improved my ability to articulate decisions I make and my expectations for my team.*

■ *It helps me focus on my "why."*

EVALUATING CURRENT ROLE AND CAREER PATH

■ *I really enjoyed the exercise to do a leadership framework. The most useful part of the exercise was to develop a life philosophy. My framework is based off of that philosophy and I use it daily! My life philosophy has helped guide my decisions on what jobs to take and has helped me prioritize my work once I've gotten new jobs. It also has kept me motivated to keep going when the job has gotten challenging. It gives me meaning beyond just self- gratification of a job well- done. My life philosophy is one sentence and has stayed true along my 4 years since I came up with it.*

■ *I realized that the new leadership role I found myself in provided very little room for me to live my values, which eventually caused me to make the decision to leave. Prior to enrolling in this program, I had honed my leadership style in smaller nonprofit organizations with strong missions. In all of those organizations it was clear from the moment I was offered my different positions that my personal values were in alignment with the mission and culture of the agency. In an organization with a mission and culture that aligns with your personal values, it is easier—but not always easy—to lead with the assurance that your leadership style is in congruence with the larger goals you are pursuing. This alignment can foster clear decision- making, strong organizational communication, and less conflict.*

SUPPORTING GROWTH

■ *The framework has been extremely useful to my leadership practice as it has remained a guiding document for me before I conduct self-reflection on how I am progressing in my leadership practice. It helps to keep me on track on my predetermined leadership path. Regular review of the framework also helps me to remember some of the leadership concepts and models, which allows me to act and speak clearly about these concepts and styles without ambiguity.*

■ *It has made me more purposeful in seeking feedback and looking for ways to improve.*

MAKING DIFFICULT DECISIONS

■ *[My core] values include ethics/ethical standards, truth, and empathy and understanding. There have been several situations where my ethics have been tested over the course of the last 2 years . . . these were difficult situations that involved complex decision-making and did not always please clients and had the possibility of becoming extremely negative public situations. In the end, I made the right decisions and feel good about them. Part of my [stakeholder group] was engaged in these situations and assisted with their feedback. These events reinforced my commitment to my value structure relating to ethics.*

WHY A FRAMEWORK IS ESSENTIAL TO THE PRACTICE OF PUBLIC HEALTH AND HEALTHCARE LEADERSHIP

The leadership framework provides an essential supporting structure for leaders. This structure, when individually and thoughtfully crafted—built upon core values, adaptation of leadership models, self-awareness, accountability, and a commitment to its renewal—provides public health and healthcare leaders, who routinely operate in complex, challenging, and often highly politicized internal and external contexts, with a solid foundation on which to stand. As those who have developed and applied the framework have described, it has given them a conceptual model from which to consider (and continuously re-evaluate) who they are as leaders, what they stand for, and how to articulate those principles. It has also guided them in making and committing to a series of choices that are essential to their leadership practice; there are many leadership theories, models, styles, and approaches from which to choose, and many other key decisions, such as identifying one's core values, that this framework elicits in the pursuit of developing one's leadership practice with intentionality and consciousness. While the accrual of these benefits is not unique to public health and healthcare leaders, their value is arguably enhanced for leaders who must routinely lead in the face of little to no information, often with many lives at stake.

The framework does not explicitly require leaders to address the issues of bias and systemic racism in their leadership contexts, but the argument can be made that taking an intentional approach to centering equity in one's leadership practice can build awareness of and a commitment to dismantling those attitudes and structures. For example, core values and, by extension, principles that explicitly include equity and equitable practices can provide a basis for setting leadership goals in this dimension, identifying and empowering stakeholders who can help inform a leader's equity practices and hold them accountable to them, and provide a basis for self-assessment against those goals.

SUMMARY

This chapter outlines a guided approach to developing a unique leadership framework, or an essential supporting structure, from which leaders can intentionally build, grow, and evergreen their leadership practice. By evaluating the choices available to them and making deliberate and conscious choices in three of six key dimensions—core values, self-reflection, theoretical bases—leaders can develop a clear sense of who they are as leaders, what they stand for, and how to articulate those principles. The remaining three dimensions of the framework—stakeholder identification and involvement, maintenance, and self-assessment—are designed to ensure that the framework evolves with a leader's needs, that key stakeholder input is considered and included in both the construction and refinement of the framework, and that leaders have the means by which to both measure their progress goals and to hold themselves accountable to those goals.

DISCUSSION QUESTIONS

1. In what ways do you think developing a leadership framework would be most beneficial to you, and why?
2. What aspect or aspects of developing the framework do you find most challenging? What strategies or resources can you identify to help you overcome those strategies?
3. Review the quote in the section titled Identifying and Defining Core Values [pp. 405-406], in which a student illustrates the integration of culture, life experience, and family influences in forming their values. Write a similar short reflection on how those factors have influenced your values. What did you learn about yourself?

ADDITIONAL RESOURCES

BOOKS

As part of the leadership course, students are asked to select and review a leadership book of their choice, to summarize it, and to indicate whether they would recommend it to their classmates. The following are some of the more popular and highly recommended titles.

- *Dare to Lead: Brave Work, Tough Consequences, Whole Hearts*, by Brené Brown
- *Daring Greatly*, by Brené Brown
- *Humble Leadership*, by Edgar Schein and Peter A. Schein
- *Mountains Beyond Mountains*, by Tracy Kidder
- *Great by Choice*, by Jim Collins
- *The Four Agreements*, by Miguel Ruiz

PODCAST

- *On Being*, by Krista Tippett: (https://onbeing.org/series)

ACKNOWLEDGMENTS

The author is grateful to her friend, colleague, and co-instructor, Ed Baker, who has a gift for bringing out the best in others. His contributions to the continued development and growth of the framework are invaluable. She is also grateful to the many UNC DrPH students and graduates who graciously and generously agreed to share their wisdom and guidance on these pages.

A robust set of instructor resources designed to supplement this text is located at http://connect.springerpub.com/content/book/978-0-8261-4924-4. Qualifying instructors may request access by emailing textbook@springerpub.com.

REFERENCES

1. Collins J, Porras JI. Building your company's vision. *Harvard Business Review*. 1996. https://hbr.org/1996/09/building-your-companys-vision
2. George B, Ibarra H, Goffee R, Jones G. *Authentic Leadership. Emotional Intelligence*. Harvard Business Review Press; 2018.
3. George B. *True North: Discover Your Authentic Leadership*. Jossey-Bass; 2007.
4. Ospina S, Foldy E. A critical review of race and ethnicity in the leadership literature: surfacing context, power and the collective dimensions of leadership. *Leadersh Q*. 2009;20:876–896. doi:10.1016/j.leaqua.2009.09.005

APPENDIX 21.1: GRADUATES' PERSPECTIVES ON THE LEADERSHIP FRAMEWORK

The author invited 70 past students to respond to an anonymous survey, distributed via email to their last known email address, regarding their experiences with the framework. Invitees must have completed the program coursework, successfully defended their dissertation, and graduated from the UNC DrPH program. While it is unclear how many intended respondents actually received the survey, 22 (or 31.4%) submitted responses. The small response numbers do not support robust statistical analysis, but they do provide helpful insights, particularly when supplemented by the comments provided by respondents.

The survey contained 10 questions. Areas of focus included:

- The frequency with which respondents read and reviewed their frameworks
- The frequency with which they had updated their frameworks
- The barriers they encountered to reading, reviewing, and updating their frameworks
- The usefulness of the framework to their leadership practice
- The ways in which they found the framework useful (or if it was not, why it was not)
- Suggestions for improving the framework
- Guidance they might offer to anyone embarking on the development of their own leadership framework
- Guidance they might offer to the author with regard to the structure or content of this chapter in order to make the framework concept as understandable, useful, and applicable as possible to students

To provide context for the frequency of updating questions, students were also asked in which year they had completed their framework.

Respondents were clustered into three categories, with most (n=6, 27.73%) having completed their frameworks in 2017 (4 years prior to when the survey was conducted), followed by 2014 and 2018 (each at n=5, 22.73%, and at 7 years and 3 years prior to when the survey was conducted). The mean elapsed time since framework completion was 5.2 years.

In terms of how often respondents had read or reviewed their frameworks since completion, almost half (9) of the respondents answered "once or twice." About a quarter (22.73%) each of respondents indicated that they reviewed it once a year or twice a year. Three respondents indicated that they had not reviewed it since completion.

Ten respondents answered "I haven't" when asked how often they had updated the framework. Just over a third (8, or 36%) indicated that they had updated it "once or twice," and four respondents (18%) indicated that they updated it annually. One respondent put it this way:

> *I have reviewed and updated the framework. One of the things that made it easier for me was the fact that it was presented to me as a framework to help me to improve as a leader rather than [using it only as] an academic work. Therefore, a lot of self-reflection went into the development of the framework and I was truthful to myself about where I was and where I want to be during the development of the framework.*

In response to what barriers to reading, reviewing, or updating their frameworks they encountered, respondents indicated that they had too many competing priorities, needed more support and tools to update it regularly, found the exercise to be too theoretical, or did not feel the need to update it regularly.

> *The framework was grounded in theory - while it was an interesting learning exercise as a way of engaging with different published leadership styles and how they might inform (or relate to) my own, I didn't see any specific value in revisiting the document per se.*

> *My framework still remains largely accurate.*

I haven't revisited the framework simply because it wasn't on the front of my radar. But I regularly apply so many of the golden nuggets that I took away from the process and from the class.

Two-thirds of respondents (14) found the framework very or extremely useful to their leadership practice. A little more than a quarter (6) found it to be moderately useful. Two respondents found it to be slightly or not at all useful. The themes are summarized and amplified by respondents' quotes in the preceding section, *Using Your Leadership Framework.*

Chapter 22

Learning From Experience

INTRODUCTION

What is "experience"? It is the process of gaining knowledge, wisdom, or skill from doing, seeing, or feeling things. It would follow, then, that more experience leads to more of all of those things. Leaders, however, especially those in the early phases of their careers, are arguably limited in their ability to collect, reflect, and act on experience. They are limited not only by the time and effort it takes to do this, but also by the breadth and depth of opportunities they have encountered.

Experience sharing is a powerful way to augment and diversify another person's knowledge. This chapter contains a series of essays from public health and healthcare leaders encapsulating a broad and diverse set of experiences and perspectives. Each leader speaks, in their own voice, to the most impactful leadership lessons they have gained through experience.

OBJECTIVES

By the end of this chapter, the reader will be able to:

- Describe experience and its value to leaders.
- Recognize a variety of leadership experiences and lessons learned.
- Perform active reflection on how to gain and share knowledge, wisdom, and skill from others (experience sharing).
- Evaluate one's own experiences and how they shape their leadership practice.

BACKGROUND

Fourteen public health and healthcare leaders were asked to respond to a total of five questions, three of which were asked of all respondents:

- *Who were some of the role models or mentors that influenced you early on? In what ways did they influence you?*
- *What is the most impactful leadership experience that you have learned from, and how did it make a difference in your subsequent leadership practice?*
- *How can students make the most of their early-career experiences in leadership?*

Respondents were also asked to choose two additional questions from the following list:

- *What attributes are important in determining leadership effectiveness?*
- *How do you select people to be on your leadership team within the organization you lead?*
- *How do you deal with a situation where someone is not a good fit or is not performing well?*
- *In relating to those to whom you report, what are some guiding principles and best practices?*
- *How do you decide when to say "yes" or "no" to a request for your time?*

- *How do you find time and ways for self-renewal and to maintain balance?*
- *How do you best prevent, or at least anticipate, unintended consequences (whether positive or negative) of your leadership decisions?*
- *What quote or statement about leadership do you have taped to your computer or tacked to your bulletin board, that you look at every day?*

The purpose of asking each leader to respond to the same questions was to expose students to a variety of leadership responses to, and reflections on, common experiences. The optional questions were offered to respondents to enable them to speak to the topics that most resonated with them.

THE ESSAYS

KAREN DESALVO AND KUSHAL KADAKIA

This essay is jointly authored by Dr. Karen DeSalvo, MD, MPH, MSc, chief health officer at Google, and former acting assistant secretary for health and New Orleans health commissioner, and Kushal Kadakia, Rhodes Scholar and current medical student at Harvard. Their experiences can offer public health students insights about the leadership opportunities and lessons across different stages of public health careers.

Who were some of the role models or mentors that influenced you early on? In what ways did they influence you?
Kushal: A common denominator for my mentors has been the ability to bridge disciplines. For example, my undergraduate advisor, Dr. Mark McClellan, combined the fields of medicine and economics to pioneer new payment and delivery models for healthcare reform. His experiences inspired me to also take an interdisciplinary approach to my training, which combined the life sciences (BS in Biology, MSc in Epidemiology) and social sciences (BA in Public Policy, MSt in U.S. History). Likewise, Ms. Jenni Owen, former policy director for Governor Roy Cooper and my internship supervisor, emphasized the importance of partnerships and public debate for translating policy research into policy impact. She modeled this ethos by moving between an academic career at Duke University and a policy career in state government. Her experiences influenced me to explore new linkages between my academic work and leadership practice, from staffing the National Academy of Medicine's COVID-19 report for public health to then working on public health issues at Google. Given the complexity of public health challenges today, the leaders of tomorrow will need to be equipped to work across sectors, and mentors with interdisciplinary careers can serve as models for developing such skills and perspectives.

What is the most impactful leadership experience that you have learned from, and how did it make a difference in your subsequent leadership practice?
Kushal: I served as student body vice president during my undergraduate career at Duke University, where I led a successful campaign to make Duke a smoke-free campus. Smoking remains the leading cause of preventable death and was a salient issue at the university and in the Durham community given both the rate of cigarette use among students and staff and the institution and region's historical legacy with tobacco. Working on the smoke-free campus initiative illustrated how academic and research interests in public health can be combined to tangibly improve the health of communities. The project also highlighted how effectuating progress requires multiple forms of engagement, from research and community engagement to identify challenges and opportunities, to activism and organizing to create momentum for change, to program administration to translate ideas into impact. The smoke-free campus project taught me many of the fundamentals of leadership and management: how to organize a team, coordinate across various stakeholders, and deliver on

short- and long-term objectives. This firsthand experience navigating communities and complex institutions to convert public health aspirations into action better positioned me to succeed in subsequent professional experiences in government and health system leadership.

How can students make the most of their early-career experiences in leadership?
Karen: A pivotal early-career experience for me was becoming the director of the Resident Internal Medicine Clinic. The role diverged from my planned career path in hospital medicine and exposed me to the structural challenges within the healthcare system, from gaps in care access to outdated information technology (IT) systems. The experience opened my eyes to the importance of strong institutional level systems to address inequities and improve quality and experience overall, often by automating processes to reduce unnecessary human error. It also broadened my perspective. I learned from thousands of patients how impactful community systems—including the social, political, and structural determinants of health—were to their overall health. These systems are often "out of scope" for medicine but are squarely in the purview of public health. This experience drove me to focus on serving the patient and their communities and pushed me to look beyond the walls of the clinic and build a career that bridged medicine and public health. I would encourage students to pursue opportunities that break them out of their siloes. The most impactful leadership experiences will be those oriented around problems and populations and that offer opportunities off the beaten path; these will provide greater flexibility for growth and development.

How do you decide when to say "yes" or "no" to a request for your time?
Karen: As leaders progress through their careers, the focus of their work will shift from operations to strategic visioning and direction. This requires developing the skills to manage others, and, in turn, becoming comfortable with delegating aspects of projects to other team members. When done with intention, delegation itself is a form of leadership, reflecting trust in fellow team members and vision about how to prioritize different tasks. Implicit in delegation is being selective about which tasks leaders say "yes" to and being thoughtful about ensuring alignment between team members and the work they are assigned to perform. Along the journey of professional growth, this means honing skills of identifying essential efforts that meet your criteria for what you absolutely must do to advance your "north star," because only you can do it. It also means people need to become expert in the gracious "no" for efforts that will not be in furtherance of key priorities. Saying "no" and setting boundaries for your time is much more difficult than saying "yes" and requires intention, clarity of purpose, and discipline. If done well, it will provide leaders with the intellectual, emotional, and physical bandwidth to be more effective.

What quote or statement about leadership do you have taped to your computer or tacked to your bulletin board, that you look at every day?
Karen and Kushal: A statement that resonates with both of us is: "When you close the gap, you raise the mean." This mantra for public health leadership and practice is a reminder to ensure all decisions, strategies, and programs are developed and executed using the lens of equity. No matter the scale at which they operate, all leaders are responsible for defining a vision for their team. Given that the goal of public health is to create the conditions where *everyone* can be healthy, it is imperative for leaders to approach their work with the explicit attention to the needs and experiences of historically marginalized populations. This statement grounded Karen's work as New Orleans health commissioner, working with community-based organizations to address health disparities and is a core principle of the current work at Google. For Kushal, his work on the Duke smoke-free campus initiative, where policy development began with outreach to the communities with the highest prevalence of cigarette use, this was a core principle. As leaders encounter challenges and obstacles in their own careers, returning to this statement can provide an internal litmus test on whether decisions are aligned with values and attuned to the ultimate aspirations of public health.

ROSS C. BROWNSON

Ross C. Brownson, PhD, is the Lipstein Distinguished Professor of Public Health at Washington University in St. Louis. He studies the translation of evidence to public health practice and policy, with a content focus on environmental and policy determinants of chronic diseases. Dr. Brownson is the author or editor of nine books and over 550 peer-reviewed articles. He is a former president of the National Association of Chronic Disease Directors and the American College of Epidemiology. Prior to joining academe, Dr. Brownson was a division director with the Missouri Department of Health.

Who were some of the role models or mentors that influenced you early on? In what ways did they influence you?

I have been fortunate to have many influential role models and mentors over my career—I will highlight two individuals. The first is Dr. John Bagby, who was my department chair when I was a graduate student at Colorado State University. John taught public health administration, which could be a boring class, but became a fascinating experience in listening to John's many stories. He had previously been the deputy director of the Centers for Disease Control and Prevention (CDC), where he led the program to eradicate malaria in the United States, and initiated smallpox eradication in Africa, Asia, and Europe. Among the many skills and attributes I have sought to model from John was his ability to be unflappable—I never saw John lose his cool no matter how tense the situation or how much he disagreed with someone. He always listened, sought common ground, and respected every person.

The other mentor that I want to highlight is Dr. Robert (Bob) Harmon. Bob was the founding director of the Missouri Department of Health when it was formed in 1986. Bob took a chance on me by appointing me as a division director in the Missouri Department of Health when I was only 30 years old. He was willing to take risks in aggressively addressing HIV/AIDS and tobacco use in a conservative state. Bob was a participatory leader who did not micromanage but entertained many ideas to foster creativity.

What is the most impactful leadership experience that you have learned from, and how did it make a difference in your subsequent leadership practice?

My most impactful leadership experiences occurred during the 8 years I spent in state government after I received my PhD. In the Missouri Department of Health, I began as an epidemiologist in the cancer program and then became a division director. Over that period, my office grew from one with three individuals to a division of 75 people. I learned many things during this period, including the crucial interface between public health practice and policy—our efforts involved working with the governor's office and the state legislature. These encounters demonstrated how political parties can effectively work together to advance public health practice. I learned how bills get written, how bills get passed, and the inner workings of the legislative process. These experiences have informed my teaching and research after moving from the practice environment to academe. I also discovered how public health agencies use (or sometimes do not use) the latest scientific evidence in their decision-making. My experiences with state and local public health practice illustrated the skill sets and organizational practices that are too often missing and require ongoing efforts to increase capacity. These practice gaps led to the start of our training program in evidence-based public health.[1] Finally, I found great value in networking with other public health professionals across the United States, primarily via the National Association of Chronic Disease Directors.[2]

How can students make the most of their early-career experiences in leadership?

My advice to students begins with the idea of being a sponge. Embrace every encounter as a learning opportunity. If we stay curious and committed to lifelong learning, there is something new to learn each day. It is also essential to take initiative—if you think you have something to contribute, volunteer to help—your peers and supervisors will notice and will appreciate your "can do" spirit. Early in your career, try to stretch yourself and take chances. It is critical to learn a broad set of skills, not only the technical skills (e.g., epidemiology, biostatistics, evaluation), but also the so-called "soft skills" that include the ability to communicate effectively, negotiate, collaborate on teams, and show the passion for your work. As you find valuable mentors and team members, it is beneficial to stay in touch and continue building your network. You are more likely to become an effective leader if you embrace the mindset of a "modular" or "scaffolded" career in which you may take on multiple, complementary jobs over your working life.

What attributes are important in determining leadership effectiveness?
Effective public health leaders should think of health from a system's mindset that addresses both proximal (downstream or directly affecting health) and distal (upstream or indirectly affecting health) factors.[3,4] Proximal determinants are often lifestyle risk behaviors such as alcohol use or tobacco use. Other proximal factors include socioeconomic conditions (e.g., wealth) or the physical environment (e.g., air pollution). Distal determinants are often more stable over time and include national, institutional, legal, and cultural factors. Success in public health leadership demands attention to both sets of factors with a central focus on health equity—a framing that moves from a deficit mindset of what society is doing poorly (disparities) to one that is positive about what society can achieve.[5] Leaders play a role in achieving health equity through a range of approaches such as engaging in strategic partnerships to address issues affecting health and quality of life, changing community-level policies, and changing practices within a public health agency. For a leader to be effective, it is also critical to remember that public health is a team sport—a mix of voices and skills leads to better health outcomes and improved health equity.

What quote or statement about leadership do you have taped to your computer or tacked to your bulletin board, that you look at every day?
I have a placard in my office that reads: "If we knew what it was we were doing, it would not be called research, would it?" This quote is from Albert Einstein and has several underlying messages for leaders. The first is that science is iterative, does not have every answer, and for many public health challenges, there are multiple rational solutions.[1] Public health is a team sport and there is a need to engage a diverse set of people across multiple disciplines to achieve public health progress. We need to be honest with our stakeholders about not only what we know about how to improve public health but also what we do not know. There are trade-offs and "gray zones" in nearly every decision we make in public health practice and policy. Humility is another concept that I connect with this quote. Just because we hold graduate degrees should not imply that we know more than a lifelong public health practitioner or a community member with lived experience. I always tell early-career colleagues to take your work very seriously but try not to take yourself too seriously.

STEPHANIE WATSON-GRANT

Stephanie Watson-Grant, DrPH, is the deputy project director for Country Health Information Systems and Data Use at John Snow Inc. She has over 17 years' experience in international health and development, starting with the Jamaican government's Agency for Community Development before working with USAID (United States Agency for International Development) and UNAIDS (Joint United Nations Programme on HIV/AIDS) in Jamaica and with the MEASURE Evaluation project, led by the University of North Carolina at Chapel Hill (UNC-CH). Dr. Watson-Grant has degrees in Political Science, International Relations, and Government from the University of the West Indies, Mona, and a DrPH from UNC-CH. Dr. Watson-Grant is an adjunct professor with Gillings School of Global Public Health at UNC-CH.

Who were some of the role models or mentors that influenced you early on? In what ways did they influence you?
I never really had a mentor. There was never one specific person I looked up to. My leadership lessons are a collection of experiences and stories from my past, from people who I admired or from people who showed me the leader I never wanted to be.

What is the most impactful leadership experience that you have learned from, and how did it make a difference in your subsequent leadership practice?

It was Tuesday morning, and the phone rang. I knew who it was, but I was not yet ready to talk to her. It was 7:30 a.m.; I had not yet had my coffee and taken a deep breath. I ignored the call. I arrived at the hotel where we were hosting a high-level regional meeting and the hotel staff were in the process of taking the door to the room that we set up as a satellite office from the hinges. It did not matter how much they explained to her I had the only key to the room; she did not listen. She wanted to get into the room and she was not interested in hearing that she could not. I watched the hotel staff's anger, acquiescence, and annoyance. I was not surprised. I had experienced many instances where she deliberately made people wait and disrespected staff and stakeholders. I had witnessed her wasting resources, and I had participated in many conversations about the organization's awareness of her abuses and its inability to address her excesses.

However, I also saw her skills, experience, and competence. I saw that her policy recommendations for HIV programming were being adopted, that she had convening power such as when she brought together a group of lawyers to work pro bono on cases related to infringements against people living with HIV and AIDS. I watched her operate among those with influence who regularly called on her for advice and input in their affairs. I saw a certain something that made me cringe yet made me sit up and take notice.

I was confused about this duality. If leadership is as Yuki describes, "the process of influencing others to understand and agree about what needs to be done and how to do it, and the process of facilitating individuals and collective efforts to accomplish shared objectives"[6]; does it matter how I feel about the individual? How they treat others? There is a safe neutrality with this definition. It is devoid of value and, in the right or wrong circumstances, can be devoid of basic decency.

Many years later, I sat before the assistant minister of health in Liberia. I was part of a team planning a research activity and the assistant minister took a keen interest in the research activity. I remember how he made time for every meeting, and how he got his staff involved in the activity. I remember him showing up at training and data analysis events. He encouraged the trainees, reminding them the activity was part of Liberian nation building; however, I mostly remember his interaction with the junior staff. I remember how he made them comfortable enough to have spirited conversations with him about data and soccer.

From these experiences, I learned two important lessons. First, people will react to a strong and confident personality. It is almost instinctive for persons to align their initial response to the demands of a strong and confident personality; however, people will see beyond the posturing to the substance or lack of substance beneath. There will be a certain something, an intangible, which gives them pause or makes them distrust the intentions of the person. This leads me to my second lesson, kindness. Kindness is meeting the constant challenge to see and listen to those around us and to treat them as well-intentioned contributors to any endeavor. It is recognizing that those we work with and lead are complex beings and not the singular beings whom we lead. Kindness builds trust. Trust allows influence, facilitation, consensus, and collective achievement.

Kindness is not talked about as a leadership principle, but it is implicit in ideas such as creating an identity, practicing self-awareness, encouraging the best in others, and listening to others. Kindness is also implicit in seeking, building, and maintaining relationships. Kindness is about seeing the people you lead and helping them with their journey toward a common goal. It is hard to be unkind and be helpful at the same time.

I have come full circle. I am no longer confused. Leadership is not neutral. I see leadership as a positive process. Negative practices are something I do not intend to spend effort defining and describing.

How can students make the most of their early-career experiences in leadership?

All of these experiences shaped my leadership experience. If I have any advice for those at the beginning of their careers or those thinking about their careers, it is to learn from all your experiences. They are all valuable, even the painful and frustrating ones. What else is life but a collection of experiences? Take time to reflect, and stop every so often to think about what you learned from the difficult experiences and from the wonderful ones.

What quote or statement about leadership do you have taped to your computer or tacked to your bulletin board, that you look at every day?
I carry with me this quote attributed to Abraham Maslow, "If all you have is a hammer, then everything will be a nail." For much of my journey, this was a reminder to me of the importance of continuous learning so that I would expand my toolbox and not take a hammer to every situation. It is also a reminder to never forget the nail. This nail represents the knowledge and experiences I started with; the ones that helped shape the leader I am today.

How do you best prevent, or at least anticipate, unintended consequences (whether positive or negative) of your leadership decisions?
I approach all leadership decisions with an attitude of grace, knowing there will be decisions I make that will have unintended consequences. I know and acknowledge I operate in a complex and dynamic environment in global health with many actors and many moving parts. What is true today may change tomorrow as others' decisions impact and change the space I work in. I apply an attitude of grace because I cannot be afraid to question or change my decisions. Public health leadership decision-making is not about smooth sailing, but it is about weathering storms you anticipate and did not anticipate, keeping the ship upright, and guiding it to port from which the ship can successfully sail again.

DAVID ADLER

David Adler, DrPH, MPA, is the deputy director of the Robert Wood Johnson Foundation's Healthy Communities theme, working to ensure that conditions in communities allow all residents to reach their best possible health and well-being. Since joining the Foundation in 2008, Adler has worked on a variety of efforts to improve the health and well-being of everyone in the United States. Adler received a BA from Swarthmore College, an MSt in Hebrew and Jewish Studies from the University of Oxford, an MPA from the University of Pennsylvania, and a DrPH in Health Leadership from the Gillings School of Global Public Health at the University of North Carolina at Chapel Hill.

Who were some of the role models or mentors that influenced you early on? In what ways did they influence you?
One mentor was Andy Hyman, the director of the Foundation's coverage team for a period of time. Andy was very different from me. I'm a rule follower and tend to play everything by the book; Andy was the exact opposite. Every rule was an opportunity for negotiation. It was a real test for me to figure out how to work with someone like that, and it taught me a few things. The first was really to think about what was the right thing to do. Andy never liked to do the expedient thing or the easy thing. He liked to do the right thing. To be fair, sometimes he made things incredibly complicated or incredibly difficult because he couldn't budge in some simple ways. That's a lesson I've tried to leave behind. But the lesson about focusing on what is right is something that sticks with me.

The second thing Andy really taught me is to not be afraid to get told no. My instinct is often to not raise ideas that I think will get shot down. While I think it's important to be strategic about what to suggest and when, I also learned that I could deal with having an idea rejected. These are both lessons in being a bit bolder than I would normally be.

What is the most impactful leadership experience that you have learned from, and how did it make a difference in your subsequent leadership practice?
One of the leadership experiences I learned the most from was one of the toughest. I moved into a role as a communications officer for the coverage team after a couple of years at the Foundation. It was an area I did not know much about, having come to the Foundation to

work on childhood obesity. It was an overwhelming change. I joined the team in the middle of the debate over the Affordable Care Act. I had to manage a team of consultants who had been working in this field for decades. It was by far the hardest learning curve I have been on. Sometimes I think about that challenge and remember that I can do some difficult things.

It was also in that role that I got some pretty harsh feedback about how I was managing my team. While the way I got the feedback wasn't ideal (someone told someone who told me), I did have to face some hard truths about how I was managing. I learned that even if feedback isn't given in the "right" or "appropriate" way, it's still worth listening to.

How can students make the most of their early-career experiences in leadership?
Early in a career, people are likely to be in a job that is not ideal for them. There is always something to learn, or someone to learn from. Focus on that. Also, go in with the attitude of a problem-solver. People appreciate a problem-solver with an orientation toward learning. It's amazing how much that attitude can make someone stand out. Together those two attitudes will help early-career professionals get the most out of early experiences.

In relating to those to whom you report, what are some guiding principles and best practices?
A guiding principle for me is to offer solutions instead of problems. I got this advice early on, and it has stuck with me. Leadership really feels like offering options and paths forward, not just saying what is wrong. This can be challenging and sometimes I don't have great ideas about what can be done. But I owe it to myself, and people I report to, to try. Giving people something to react to is often a way to get the best information or thinking out of them as opposed to going with a blank slate or a list of complaints.

I also try to put myself in the position of the people I report to and think about what they are balancing. I try to understand why they might be doing or suggesting something that seems different from what I think I would do in their situation. Along those lines, I also try to remember to let them know when they've done something really helpful.

What quote or statement about leadership do you have taped to your computer or tacked to your bulletin board, that you look at every day?
"Do the next right thing." There are a lot of decisions to make on any given day. I often make the wrong decision or do the wrong thing. No matter how many times I have tried, I have never once been able to change what has happened in the past. Focusing on the next thing I can do is all I can do.

ELIZABETH (LIZ) MAGUIRE

Elizabeth (Liz) Maguire, MA, worked for over 45 years in the international sexual and reproductive health and rights field. Her senior leadership positions included 16 years as CEO of the international nonprofit Ipas and 22 years at USAID where she was the first woman director of the global reproductive health program during the 1990s. During her career, Maguire traveled to 85 countries. She is now a senior advisor, mentor, guest lecturer, and writer. Maguire has won multiple awards for her distinguished service as well as for her memoir Advancing Reproductive Choice: Leading With Conviction and Compassion, *published in 2020.*

Who were some of the role models or mentors that influenced you early on? In what ways did they influence you?
In the 1970s, at the beginning of my international career, I was privileged to meet with many of the great pioneers in family planning and reproductive health in each region. They were mostly male obstetrician–gynecologists since there were few women in prominent positions at that time.

I would like to highlight four extraordinary individuals who played a major role on the global stage: the late Dr. Allan Rosenfield, former dean of Columbia University Mailman School of Public Health; the late Professor Fred Sai of Ghana, former president of the International Planned Parenthood Federation, among his long list of important titles; Dr. Nafis Sadik of Pakistan, former executive director of the United Nations Population Fund; and Professor Mahmoud Fathalla of Egypt, whose many distinguished positions included president of the International Federation of Gynecology and Obstetrics. They served as my role models and mentors for over three decades.

These brilliant, charismatic, and courageous leaders inspired me during my career in championing the sexual and reproductive health and rights of women and girls in developing countries. Fighting for these fundamental rights requires bold action, addressing stigma and controversy, securing the commitment of senior government officials and civil society representatives, extensive use of the media, and building broad coalitions for change.

What is the most impactful leadership experience that you have learned from, and how did it make a difference in your subsequent leadership practice?
In January 1993, approximately two decades after starting my career, I was appointed the first woman director of the global family planning and reproductive health program of the U.S. Agency for International Development. The additional skills and experience I developed during my 6 years in this position had an important impact on my leadership practice for the remainder of my 45-year career.

In September 1994, I served as one of the lead negotiators on the U.S. delegation to the historic International Conference on Population and Development in Cairo where there was a major paradigm shift to "woman-centered" reproductive healthcare. With this significant development, my staff and I worked on designing and implementing groundbreaking policy and program initiatives along with an innovative communications and outreach strategy. During this period, we also dealt with challenging Congressional restrictions as well as bureaucratic obstacles.

Throughout my tenure, I focused on implementing good leadership practices. I led with my core values; identified, supported, and empowered talented staff; provided a positive, rewarding, and participatory work environment; engaged staff in strategic planning exercises and coalesced around a shared vision; and convened experts to brainstorm innovations and ways to increase impact. I remained focused on achieving key milestones and maximizing results, problem-solving, and providing open communications, support, and positive feedback to staff.

I introduced these and other leadership practices during my 16 years as CEO of Ipas. With a committed and talented team, the organization became a global leader in advancing women's reproductive health and rights, including access to safe abortion. We increased our annual funding seven-fold and greatly expanded Ipas's geographic reach and impact on saving and enhancing women's lives.

How can students make the most of their early-career experiences in leadership?
Guiding, supporting, and empowering young leaders has been a lifelong passion. I find it most rewarding to work with individuals with whom I share a common vision, commitment, and set of core values.

For those in the early stages of their career who want to be leaders, I underscore the importance of: identifying personal strengths and weaknesses as well as activities that provide the greatest satisfaction; gaining new skills, knowledge, and experience along with seeking opportunities for continuous personal and professional growth; working with mentors and coaches; creating strong relationships with peers and supervisors; building confidence, self-esteem, and new perspectives by doing new activities and implementing innovations; working hard and persevering through challenging times; never being afraid to make mistakes as these provide valuable learning opportunities; maintaining a positive attitude even in the face of challenges; strengthening oral and written communication skills; learning how to be an effective advocate for yourself and how to motivate and empower others; expanding your network of supporters and influencers; and changing jobs and/or organizations in order to assume higher levels of responsibility and climb the leadership ladder.

What attributes are important in determining leadership effectiveness?
There is no perfect leadership type; each leader is unique. In my opinion, great leadership starts with strong moral and ethical values. I believe that passion, compassion, perseverance, courage, resilience, flexibility, honesty, integrity, optimism, kindness, generosity, gratitude, and humility are among the important core values of a successful leader. Also critical is the ability to communicate effectively and listen openly to the views of all staff. First and foremost, leaders must gain the trust and respect of all team members and focus on building and maintaining strong relationships and expressing appreciation. Emotional intelligence is an essential attribute.

In creating effective teams, leaders must be able to attract, support, and reward great staff who bring complementary skills. They must provide a supportive and stimulating work environment where the roles, responsibilities, and expectations of all members are clear. Other responsibilities encompass developing with their staff a shared vision, mission, and strategy along with annual action plans and effective systems that are evaluated regularly and modified as needed. Evidence-based decision-making is imperative. The ability to think big, take bold action, and ensure continuous innovation and improvement is also key to maximizing impact. Leaders must be able to multi-task, delegate well, make sound decisions, remain open-minded and adaptable, manage conflict, ensure accountability, take corrective actions, and lead staff effectively through complex and often challenging situations.

Leaders must empower and guide staff to reach their full potential. They must also prioritize developing new leaders.

What quote or statement about leadership do you have taped to your computer or tacked to your bulletin board, that you look at every day?
The following inspirational quotes address what I believe are some of the most important characteristics of leadership:

- "Great leadership usually starts with a willing heart, a positive attitude, and a desire to make a difference." – Mac Anderson
- "The greatest leaders mobilize others by coalescing people around a shared vision." – Ken Blanchard
- "Leadership is about empathy. It is about having the ability to relate to and connect with people for the purpose of inspiring and empowering their lives." – Oprah Winfrey
- "Leaders don't create followers, they create more leaders." – Tom Peters

DAVE CHANG

As a clinical assistant professor at Stanford University, Dave Chang, MD, DrPH, teaches classes on population health, health equity, and community engagement. He has a joint appointment as assistant health officer in San Mateo County (CA), and previously served as a local public health director in Virginia. He received his undergraduate degree from Duke, his medical degree from Tufts, and his doctorate in public health degree from UNC-Chapel Hill, giving him the distinction of being both a Blue Devil and a Tar Heel. He lives in the Bay Area with his wife, an ophthalmologist, and their four children, dog, cat, and fish.

Who were some of the role models or mentors that influenced you early on? In what ways did they influence you?
Before seeking out a mentor, spend time to identify your unique personal and professional leadership values, understanding that no leader can "do it all." Then look for role models who live out your core values.

One role model, a professor of medicine at Johns Hopkins, modeled living out a work–life balance that was not marked by obligation but by intention. When at work, he was fully present and intentional in creating a healthy team culture, by routinely sharing poems and other works of literature for us to reflect on as we treated sick patients. Yet he was always unapologetic about giving time to his family, whom he called regularly in front of our team. He never made his time with us feel hurried, but he was always gone by mid-day to attend to things at home or other work responsibilities.

Another role model, a public health officer of a large city, demonstrated the importance of cultural humility. Thoughtful, soft-spoken, and kind, this mentor provided a counterpoint to the common view of a leader as being physically intimidating, loud, and dominating. He taught me that in any situation, a leader's first job is to intentionally create a safe space for all team members, one that is marked by mutual respect. This safe space is the foundation for trust that ultimately results in interdependence and opportunities to discover new ways of doing work together.

What is the most impactful leadership experience that you have learned from, and how did it make a difference in your subsequent leadership practice?
Leading our local health department through our initial public health accreditation process taught me what is required to sustain a complex multi-year process of systemic change in an organization. This experience also allowed me to regularly test, apply, and reassess leadership behaviors and frameworks. One framework I used often during the accreditation process is the Center for Creative Leadership's Direction-Alignment-Commitment (DAC) approach. In the midst of leadership challenges now, I periodically step back to make sure that we are in agreement as to what we are trying to achieve (direction), we are working in coordination (alignment), and we are committed to the success of the collective (commitment.)

How can students make the most of their early-career experiences in leadership?
As an early-career leader, avoid falling into the trap of trying to assume a persona or identity of what you envision a leader should be or act like. Instead, start by taking an inventory of your key values, the types of leadership behaviors you admire, and then develop your own personalized framework of leadership. Ask for help from your role models and mentors (who could be professional colleagues who are farther along in their journeys, or, in my case, my father-in-law, who was a department chair at a university). Read about models of leadership that appeal to you. Then adopt a quality improvement mindset of growing in your leadership behaviors. As you read and engage with your team, continuously test out new leadership behaviors and actions, and then reflect and reassess if those behaviors were effective. Also take time to write down and translate what you are observing and learning into models that are simple for you to apply on a day-to-day basis. Remember that leadership is not inherited or something you achieve; rather, leadership is learned, adapted, personal, and practiced.

How do you decide when to say "yes" or "no" to a request for your time?
When I worked in a public health department, I oftentimes approached requests for my involvement in new opportunities by asking these three questions: "Tell me more?", "Why not?", and "Who else needs to be here?" Oftentimes, the challenge in working in government is moving beyond the morass of day-to-day internal administrative tasks to welcoming new opportunities to think and do things differently.

Working at a large academic center where innovation is already valued has meant adjusting the questions that I ask myself when approached with a request for my time. Before coming to Stanford, I clearly articulated two overarching goals for my time. The question I ask now is, "How well does this request align with my primary aims for being here?" If there is alignment with both goals, I typically say "Yes," and if none, then usually "No."

How do you find time and ways for self-renewal and to maintain balance?
Maintaining balance is somewhat of a misnomer as it implies a constant state of tension while juggling many tasks. Instead, I find priority-setting and the image of filling a cup first with large stones (people and activities most important to you), before moving onto smaller stones (e.g., less important activities) more in line with how to maintain a healthy lifestyle, and one that must acknowledge limits.

Like many of you, both my partner and I work while still having kids at home, often depending on each other for childcare. We have needed to create rhythms in our life for space, rest, and reflection. We put on the TV twice a week for the kids in the evenings so we can go for a walk to catch up on life. We give each other at least 30 to 45 minutes to exercise 5 to 7 days a week. Also, once a month we give each other a day to go on a personal retreat, during which we can read, sleep, write, and exercise.

Similar to the words "family" or "faith," the word "leadership" may evoke a whole set of emotions, many conflicting, but oftentimes deeply personal and complex. I suspect some of our readers are like me: we take our work leading teams seriously, but we may still care to have home and community lives that are healthy and balanced.

My own experience as a husband, father of four children, committed friend and neighbor, physician, teacher, and public health leader, and my observations of other physician and public health leaders who are committed to "being there" in both personal and professional spheres of life has shown me that it is impossible to "do it all." Unfortunately, our books, podcasts, and movies continue to promote the archetype of a hero–leader who works 24/7, makes all the right leadership calls at work, and remains committed and available to family and friends. Those who are driven to achieve this standard of leadership often spiral into toxicity, judgement of others, or depression and anxiety from overwork.

ALYSON ROSE-WOOD

Alyson Rose-Wood is an officer in the U.S. Public Health Service assigned to the CDC. Commander Rose-Wood's career focuses on global health workforce development, harm reduction, hepatitis elimination, migrant health, and vector-borne diseases. For 5 years she had responsibility for the Americas regional portfolio in the Office of the Secretary of the U.S. Department of Health and Human Services. A graduate of Trinity University (2003), Harvard (2009), and the University of North Carolina at Chapel Hill (2020), Alyson was a Peace Corps Volunteer in Morocco and spent her childhood in Botswana, Ethiopia, Honduras, and Mali.

Who were some of the role models or mentors that influenced you early on? In what ways did they influence you?
A great strength you can have as a leader is your ability to think about others. When I recall the mentors who have influenced me in my career, the defining characteristics they each had were their humility and their compassion. While they each had a sense of their legacy and worked to build it, the means they used to reach their goals were grounded in kindness. Thanks to working for these mentors, I've experienced workplaces with competent leadership and where people liked their jobs. In those conditions, you can grow as a leader.

What is the most impactful leadership experience that you have learned from, and how did it make a difference in your subsequent leadership practice?
Between the ages of 18 to 24 years, I worked seasonally as an international white-water raft guide, leading boats of paying guests down rivers that were new to me like the Omo River (Ethiopia). At the time, I didn't recognize the value of early-career leadership opportunities, especially the ones that weren't pitched to me as leadership opportunities. But those years as a river guide have had an incalculable impact on me professionally and have reverberated

through each phase of my career. The river guide job meant I was voluntarily putting myself in unchartered waters and coming face-to-face with uncomfortable situations on a daily basis. Sometimes those uncomfortable situations involved territorial hippopotamuses or biting tsetse flies. But more often than not, those uncomfortable situations involved people. Every day I was taking people down the river I was honing my leadership skills: communication, conflict resolution, coping under pressure, preparing for the worst-case scenario, problem-solving. I learned quickly what a gift a sense of humor can be. I became skilled at reading people, knowing whom I could trust in the front of the boat to set the paddling pace. I discovered that when I was physically and emotionally spent, I was still able to find the energy to dig down and keep going.

How can students make the most of their early-career experiences in leadership?
Demonstrating leadership is about recognizing the value of your experiences and using the transferrable skills. In my early career years, I didn't know what experiences would wind up mattering to me, affecting me, educating me. So, I had to be open to trying things—to saying yes. I paid attention to what lifted me and what drained me and I sought to organize my life to do more of the first and less of the second. I discovered I had to say "no" to asks of my time in order to be able to focus on the first. This has meant doing things that didn't fit with my original career plan. Sometimes it's meant saying no to a great-sounding position. But I've never regretted it.

How do you select people to be on your leadership team within the organization you lead?
My father was a career diplomat with the U.S. Department of State. When I was 8 years old and we were living in the country of Mali, I remember asking him what he did every day at work. He was the deputy to the U.S. ambassador at the time. I recall him telling me, "I tell people no and make sure they leave my office with a smile. But the most important part of my day is turning on the ambassador's air conditioner."

My father laughed in hearing this anecdote relayed to him decades later. "I don't think I said no to everyone," he explained. "If anything, I tried to say yes. But I cannot underscore enough how important it was to turn on the ambassador's air conditioner before she arrived at the office!"

As I've progressed in my career and worked under different leaders—and grown in my leadership as well—I've realized that being a successful leader includes managing the intangibles such as esprit de corps, office tone, and ensuring that staff understand that their work matters and is contributing to the overall vision.

But being a leader also includes carefully hiring your deputy who will be doing the day-to-day management, including "turning on your air conditioner." I've been told that the deputy's job is to be the "thermostat" to quote a cliché, both sensing the existing temperature and also adjusting the system to a new temperature as needed. This has been something I've aimed to accomplish while working in deputy leadership positions.

What has been challenging for me is the transition from a management to a leadership role. It requires a shift in perspective; there are different skills and different expectations that come with a leadership position. What's more, I've learned that there is a lot of cultural specificity to how leadership is received and what is expected of a leader, especially in my field of global public health.

The transition in roles from day-to-day management to leadership has required me to have the self-awareness to say, "I have blind spots." Because I have found leadership to almost never be a solitary endeavor, I have surrounded myself with people who think differently from me and who complement some of my own weaknesses. For me, this has meant selecting a diverse team (e.g., gender, national origin, race, sexual orientation, thought). Because whatever bias any member of the team has, and we all have biases, they will be neutralized by other people.

What quote or statement about leadership do you have taped to your computer or tacked to your bulletin board, that you look at every day?

In 2015 I received the following message from one of my mentors who was retiring from his leadership role in the World Health Organization. I keep his message next to me at work as it is a reminder to me of the type of colleague, manager, and leader I want to be and how I want to be remembered:

> *Over my career, I am constantly reminded of an old adage, "Be kind to people as you go up the ladder, because they will be the same ones you encounter as you come down." Public health is about change, and how to adapt to change, whether you are going up, staying the same, or coming down the ladder. But, as my dad used to say, "Kindness begets kindness." People will always appreciate that and you will still be able to get things done.*

His message that kindness will not get in the way of reaching my leadership goals continues to resonate with me.

INNOCENT NDUBUISI IBEGBUNAM

Innocent Ndubuisi Ibegbunam, DrPH, MPH, is a visionary leader, working in International Health Development for over 15 years. He had worked with various international development partners (with funding from USAID, US-CDC, The Global Fund) to improve health systems through design and implementation in low- and middle-income countries. These are all geared toward improving access to quality health services for the vulnerable population. Dr. Ibegbunam obtained his doctor of public health (DrPH) from the University of North Carolina at Chapel Hill, master of public health (MPH) from the University of Liverpool, United Kingdom, and bachelor of pharmacy from the University of Nigeria, Nsukka. He is married with children.

Who were some of the role models or mentors that influenced you early on? In what ways did they influence you?

My leadership role model growing up was my mother (Josephine Ibegbunam); though she only had attained a basic level of education, she was an astute leader in her own right. She held court in our home with many women, and even men, coming to consult her on leadership topics within the community. This was further brought to life for me early on when I read different novels with leadership characters supporting others. These experiences very early in life helped shape my perspective of a leader as someone who is self-confident, independent, and always willing to assist others in resolving challenges through their influence within the community.

For my secondary school education (grades 7–12), living in a boarding school was an opportunity to start exhibiting some of those traits of self-confidence, independence, counseling others, and helping to solve problems through my influence, which I learned via observations and readings, without giving thought to it as leadership. For me, it was more about being satisfied with the little I had while assisting others through my knowledge and influence. That spirit of contentment and desire to assist, which I learned from my mother, attracted "followers" who were influenced by my strong character and willingness to drive a defined and morally sound agenda.

What is the most impactful leadership experience that you have learned from, and how did it make a difference in your subsequent leadership practice?

During my undergraduate studies at the University of Nigeria, Nsukka, I was exposed to my first major leadership role via appointment. I was appointed to lead the affairs of my classmates by coordinating activities of a Christian group for the class. That was how I started informal leadership and from then it was one leadership responsibility after another, with the peak in my penultimate year in the University when I was leading the largest group in the Church (Guild of St. Anthony of Padua). I was also elected the student union speaker of the Parliament for my Department, while also serving as the class captain for my class.

Holding all these responsibilities simultaneously brought so much limelight and kept me on my toes to clearly communicate, influence, and meet expectations of my peers and teams. The experiences I had growing up, with reminders on humility and how transient "power" and leadership positions were, helped to keep my feet on the ground despite the limelight. Self-awareness and opportunities for personal reflection on the moral soundness of my actions kept me going during difficult moments.

Furthermore, the level of influence I had on my peers both in affairs of the class, the student union political environment, and responsibility within the church groups, were guided by continuous self-reflections. Other major attributes that kept me afloat included my oratory skills, which was a major attribute to keep students focused, and my steadfastness and level-headedness in crises, which enabled me to command unplanned followership. I was also strong-willed and determined to make my own decisions rather than allow others to dictate for me, which was a double-edged sword, as some people wanted to push me in a different direction with the trust that I had more leadership potential than I was offering. However, I insisted on not going beyond what I had mapped out for myself 2 years earlier around my leadership in student government unionism via the legislative rather than the executive branch.

How can students make the most of their early-career experiences in leadership?

Students can benefit significantly from early leadership opportunities by volunteering to go the extra mile in the quest for consistency and excellence. This may be very challenging and painful, especially when you are the only person who believes in your cause of action or when you seem to be in opposition to the popular opinion. Even if you do not end up getting your way, and even if you were wrong, you will have learned a lesson on how to stand firm on your own and influence others. It is a big lesson on strength of character and how to communicate your views to others. Furthermore, identifying and following early mentors in leadership, and making efforts to understand their approach, will help keep you on the right path. For me, my mother had a photographic memory and was able to use storytelling to put things in perspective in her quest to influence followers, a technique that I have also used.

What attributes are important in determining leadership effectiveness?

Key attributes of leadership effectiveness, from my perspective, revolve around clear communication of the vision and mission to the team, in addition to setting clear deliverables with timelines, and providing required resources (capacity building, financial and material resources) to meet the deliverable within the desired timeline. Furthermore, demonstrating empathy and connecting with the team at a personal level is vital in boosting team morale and drive for results. Effective leadership also requires personal credibility and drive from the leader. These help to engender trust among the team, even when there are unplanned setbacks, and to encourage the quest for excellence. From my personal experience, teams are easily influenced when they see that the leader is truly empathic and can be trusted to lead the team in the right direction even in difficult circumstances. Also, being fair in the treatment of team members, periodically celebrating success, acknowledging achievements, resolving conflicts, and knowing the right time to address such conflicts are other vital leadership effectiveness attributes I have utilized. These attributes have assisted me in keeping the team focused and maintaining morale that will ensure desired results were achieved.

How do you select people to be on your leadership team within the organization you lead?

The key characteristics I consider in selection of members of my leadership team include knowledge of the subject matter, strong and clear communication skills, honesty on personal limitations, and fit within the team dynamics. Other considerations include self-confidence, personal drive, willingness to take risks, not being afraid of making mistakes, and willingness to accept responsibility for the team's poor performance (with a pathway toward reversing the trend), while acknowledging success as collective effort. Also, responsiveness, consistency, and continuous learning are other key attributes that have kept me going for a long time, and I require these from my leadership team. I always tell my teams not to allow the perfect to be the enemy of the good, but to keep communication lines constantly open with the clients and stakeholders, while being adaptive to changes based on new evidence. I explain to my teams that responsiveness and proactive communication will enable us to continue to share our progress and successes: I encourage them to highlight challenges and opportunities for improvement, while seeking assistance at the right time to achieve the desired outcome. Combining these attributes has made me successful in my leadership experience, and I encourage those around me to explore them.

NANCY MCGEE

Nancy McGee, JD, MPH, DrPH, is a member of the Healthcare and Life Sciences Practice at Heidrick & Struggles. With over 25 years' experience working with life sciences companies, Nancy has a deep understanding of the healthcare ecosystem and a strong background in overseeing the strategic direction of large organizations and shaping their leadership teams. Previously, Nancy served as the executive vice president at Avalere Health. She held positions at Castlight Health; Manatt, Phelps & Phillips; and she served as the chief operating officer for Lash Group at AmerisourceBergen Corporation. She began her consulting career at The Lewin Group.

Who were some of the role models or mentors that influenced you early on? In what ways did they influence you?
Role models can emerge from unexpected places. I grew up in San Diego, California, in the early 1970s. Prior to going to kindergarten, I went everywhere with my mother. Mom was a housewife, and her passion was art. She became a Docent at the San Diego Museum of Art and served on a number of museum committees focused on fundraising activities, acquisition of works of art, and the overall management of the museum. While the committees could make recommendations, they were not the final decision-maker. It was necessary to cooperate with the operational management of the museum in order to get things done.

Volunteers often do not have power as we think of it in the traditional workplace. Instead, it is necessary to influence others in order to structure and drive action. It was in this room at an early age that I met a team of role models. I learned that each person had their own way of expressing and achieving influence. For example, one person was very quiet and reserved. I noticed that when she spoke up her thoughts were consistently well organized, concise, and precise. As a result, her words were given particular weight in meetings with operational management. Just because she was soft-spoken did not mean she was not powerful. Another person was extremely direct. She could cut conflict quickly and set direction. Mom was regarded as the operator. She was the one who the team relied on for her organizational skills.

By learning about different influencing approaches as a child, it shaped the way I lead today. The ability to use multiple influencing strategies has helped me to be a successful leader when facing diverse audiences, challenges, and environments.

What is the most impactful leadership experience that you have learned from, and how did it make a difference in your subsequent leadership practice?
In 2008, I served as the senior vice president and chief of operations for a division of a Fortune 50 company. The national financial crisis occurred during my tenure. No one knew how long it would last. As each month passed, headlines announced companies that were laying off hundreds, then thousands, of employees. Businesses went bankrupt. There was a great deal of fear.

Our senior leadership team felt that every job was precious. We were going to honor our employees by trying our best to keep their jobs safe. We worked together to determine how we needed to modify our operations in order to achieve our objective. We reviewed the impact of the recession in each of the states where we had a geographical operating presence. We heard from our human resources team about the rising number of spouses of our employees who had lost their jobs, which made holding on to jobs even more important. We listened to a report from our finance team regarding our profitability. We reviewed every program we operated to determine if we could share our work more efficiently across existing teams.

Our bold plan required everyone in the company to work together. We decided that we would share our objective, analysis, and path forward with the entire company as we would all need to take on more in order to make it work. We had a unified team, not only at the top, but through the entirety of the company. It is one of the greatest highlights of my career that we not only preserved jobs during the recession, but our ability to change how we worked created additional job opportunities and we were able to hire people. The power of collaboration, creative thinking, and transparency are the lessons I learned during this experience and have carried forward as a leader.

How can students make the most of their early-career experiences in leadership?
Feedback can feel like an unwanted, irritating guest. It can be particularly excruciating when received early in our career when we are trying so hard to be perfect. Who wants to hear that our efforts did not measure up, particularly from those that we are trying to impress?

One of the leaders I worked for early on in my career made it a firm-wide rule that we were to give each other timely feedback. The person receiving feedback could only respond with two words: "thank you." The receiver would need to think seriously about the feedback for 24 hours. After the 24-hour period, they could then ask questions about the feedback and engage in a discussion. It worked; feedback was offered, it was embraced, behaviors changed for the positive, and our culture thrived.

The early part of a career is the time when we are open to learning from our environment and are often experimenting with different leadership styles. As a result, the receipt of feedback is critical to hone leadership skills. Thinking about it for 24 hours takes away the ability to get defensive and promotes positive introspection. As a result, when you receive a gift of feedback, give thanks, think about it overnight, and consider what you could learn by trying something different.

How do you deal with a situation where someone is not a good fit or is not performing well?
When someone is not performing well, they know. It's the rare person who wants to fail at work. What is more common is that people who are failing do not know how to ask for help. It is the job of a leader to deliver feedback early and often. If someone is struggling, don't ignore it; engage the discussion. There is usually a reason why someone is not performing well. Sometimes it can be addressed. Other times, the position is simply not a good fit and it's important to act with integrity and quickly let that person go. The people that I have had to let go often express relief.

How do you find time and ways for self-renewal and to maintain balance?
Meetings are like pistachios; when there is a bowl, it's difficult to only eat one. As meeting invites flood our collective inboxes, it's easy to give away time without thinking about it.

I ask myself questions before accepting invitations: "Do I need to be in this meeting?", "Do I have anything to contribute?", and "Is it a critical meeting for me to do my job?" If the answer to any of these questions is "No," then I decline the invitation.

Developing a discipline around meetings helped me to be able to do the things I need to feel refreshed and at my best.

MAX MICHAEL

Max Michael, MD, has served in a variety of leadership positions including medical director for two federally qualified health centers, director of outpatient services, chair of the department of medicine, CEO/medical director of a public hospital, and dean of a school of public health. He created the Community Care Plan, the nation's first HMO for uninsured persons, for residents in two local housing communities. He continues to practice internal medicine and lives in Birmingham, Alabama.

Who were some of the role models or mentors that influenced you early on? In what ways did they influence you?
The mentors that influenced me early on were experiences whose lessons stayed with me throughout my career. For example, when I was about 13 or 14 years old, I spent many hours working with the Bohannon brothers who ran a small engine repair shop inside an old gas station at Goodby's Lake. It was about a mile bike ride from our house down Old Saint Augustine Road. I helped out in the garage bay filled with lawnmower engines and parts scattered all over the floor. Every repair was a challenge, figuring out what was wrong, slowly taking it apart, and finding the right part. All this while sitting on the floor in a poorly lighted space, with greasy tools, oily engine parts, dirty rags, oil and gas cans, and empty Coke bottles.

I helped loosen flywheels, grabbing parts, tightening nuts, and pulling starter cords. Each time an engine cranked we laughed at our success and enjoyed the acrid smell of exhaust. Together we scooted across the floor to wrestle with the next broken engine; scooted because the Bohannon brothers couldn't walk, were difficult to understand, and struggled with holding tools and parts steady because of their cerebral palsy. Working with the Bohannon brothers I learned the importance of helping others reach their goals, patience, and the sheer joy of fixing a broken lawnmower.

What is the most impactful leadership experience that you have learned from, and how did it make a difference in your subsequent leadership practice?
Several summers in high school I worked at the local health department doing a variety of odd tasks, including logging in confiscated moonshine. I started out opening small glass bottles with stool samples sent in by food handlers to test for enteric pathogens. By the time the cardboard tubes got to me, the Florida heat turned the bottles into time bombs. Invariably the sender interpreted "small stool sample" to mean filling the bottle to the top, so when I tried to twist the bottle open a veritable shitstorm erupted all over me. I wondered what part of "small" didn't folks understand; I needed just enough for the wire inoculating hook. But then I would have to smile when in some bottles I would find dimes or a quarter on top of the stool to cover the costs of mailing, I guess.

Even now I can't help but smile at what I learned opening those bottles. It is important to know your organization from bottom to top, even if it means getting dirty. It is hard to lead if you don't have a feel for the jobs you are asking people to do. I don't know what the food handlers were told to do with the glass bottles, but certainly the communication was less than ideal; know your audience so you can be certain they understand your message. And the coins on the top of the bottle taught me people are by and large kind and thoughtful.

Finally, as a college junior I well remember the anonymous caller who told me I was being inducted into the secret society. I was to rent a tux, pack a small suitcase for a possible trip, and show up at a local hotel Sunday afternoon without my four roommates knowing. The ballroom was crowded, including the 25 or so juniors, reveling in the excitement of possible travel to Japan or England on behalf of the university. We were blindfolded before the ceremony started, then led through the recitation of secret oaths and listened intently about the importance of the society to the university. The ceremony ended with a flourish as a senior stood in front of me, removed my blindfold, and said, "Do you *really* think you are *that* important?"

The enduring lessons for me were humility—don't take yourself too seriously, no matter how important the job; always maintain your sense of humor about the world around you; and learn to laugh at yourself.

One of my most impactful leadership experiences came early in my tenure as CEO of our local county hospital. Excited about starting on a program to improve culture and morale, I contracted with two experts from the university who had decades of experience with organizational change. After less than 2 weeks of meetings with staff on all three shifts, they reminded me that culture change required that about 10% of the staff needed to be on board at the beginning of the process. They told me less than 1% of any shift attended their meetings. Ideas are exciting, a dime a dozen, and useless if the leader gets too far ahead of the staff. I didn't do the hard work of hearing from staff about their ideas before trying to implement the program across the organization. Sharing ideas to get buy-in takes time and repetition; it is easy to forget you have lived with your idea day and night for weeks and months. You have a vested interest in the idea; give your staff time to process the idea and eventually share your enthusiasm.

How can students make the most of their early-career experiences in leadership?
Students can make the most of their early career experiences in leadership by closely watching the different leaders they interact with all the time, from their classroom instructors, program directors, club presidents, deans, and the like. Watch how each of them uses their position to lead in each particular setting; keep a diary of how each motivates and inspires students and how they handle mistakes and failures. Note how often you hear from the good leader, "I'm sorry," "I was wrong," or "I made a mistake."

In relating to those to whom you report, what are some guiding principles and best practices?
We all have bosses. Be sensitive to the pressures and demands the person to whom you report is under. Try to understand those pressures and motivations to better serve them while accomplishing your own goals.

What quote or statement about leadership do you have taped to your computer or tacked to your bulletin board, that you look at every day?
"And now," cried Max, "let the wild rumpus start!"

KATIE KANEY

Katie Kaney, DrPH, has over 25 years of experience in healthcare strategy and operations, and has been responsible for portfolios spanning thousands of employees, physicians, and services with earnings in excess of $5B. Achievements include cutting edge development in physician partnership/ integration, mobile medicine, community health, and virtual health. Katie is dedicated to community service, including serving as past board president of Mecklenburg County EMS, Loaves & Fishes, Healthy Charlotte, and Leadership Charlotte; and as a board member on The Gillings School of Global Public Health Foundation, the National Research Institute, and the Advisory Board for Pfizer. She holds a BA in Biology and an MBA from the University at Buffalo, and a DrPH from the UNC Gillings School of Global Public Health.

Who were some of the role models or mentors that influenced you early on? In what ways did they influence you?
Early on, my greatest role models were my grandparents and parents. I was raised to value an education, work hard, and make a difference in the community. The essence of servant leadership was instilled in me at an early age; I was taught to find my passion, to be resilient, to not be discouraged by barriers, and to make the world a better place. Their actions underscored their lessons; each had a rich history of serving in community-based organizations, giving generously to causes such as food insecurity and access to education, and engaging in philanthropy.

What is the most impactful leadership experience that you have learned from, and how did it make a difference in your subsequent leadership practice?
Upon my arrival in North Carolina, armed with a BA in Biology and MBA, I had little real work experience, but I didn't let that slow me down. While I started my career at an entry level job at a large healthcare system, promotions came quickly into roles which, frankly, on paper I was not qualified for. Within 3 years, I was serving as a vice president at a large tertiary/quaternary academic medical center, responsible for the 25th busiest emergency department in the United States and one of the busiest, most respected trauma centers.

Finding myself surrounded by the best clinicians, researchers, and academicians created a foundational element in my leadership practice—continuous learning and improvement. As an executive, I was invited by my physician leaders to sit in on several M&M (morbidity & mortality) conferences. The conversation centered on what went wrong and how to fix it, not on making excuses or downplaying the amount of responsibility each individual and the collective team held for each patient entrusted to us.

Watching direct conversations play out in a respectful manner, using data and evidence to validate right and wrong decisions, and seeing the vulnerability the team showed, supported by their chairs and chiefs, impacted me profoundly. It also showed me how many times systems issues were key factors in problematic outcomes and helped me see that my key role in leading efforts to fix the problems was to foster an environment which supported the reliability of individuals and teams. Based upon this, I incorporated continuous learning and improvement as a key leadership attribute for me and my team, along with the constant reminder that the teams we work with every day hold immense responsibility and accountability for life; for this I hold unyielding respect and gratitude. Always remembering that our decisions impact people, patients, and communities has been a foundational element of my leadership practice. It often serves as common ground to rally various leaders and differing perspectives to align in service of the mission through the decisions we make and support.

How can students make the most of their early-career experiences in leadership?
Gaining trust and learning from others is highly undervalued. Take the opportunity early in your career to ask questions, shadow others, ask to participate in projects, or sit in on meetings with executive leaders; in essence, do your job and ask for more. Expose yourself to as much as you can and use your inexperience as an advantage. Through this you will also find the leaders with whom you wish to develop an even deeper connection as a mentor and a sponsor. In my career, I have learned as much from ineffective leaders as I have from effective ones, assimilating best practices and augmenting my authentic style. Do the same early on, and you will have the opportunity to use your "early" as an advantage. Take it!

How do you deal with a situation where someone is not a good fit or is not performing well?
Some of the best advice I ever got is that I should never have to fire anyone. If I did a good job setting expectations, measuring/managing performance, and constantly communicating, then if underperformance happens, it is not a surprise. In my experience, most people do not want to stay in a job if they are unable to meet the standards set. As a leader, it is essential to be clear about your expectations, and to support your team to achieve expectations; it is equally essential to provide transparent feedback if the job cannot be accomplished.

In relating to those to whom you report, what are some guiding principles and best practices?
The saying goes that if you make your boss look good, then you look good! Overall, I have found that to be true. However, as I have been afforded more choices as my experience expanded and I matured as a leader, my guiding principle is to work for someone you respect and who has integrity. This does not mean you must have the same leadership style / approach or even the same skill set; I have found the common denominator of mutual respect and integrity allows for you to be your best self and your true self at work. For me, I also have found I can't compromise on my true alignment to the mission of healthcare, which is the greater calling to help others.

UGBEDE ABU

Ugbede Abu, DrPH, MPH, is a senior supply chain advisor at Social Solutions International, Washington, DC, deployed to the President's Malaria Initiative (PMI), the U.S. Government's flagship global malaria initiative led by USAID and implemented with the CDC. Ugbede is a public health professional with over 25 years of specialized experience in health and pharmaceutical systems program planning and implementation in international settings, including Ethiopia, Guinea, Malawi, Nigeria, and Uganda. Ugbede earned his doctor of public health (DrPH) from the University of North Carolina, USA; MPH from the University of Limpopo, South Africa; and pharmacy degree from Ahmadu Bello University, Nigeria.

Who were some of the role models or mentors that influenced you early on? In what ways did they influence you?

My role model was my late father, James Ojonugwa Abu. I grew to know him as my biologic father and later discovered he was much more than a father; he was a role model to me. He influenced every facet of my life from a young age to adulthood—he gave me the best advice I have ever received regarding goal setting, career, faith, human relations, work, play, and resilience. His advice and counsel helped me to discover my potential, envision my career, and adopt traits that have enabled me to flourish in life.

My father was a strong advocate for continuous learning, and he was my cheerleader. He encouraged me to look beyond a college education. I started and completed my graduate and doctorate degrees in public health against all odds with his exceptional support. Looking back, I am proud to mention that his exemplary lifestyle and wise counsel influenced my life and helped me navigate the complex issues I have experienced. He was an incredible role model because of his principles, social skills, sterling leadership qualities, and approach to life. He was a visionary and selfless leader, passionate about mentoring, serving others, and community development. I am fortunate that our paths crossed. I gained lifelong lessons from him that have helped me approach life with a deep sense of responsibility, humility, hope, and positivity.

What is the most impactful leadership experience that you have learned from, and how did it make a difference in your subsequent leadership practice?

My father exposed me to the concept of strategic thinking very early in life. He taught me to appreciate the value of self-awareness and goal setting. Depending on the context, he was always quick to work me through his mantra of "looking ahead" based on his understanding of the current and future state. I realized his views and penchant for strategic planning were rooted in very sound leadership principles. I had the opportunity to see my father step into leadership roles in our extended family, community, business, and church.

Over the years, I have applied my father's strategic planning experience to enhance my leadership practice in different areas. As a result, I supported my teams in Nigeria, Malawi, and the United States to design and implement innovative and impactful public health programs successfully. By approaching leadership from a strategic standpoint, I have gained the confidence to articulate ideas holistically and influence my team to look at the "big picture," which is a critical attribute for a well-performing team.

How can students make the most of their early-career experiences in leadership?

Leadership is a puzzle with several interrelated components. I would encourage students to lay a rock-solid foundation for their leadership journey and build on it incrementally. They should not be shy about seeking input from their peers, mentors, and role models as they think through their leadership goals. One of the most valuable initial steps is to identify their leadership trajectory with clear objectives and what it will take to achieve them—a game plan. It always pays to have a plan "B" or "C" if possible. That way, one can quickly adapt to changes along the way without getting stuck at any point.

Leadership students should consistently develop a culture of self-evaluation. Honest self-evaluation is critical for identifying progress, successes, and challenges. Such assessment will reinforce the need to stay on course or pivot to another direction. However, self-evaluation is excellent but not sufficient; students should also look on the flip side by soliciting external feedback from colleagues, family, and people familiar with their work or exposed to it. I see value in both internal and external evaluation.

We live in a very interconnected world, full of opportunities and challenges. Aspiring leaders should develop sound principles that will help them stay focused without distraction. They should take bold steps to let go of things that might hinder progress, including ad hoc and distracting meetings or events.

What attributes are important in determining leadership effectiveness?
Effective leaders are mission-driven and result-oriented. They must possess the following attributes in their toolkit to remain effective and on track.

The ability to influence others is critical in determining leadership effectiveness because leaders must work with their teams and external partners to achieve organizational goals. Leaders need to deploy tact and soft skills to get people aligned with their visions and missions.

Clear communication is another critical attribute for determining leadership effectiveness. Leaders need to share clear information with their teams to keep everyone engaged and motivated. On the other hand, effective leaders must also be ready to listen to their teams and other stakeholders to gain trust and followership.

Work ethic is another incredible attribute that can determine leadership effectiveness. By demonstrating a solid work ethic, leaders can set the tone and influence their team to achieve desirable standards in a workplace. Leaders who "walk the talk" can genuinely promote the culture of accountability and equity in their organization.

In relating to those to whom you report, what are some guiding principles and best practices?
A productive working relationship between a supervisee and supervisor in a workplace is critical for productivity and professional development. Supervisees should take deliberate steps to apply some of these guiding principles:

1. Understand their supervisors' leadership styles. It will help them get along with their supervisors.
2. Identify their boss' priority within the organization, what keeps them up at night, and how they can support their supervisor to achieve their priorities, especially those related to the broader organizational goals.
3. Aim to gain the trust of their supervisors by exhibiting a sound work ethic and a deep sense of professionalism.
4. Establish an excellent communication channel with their supervisor. They should exercise judgment in deciding what, when, and how to communicate with their supervisors—most bosses want to know when issues are brewing in their team before they blow up. Be sure to avoid taking your supervisor by surprise; give your supervisor a heads-up on any critical incident, even if you do not yet have the full details.

LISA M. KOONIN

Lisa M. Koonin, DrPH, MN, MPH, founded Health Preparedness Partners to advise organizations on how to prepare for and respond to pandemics. After 30+ years with the CDC, she is recognized as an international expert in pandemic countermeasures. Dr. Koonin is an epidemiologist and family nurse practitioner; she earned a master of nursing and MPH degrees from Emory University, and a public health doctorate degree from the University of North Carolina–Chapel Hill (UNC). She also serves as an adjunct assistant professor at the UNC Gillings School of Global Public Health.

Who were some of the role models or mentors that influenced you early on? In what ways did they influence you?
The first time I accepted a leadership position, I wasn't sure if I "had what it takes" to lead a team with a critical mission. I called my mentor for advice. She counseled me to ". . . be sure the next job you take is appropriate for you but is a 'stretch' beyond where you are now. You will quickly grow into that role and forever be transformed." Her words gave me the

courage to accept that new role and I quickly adapted. For every career change after that, I heard her voice in my ear that encouraged me to consider leadership positions with greater responsibility. When I look back, I see my fears were unfounded and I remain grateful for her advice.

What is the most impactful leadership experience that you have learned from, and how did it make a difference in your subsequent leadership practice?
I served 30+ years at the CDC, much of it involved in planning for, leading teams focused on, and responding to infectious disease threats, like pandemic influenza. In 2006, I began working with a small group from the White House and CDC to develop a new national policy for reducing the spread of influenza during a severe pandemic using nonpharmacologic measures. The most impactful leadership experiences I have had in my career were during that time when we were developing these social distancing policies.

Here's the story: We knew that vaccine would not be available at the beginning of a pandemic and that some immediate strategies would be needed to reduce the spread of the disease and limit morbidity and mortality. Because people who are infected with a pandemic respiratory disease can be contagious before they are symptomatic or could be asymptomatic but contagious, the strategy we developed was social distancing—keeping people physically apart, to reduce onward disease transmission. However, there were many obstacles to ensure this strategy would be accepted by federal, state, and local public health officials. Although the measure would likely be effective at reducing disease transmission, it could also be disruptive to society (e.g., school closure, cancelling mass gatherings). We could only estimate effectiveness through modeling studies and historical analyses, because then, there were no real-world data. Several prominent public health officials opposed this strategy, stating that it would never work, that a future pandemic would never be so severe as to warrant these interventions, and that they would create more harm than good. Their vigorous opposition caused our small team to consider their concerns and rigorously evaluate alternative approaches, only to reinforce our commitment to the concept. Based on exhaustive research and historical analyses, social distancing seemed to be the best strategy. No other effective strategy could be identified for use before a vaccine could be developed. We believed that one day, these measures would be needed to save lives, so we persisted.[7]

After a year of stakeholder engagement, experimenting with ideas, and conducting public polls, we finally arrived at a consensus and published the CDC's Community Mitigation guidance in February 2007.[8] Without the team's courage and tenacity, this strategy would have never been adapted as policy by the Department of Health and Human Services (HHS) and CDC, and ultimately incorporated into pandemic plans by many countries around the world. These social distancing strategies have served as a key component of the COVID-19 emergency response.

How can students make the most of their early-career experiences in leadership?
When starting a new leadership position, it is extremely important to be a good listener. The first month or more of a new position, the new leader should be actively listening; absorbing the workplace culture and learning about the organization and staff (as individuals and how everyone fits into the team, including their aspirations and goals). In addition, understand what has and has not worked in the past, and why. Early in one's career, leaders can improve their chances of success by listening to and learning from those they lead.

What attributes are important in determining leadership effectiveness?
To be a successful leader I had to incorporate the traits and behaviors that are widely described as "essential leadership qualities" including: *integrity, honesty, compassion, humility, kindness, generosity, decisiveness, and inclusiveness, plus the ability to trust and delegate to others.* However, the two critical characteristics that have most led to my growth and success as a leader have been *courage* and *perseverance*—I can weather almost any storm by summoning courage and by staying tenacious.

What quote or statement about leadership do you have taped to your computer or tacked to your bulletin board, that you look at every day?
Years ago, I came across a simple statement—"Perseverance Furthers"—taken from the Chinese *I Ching*. I have those words where I can see them every day. The passage actually reads: "The creative works sublime success, furthering through perseverance."[9(p56)] In their interpretation, Wilhelm and Baynes explain: "In relation to the human world, it denotes the creative action of the . . . Leader . . . , who through his (her) power awakens and develops their higher nature."[(9p56)] As the statement describes, I learned my role as a leader is to persist when needed, and to inspire and support others so they can achieve their goals.

Many times, these qualities of courage and perseverance enabled me to establish and achieve significant objectives. They enabled me to set audacious goals, and even though I might not achieve them all, I tried. I stretched beyond my comfort zone, was flexible but persistent, and was forgiving of myself and others. However, perseverance doesn't mean doggedly pursuing a goal without checking in constantly about the feasibility and acceptability of the goal. It is critical to iterate, solicit new input and ideas, and alter or amend the methods to get there—or even change the goal itself. To solve thorny public health problems, the leader has to generate and test multiple solutions; some just won't work. It takes significant courage to persist, to be brave in the face of failure, to change course and try again if the first ideas do not succeed.

SUMMARY

These leadership experiences are rich with great breadth and depth of meaning. Among the three common questions addressed are many life-molding examples. First, mentors and their impact on these leaders are significant in leadership development. The mentor–mentee relationships described here are not haphazard or random, but rather indicate an important degree of intentionality. A meaningful starting place is to look within, and then search for role models "who live out your values" and who then help to discover the leadership potential that can be nurtured. A common theme among these leaders' early mentors is respect—respect for every individual in the workplace and conveying to each that their work matters.

Second, the leadership experiences that were identified as most impactful were often ones that were particularly challenging and sometimes uncomfortable, causing these leaders to "stretch" early in their leadership development. The lessons learned from those experiences imbued a new sense of resiliency, through finding the energy, digging down, and learning continuously. Taking the time to reflect on that learning is as important as the experience itself.

And third, students can make the most of their early-career experiences in leadership by embracing every opportunity to learn, to get feedback, and to write this down for further reflection. These leaders urged those just beginning on their leadership paths to pursue opportunities that "break them out of their silos," to be open to trying new things, to saying "Yes" much more often than saying "No": "Do your job and ask for more." Students should circle back again and again with mentors as they build their own networks. All these early experiences are valuable, "even the painful and frustrating ones. What else is life but a collection of experiences?"

DISCUSSION QUESTIONS

1. Answer the five questions (three required of all respondents and two more from the optional list). What did you learn about yourself in the process?
2. Interview a classmate. Use the three required questions and ask your classmate to choose two additional questions from the list. What did you learn about yourself and your classmate?

3. Choose a leader that you admire. Which questions would you like them to answer and why?
4. Which of the answers in the chapter most resonated with you? Why?
5. Did you have any negative reactions to any of the responses? What were they and why?

REFERENCES

1. Brownson RC, Baker EA, Deshpande AD, Gillespie KN. *Evidence-Based Public Health*. 3rd ed. Oxford University Press; 2018.
2. National Association of Chronic Disease Directors. About NACDD. 2021. https://chronicdisease.org/page/about_nacdd
3. Arah OA, Westert GP, Delnoij DM, Klazinga NS. Health system outcomes and determinants amenable to public health in industrialized countries: a pooled, cross-sectional time series analysis. *BMC Public Health*. 2005;5:81. doi:10.1186/1471-2458-5-81
4. Erwin PC, Brownson RC. The public health practitioner of the future. *Am J Public Health*. 2017;107(8):1227–1232. doi:10.2105/AJPH.2017.303823
5. Brownson RC, Kumanyika SK, Kreuter MW, Haire-Joshu D. Implementation science should give higher priority to health equity. *Implement Sci*. 2021;16(1):28. doi:10.1186/s13012-021-01097-0
6. Yukl G. *Leadership in Organizations*. Pearson Prentice Hall; 2010.
7. Our experiences were described in more detail by author Michael Lewis in his book, *The Premonition*, published in May, 2021. https://wwnorton.com/books/9780393881554 and by Eric Lipton in his *New York Times* article published in April, 2020. https://www.nytimes.com/2020/04/22/us/politics/social-distancing-coronavirus.html
8. Centers for Disease Control and Prevention. Interim pre-pandemic planning guidance: community strategy for pandemic influenza mitigation in the United States—early, targeted, layered use of nonpharmaceutical interventions. 2007. https://www.cdc.gov/flu/pandemic-resources/pdf/community_mitigation-sm.pdf
9. Wilhelm R, Baynes CF, trans. *I Ching: Or, Book of Changes*. 3rd ed., Bollingen Series XIX. Princeton University Press; 1967. 1st ed. 1950.

Index